ry

For Churchill Livingstone

Publisher Laurence Hunter
Project Editor Jane Shanks
Project Controller Kay Hunston
Design Direction Erik Bigland

SCOTT
An Aid to Clinical Surgery

EDITED BY

Robin C. N. Williamson

MA MD MChir FRCS Hon FRCS (Thailand) Hon PhD (Mahidol)
Professor of Surgery, Imperial College School of Medicine, University of London;
Consultant Surgeon, Hammersmith Hospital, London, UK

Bruce P. Waxman

BMedSc MBBS FRACS FRCS (Eng) FACS
Associate Professor and Director, Academic Surgical Unit, Monash University,
Dandenong Hospital, Southern HealthCare Network, Melbourne, Australia

SIXTH EDITION

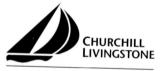
CHURCHILL
LIVINGSTONE

EDINBURGH LONDON NEW YORK PHILADELPHIA SYDNEY TORONTO 1998

CHURCHILL LIVINGSTONE
An imprint of Elsevier Science Limited

Robert Stevenson House, 1–3 Baxter's Place, Leith Walk,
Edinburgh EH1 3AF, UK

First edition 1971
Second edition 1979
Third edition 1984
Fourth edition 1989
Fifth edition 1994
Sixth edition 1998
  Reprinted 1999
  Reprinted 2002

ISBN 0 443 05603 X
International edition ISBN 0 443 05609 9
  Reprinted 1999
  Reprinted 2002

British Library Cataloguing in Publication Data
A catalogue record for this book is available from the British
Library.

Library of Congress Cataloging in Publication Data
A catalog record for this book is available from the Library of
Congress.

Medical knowledge is constantly changing. As new information
becomes available, changes in treatment, procedures, equipment
and the use of drugs become necessary. The editors, contributors
and the publishers have, as far as it is possible, taken care to ensure
that the information given in this text is accurate and up to date.
However, readers are strongly advised to confirm that the
information, especially with regard to drug usage, complies with
current legislation and standards of practice.

The
publisher's
policy is to use
**paper manufactured
from sustainable forests**

Printed in China by RDC Group Limited
N/03

Preface

This book is an aid to clinical surgery and should not be regarded as a comprehensive surgical text. The objective is to provide medical students with nearly all the factual information they require to pass their standard examinations. It is our hope that enough material will be available on 'mainstream' surgical specialties to avoid the need for separate texts in each of these.

We retain our triple objectives: (1) to introduce the basic vocabulary and surgical principles for students to feel at ease on the surgical ward; (2) to provide the essential information on common surgical conditions, enabling students to tackle the major task of analysing clinical problems; (3) to speed the student on his or her passage through the various surgical examinations. It was not our objective to supply detail of surgical operations; where needed, this information is readily available from specialist manuals.

With this sixth edition of the book we have introduced a number of changes. Chapters are now grouped together in nine major sections. Like modern surgical practice these groupings are elastic, but they may help to orientate students and trainees attached to a particular specialty unit. Thus trauma has been emphasized by grouping the six chapters that cover the field. Three separate chapters on infection in the fifth edition have been amalgamated into a new Chapter 6 (Surgical infection). Conditions of the face, lip, tongue and mouth have been combined with neck swellings in a new Chapter 19 (Head and Neck). The important growth areas of minimal access surgery, surgical oncology and transplantation now have their own chapters (9 to 11) in the first section. The metabolic

response to injury has been expanded to include all aspects of surgical nutrition and metabolism (Chapter 4), while postoperative complications are now set in the context of the total care of the surgical patient before, during and after operation (Chapter 8).

Our objective in this revision has been to make the book more attractive without upsetting the popular style that Peter Scott used in the first edition. There are now many more illustrations, and the lay-out has been updated in terms of headings and the arrangement of the text. Each chapter now starts with an overview that highlights the main topics covered and ends with a list of key references. These references are not designed to be comprehensive but to provide an entree into the surgical literature, guiding the student towards salient journal articles and book chapters where some important subjects are considered in greater detail.

These several alterations have meant a certain number of changes to the team of authors, although the two Editors are unchanged from the fifth edition. The Australasian origins of the book have been strengthened by the inclusion of some New Zealanders, while we welcome several British contributors, many based at the newly-formed Imperial College School of Medicine in London. The pace of change in surgery has been as rapid as in other clinical disciplines, so the Editors are glad to acknowledge their debt to the authors who have updated their text.

It is a pleasure to note the continuing contribution from Professor Hugh Dudley (Chapter 1), who held Chairs of Surgery in Melbourne and London during the course of a distinguished professional career and whose involvement with the book is described in a new tribute. His guiding principles remain in force.

Although this book can be no substitute for knowledge gained directly from the ward, clinic or operating theatre, we trust that it may still serve to illuminate your understanding of the surgical patients you encounter.

Robin Williamson   Bruce Waxman
London, UK   Melbourne, Australia

Contributors

Paul D. Abel ChM FRCS FRCS (Eng)
Senior Lecturer, Honorary Consultant Urologist,
Department of Surgery, Imperial College School of
Medicine, Hammersmith Hospital, London, UK

Paul C. B. Anderson BSc MBChB (Hons)
Surgical Senior House Officer, Fazakerley Hospital,
Liverpool, UK

Graeme Brazenor BMedSc MBBS FRACS
Consultant Neurosurgeon, Austin Hospital, Melbourne,
Australia

Steven T. F. Chan MBBS PhD FRACS FRCS (Edin) FAMS
Associate Professor of Surgery, National University of
Singapore, Singapore

Hugh Dudley CBE ChM FRCS (Edin) FRACS FRCS (Eng)
Emeritus Professor, University of London, London, UK

Colin Goodchild MA MB BChir PhD FRCA FANZCA
Professor and Head, University Department of Anaesthesia,
Monash Medical Centre, Melbourne, Australia

David Gotley MD FRACS
Senior Lecturer, University of Queensland, Department of
Surgery, Princess Alexandra Hospital, Brisbane, Australia

Donald W. Howie MBBS PhD FRACS FAOA
Professor of Orthopaedics and Trauma, University of
Adelaide and Clinical Director of Service and Head of
Department of Orthopaedics and Trauma, Royal Adelaide
Hospital, Adelaide, Australia

Mark W. Kissin MA MB MChir FRCS
Consultant Breast and General Surgeon, Royal Surrey
County Hospital, St Luke's Hospital Trust and Tarvis Breast
Screening Centre, Guildford, Surrey; Regional
Co-ordinator for Breast Screening, South West Thames
Region, UK

Witold A. Kmiot MS FRCS (Gen)
Honorary Senior Lecturer and Consultant Colorectal
Surgeon, Department of Surgery, Imperial College School
of Medicine, Hammersmith Hospital, London, UK

Mark Laniado BSc (Hons) FRCS
Research Fellow in Urology, Imperial College School of
Medicine, Hammersmith Hospital, London, UK

Villis R. Marshall MD FRACS
Professor and Chairman, Flinders University Department of
Surgery, Flinders Medical Centre, Bedford Park, Adelaide,
Australia

John P. Masterton AM MBChB FRCS FRACS
Associate Professor, Monash University, Department of
Surgery and Formerly Head of Burns Unit, Alfred Hospital,
Melbourne, Australia

Michael L. Nicholson MD FRCS
Professor of Transplant Surgery, University of Leicester,
Leicester General Hospital, Leicester, UK

Paul O'Brien MBBS MD FRACS
Professor of Surgery, Monash University; Head of
Department of General Surgery, Alfred Hospital,
Melbourne, Australia

Robin K. S. Phillips MBBS MS FRCS
Consultant Surgeon, St Mark's Hospital, London; Dean,
St Mark's Academic Institute, London, UK

David M. Scott-Coombes MS FRCS
Consultant Surgeon, King's College Hospital, London, UK

James Shaw DSc MD FRACS
Associate Professor of Surgery and Vascular, Oncology and Endocrine Surgeon, Auckland Hospital, Auckland, New Zealand

Peter L. Smith MBBS FRCP FRCS
Consultant Cardiothoracic Surgeon, Hammersmith Hospital, London; Senior Lecturer, Cardiothoracic Surgery, Imperial College School of Medicine, London, UK

Gerard Stansby MA MChir FRCS
Senior Lecturer and Honorary Consultant Surgeon, Imperial College School of Medicine, St Mary's Hospital, London, UK

Jeremy N. Thompson MChir FRCS
Consultant Surgeon, Chelsea and Westminster and Royal Marsden Hospitals, London, UK

John D. Turnidge MBBS FRACP FRCPA
Associate Professor of Microbiology, Monash University; Director, Microbiology and Infectious Diseases Department, Women's and Children's Hospital, Adelaide, Australia

Andre van Rij MBChB BMedSc MD FRACS
Ralph Barnett Professor of Surgery, Head of Surgery, Dunedin School of Medicine, University of Otago, New Zealand

Bruce P. Waxman BMedSc MBBS FRACS FRCS (Eng) FACS
Associate Professor and Director, Academic Surgical Unit, Monash University, Dandenong Hospital, Southern Health Care Network, Melbourne, Australia

A. John Webb MB ChM FRCS (Eng) FIAC
Senior Research Fellow, Department of Surgery, Bristol Royal Infirmary, Bristol, UK

Robin C. N. Williamson MA MD MChir FRCS Hon FRCS (Thailand) Hon PhD (Mahidol)
Professor of Surgery, Imperial College School of Medicine, Hammersmith Hospital, London, UK

John H. N. Wolfe MS FRCS
Consultant Vascular Surgeon, St Mary's Hospital Regional Vascular Unit; Honorary Senior Lecturer, Royal Postgraduate Medical School, London, UK

Andrew Zbar MB BS FRCS FRACS
Surgical Research Fellow Department of Surgery, Imperial College School of Medicine, Hammersmith Hospital, London, UK

Tribute to previous editors

Peter R. Scott
MBBS FRCS (Eng) FRCS (Edin) FRACS FACS

Peter Robert Scott was the author and editor of the first edition of *An Aid to Clinical Surgery*, published in 1971. Peter Scott was born in Geelong, Victoria, Australia on 24 March 1931 and was raised in suburban Melbourne, attended Melbourne High School, and graduated MBBS with honours from the University of Melbourne. He completed surgical training at the Royal Melbourne Hospital (RMH) and underwent further training in the UK at Kingston Hospital, Surrey; Southend General Hospital, Essex; St Thomas Hospital, London; and the Royal Postgraduate Medical School, Hammersmith. He also worked in the USA at the Lahey and Mayo Clinic. Returning to RMH he became successively Acting Surgeon to Outpatients; Surgeon to Outpatients; and Head of a General Surgery Unit at that hospital until his retirement in 1996 and subsequent appointment as Honorary Senior Consultant Surgeon. He led the RMH civilian surgical team to Long Xuyen, South Vietnam during the Vietnam war in 1966. He also held appointments as Consultant Surgeon to the Essendon District Hospital and Frankston Community Hospital. His major area of surgical interest was upper gastrointestinal surgery. He has published many articles in surgical journals and outside medicine through his interest in genealogy.

Peter Scott's most valuable contribution to medical education is his unique ability to impart knowledge to medical students and aspiring surgical trainees. His lectures and tutorials to final year medical students at RMH became legendary and were attended by students from all clinical years and indeed by medical students from all over Melbourne. Many of the lectures and line diagrams were incorporated into the first edition of this book, and although there have been many subsequent editions and editors, the style and vision that originated will always remain in *Scott*.

Hugh A. F. Dudley
CBE ChM FRACS (Eng) FRCS (Eng) FRACS

Hugh Arnold Freeman Dudley was invited by the publishers to become editor of the second edition of *Scott*, which was published in 1979. He subsequently was editor of the third and fourth editions, inviting Bruce Waxman as associate editor for the third edition to maintain an Anglo-Australian input. He invited Robin Williamson to take over as editor for the fifth edition. Hugh has continued to contribute as chapter author but this sixth edition will be his last. Without his input *Scott* would not have survived.

Hugh Dudley was born in Dublin of Anglo-Irish parents on 1 July 1925. His secondary education was in the West Riding of Yorkshire, England, and he qualified MB, ChB from Edinburgh University in 1947. He completed surgical training at the Royal Infirmary of Edinburgh, Scotland under the late Sir James Learmonth and at Harvard Medical School with Dr Francis Moore. He returned to Scotland as Senior Lecturer at Aberdeen, and from there was appointed by Monash University as the Foundation Professor of Surgery, at Alfred Hospital, Melbourne, Australia in 1963. He led two surgical teams from that hospital into Vietnam in 1967 and 1969. He returned to England in 1972 as Professor of Surgery and Director of the Academic Surgical Unit, St Mary's Hospital Medical School, London, where he remained until his retirement in 1988. He was Chairman of the

British Journal of Surgery (1980–88) and was responsible for a major reorganisation of the administrative structure of that journal during that period. He was also the President of the Surgical Research Society of Australasia (1968–70) and of the Surgical Research Society of Great Britain and Ireland (1981). He was President of the Biological Society of Great Britain (1978–80) and holds Honorary Fellowships of the American Surgical Association; the American Society for the Surgery of Trauma; and the South African College of Surgeons.

Professor Dudley has been a prolific writer of surgical journal articles and gained international renown as author, editor and co-editor of a number of surgical texts. Many medical students and surgical trainees, in both the UK and Australasia, have been influenced by his incisive comments and thorough and systematic approach to academic and clinical surgery. Several members of the 'Dudley school' have gone on to be appointed to either Chairs in Surgery or other major academic positions throughout the UK, South-East Asia and Australasia, and owe much to his influence, academic philosophies and teachings, and surgical principles.

Contents

SECTION 8: Vascular surgery

SECTION 9: General disorders

General principles of surgery

Clinical methods

Hugh Dudley

OVERVIEW

This chapter provides a background to the way that clinical surgery is *practised* which is frequently somewhat different from the way it is taught. The objective is to explain some of the reasons for the way things happen in surgical diagnosis and management and, in particular, to introduce methods of reasoning which are commonly used but rarely explained. A list is also given of some axioms that are particularly useful in (although not exclusive to) clinical behaviour. It is intended to encourage the student to look beyond the conventional ways of analysis of the clinical task and to encourage clear thinking about objectives.

The common meaning of 'clinical methods' is the practical details of how to take a history and make a physical and mental examination of your patient. This chapter is not about such matters, details of which are touched on elsewhere in this book. Instead it covers the general way that we go about clinical work. There is a gradual change in the way surgical (and indeed medical) problems are approached and we would like to give students some basis upon which to build when, as we expect, the ideas which follow become more a part of the vocabulary and tools of medicine.

You can be fairly certain that you will not be examined directly on the subjects that are discussed and this may tempt you to skip the chapter. Please do not – it may be useful to you when all the exams are over. It can also give you some insight into the ways you see your teachers tackle problems on the wards and in the outpatient clinics.

DIFFERENT CLINICAL METHODS

There are three modes used in clinical work, although these are often intermingled in any encounter with a patient:

- diagnostic/decision-making – we identify and analyse the patient's problem.
- data base – we get all the information possible on a patient either to help diagnosis or to have items available which may be useful now or in the future; in textbooks this is usually the instruction to 'take a full history and make a complete clinical examination'.
- management – we move to a series of tasks aimed at solving the problem. Further decision-making may be involved.

DIAGNOSTIC/DECISION-MAKING

A good example is the surgeon in the accident and emergency department confronted with a patient with acute abdominal pain. The history that is taken and the examination that is made are (initially) focused on identifying the cause. Neither is aimed at being exhaustive and one question or one item of examination and its result leads on to the next. For instance, learning that there is acute upper abdominal pain could lead to a further question about the presence or absence of shoulder tip pain (perforated ulcer or acute cholecystitis?); or to find tenderness and guarding low in the right iliac fossa may indicate that the next thing to do is a rectal examination or, in a female, a pelvic examination (acute appendicitis or right salpingitis?). As information emerges, the surgeon quickly develops an hypothesis about the likely cause and uses the next question or examination to test the hypothesis by getting information that either contradicts or supports it. The objective is to narrow the range of possibilities and concentrate on reaching an answer to the problem which can then be the basis for action. Such a method is sometimes called *heuristic* or goal-seeking. It is frequently driven by the urgency of the problem – the presence of an acute disturbance which threatens life.

Three points should be remembered. First, the aim is to make a diagnosis in a *frame* that can be acted on. A woman with a hard irregular lump in the breast tethered to the overlying skin almost certainly has breast cancer (see 'pattern recognition' below), but the clinical diagnostic frame is not suitable for action and further information from a biopsy is necessary to reach a pathological diagnosis before definitive treatment can be undertaken.

Second, and by contrast, action can (and should) sometimes be undertaken when the diagnosis is not completely defined pathologically. Diffuse tenderness and guarding in the abdomen plus circulatory disturbance imply an acute abdominal condition – peritoneal irritation – which nearly always requires an operation to treat the cause, even though this is not exactly known. However, it is an axiom that the more precise the diagnosis, the better is the treatment planned.

Third, diagnosis of this kind is largely achieved, as the examples given indicate, by *pattern recognition*. What is reasoned is that if A and B and C, etc. are present then it is *likely* that condition X or disease Y exists because A, B, C, etc. make up a pattern that we have seen before in association with X or Y. The more items that are present that we have known to be associated with X or Y in the past, the more likely it is that X or Y is present. Most of the time these likelihoods have been learnt from experience or from textbooks and applied by intuitive mental processes. However, it is possible to program a computer to sum up the likelihoods to give a mathematical expression of the probability of a given condition given certain attributes – symptoms, signs or tests. This has been particularly useful in improving the diagnosis of acute abdominal pain. There are two reasons for the computer's success: it can do the sums better and faster than the brain; and the clinical features the computer needs must be precisely recorded, which encourages more disciplined collection of information. Such *computer-assisted* diagnosis (the machine is not making the diagnosis, only pointing out probabilities that should be borne in mind) can be applied to other conditions as long as there is enough prior information to generate the probabilities of

association between a symptom or sign and the occurrence of a disease or disorder.

Diagnostic threshold

If we cannot, using probabilities and pattern recognition, always be certain of a diagnosis, some level of probability must be set at which we are going to accept and act on the premise that a particular disorder is present even though the evidence is incomplete. This is sometimes given the rather fancy title of 'decision-making under uncertainty', which most students will more easily recognise as 'that's life'. More seriously, we are constantly making such uncertain decisions; clearly the more serious the decision for the patient, the higher is the degree of certainty that we would like to have before taking the plunge of accepting it and going on to take action. Setting diagnostic thresholds is at the moment largely a subjective matter but will become increasingly externalised for reasons connected with the cost–benefit analysis now common in organised health services based on public funds.

Differential diagnosis

There may be a point in the clinical analysis when we have facts that partially support any of a number of diagnoses. Suppose that, after we have taken what we think to be a diagnostically relevant history and have carried out the appropriate physical examination in a patient with acute upper abdominal pain, we are left with three possibilities that would all fit the available facts equally well. We cannot, at this stage, distinguish between perforated peptic ulcer, acute pancreatitis and acute cholecystitis. Then we say that

$$P(\mathrm{D}_1) = P(\mathrm{D}_2) = P(\mathrm{D}_3)$$

where D_1, D_2 and D_3 are our three conditions. The probabilities are equal and their sum of course is 1. Differentiation between them is done by trying in some way to reduce the probability of one or other of the conditions and so to increase the probabilities of the others. Alternatively, we might try to find some information which increases the probability of one at the expense of the other two. As an example, gas under the diaphragm on a chest X-ray only occurs in the case of a perforated ulcer, so that, given that gas is found, the probability of this is greatly increased (virtually to 1) as compared with the other two. Similarly a *markedly* raised serum amylase concentration increases the probability of acute pancreatitis and lowers that of the other two conditions; although a *slight* rise does sometimes take place in both of them and we have to settle for a threshold value which separates *slight* from *marked*.

Mechanisms

Students learn about the mechanisms of disease in their basic science studies. Knowledge of mechanisms can be of use in diagnosis and it is always worthwhile asking the question: 'what mechanism could be the cause of this symptom or sign, or of this combination of symptoms and signs?' Pain over the shoulder tip in the context given above is a consequence of the common innervation of the skin and the diaphragm, which is in turn a consequence of their development. It would be possible to recognise the pattern without knowing the mechanism but, particularly in dealing with clinical observations that are difficult to analyse, thinking about mechanisms can help in reaching a conclusion about whether or not a postulated cause is *feasible* (see also 'Clinical behaviour' p. 4).

DATA BASE

Facts are usually collected on a structured basis – history, physical findings and investigations – or, what amounts to almost the same thing, by using a check list. What is implied is that there should be no thinking of the focused kind already discussed until all the possible facts have been gathered in. Although we should try during this exercise to be as objective as possible, only a computer can be truly so, and inevitably some mental processing goes on while the data base is being collected.

There are three main reasons for getting as many of the medical facts about a patient as possible, given that there are always limits to time and resources:

- First, we can never be quite certain when an isolated fact is or is not important in solving a problem.
- Second, facts which are not directly relevant to the solution of the problem may have a bearing on subsequent management – for example, it is very important to know that a patient upon whom you are thinking of performing a major operation has a history of coronary artery disease, or that routine examination produces evidence of urinary tract or respiratory disorder.

- Third, facts about an individual patient may not necessarily be personally beneficial but, when put together with similar ones from other patients, they may advance medical understanding and so make our subsequent care more effective.

Diagnostic/decision-making and data base modes overlap. In one circumstance, to reach a quick decision based on focused enquiry and examination may be in the patient's best interests; in another, an exhaustive enquiry may be necessary to obtain as many pieces of a complex jigsaw before trying to fit them together. You will see clinicians switch between both and it is important to remember not to be slavishly attached to one or the other.

MANAGEMENT

Having got a diagnosis, or a decision about action (e.g. that a patient has an acute abdomen which requires operation), the surgical team begins to do things, such as make further investigations or preparations for a surgical procedure. As matters develop (the *clinical course* of the patient), some actions can produce changes in the patient (e.g. those that constitute the metabolic response to injury – see Chapter 4 – or postoperative changes in respiratory function). The management process is a continuous one in which updates on the patient's status begin a new process of considering what to do next. In order that management can be soundly based, information of two kinds is needed:

- What was the nature of the patient at the outset, i.e. from what baseline did we start?
- What changes have subsequently taken place?

Both of these questions are answered by the use of repeated examinations and investigations. To understand this, it is necessary to look a little more closely at investigation and its purposes.

INVESTIGATIONS

Although we tend to talk about investigations as being different from history-taking and clinical examination, they are just another class of information. However, they have a number of special features which need to be kept in mind.

Discriminatory investigations are designed to help diagnosis, and particularly differential diagnosis. The chest X-ray mentioned previously which may show gas under the diaphragm is a very good example – it discriminates well between the three possibilities. It is not, however, symmetrical: it is diagnostic if positive, but unhelpful if negative. Also, when thinking about a discriminatory investigation we must have some prior view about how likely it is to be effective. This depends on its *specificity*, i.e. how frequently it is found to be positive in patients suffering from the condition, and how infrequently it is also positive in those who do not. Specificity contrasts with *sensitivity*: a sensitive test may be positive in a large number of patients with the diagnosis we seek, but it may also be positive in a large number of those who have other conditions. An example is testing for occult blood in the stool. The test can be made variably sensitive to the presence of blood, but it lacks specificity in that blood in the stool can be caused by anything from bleeding gums through duodenal ulcer to colon cancer or haemorrhoids. In general, the more sensitive a test is, the less likely it is to be specific.

In diagnostic/decision-making we use the most discriminatory tests. However, before a test is chosen there are two other factors to consider:

- invasiveness
- cost.

Invasiveness is an ill-defined term. In some circumstances saying 'good morning' to someone can be highly invasive. However, it usually means the amount of risk from the investigation to the body or psyche of the patient, which is roughly correlated with the degree of intervention required. A venepuncture is usually easy and without danger, but an arterial puncture may be more difficult, more likely to cause complications, such as a periarterial haematoma, and more prone to be associated with pain and distress. The arterial puncture is thus said to be more invasive. The less invasive a test which can achieve a diagnosis, the better.

A complicated investigation is likely to incur a greater *cost* than a simple one. Cost and invasiveness are often loosely associated. Thus in a patient with obstructive jaundice a high quality ultrasound investigation that shows a dilated duct and a stone at the lower end is cheap and also relatively non-invasive compared with an endoscopic retrograde cholangiopancreatogram or a percutaneous cholegram. However, we have very little idea of real economic costs, and the subject is a minefield for clinicians and administrators. The right view to take is that the quickest, cheapest and least taxing way for the patient is the best.

Investigations other than those that are discriminatory fall into two categories: screening and baseline.

Screening. An investigation such as an exercise ECG or a mammogram (see p. 206) can be done on a population at large or on a selected group within it, so that a condition such as myocardial ischaemia or breast cancer may be identified before it causes symptoms. The merits and demerits of screening are largely beyond the scope of this book, but an example is given later on (p. 212) where it may alter prognosis in surgical disease. Screening can also be 'opportunistic'. If a patient presents to the doctor because of *any* symptom or disorder and is in a group at risk of another condition (defined by age or known risk factors), the opportunity can be taken to test for this. There is a strong body of opinion that supports opportunistic rather than population screening.

Baseline. As mentioned above, when operations or other forms of management are undertaken, things alter. To understand change it is necessary to know where the patient started from, and for this certain baseline investigations are needed. A preoperative chest X-ray or an ECG is a *template* against which postoperative changes, such as the development of respiratory complications or chest pain, can be judged. Clearly, different age groups and different types of operation require different sets of baseline investigations.

CLINICAL BEHAVIOUR

Students come into clinical medicine firstly as spectators of the working methods of the clinical team. They can be excused for feeling somewhat confused. They have to learn a completely new vocabulary, and most of what they have been taught in basic medical science seems irrelevant as surgeons go about their work using pattern recognition, short cuts of intuition and a verbal repertoire which is often terse and jargon-ridden. Most clinical texts communicate more about facts than about behaviour and it is for this reason that we append a few notes here:

- In approaching a problem do not be afraid to guess – most of clinical medicine is intelligent guesswork (based on accepting threshold levels of probability), although surgeons in particular tend to give the impression that they are omnipotent which can reassure anxious patients as well as bolstering the surgical ego. While you are a student, your guesses do not carry any costs for the patient. However, do not make unintelligent guesses; what you conclude must be consistent with the facts that you have and your background knowledge of mechanisms. Do not, for example, diagnose haemophilia in a female or colitis in someone who has had their colon and rectum removed. These examples may sound silly but we have heard students do both, simply through not thinking about context and logic.

• Do not reason beyond the available facts, but try and use all those that are available. This is nearly the same as saying, do not think along the lines 'if such and such were present and so and so were not then it would be reasonable to say that this or that would be present'. Statements of this type are conjectural rather than being based on evidence.

• Remember Occam's razor – the concept that you should not postulate things to exist that are not necessary to provide a unified explanation of the facts in front of you. More specifically, in acute surgery or medicine it is rare for two diagnoses to coexist as the cause for the patient's presentation. This is not to say that there may not be more than one thing wrong with the patient – those with acute cholecystitis can have coronary artery disease but the symptoms and signs at any one moment usually have a single cause.

• Professionalise your vocabulary by using terms that are as precise as possible. Language is an important and neglected part of the technology of medicine; for example, when you say a lump is 'hard', be prepared to define what you mean (the subcutaneous surface of the distal third of the ulna is an appropriate yardstick). Do not talk about 'chaps', 'blokes', 'lasses', 'lads', 'cases' or use any other patronising descriptions. Human beings are human beings and should be discussed in terms that you would like used about yourself.

• Seek, as already indicated above, mechanisms whenever possible even if you can make a decision on pattern recognition alone. The intellectual exercise is invigorating and at some time or other you will encounter a problem that can be solved only in this way. Moreover, to try and explain symptoms and signs on the basis of a postulated disease process sometimes leads to the conclusion that one cannot do so; the mechanism is inconsistent with the facts and therefore the cause must lie in something else. For example, in a patient known to have gallstones, symptoms and signs must conform to those given on page 258 before it is justifiable to ascribe them to the presence of the stones, which are common and do not necessarily cause symptoms. (In this example many patients are not relieved of their problem by the removal of such stones, and not only is harm caused to the individual but also resources are wasted).

• You will need to think and learn laterally. Obstruction of hollow tubes has some of the same effects wherever it occurs in the body. The complications of gastrointestinal disease that need surgical care are mostly the same whatever that disease – haemorrhage, perforation, obstruction and (sometimes) malignant change.

• You must get your priorities right. Do not take a family history from the man in casualty with a sucking chest wound, at least until after the acute problem has been dealt with. Urgency overrides formal clinical rigour.

• You should develop and use rubrics (frameworks against which you can analyse a problem). For example, a lump can be described by its position, size, shape, consistency, surface contour and fixity to deep and superficial structures, and by any special features that it may have such as fluctuation, tenderness, heat, colour change, pulsation, thrill or bruit. An ulcer can be categorised in a similar way. By doing this you not only become more consistent in what you do, but you will also not miss out things that are of importance.

• Do not feel that you have to exclude a physical cause for the patient's symptoms and signs completely and utterly before you dare resort to a psychological explanation. When faced with a problem that does not seem to fit a well-recognised physical pattern, or for which you cannot see a clear-cut physiological, pathological or other mechanism, try and keep two parallel lines of reasoning going – the physical and the psychological.

• Always remember that the patient interprets clinical features without having your expert knowledge of mechanisms, but that nevertheless what is experienced is real for the patient even if abstract or irrelevant to you.

• Distinguish between solving the patient's problem and dealing with the disease as *you* see it. The patient consults the surgeon because there is a problem or illness that is personal even though you interpret it in medical and in general terms.

FURTHER READING

de Dombal F T 1993 Surgical decision making. Butterworth-Heinemann, Oxford

Phillips C I (ed) 1995 Logic in medicine, 2nd edn. BMJ Publishing Group, London

2

Principles of anaesthesia, pain management and respiratory management in surgery

Colin Goodchild

OVERVIEW

This chapter deals with the responsibilities of the anaesthetist and intensivist in managing those patients who will require anaesthesia for operative intervention, the ongoing control of their pain in the postoperative period, and those selected patients who require special forms of prolonged airway management and ventilation because of respiratory complications following surgery. The different components of anaesthesia are covered, including a discussion of the different drugs, in both general anaesthesia and local anaesthesia.

The mechanisms and causes of pain are presented, as are the common analgesic agents, particularly opioids, local anaesthetics and non-steroidal anti-inflammatories. The ventilatory management of patients with either upper airway obstruction or ineffective ventilation requires consideration of preventative technique and treatment involving airway management and ventilatory support often occurring in the intensive care/therapy unit.

PRINCIPLES OF ANAESTHESIA

Anaesthesia involves the abolition of all sensation, touch, posture, temperature and pain, and is the term normally reserved for states in which the patient is unconscious. Many modern anaesthetic techniques are complex with respect to both the range of drugs and the equipment used. It is possible to produce the anaesthetic state with the simple traditional method using a single drug. A large number of drugs are capable of abolishing all sensations but some (e.g. methyl alcohol) produce tissue damage whilst others (ethyl alcohol) cause less damage to tissues but are associated with prolonged and unpleasant recovery. A small group of drugs known as the inhalational anaesthetics (e.g. halothane, enflurane, isoflurane or sevoflurane) cause reversible depression of the central nervous system with an acceptable quality of recovery.

General anaesthetic agents are not often used alone in modern anaesthetic practice, but are combined with muscle relaxants and analgesics to produce balanced general anaesthesia. These latter two classes of drugs reduce the dose of general anaesthetic needed to keep the patient unconscious and in a state where surgery is possible. The pain of surgery usually persists into the postoperative period and thus the anaesthetist is often responsible for initiating postoperative pain treatment regimens. Like the conduct of general anaesthesia, the treatment of postoperative pain in modern practice often involves combinations of different classes of drugs that potentiate each other's actions.

THE COMPONENTS OF ANAESTHESIA

Anaesthesia has three components: hypnosis, analgesia and muscular relaxation. In the past it was common practice to produce all three by the administration of potent inhalational agents such as diethyl ether, and it is possible to do this with more modern agents such as halothane or isoflurane. However, with the introduction of tubocurarine in 1942 by Griffith and Johnson of Montreal, Gray in Liverpool in the UK suggested the concept of balanced general anaesthesia. Since the unconscious patient does not feel pain in the normally accepted sense but shows reflex responses to stimuli which could normally be regarded as painful, the term analgesia is replaced by suppression of reflex activity when describing drugs used to produce balanced general anaesthesia. Modern anaesthetists use small doses of specific drugs to produce three components: hypnosis or sleep, antinociception ('analgesia') and muscular relaxation. Although the drugs used for these three components have one main component as their primary action, drugs in each class do potentiate the actions of drugs in other classes.

Hypnosis

Commonly, hypnosis is induced by intravenous injection of a drug which has a short duration of action. Thiopentone (a thiobarbiturate) has been the commonest agent used for this, but now more modern drugs such as diisopropyl phenol (propofol) are also used commonly for induction of anaesthesia. Alternatively, one may induce unconsciousness by inhalation of a gas such as nitrous oxide combined with a vapour, e.g. halothane or isoflurane. During anaesthesia, hypnosis is maintained by inhalation of gases and vapours that have as their primary pharmacological action general central nervous system depression and depression of the level of consciousness. Alternatively, unconsciousness may be maintained by continuous intravenous infusion of a barbiturate (e.g. methohexitone) or propofol. Recovery from the effects of this maintenance regime is by exhalation of inhaled anaesthetics through the lungs or by metabolism of drugs given intravenously. Slower recovery follows from the use of very fat-soluble inhalational agents or intravenous drugs with a long half-life (e.g. thiopentone).

Analgesia

Inhalation of nitrous oxide produces a significant degree of analgesia but this may be supplemented by the addition of intravenous analgesics such as morphine or fentanyl. These drugs are powerful respiratory depressants and so they have to be used judiciously when the patient is breathing spontaneously under general anaesthesia. Higher doses may be used in patients who are being artificially ventilated. There is a modern trend towards the use of higher doses of very short-acting opioids (e.g. remifentanil) to produce intense analgesia during surgery. The actions of these drugs wear off quickly and are supplanted in the recovery phase with more usual doses of longer acting opioids such as morphine.

Muscular relaxation

Some muscle relaxation is necessary for most operations. This varies from simple relaxation of forearm muscles during the manipulation of a Colles' fracture to the more profound muscular relaxation needed for upper abdominal and intrathoracic operations. Some muscle relaxation is produced by using potent volatile anaesthetic agents but the dose of these needed for this effect is quite high, thus leading to prolonged recovery. To reduce this dose, neuromuscular blocking agents have been introduced into modern balanced general anaesthesia. These drugs (e.g. curare, vecuronium and atracurium) act by antagonising the effect of acetyl choline at the muscle end plate. Thus, all striated muscles are affected including respiratory muscles. Artificial ventilation therefore has to be instituted by intermittent positive pressure via an endotracheal tube.

MODE OF ACTION OF ANAESTHETICS

Even though it is now more than 150 years since the first anaesthetic was given, it is still unknown how such a wide variety of drugs produce general anaesthesia. To explain the production of the anaesthetic state by such a wide variety of compounds, a number of theories have been proposed. No one knows precisely how the drugs act or whether they indeed all act at the same site or sites within the central nervous system. Many theories were proposed on the basis of physical properties of drugs. For instance, the Meyer and Overton theory suggested that anaesthetic potency was related to the oil/water solubility partition coefficient of the drugs. Thus the common mode of action of all of these drugs was that they dissolved in membranes of neurones in the central nervous system and caused general disruption of neural function. However, many anaesthetic drugs did not follow this rule. We now know that a wide variety of inhalational and intravenous agents potentiate the actions of gamma-aminobutyric acid (GABA) within the central nervous system. GABA is an amino acid inhibitory neurotransmitter widely distributed throughout the central nervous system in 30–40% of all synapses. Its inhibitory actions include depression of consciousness, inhibition of memory, anticonvulsant and analgesic actions. Elucidation of this complex problem remains one of the great challenges to medical science and it is the subject of active research programmes by many anaesthetists, pharmacologists and molecular biologists throughout the world.

Local anaesthetics

The passage of impulses along nerves is associated with electrical depolarisation of the neuronal membrane. Sodium and potassium ions enter and leave the nerve during different phases of depolarisation and conduction. Local anaesthetic drugs (e.g. lignocaine, bupivacaine and ropivacaine) interfere with conduction along nerves of all types by inhibiting the passage of sodium ions through membrane channels. Local anaesthetic solutions are stored for injection as water-soluble salts, usually the hydrochloride. These solutions are acid with a low pH. However, when they are injected into tissues which are alkaline (pH 7.4), a reaction is caused which liberates the base of the local anaesthetic. This does not occur if the solution is injected into infected tissues where the pH may be low (possible 5–6). The salt will fail to liberate the base, and local anaesthetics do not produce their effect at sites of infection. It is the anaesthetic base that dissolves in membrane lipid to produce the local anaesthetic action.

EMLA is the commercial name given to a eutectic mixture of lignocaine and prilocaine. When this is held in contact with the skin by a special adhesive pad, there is a slow onset of anaesthesia in that area of skin over a period of 1 hour. This is useful for preparing a site for venepuncture, particularly in children.

Fibre-selective block. High concentrations of all local anaesthetics cause a total block of conduction in all nerve fibre types: somatic motor fibres used for movement of skeletal muscles; autonomic motor fibres, e.g. sympathetic, used for control of vasomotor tone and blood pressure; large myelinated fibres used for general sensations such as light touch, vibration sense and pressure and joint position sense; and small diameter fibres ($A\delta$ and C) that mediate general sensations as well as pain. However, more dilute solutions of local anaesthetics tend to block conduction in the smaller diameter $A\delta$ and C fibres, leaving only large myelinated nerve fibre function intact. Furthermore, very dilute solutions of local anaesthetics tend to block conduction only in C fibres that are firing at high frequency, e.g. pain fibres that have been sensitised by the release of inflammatory mediators following injury. Thus higher concentrations of local anaesthetics tend to be used for surgical anaesthesia, whilst more dilute solutions tend to be used for the treatment of postoperative pain.

Applications. Local anaesthetics may be used topically, i.e. painted or sprayed on mucous membranes and wound surfaces so that they are absorbed locally to produce analgesia of that area. Topical analgesia is used commonly for examinations or minor surgical procedures of the urethra, eye, nose, throat and bronchial tree. A tissue may also be anaesthetised by local infiltration, by injection of a dilute local anaesthetic solution in the area of a proposed operation. This is used widely for minor surgical operations. Local anaesthetic solution may also be injected in close proximity to a nerve innervating the surgical area. Bier's or intravenous regional block involves applying a tourniquet to an arm or a leg and subsequently filling the veins of the limb with local anaesthetic. This technique is particularly useful for the manipulation of fractures in the distal part of the limb as well as invasive surgery such as carpal tunnel release.

More extensive surgery in the abdomen or thorax requires a central block, i.e. introduction of local anaesthetic into the cerebrospinal fluid (spinal or subarachnoid analgesia) or into the epidural space. The epidural space lies between the dura and the periosteum of the vertebral canal through which all the spinal nerves pass in travelling from the spinal cord to the intervertebral foramen. Both of these blocks suffer from one major disadvantage – the possibility of severe hypotension due to blockade of conduction in sympathetic nerves. Both intrathecal and extradural anaesthesia/analgesia may be maintained by the introduction of a small catheter into the relevant space to allow repeated intermittent injections or continuous infusions of analgesic/anaesthetic agents. These techniques are commonly used for postoperative pain relief.

PAIN MANAGEMENT

A general definition of pain is that it is a sensory and emotional experience associated with potential or actual tissue damage or one that can be interpreted as such. This definition covers chronic pain syndromes as well as acute postoperative pain.

BASIC MECHANISMS

The clinical features of surgical and postoperative pain

are local pain at rest, the characteristics of which vary with the site and type of diseased tissues, and pain initiated by or exacerbated by movement with attendant local muscle spasm. This latter symptom and sign are associated with tissue inflammation. These two features are caused by different pathophysiological mechanisms. Tissue damage caused by trauma or infection stimulates pain receptors attached to small myelinated (Aδ) and unmyelinated (C) fibres. These cause pain and reflex sympathetic nerve discharge in the region of injury. This sympathetic discharge and the tissue damage cause the release of a number of inflammatory mediators: prostaglandins, bradykinin, neurokinin, nerve growth factor and interleukins. These substances sensitise tissue pain receptors so that they fire off action potentials and signal pain from the area of injury even when stimuli that are not normally painful are applied. Thus, touching a surgical wound induces pain. This is called primary hyperalgesia. When the frequency of firing of afferent C pain fibres reaches a critical frequency, the target neurones in the spinal cord become sensitised so that they fire off more action potentials for a given input. This general sensitisation, sometimes called wind-up, leads to exaggerated spinal cord reflexes, which in turn cause reflex muscle contraction (guarding) and greater pain sensation associated with movement.

PAIN MEASUREMENT

There are a number of methods for the measurement of different aspects of the pain experience. The commonest is a visual analogue scale. This is a 10 cm line on which the patient is asked to mark what most closely represents the pain experience. By changing the words at the ends of the line, one may assess the sensory (no pain to intense pain) or affect components (no pain to unpleasant pain). Lists of words ranked for severity describing sensory or affect components of the pain experience may also be used (verbal descriptor scales). The patient is asked to mark which word most closely represents their pain experience. Regular measurements will indicate when drug effects wear off and may also suggest that drugs of a different type might be more appropriate. For instance, a patient recording low scores on the sensory component but high scores on the affect may respond well to sympathetic personal handling or a mild sedative rather than increased doses of opioid. There are a number of therapies primarily directed towards the sensory components of the pain experience that work at a number of different

sites in the pain pathway. Local anaesthetics have already been mentioned as a way of interrupting pain impulse traffic travelling towards the central nervous system. More dilute solutions of local anaesthetics will interrupt transmission in high-frequency firing C fibres and thus tend to prevent spinal cord sensitisation and improve movement pain control. However, such dilute solutions, used alone, are not sufficient to produce pain relief at rest. Rather than use high concentrations of local anaesthetics producing numbness and other side-effects, they are often used in combination with other drugs, particularly opioids.

OPIOIDS

Opioids are synthetic and naturally occurring substances with actions like morphine that can be blocked by naloxone (the opioid antagonist). Members of this group are morphine, diamorphine (heroin), pethidine and codeine. Once inside the body these compounds bind with opioid receptors on the surface of neurones in the central and peripheral nervous systems. The drug receptor interaction explains all of the therapeutic effects as well as the side-effects effects of these compounds. Endogenous opioid neurotransmitter systems are normally the agonists at these receptors. They are involved in sensory pain processing in the spinal cord and brain stem (sensory component of the pain experience) and in the control of mood in the limbic system (affect component of the pain experience).

The treatment of postoperative pain with opioids alone is not very effective and may cause harm. It is well known that rest pain may be relieved very easily with small doses of opioids, but pain associated with movement (due to spinal cord sensitisation; see above) is not very sensitive to opioid therapy. Thus a patient will report abolition of rest pain by small doses of opioid but will require very high doses of opioid to relieve the pain of movement. Even then the patient will report that the movement pain persists but is now tolerable. This word describes the change in the affect component of the pain experience caused by larger doses of morphine altering the mood after binding with receptors in the limbic system. These higher doses are accompanied by a number of troublesome and potentially serious side-effects. The side-effects of these drugs are respiratory depression and nausea, and vomiting due to actions of the drugs in the medulla oblongata. Constipation is caused by combination with opioid receptors in the myenteric plexus of the

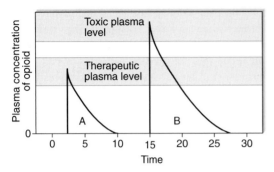

Fig. 2.1 Plasma concentration vs time effect of single-dose intramuscular injection of opioid. A. Therapeutic dose. **B.** Higher dose.

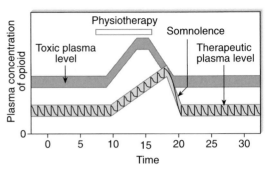

Fig. 2.2 Plasma concentration of opioid in patient-controlled intravenous analgesia.

gastrointestinal tract. Binding of morphine with these receptors increases gut intraluminal pressure. Many authorities regard this as a contraindication for morphine use in postoperative analgesia after laparotomy and bowel anastomosis.

Figure 2.1 shows what happens when a single dose of intramuscular opioid (e.g. morphine) is given for postoperative pain relief. Dose A is well chosen in that a therapeutic level for pain relief is achieved quickly and the dose is not high enough to cause respiratory depression. However, such a small dose is quickly cleared from the body and the patient begins to feel pain very soon after the dose as the blood level falls.

In order to achieve a longer period in the therapeutic range, conventional intramuscular opioid therapy ('PRN' or as required) involves a much higher dose such as dose B (see Fig. 2.1). The blood level after dose B remains above the therapeutic level for much longer but at the cost of the peak going into the range of respiratory depression. There are two ways of solving this problem. The first approach is continuous intravenous infusion of opioid to maintain a constant blood level. However, the plasma level required for adequate analgesia varies with activity, a much higher blood level of opioid being needed to maintain analgesia to cooperate with the physiotherapist. Once physiotherapy is completed, the blood level required for adequate analgesia at rest is low. Thus a common approach when using an opioid as the sole analgesic agent is to use patient-controlled analgesia (PCA). Small doses of opioid are given intravenously to the patient on demand by the press of a button. This allows the patient to vary the plasma concentration of drug according to the pain experience (Fig. 2.2). This has the advantage of overcoming inter-

patient variability as well as being able to vary the plasma level according to activity and type of operation. Nursing work is decreased by reducing the frequency of checking controlled drugs and it has a high patient acceptance.

However, PCA with opioids suffers from the philosophical problem of using the wrong drug for movement pain. The extra demands taken to cover physiotherapy may cause somnolence when the physiotherapist leaves, because the blood level exceeds that required for analgesia at rest (zone marked somnolence in Fig. 2.2). Nausea and vomiting are a major problem with PCA opioids. Thus, simultaneous administration of another analgesic drug to decrease spinal cord sensitisation is more logical to improve the pain relief profile whilst at the same time reducing opioid requirements and attendant opioid side-effects.

Combination with local anaesthetics

A modern approach to postoperative pain relief after laparotomy or thoracotomy is continuous epidural or intrathecal infusion of dilute local anaesthetic solutions combined with an opioid such as fentanyl, phenoperidine or diamorphine. The opioids bind with opioid receptors in the spinal cord to produce pain relief at rest whilst the dilute local anaesthetics interrupt incoming high-frequency C fibre discharge so that spinal cord sensitisation is reduced. The doses of opioid required are very small and thus opioid side-effects are much less common and the dilute local anaesthetic solution produces less or no paralysis of skeletal muscles and minimal disturbance of autonomic function. Other drugs may be used in these spinal solutions to decrease spinal cord sensitisation, such as benzodiazepines (e.g. midazolam) that bind with spinal cord $GABA_A$ receptors.

Combination with NSAIDs

Another logical combination is the addition of a non-steroidal anti-inflammatory drug (NSAID) that can be given intramuscularly, rectally or orally. A drug such as ketorolac or naproxen reduces the production of prostaglandins induced by surgical tissue damage. These are responsible for sensitisation of peripheral nerves, and so inhibition of their production decreases the frequency of firing afferent C fibres and thus improves movement pain relief by preventing spinal cord sensitisation. Provided there are no contraindications to the use of these drugs, e.g. danger of bleeding, peptic ulceration or compromised renal function, they can be used successfully to improve the pain relief profile of opioids and at the same time reduce the doses of opioids needed for adequate pain relief.

CONCLUSION

Modern anaesthesia and postoperative pain relief involves the choice of drugs that have selective actions within the nervous system, both peripheral and central. Combinations are used that maximise potentiation of the therapeutic effect of one drug by another, thus reducing the dose of individual component drugs and their side-effects.

RESPIRATORY MANAGEMENT IN SURGERY

Surgical patients require respiratory management – insertion of an endotracheal tube or tracheostomy, with or without mechanical ventilation of the lungs – in the following circumstances:

- respiratory obstruction in the upper airways
- ineffective mechanical performance, including paralysis
- lung disorders that interfere with gas exchange.

UPPER AIRWAYS OBSTRUCTION

There is a long list of causes, among which are the following:

- oedema – infections in the neck such as subfascial cellulitis, angioneurotic oedema, smoke inhalation, acute laryngotracheitis, acute epiglottitis
- foreign body, e.g. dentures, peanuts, meat (steakhouse syndrome)
- potential for inhalation of vomit/aspiration, such as emergency surgery in a patient with delayed gastric emptying and possibly large volumes of intragastric contents
- tumours (and their treatment), e.g. laryngeal carcinoma, thyroid carcinoma.

Diagnosis

The history may make this obvious. On examination there may be:

- an obvious cause in the neck
- cyanosis
- laboured breathing
- stridor, usually during inspiration, which is by far the most important observation and an indication of very high-grade obstruction.

In acute impaction of a foreign body there are convulsive respiratory movements, rapidly deepening cyanosis and indrawing of the intercostal spaces on inspiration.

Treatment

This depends on the cause. Occasionally it may be possible to tide the patient over an acute infection or to drain any pus that is present. Caution is needed in anaesthetising the patient because the respiratory state may worsen.

Endotracheal intubation may often be possible as a temporary measure until either the problem resolves or definitive treatment is carried out. It is relatively easy to do, does not create a wound and provides a reasonable pathway for aspiration of secretions. However, it is uncomfortable for the patient, can cause damage to the vocal cords and provides a pathway for infection into the lungs.

Tracheostomy should not, if at all possible, be done as an emergency in upper airways obstruction, although it may be required for long-term management (e.g. following laryngectomy).

In foreign body impaction, the patient is turned face down and, if at all possible, the foreign body is immediately removed. Meat or a peanut impacted in the larynx can often be driven out by getting behind the patient and forcibly compressing the upper abdomen and encircling the arms – the 'bear hug' or Heimlich manoeuvre. Failure to expel a foreign body or to overcome upper airway obstruction with endotracheal intubation is indication for emergency tracheostomy.

Tracheostomy. The operation is not performed very often, but the common indications are as follows:

- after radical surgery on the head and neck
- for *prolonged* IPPR (intermittent positive pressure respiration)
- occasionally in disorders such as myasthenia gravis and in the management of *prolonged* unconsciousness
- occasionally in acute or chronic pulmonary conditions, when reduction in anatomical dead space is needed as well as good access for tracheal suction. A tracheostomy in such circumstances is very much a double-edged weapon.

Tracheostomy is carried out electively after endotracheal intubation. The operator approaches the trachea through a transverse incision, retracting the thyroid isthmus upwards and making an incision at the level of the second, third or fourth tracheal ring.

Various types of incisions in the trachea are performed. In the emergency situation, a vertical incision is performed, carrying the incision straight down on the trachea. Percutaneous tracheostomy using a needle/guide wire technique is now performed in patients in intensive care (therapy) units.

Management. Humidification of the air is vital to prevent crusting, but the trachea adapts in the long term to obviate the need for humidification. Adequate atraumatic suction is required and saline lavage may be helpful to clear secretions. Mucolytic agents will help to loosen tenacious sputum.

INEFFECTIVE MECHANICS OF VENTILATION

Pain, mechanical disorganisation (flail chest), a stiff chest wall or lungs, and inadequate respiratory drive (e.g. head injury) may all cause hypoventilation and failure to clear bronchial secretions. The problem is aggravated if there is abdominal distension, which pushes the diaphragm up or impedes its descent. Any or all of these factors may be made worse by opioids or muscle relaxants.

There are three consequences:

- hypoventilation to the point of respiratory failure
- compressed basal alveoli may be closed during part or all of the respiratory cycle, so that blood flowing

through them is not oxygenated; this intrapulmonary shunt contributes to hypoxia
- retained secretions plug the bronchi causing the classical sequence of collapse–consolidation–infection; again these collapsed segments constitute an intrapulmonary shunt.

All these phenomena are seen in their clearest form in the patient after abdominal surgery, but they may also occur in acute chest diseases, neurological diseases and head injury.

Diagnosis of mechanical failure

The signs of impending respiratory failure can be difficult to elicit, but the following are indicative:

- patient complains of fatigue; as hypoxia develops, there is often confusion (acute brain syndrome)
- laboured breathing, usually shallow
- central cyanosis
- deterioration in blood gas tensions – a low P_aO_2 and high P_aCO_2 with respiratory acidosis characteristics.

Management

Prophylaxis. As always, prevention is better than cure. Elective operation should not be done on patients with active acute lung disease. Prophylactic antibiotics should be given to such patients who are in remission. Pain must be relieved as completely as possible whilst avoiding the use of high doses of opioids which may depress consciousness and respiratory drive.

Irritant anaesthetic agents are to be avoided, as is abdominal distension, and vigorous physiotherapy should be used. Patients with head and chest injury should be intubated and, if necessary, ventilated early before frank hypoxia has developed.

Treatment. The airway should be cleared of any accumulated secretions by physiotherapy, tracheal suction or bronchoscopy, and any contributing factors should be relieved. Institute mechanical support by intubation and IPPV.

LUNG DISORDERS

Any disease that destroys or damages the lung parenchyma may make surgical management more difficult, but two special circumstances are common in a surgical context: aspiration of vomit, and adult respiratory distress syndrome (ARDS).

Aspiration of vomit (syn. 'inhalation')

Patients with a full stomach vomit. Normally this invokes a protective reflex which closes off the larynx by cord apposition and the flap action of the epiglottis. This reflex may fail in:

- cord paralysis, e.g. bilateral recurrent nerve damage, say, at thyroidectomy
- unconscious patients
- use of muscle relaxants at induction of anaesthesia
- weakened patients such as those with profound hypotension.

The pathophysiological effect of aspirations produces an intense inflammation of the lungs with failure of gas exchange in the affected segment. Usually the right side is more affected than the left, perhaps because of the steeper angulation of the right bronchi. The degree of respiratory failure is proportional to the area involved.

Prophylaxis. In circumstances such as intestinal obstruction, the stomach should be kept empty with nasogastric intubation suction. In high-risk patients, such as those who are unconscious after head injury, the airway should be protected by endotracheal intubation or tracheostomy. At induction of anaesthetic, additional protection should be provided by compression of the oesophagus against the cervical cord, using pressure on the cricoid cartilage ('cricoid pressure').

Treatment. This is by:

- bronchoscopy and bronchial lavage
- respiratory support
- antibiotics
- steroids.

The use of steroids is controversial, although the majority view now is that their use has little place in the treatment of this condition.

Adult respiratory distress syndrome (ARDS)

This condition occurs commonly in seriously ill surgical patients. The major contributing cause is usually overwhelming sepsis, particularly severe Gram-negative sepsis. The typical clinical picture is the patient who develops a septic complication of the abdomen such as peritonitis or residual abscess. Hypoxia and respiratory failure with stiff lungs follow within 24–48 hours. There is nothing typical to be made out on chest examination, but a chest X-ray shows fluffy and patchy consolidation. Autopsy shows consolidation with interstitial oedema.

The current view is that the condition is predominantly caused by the deposition of endotoxin-activated leucocytes in the capillary bed of the lungs. These cells 'explode' biochemically, producing free oxygen radicals and perhaps cyclo-oxygenase activators.

Prophylaxis. Avoid or treat severe sepsis as early as possible.

Treatment. This is supportive:

- control sepsis; incipient ARDS is an indication of operation to locate and drain pus in the patient with abdominal sepsis
- institute and maintain IPPV with positive and expiratory pressure (PEEP) until the condition has resolved.

The condition may improve if the primary focus of sepsis is adequately treated. Return to the operating theatre for exploratory laparotomy is required. These patients are often too sick *not* to have an operation.

FURTHER READING

Komesaroff D 1985 Anaesthesia for the non-specialist. Williams and Wilkins, London
Lunn J N 1979 Lecture notes on anaesthetics. Blackwell Scientific, Oxford
Nimmo W S, Smith G (eds) 1996 Anaesthesia. Blackwell Scientific, Oxford

3

Body water and electrolytes in surgery
Andre van Rij

OVERVIEW

A thorough knowledge of the effects of illness, injury and surgery on the balance of water and electrolytes within the body and their losses from it is essential in surgical care. Maintaining their balance is one of the most common tasks in the day-to-day management of the surgical patient, especially when normal oral intakes are not possible.

Surgery as well as injury and acute illness interfere with normal water and electrolyte balance in the body and frequently pose problems in maintaining or correcting the balance. For this reason a good understanding of the normal organisation and distribution of body fluids is essential. Some of the essential quantitative data are given in Tables 3.1 and 3.2.

ORGANISATION AND DISTRIBUTION

In healthy adults, water constitutes approximately 60% of body weight. Although water is distributed throughout the body, it can be divided into two subvolumes separated by the cell membrane: intracellular fluid (ICF) and extracellular fluid (ECF) (Fig. 3.1). The ECF can be further divided into *intravascular* and *extravascular* (interstitial) compartments. In addition to these compartments, a certain amount of water is always present in the body cavities – gastrointestinal tract, CSF, aqueous humour. Such water has been processed through cells to reach these sites and is thus called *transcellular* water. The volume of transcellular water is usually small (about 0.5 L in

Table 3.1 Normal chemical composition and fluid volumes for a man weighing 65 kg

	Litres
Total body water (TBW)	40.0
Intracellular fluid (ICF)	24.0
Extracellular fluid (ECF)	15.0
Plasma volume (PV)	3.0
Interstitial fluid (IF)	12.0
Transcellular water (CSF, pleural, peritoneal, intestinal)	0.5–1.0
Daily volume of:	
• saliva	1.5
• gastric juice	2.5
• bile	0.5
• pancreatic juice	0.7
• succus entericus	3.0
Daily water losses in:	
• expired air	0.4
• faeces	0.1
• skin (insensible)	0.3
• urine (obligatory)	0.5
• **total**	**1.3**
Daily losses in urine of:	
• urea	25 g
• nitrogen	12 g
• sodium	150–200 mmol
• potassium	100 mmol
Total body:	
• protein	11.0 kg
• fat	9.0 kg
• carbohydrates	0.5 kg
• minerals	4.5 kg

an adult), but in certain sites, such as the gastrointestinal tract and kidney tubules, turnover is so rapid that many litres are processed each day. If the return pathway is

Table 3.2 Important ionic concentrations (mmol/L)

	ICF	ECF	
Na	10	135	
K	150	4	
Ca	2.5	2.5	
Mg	7.5	1	
Cl	10	100	
PO$_4$	45	1	
HCO$_3$	10	27	
	Na	K	Cl
Gastric aspirate	110	5	100
Intestinal aspirate	120	10	100

the ECF is mainly sodium chloride and sodium bicarbonate. The osmolality is equal in both the ECF and ICF as water moves freely across the cell membrane. Active transport mechanisms also exist to maintain the differential in sodium and potassium concentrations within the ECF and ICF. Thus, changes in osmotic pressure (tonicity) within either the ECF or ICF by solute confined to this compartment are equilibrated by the movement of water across the cell membrane. Usually, the osmolality of body fluids is maintained within the narrow range of 285–295 mosm/kg by adjustments in antidiuretic hormone (ADH) secretion and thirst-mediated water intake. Any excessive water intake and hypo-osmolality are countered by suppression of ADH and the excretion of a dilute urine. Inadequate water intake and hyperosmolality will stimulate ADH secretion and thirst. The resulting increased water intake and decreased water loss will restore the osmolality of body fluids to normal.

The main factor determining the size of the ECF is its sodium content. An increase in sodium with its attendant water results in an increase in the ECF, while sodium loss results in a reduction in ECF volume. Because of the close relationship between the sodium content and the volume of the ECF, it is no surprise that the major factor controlling renal sodium excretion is the size of the extracellular space. Expansion of the ECF enhances urinary sodium excretion, whereas volume contraction, even to a mild degree, results in limited sodium excretion; in some cases a virtually sodium-free urine may be excreted.

blocked or the production increased (e.g. in small bowel obstruction), then quite large volumes can be lost from the ECF volume into the transcellular water. Significant shifts like this of fluids into or from any of these compartments may seriously affect critical body functions. Maintaining the intravascular compartment for adequate circulation is the most immediate priority when shifts in distribution occur.

SODIUM AND WATER DISTRIBUTION

Sodium (Na$^+$) and potassium (K$^+$) are the main cations in body fluids, with sodium almost completely restricted to the ECF and potassium to the ICF. The composition of

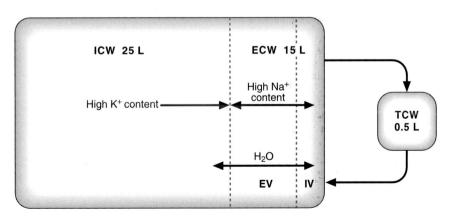

EV = extravascular
IV = intravascular

Fig. 3.1 Normal body fluid compartments. ICW, intracellular water; ECW, extracellular water; TCW, transcellular water.

Sodium turnover

In temperate regions sodium losses are almost entirely in the urine and intake is directly proportional to urinary output. Normal intake of sodium in the Western world is between 100–200 mmol/day, but with sodium restriction renal output can fall to 5 mmol/day. When extra renal losses of sodium are substantial as with persistent vomiting or diarrhoea, urinary sodium losses are dramatically minimised. Urinary conservation of sodium also occurs following injury and surgery.

Potassium turnover

Potassium is the most abundant intracellular cation, with total body stores of approximately 3500 mmol in a 70 kg man. In contrast, the extracellular potassium is only 2% of this but is finely tuned to a concentration of 3.5–5 mmol/L. The concentration of potassium across cellular membranes has a critical effect on the transmembrane potential. Even small changes in extracellular potassium have critical effects on cardiac, skeletal and smooth muscle function. Transport of potassium into cells occurs along with glucose and amino acid as regulated particularly by insulin. Intracellular potassium loss increases with cellular catabolism. This is increased with the stress of injury and surgery. Changes in acid–base balance have important effects on potassium turnover.

Most potassium is excreted in the urine. Losses are not well controlled. Many drugs and renal diseases interfere with this system. Extrarenal losses of potassium are normally minimal, but with continued diarrhoea, vomiting or fistula fluid losses quite large deficits may occur. Unfortunately a considerable depletion of body potassium may result before the serum potassium becomes abnormally low.

PRINCIPLES OF FLUID MANAGEMENT

Often surgical patients are not able to take in adequate volumes of fluid. In addition, the normal physiological control of fluid and electrolyte exchange and of body losses are impaired. The goal of fluid management is to provide adequate volumes of the correct fluids to assist the body to achieve balance amongst the various compartments. This can be conveniently divided into:

- Correction of existing abnormalities.
- Maintenance of daily requirements. In the first few days this is based on usual intakes of water, sodium and potassium. For more prolonged periods other cations such as calcium and magnesium will be considered. Eventually nutrients are also included in these fluids.
- Replacement of ongoing losses. These are estimated by measuring the volumes lost where possible and by having a knowledge of their content (Tables 3.1 and 3.2).

Some knowledge of the content of suitable solutions for intravenous use is essential – 'normal saline' or '1/5 normal saline with dextrose' with or without added potassium suffice for most circumstances of daily maintenance or replacement of losses. Hartmann's solution is an alternative to normal saline for the latter (Table 3.3). More complex solutions may be preferred in special circumstances.

The main *disorders* of surgical relevance are:

- ECF depletion
- ECF expansion
- hyponatraemia
- hypernatraemia
- hypokalaemia
- hyperkalaemia.

Table 3.3	Solutions that may be used for fluid management
Component	Quantity
Maintenance (daily)	
Normal saline:	
• sodium	90–100 mmol
• potassium	60–100 mmol
• water	2–3 L
1/5 normal saline with dextrose:	
• sodium	30 mmol/L
• potassium	20 mmol/L
• dextrose*	42 g/L
Replacement of ECF	
Normal or 9% saline:	
• sodium	154 mmol/L
• chloride	154 mmol/L
Hartmann's balanced salt:	
• sodium	131 mmol/L
• chloride	111 mmol/L
• lactate†	29 mmol/L
• potassium may be added	5 mmol/L
• calcium	4 mmol/L

*Dextrose is added for isotonicity but it is also protein sparing.
†Lactate is metabolised to provide carbonate.

EXTRACELLULAR FLUID DEPLETION (dehydration – the loss of salt and water)

ECF depletion is the most common and most important abnormality of body fluids and is best known as dehydration.

Pathogenesis

Generally, the loss of excessive body fluids such as perspiration or gastrointestinal fluids, e.g. diarrhoea, occurs as salt and water, which to all intents and purpose are in the same concentration as the ECF. The ECF shrinks without significant adjustment from the ICF (Fig 3.2). Shifts occur within the ECF to maintain the intravascular compartment and the circulation. In due course, the circulating volume shrinks and compensatory tachycardia helps to maintain body perfusion. If losses continue, hypotension and collapse with hypovolaemic shock and death may supervene.

Similar changes occur when isotonic salt and water are sequestrated within the body. Surprisingly large volumes of fluid can be 'lost' in the gut lumen with bowel obstruction, in cases of oedema in injured tissues and from leaky capillaries. The stress of injury or surgery may cause an elusive loss of effective ECF into the so-called 'third space'.

Clinical features

A history of excessive or abnormal fluid losses, particularly with diminished intakes, are important clues. Apathy and weakness and sunken eyes may be apparent. Thirst is an early feature, while a dry tongue and poor skin turgor are later features. Decreased urine output and increased specific gravity are the best simple indicators of dehydration as measures of the kidneys' attempt to protect a shrinking ECF. A dropping jugular venous pressure, tachycardia and low blood pressure mark serious deficits. Isotonic losses of salt and water have no effect on the serum sodium.

Management

Prevention is better than cure and this is achieved by good maintenance and replacement fluid therapy. Treatment is to replace the ECF deficit, using an isotonic solution with a comparable sodium concentration. 'Normal' saline suffices in almost every circumstance. The body has considerable agility in making the finer readjustments once the basis for resuscitation has been provided. Additional potassium may be added subsequently if this is also low.

The correct rate and amount of infusion depend on the severity of the deficit, the urgency if surgery is contemplated and the patient's cardiovascular status. The best

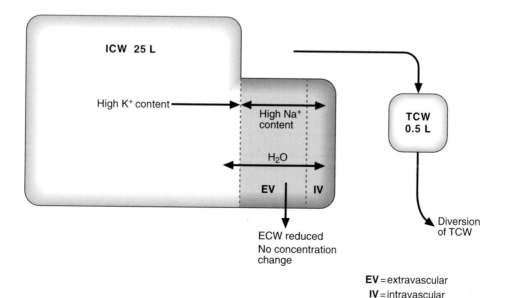

Fig. 3.2 Change of body fluid compartments in extracellular fluid depletion. ECW, extracellular water; TCW, transcellular water.

measure is the response observed in the central venous pressure, pulse and blood pressure, as well as hourly urine volume. Too much can precipitate fluid overload.

It is important to take into account the fact that, as a patient recovers from their illness, any previously sequestrated ECF volume is mobilised and may further re-expand the ECF.

EXTRACELLULAR FLUID EXPANSION
(volume overload – salt and water excess)

ECF overload is a common problem with the increasing number of older surgical patients with fragile cardiovascular status. The problem in a surgical ward is often iatrogenic.

Pathogenesis

This disorder arises when there is too much salt and water with an overexpansion of the ECF volume. This occurs with impairment of renal excretion resulting from hormonal and various circulatory factors as well as deterioration in kidney function. Therapeutic infusion of saline in the presence of underlying cardiac, hepatic or renal insufficiency may precipitate overload. In addition, trauma and surgery induce some water and salt retention. This is more marked in the elderly and makes them more vulnerable to overload with infusions. The intravascular compartment enlarges and interstitial fluid accumulates as oedema and leaks out into transcellular spaces as in pleural effusion and pulmonary oedema (Fig. 3.3).

Clinical features

There may be a history of sudden weight gain or an accumulating positive balance on the fluid chart. Peripheral oedema, raised central venous pressure, dyspnoea, basal lung crepitations and pulmonary oedema may all be observed. A history and other features of heart failure or hepatic or renal failure may alert to the problem.

Management

Prevention by being alert to at-risk patients is important. Restriction of further sodium and water infusion prevents further deterioration. Diuretics help to shrink the ECF. Support for frank pulmonary oedema may be required with oxygen, morphine and, rarely, ventilation assistance. Underlying cardiac and renal disease may require more intensive therapy.

HYPONATRAEMIA (water overload, hypo-osmolality)

This is the most common iatrogenic fluid and electrolyte disorder in the surgical ward.

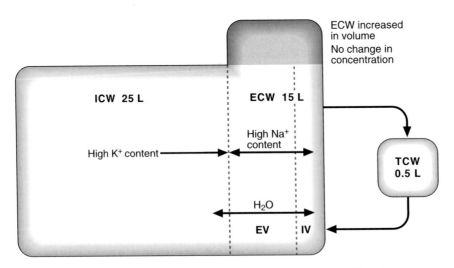

Fig. 3.3 Change of body fluid compartments in sodium and water (ECF) excess. ICW, intracellular water; ECW, extracellular water; TCW, transcellular water.

Pathogenesis

By far the most common cause of hyponatraemia is an excess of water rather than a deficit of sodium. This occurs particularly when renal clearance of free water is impaired. Free water clearance is often reduced in the elderly and in those with cardiac and renal disease. In addition, the transient increase of ADH secretion associated with surgical stress reduces free water clearance. Inappropriate ADH secretion sometimes occurs with some tumours, pulmonary diseases and central nervous disorders. In these circumstances the infusion of usual volumes of maintenance fluids provides more water than can be coped with.

Hyponatraemia may also occur when salt and water loss of dehydration is replaced by water. Less commonly, hyponatraemia results when other osmotically active molecules contribute, as in hyperglycaemia.

Clinical features

Most hyponatraemia is asymptomatic and self-limiting. A history of predisposing conditions and the presence of an intravenous infusion should be looked for. Once the serum sodium drops to 120 mmol/L symptoms of water intoxication occur with weakness cramps and confusion. Coma may occur.

Management

Water restriction is sufficient for both prevention and treatment in most instances. When there has been associated dehydration and decreased ECF volume, isotonic saline may be used. Symptomatic hyponatraemia is treated similarly and hypertonic saline should rarely be used. Rapid correction may be dangerous.

HYPERNATRAEMIA (hyperosmolality)

This is uncommon but requires prompt treatment.

Pathogenesis

A high serum sodium always indicates a deficit in total body water relative to solute. It can arise as a result of either inadequate water intake or excessive water loss; the loss may be either renal (e.g. concentrating defect) or extrarenal (e.g. sweat and respiratory losses). Excessive intakes of sodium in some infusions can result in hypernatraemia.

Clinical features

Central nervous system effects predominate as water is drawn out of the cells. Restlessness, spasms and fitting occur when serum sodium is about 160 mmol/L.

Management

Judicious replacement of water is required. If this is too rapid, the fluid shifts may result in cerebral oedema.

HYPOKALAEMIA

This is a problem frequently diagnosed prior to surgery because of the widespread use of cardiovascular drugs and diuretics in particular. Operative risk with cardiac arrhythmias is increased.

Pathogenesis

Potassium loss in the urine occurs when sodium is conserved (as in starvation, after injury or with dehydration). Alkalosis accentuates hypokalaemia by increasing renal losses and shifting potassium into cells in exchange for hydrogen ions. Losses induced by potassium-wasting diuretics are also important. Extrarenal losses are increased with persistent vomiting, diarrhoea or fistula losses. Mucous diarrhoea (as occurs with villous adenoma of the rectum) contains 10 times the plasma concentration of potassium. Small daily deficits have to accumulate as much as 400 mmol before serum potassium is affected.

Clinical features

These are lethargy, disorientation, decreased striated and smooth muscle tone with consequent ptosis, ileus and cardiac arrhythmia. Low serum potassium, alkalosis and ECG changes (low T waves, prolonged QT interval and presence of U waves) are confirmatory. Digoxin toxicity may occur.

Management

Daily potassium supplement and, where possible, treatment of the underlying cause suffice. In severe hypokalaemia, intravenous infusion of potassium is required. This should be done with care for, if given too quickly, it may cause fatal arrhythmia. In emergencies more rapid administration should be monitored with an ECG.

HYPERKALAEMIA

This is less common but may need to be treated with greater urgency.

Pathogenesis

Impaired renal excretion of potassium is the most frequent factor leading to hyperkalaemia. Increased loss of intracellular potassium into the ECF occurs with tissue catabolism (with starvation, surgical stress or sepsis) and direct tissue injury (crush injury) as well as with acidosis (in exchange for hydrogen ion). When these occur in patients with some renal impairment, hyperkalaemia is far more likely.

Clinical features

The most serious effects are cardiac arrhythmias including ventricular fibrillation and sudden asystole. Neuromuscular effects include anxiety, paraesthesia and weakness progressing to flaccid paralysis. High serum potassium and ECG changes – peaked T waves, loss of P waves and widening QRS complex – are diagnostic.

Management

With chronic renal impairment, dietary restriction and (when indicated) dialysis prevent hyperkalaemia. Severe hyperkalaemia is an emergency. Cardiac toxicity is minimised by intravenous calcium infusion. The prompt infusion of glucose and insulin shifts ECF potassium out into the ICF. Some potassium excess can be removed with exchange resins in the gastrointestinal tract. In severe cases haemofiltration or renal dialysis may be required.

ACID–BASE BALANCE

The difficulty for the student in understanding acid–base balance is the many confusing ways it is explained. It is, however, important to have a grasp of how the body maintains this balance. Small changes in pH (more correctly hydrogen ion activity) have considerable impact on metabolic functions. The control of the balance is closely linked to electrolytes (especially potassium and bicarbonate) and of course renal function (acid clearance and bicarbonate regeneration) and respiratory function (CO_2 washout). In addition, there is the system of acid and base buffers which stabilise pH in both the ICF and ECF.

Disturbances of acid–base are important, especially in the more critically ill patient. They are conveniently divided into four types:

- respiratory alkalosis
- respiratory acidosis
- metabolic acidosis
- metabolic alkalosis.

Respiratory alkalosis occurs with hyperventilation, often induced by hypoxia or anxiety. The P_{CO_2} drops, bicarbonate falls and the pH rises. It is common in the early postoperative period when it is usually asymptomatic. If severe, however, dizziness and paraesthesia result. Treatment is by controlling the cause. Rebreathing can give temporary relief.

Respiratory acidosis occurs with hypoventilation. Respiratory depression with drugs (anaesthetics, narcotics), impairment of chest movement (as with abdominal or chest pain) and chronic respiratory disease all commonly predispose to this in the surgical ward. The P_{CO_2} increases and pH falls and blood buffers are unaffected. If severe, drowsiness, flapping tremor and coma may ensue. Prevention is achieved by good attention to pain relief and respiratory cares. Ventilatory support may be needed at times.

Metabolic acidosis is the result of too much acid production (ketoacidosis, lactic acidosis), the inability to clear this (renal impairment), the loss of buffer (diarrhoea, pancreatic fistula) or the inability to replace buffer (renal impairment). The buffer, especially bicarbonate, is used up and the pH falls. The P_{CO_2} may drop as compensatory hyperventilation occurs. Peripheral vasodilatation and increased cardiac output result, but this may go on to depressed cardiac contractility and collapse. Oxygen delivery is also impaired. Metabolic acidosis of particular surgical relevance occurs where there is underperfused tissue. This occurs with shock when the whole body is underperfused and when large areas of ischaemia occur in the gut or limb. Management is to resuscitate and ensure good reperfusion. Replacement of bicarbonate is required only in severe acidosis.

Metabolic alkalosis is relatively uncommon. Depletion of acid results in a rising pH and increase in base buffer.

This occurs with persistent vomiting, e.g. with pyloric stenosis. A similar rise in pH occurs with hypokalaemia as intracellular potassium is shifted into ECF in exchange for hydrogen. Metabolic acidosis may also result with excessive intake of bicarbonate or lactate (converted to bicarbonate). This is usually asymptomatic, but if severe, confusion, tetany and coma may occur. Good fluid and electrolyte management of the underlying cause is sufficient to correct this disorder.

FURTHER READING

Hill G L, Farndon J R 1994 IV fluid therapy. In: Guide for house surgeons and interns in the surgical unit, 9th edn. Butterworth-Heinemann, Oxford, p 92–106

Wait R B, Kahng K M, Dresner L S 1996 Fluids and electrolytes and acid–base balance. In: Greenfield L J, Mulholland M, Oldham K T, Zelenock G B, Lillemoe K D (eds) Surgery: scientific principles and practice, 2nd edn. Lippincott-Raven, Philadelphia, p 242–266

4 Surgical nutrition and metabolism
Andre van Rij Bruce Waxman

OVERVIEW

Injury, sepsis and surgery induce a well orchestrated response from the body which impacts on fluid balance, energy requirements, defence mechanisms and eventually the healing process. When this process is prolonged, devastating depletion of body reserves occurs, with resulting malnutrition and increased complications. Understanding these processes and the measures to control their effects is central to the care of the surgical patient. This chapter covers the metabolic responses to injury, ways of modifying the response, and assessing and treating the effects of nutrition.

METABOLIC RESPONSE TO INJURY

The goal is to preserve body composition and functional integrity and to carry out repairs and rehabilitation.

Injury in its broadest sense encompasses trauma, surgery and sepsis. Their effects on the metabolic response are similar. Indeed, any significant acute illness, e.g. pancreatitis or toxic megacolon, may show the same response. The severity of the response is related to the level of the stress and its duration. Sepsis is a particularly potent stimulus.

While almost every aspect of the body participates, the following are particularly important:

- cardiovascular system
- water and electrolyte balance
- energy metabolism
- protein metabolism
- the metabolic messengers and modulators.

CARDIOVASCULAR SYSTEM

The more immediate responses to injury in the circulatory system are discussed in Chapter 5.

WATER AND ELECTROLYTE BALANCE

Urinary volume is decreased and sodium excretion diminished to preserve ECF volume. Within minutes of injury, there is a marked increase in antidiuretic hormone (ADH) secretion (mainly pain-induced) lasting 24–36 hours. During this time the volume of urine secreted is the *volume obligatore* – that necessary to excrete the solute load at the highest attainable concentration (down to 0.4 ml/min).

Aldosterone secretion increases partly as a result of increased adrenocorticotrophic hormone (ACTH) – for about 24 hours – but more as a result of increased renin levels secondary to a fall in circulatory blood volume and pressure. Urinary sodium excretion diminishes and potassium losses increase both in exchange for the sodium and also with the increased release of intracellular potassium. In simple terms, for the first day or two at least, sodium losses halve (50 mmol/day) and potassium losses double (100 mmol/day).

ENERGY METABOLISM

Following injury, food intake is stopped for a period and yet the energy demands continue. These requirements, as shown by measurements of oxygen consumption and metabolic rate, increase as the severity of the injury increases. The energy required for this is primarily supplied by mobilisation of fat, of which there are usually considerable reserves. The triglycerides are converted by hormone-sensitive lipase stimulated by increased catecholamines (as well as glucagon, growth hormone and glucocorticoids), providing fatty acids for release into the blood. These fatty acids are particularly useful for the heart, liver and skeletal muscle.

For other vital tissues such as white cells, brain and kidney, glucose is an essential energy source. However, reserves in the form of glycogen are limited and short-lived (24–48h). Thereafter, the only alternative source is the conversion of protein to amino acids and their conversion by the pathway of gluconeogenesis to glucose. Following more severe injury, blood glucose turnover is increased. At the same time there is some resistance to the effects of insulin on glucose uptake. Raised blood sugar, especially in diabetics, may be an early indicator of stress.

PROTEIN METABOLISM

An early observation made in patients following surgery was that the nitrogen in the urine increased despite no nitrogen (protein) intake. This was most apparent after severe injury or sepsis. The increase in urinary nitrogen was largely the result of increased protein breakdown to amino acids for gluconeogenesis. The released ammonium is detoxified in the liver and converted to urea which is readily measured in the urine. All of this coincided with increased energy demands shown by increased oxygen requirements and metabolic rate.

In addition to this protein breakdown (catabolism), there is also prompt requirement for new proteins to be produced, e.g. as a result of the following: the wound is invaded by an orchestration of different proteins and proliferating cells to initiate repair; white cell population turnover increases; the liver becomes a powerhouse of activity with the induction of protein synthesis to provide enzymes for detoxification and an array of proteins to be secreted into the blood (acute reactive proteins). All this also requires amino acids to be made available.

The proteolysis, to provide a source of amino acids, can occur at a great rate and reserves of protein are limited. Skeletal muscle supplies much of this, as well as the gut and liver. If the stress of injury is protracted, some critical processes are eventually affected, e.g. impaired healing, impaired immunity, muscle wasting and weakness, breakdown of the gut–mucosal barrier.

Subsequently, when the stress subsides and the patient begins to recover, protein synthesis dominates (anabolic phase). Recovery of fat occurs a little later in this phase.

THE METABOLIC MESSENGERS AND MODULATORS

The response to injury is initiated in a variety of ways through pain, cardiovascular stress and instability, or chemical factors released by bacteria or inflammation. These switch on the two major messenger systems that regulate the ensuing events:

- the neurohormonal pathway
- the inflammatory pathway.

The neurohormonal pathway is that whereby sensory input (pain, fear) connects with the hypothalamo-pituitary axis leading to increased secretion of corticotrophin-releasing factor to stimulate ACTH production (and thereby cortisol and aldosterone), as well as through sympathetic outflow to induce increased catecholamine release. Flow-on effects include increased levels of glucagon. These are the initiators of the catabolic phase. About 3 days after an uncomplicated operation, this fades out and the efficacy of other hormones increases, in particular insulin and growth hormone (anabolic phase). This lasts a lot longer.

The inflammatory pathway messengers are a number of cellular products, in particular cytokines (such as tumour necrosis factor and the interleukins 1 and 6) released locally at the time of injury, which have important local effects. When produced in larger amounts with more severe injury they spill over and are circulated systemically. The production of these molecules may then be amplified in other tissues and go on to have widespread metabolic effects such as, among many others, inducing ecosanoid and complement cascades, acute phase protein production, upregulating cellular adhesion molecule expression, and increasing muscle amino acid mobilisation. They are also responsible for anorexia, fever and, in excess, hypotension.

MODIFYING THE RESPONSE

The severity of the metabolic response varies markedly. In an elective uncomplicated operation the metabolic changes are hardly noticeable and of little consequence. After more significant injury there may be a brisk response, but this is short-lived with an uncomplicated recovery. The metabolic adaptations have been to good effect. By contrast, after a major 30% burn or ongoing abdominal infection, the response is severe and prolonged and components of it exceed the body reserves. Accelerated starvation, immune suppression and malnutrition supervene to threaten the outcome. If the patient survives, recovery will be a protracted affair. Measures to avoid these 'harmful' consequences of the metabolic response are vital in the care of these patients. These measures are described below.

Injury prevention. This needs to take place within the community.

Minimising the injury. This is by good first aid, resuscitation and trauma management, with prompt surgery to remove the ongoing stimulus. Similarly, prompt treatment of infection and illnesses is an important measure. At operation, good surgical skills with gentle handling of tissue reduce inflammatory reaction.

Prevention of complications. Complications are avoided by using measures such as antibiotic prophylaxis to avoid postoperative infection and by the use of sound surgical principles.

Optimal general patient care before and after surgery. The relief of anxiety and optimal pain relief reduce neurohumoral pathway activity. Epidural anaesthesia, in particular, has a salutary effect on the catabolic phase. Other medical problems are often present, especially in the elderly, and these need to be well controlled otherwise they add to the stress of the surgical injury.

Nutrient replacement. This is important and yet, surprisingly, is all too often neglected. Most patients undergoing surgery are well nourished and can tolerate 3–4 days without food. With more severe injury, when nutrient reserves are being used at a great pace, replacement becomes more important, especially the longer the stress is present. Providing nutrition by mouth is the obvious approach. Unfortunately, sick patients are often anorexic and do not tolerate oral food well. After abdominal surgery this may be even more unlikely. Even then the intestine can be accessed by a tube placed into the stomach (nasogastric tube or feeding gastrostomy) or the small bowel (jejunostomy tube). This enteral feeding is the preferred route and can be well tolerated quite soon after injury.

At times the enteral route is not safe (regurgitation),

not suitable (small bowel fistula) or not possible (small bowel ileus) and nutrients then have to be given intravenously (parenteral feeding). The regular infusion of dextrose in 1/5 normal saline with dextrose (hydrated glucose 3.4 kcal/g) to maintain fluid balance (see Ch. 3) provides less than 500 kcal/day. While well below daily energy requirement, this does have some useful protein-sparing effect (in the place of glucose from gluconeogenesis). However, it is a mistake to accept this as sufficient nutrient replacement when the absence of food has exceeded 5 days. In the face of a major catabolic decline this small dose of dextrose has minimal impact. In these circumstances a full complement of nutrients is required, i.e. total parenteral nutrition (TPN). Some knowledge of the daily requirements is necessary (Table 4.1).

TPN solutions that provide all these components in the right form, proportions and amounts are complex and costly, comprising 50% dextrose, amino acids (Synthamin or Vamin), fats (Intralipid), electrolytes and vitamins. They are also hypertonic and extremely irritating in peripheral veins and must be infused through a catheter (e.g. via the subclavian vein) into the superior vena cava where the solution is diluted rapidly. Some TPN solutions with a modified composition containing predominantly Intralipid may be given by the peripheral vein. TPN is not without hazard, with infection (line sepsis) and metabolic complications resulting from too much or too little. TPN alone cannot reverse the catabolic losses in the seriously ill patient but can make the difference that alters the outcome and shortens convalescence.

Manipulation of the messengers. Attempts to switch

Table 4.1 Fuel reserves in a 70 kg man and the intravenous nutrient requirements 7 days after an uncomplicated partial gastrectomy (except for a prolonged ileus)

	Weight (kg)	Energy (kcal)
Fat	14	125 000
Protein		
— skeletal muscle	6	24 000
— other	6	24 000
Glycogen	0.25	900
Free glucose	0.02	80

Daily requirement: energy, 1500–1700 kcal primarily as 20% dextrose; protein as amino acids, 0.8 g/kg; fat, 20–30% of energy; 'maintenance' water and electrolytes (Ch. 3); calcium, magnesium, phosphate and trace elements, e.g. zinc, copper and vitamins.

off the undesirable effects of the catabolic response (e.g. anti-TNF antibody, catecholamine blockers) or to switch on the anabolic phase (e.g. anabolic steriods) by this means have been generally disappointing. Insulin in TPN improves the uptake of additional glucose but has little impact on overall protein status. Some promise exists with recombinant growth hormone infusion but costs preclude this at present. Addition of glutamine to TPN solutions may also have benefits.

NUTRITION OF THE SURGICAL PATIENT

It is important to be aware that many patients coming to surgery are already nutritionally compromised, either because of prolonged or intermittent starvation or because of the effect of the underlying disease process. It is well recognised that malnutrition, e.g. 10–15% loss of body weight, significantly increases surgical morbidity and mortality.

Anorexia is commonly experienced and is accentuated by poor food palatability and impaired taste; inability to eat or to keep food down; the unavailability of food at home as a result of socioeconomic factors; or physical disability. Catabolic effects of existing disease and other comorbidities – which include cancer, severe respiratory and cardiac disease and malabsorptive disorders – accentuate the poor nutritional state.

In addition to taking a full medical history to ascertain these problems, it is also important to assess the nutritional state of the patient by taking a careful dietary history. The physical examination may reveal evidence of muscle wasting, but should be complemented by anthropometric measurements, including body weight and height – to calculate the body mass index: BMI = weight $(kg)/[height (m)]^2$ – and skin fold thickness. Blood tests including lymphocyte count, serum albumin and serum transferrin, and antigen skin reactivity – a test of cellular immunity – provide further information to assess the degree of malnutrition. All these parameters may be used to calculate a nutrition index.

Some correction of nutritional deficits is obviously desirable before surgery. As a first option, enteral feeding is used. There are a variety of manufactured balanced liquid diets with low residue or with food in its elemental components to facilitate nutrient availability to the gut (e.g. Ensure, Traumacol). At times TPN may be required. To fully achieve the benefits of aggressive nutritional support may require some considerable time. In surgical patients where there is urgency, that time is not available. Even if it were, the continued presence of the catabolism caused by the surgical problem counters the benefit of nutritional interventions. Prompt surgery with attention to nutritional support in the postoperative period is then more sensible.

Nutritional support of the surgical patient requires a team approach. This may involve a clinical nutritional support unit comprising physicians or surgeons with an interest in nutrition, dietitians, pharmacists and biochemists. Regular, often daily, review of the patient and appropriate blood tests and nutritional assessment are necessary to produce the best outcome.

FURTHER READING

Fischer J E 1997 Metabolism in surgical patients. In: Sabiston D C, Jr, Lyerly H K (eds) Textbook of surgery: the biological basis of modern surgical practice, 15th edn. WB Saunders, Philadelphia, p 137–175

Gann D S, Cross J S 1993 The neuroendocrine response to critical illness. In: Barie P S, Shires G T (eds) Surgical intensive care. Little, Brown, Boston, p 93–134

Hill G L (ed) 1992 Disorders of nutrition and metabolism in clinical surgery: understanding and management. Churchill Livingstone, Edinburgh

Moran B J 1996 Recent advances in nutritional support of surgical patients. In: Johnson C D, Taylor I (eds) Recent advances in surgery 19. Churchill Livingstone, Edinburgh

5

Shock
Steven Chan

OVERVIEW

An understanding of the physiology of the body's response to a reduced effective circulating blood volume is essential to the management of the clinical shock state. Although the clinical causes of shock may be varied, the general principles of management should include immediate action, assessment and definitive treatment. In surgical patients, in particular, septic shock is not uncommonly encountered. Major and continuing advances in the common pathway of injury in septic shock are the cornerstone to successful treatment in subsets of these patients. Complex interactions of cells, cytokines and humoral pathways are involved in the systemic inflammatory response syndrome and multiple organ dysfunction syndrome, and more precise delineation of these mechanisms will guide the development of additional approaches to prevention and treatment.

Shock is a useful but imprecise term: useful because it describes a clinical appearance of circulatory collapse; imprecise as it gives neither information about aetiology nor guidance for a plan of treatment.

Shock may be defined in physiological terms as the body's response to a reduced effective circulating blood volume, but in everyday practice the word is used to describe the clinical state of affairs of reduced peripheral blood flow and resultant peripheral tissue hypoxia. It is these two mechanisms that explain most of the clinical manifestations of the shock syndromes: pallor; cold, clammy periphery; peripheral cyanosis; and mental confusion.

The method of production of reduced perfusion will vary from instance to instance, so when summoned to a patient said to be 'in shock', the first question to be asked is: 'What is the cause?'. Only in this way can a plan of treatment be arrived at.

The five major causes of 'shock' are:

- fainting and neural phenomena
- loss of circulating volume
- 'pump failure'
- massive sepsis
- metabolic and immunological disorders.

The general principles of treatment are in three phases:

- immediate action
- assessment
- definitive treatment.

FAINTING AND NEURAL PHENOMENA

The fainting of emotional stress, also referred to as a 'vasovagal attack' because of the associated bradycardia, hypotension and hyperpnoea, has in the past been included under the heading of shock.

The physiological disturbances are:

- bradycardia – reduction in cardiac output
- peripheral vasodilatation in skeletal muscle (cholinergic) – fall in blood pressure
- ADH secretion – cutaneous vasoconstriction and pallor.

Certainly this is the case to the layman who habitually describes as 'shocked' anyone who has had a fright. The term 'neurogenic shock' is best not used, although periph-eral tissue hypoxia in the brain is characteristic of fainting which has a neurogenic basis. It is important to remember that other factors such as blood loss can, if the patient is upright, lead to the development of the physiological chain of events – adrenaline secretion, muscular vasodilatation, bradycardia and cerebral hypoxia – which leads to faint-ing. Thus, fainting may be a component of some particular circumstances of blood loss. Perhaps the most frequently encountered in civilian practice is the patient who has a major gastrointestinal haemorrhage and then either defae-cates or vomits. The Valsalva effect so produced reduces venous return to the heart and precipitates a faint.

It is also important to remember that, if when a patient faints he is prevented from falling, the cerebral hypoxia is self-perpetuating and may result in irreversible brain damage and/or a cardiac arrest. Death under light general anaesthesia in the dentist's chair and possibly some fatal-ities in elderly patients propped upright in bed in hospital may be assigned to this cause.

Management

Lay the patient flat, preferably with the legs elevated; spontaneous recovery follows. Seek causes of bleeding.

Spinal shock

This is the clinical syndrome that may develop following damage of the spinal cord. It is discussed in detail in Chapter 12.

SHOCK FROM REDUCTION OF CIRCULATING VOLUME

There are three major causes of volume reduction:

- whole blood loss
- plasma loss
- loss of extracellular (ECF) fluid.

Whole blood loss may be either external, e.g. from the body surface or the gastrointestinal or genitourinary tracts, or internal into damaged tissues (e.g. a fracture haematoma or an infarcted organ) or a body cavity (e.g. intraperitoneal haemorrhage from a ruptured aortic aneurysm or ectopic pregnancy). The effects of external or internal haemorrhage are the same, although the rate of loss may be slow and progressive into tissues where tension increases gradually.

Plasma loss occurs in burns as a consequence of leak-age of protein and exudate through damaged capillaries. Dilute plasma is also lost into an area of inflammation or tissue damage, but the protein content of such loss is rarely important in considering fluid replacement, except in the case of fulminant pancreatitis.

Loss of extracellular fluid (ECF) is a consequence of three situations. Firstly, it can occur as a result of devia-tions of the normal exchange mechanism (loss of trans-cellular water). Extracellular fluid is in a constant state of exchange across the gastrointestinal tract and the nephron. Normally, although large quantities are moved every day in this manner, the net amount of extracellular water that is 'transcellular' (mainly in the lumen of the gut) at any instant is quite small. However, by interfer-ence with reabsorption, the extracellular fluid can be con-tinuously drained from its normal site. Such losses occur in vomiting, diarrhoea, fistulae and failure of tubular reabsorption of urine. In each instance, the fluid lost varies in composition, but basically it is rich in sodium ions. Big losses are accompanied by shrinkage of plasma volume and the onset of shock (Fig. 3.1, p. 15).

Second, there can be an increased loss of ECF along a normal pathway. The best single example of this situa-tion is excessive sweating without replacement in a non-acclimatised individual. Sufficient dilute extracellular fluid may be leached out to produce a profound reduction in ECF and a shock state but this is rare in temperate cli-mates.

Finally, ECF can be lost as a result of disruption to the anatomical boundaries of fluid compartments (the 'third space phenomenon'). There are two kinds of disruption:

- loss of biochemical integrity of a cell membrane (e.g. by hypoxia with leakage of sodium into the cell and thus a reduction in 'effective extracellular volume') – probably uncommon
- increased capillary permeability, as in an inflamed area (see the description of plasma loss above).

PHYSIOLOGICAL ADJUSTMENTS TO LOSS OF CIRCULATORY VOLUME

Two major physiological adjustments occur: peripheral vasoconstriction, and an ingress of extracellular water into the circulation which produces haemodilution.

Peripheral vasoconstriction adapts the volume of the vascular tree to the reduced volume of blood it contains (it should be noted that a phrase beloved of many writers on shock – 'discrepancy between volume of blood and the capacity of the vascular tree' – is a physical impossibility). The vasoconstriction is widespread, affecting the capacitance vessels on the venous side of the circulation as well as arterioles. In both instances, as the vascular network shrinks the pressure tends to fall, but initially, because of increased resistance to flow, it is maintained on the arterial side, with or without a mild increase in heart rate. Measurements of intravascular pressure are thus usefully made on both the arterial and venous side of the circulation, particularly the latter (i.e. by measuring central venous pressure or pulmonary artery pressure).

The ingress of extracellular water into the circulation occurs by virtue of the altered pressure relations in the arteriole–capillary–venule loop. As mentioned above, this produces haemodilution. The phenomenon is known as transcapillary refilling. Initially, this is quite a rapid process and after a haemorrhage of 1.5–2.0 L, three-quarters of the resulting haemodilution is over in 6–8 hours; this is of importance in the management of patients with suspected continued bleeding into, say, the gastrointestinal tract. Repeated determinations over some hours indicating a progressively falling haemoglobin, haematocrit or red cell count (all rough indications of haemodilution) are more often than not indications of continued haemorrhage.

REDUCTION IN CIRCULATING VOLUME: CORRELATION WITH PHYSICAL FINDINGS

Computation of blood volume deficits is difficult, and even direct measurement of blood volume is only accurate to about 5% (± 300 ml in an average man). No single measurement should be relied up on, but rather a summation of the data as shown in Tables 5.1 and 5.2.

In some circumstances it may be possible to correlate the clinical assessment with measured loss, e.g. blood during the course of an operation, or ECF from a fistula. Even if the measurement lacks refinement (as does simple swab weighing), it is more useful than an ill-educated guess. Historical evidence may also be useful, although lay people and members of the medical and nursing profession all tend to exaggerate visible blood loss (except surgeons, who always underestimate the amount of blood they spill). Finally, semi-objective assessment may be possible by seeing the extent of injury and referring to previously established figures.

When an assessment of whole blood loss has been made, a decision must also be reached on the extent of additional 'third space' requirements.

Table 5.1 Physical findings related to reduction in circulating volume (reproduced from Bailey H 1985 Emergency surgery, 11th edn, by permission of John Wright, Bristol)

Clinical status	Vital signs	Intravascular deficit in adult
Patient well, not anxious	Pulse 70–80 BP 120 systolic Central venous pressure 5–10 cm water Urine volume at least 40–50 ml/h	Less than 700 ml
Mild anxiety, restlessness, pallor, coldness, possibly sweating; thirst; fainting in upright position	Pulse 90–100 BP 90–100 CVP 0–5 Urine volume less than 30 ml/h	1–2 L
Great anxiety, disorientation; air hunger, icy extremities, fall in body temperature; severe thirst	Pulse 130+ BP 70 CVP –5 Urine volume nil	2–3.5 L

Table 5.2 Points of differentiation between whole blood, plasma and ECF loss

	Whole blood	Plasma	ECF
Haematocrit	Normal initially; falls some hours	Rises	Rises
Skin colour	Pallor	Usually unchanged	Usually unchanged
Tongue	Moist	Moist	Dry

MANAGEMENT OF THE LOSS

A volume appropriate to the loss should be replaced with the type of fluid that is lost; for example, ECF losses are replaced with Hartmann's solution. Crystalloids are the fluids of choice in the initial replacement of all types of fluid losses until blood or plasma is available.

This is because volume replacement is primarily more important than oxygen-carrying capacity, because if cardiac output is maintained, enough oxygen can still be delivered to the tissues down to a haemoglobin level of 8 g/dl. Care should be exercised in using large volumes of plasma or albumin, particularly when sepsis is present, as these forms of fluid replacement may be related to the cause of adult respiratory distress syndrome, so-called 'shock lung'.

The loss must be stopped. Normally, replacement precedes stopping of the loss, but occasionally replacement will be ineffective until the loss is stopped (e.g. massive arterial bleeding).

PUMP FAILURE (syn. cardiogenic shock)

The causes of pump failure are:

- *myocardial* – infarction, valvular damage or rupture, and arrythmias
- *pericardial* – cardiac tamponade or constrictive pericarditis
- *outflow obstruction* – pulmonary embolism causing pulmonary artery obstruction, and dissecting aneurysm causing aortic obstruction may result in secondary pump failure.

Cardiogenic shock is differentiated from low volume states by the following:

- no history and no signs of blood loss
- raised rather than lowered venous pressure (jugular venous or CVP)
- evidence of a focal lesion on ECG.

Treatment

Cardiac tamponade is an emergency requiring specific treatment by drainage of blood from the pericardial sac. Other varieties of cardiogenic shock are managed by cardiologists with inotropic agents, transvenous pacing, correction of arrythmias, and occasionally intra-aortic balloon counter-pulsation which may be particularly useful in cardiogenic shock before or after cardiac surgery.

MASSIVE SEPSIS (syn. septic shock, bacteraemic shock, bacterial shock)

Definition. The term massive sepsis is preferred to septicaemia because the latter is, in fact, a bateriological diagnosis which may be achieved only in retrospect, if at all. Furthermore, there is evidence that an acute local process may throw off not organisms but products of infection which cause the shock state.

BACTERIA AND TOXINS

Gram-negative bacteria and endotoxins

The common pathogens are the aerobic *Escherichia coli*, *Klebsiella*, *Pseudomonas* and *Proteus* species and the anaerobic *Bacteroides* species. An endotoxin is a lipopolysaccharide released from the structural component of the outer membrane of Gram-negative organisms following the death of bacteria which is destroyed by the reticuloendothelial system (RES). Gram-negative sepsis and endotoxaemia are favoured by factors that impair host resistance and RES function, such as severe illness, diabetes, steroids and immunosuppressive therapy.

During critical illness, the gastrointestinal mucosal barrier may be sufficiently compromised to allow translocation of luminal bacteria and their products thus perpetuating the septic state (Wilmore et al 1988).

Gram-positive bacteria and exotoxins

Exotoxins are secreted by living bacteria and are generally more toxic than endotoxins. Clostridial species secrete potent exotoxins which may cause massive local tissue destruction and also have cardiogenic and neurological effects. The more common Gram-positive bacteria, staphylococci and streptococci, rarely cause massive sepsis. The 'toxic shock' syndrome is one exception. This occurs in women using vaginal tampons and has typical clinical features: high fever, erythematous rash followed by desquamation, and hypotension. The causative organism is a penicillin-resistant toxigenic *Staphylococcus aureus* (TSST-1 exotoxin).

SURGICAL PATHOLOGY

The common pathway of injury in sepsis is shown in Figure 5.1. It is customary and desirable to distinguish two pathological forms of shock in massive sepsis: instances with and without a focus. In the latter, the prognosis is worse than in the former and common portals of entry are the urinary tract, the portal tract and badly managed intravenous therapy.

In both cases, microorganisms invade the bloodstream releasing large amounts of mediators. These mediators may consist of exotoxins, structural component (lipopolysaccharide) endotoxins or teichoic acid antigens, or host-manufactured products such as cytokines (tumour necrosis factor, interleukin-1 from leucocytes) or complement activation. These in turn mediate the car-

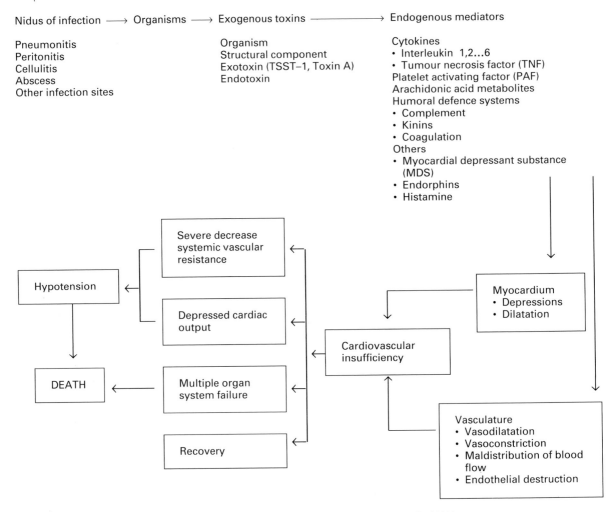

Nidus of infection ⟶ Organisms ⟶ Exogenous toxins ⟶ Endogenous mediators

Pneumonitis
Peritonitis
Cellulitis
Abscess
Other infection sites

Organism
Structural component
Exotoxin (TSST–1, Toxin A)
Endotoxin

Cytokines
• Interleukin 1,2...6
• Tumour necrosis factor (TNF)
Platelet activating factor (PAF)
Arachidonic acid metabolites
Humoral defence systems
• Complement
• Kinins
• Coagulation
Others
• Myocardial depressant substance
  (MDS)
• Endorphins
• Histamine

Severe decrease systemic vascular resistance

Hypotension

Depressed cardiac output

DEATH

Multiple organ system failure

Recovery

Cardiovascular insufficiency

Myocardium
• Depressions
• Dilatation

Vasculature
• Vasodilatation
• Vasoconstriction
• Maldistribution of blood flow
• Endothelial destruction

Fig. 5.1 The common pathway of injury in sepsis. (Reproduced with permission from Parrillo 1990.)

diovascular pattern seen in septic shock (Parrillo 1990). Early features are those of a decrease in systemic vascular resistance with a normal or high cardiac output. This phase is usually transient and followed by predominantly intense arteriolar and possibly venular vasocontriction, perhaps the consequence of catecholamine and catecholamine-like substances. The arteriolar vasocontriction reduces or abolishes peripheral blood flow, and the venous effects reduce the blood available for venous return. Thus, cardiac output falls, further aggravating the peripheral hypoxia.

There is controversy over the presence of myocardial depressant substance or a direct effect of bacterial toxins on the heart. Many other factors may contribute to the individual circumstances of a patient who presents with a presumed diagnosis of shock with sepsis. Acute ECF reduction, blood loss, respiratory insufficiency, metabolic acidosis and adrenocortical failure may complicate the picture and call for treatment in their own right. Non-survivors develop either unresponsive hypotension or progressive, *multiple organ system failure* which commonly affects the kidneys, liver, central nervous system, lungs and heart.

CLINICAL FEATURES AND DIAGNOSIS

Causes of blood volume reduction sufficient to account for the profound clinical disturbances are absent, but there may be a history of predisposing drug ingestion (e.g. steroids) or of a febrile illness. In favourable circumstances, the diagnosis is made easy by the presence of obvious sepsis or of a portal of entry. On examination, the patient is anxious, cyanosed, and has an extremely sluggish capillary return, a cold periphery and tightly constricted veins. Arterial blood pressure and central venous pressure are both low. This is the common syndrome of 'cold hypotension'. It may be preceded by a milder state of 'warm hypotension' in which there is peripheral vasodilatation.

Although blood cultures should be taken repeatedly in instances of shock thought to be associated with sepsis, they are more useful in retrospective evaluation and in the refinement of a chemotherapeutic regimen than for urgent diagnosis. An important investigation is a peripheral blood smear. With rare exceptions this will show a leucocytosis and, of much greater importance, the neutrophils will usually contain toxic granulations and Dohle bodies. Both of these are manifestations of severe infection and greatly strengthen the diagnosis. Profound disturbances in clotting and disseminated intravascular coagulation may follow massive sepsis and be part of the clinical picture.

MANAGEMENT

Sepsis should be treated in the following way:

- Administer systemic antibiotics, making a 'best guess' on the likely organisms.
- Drain any focal collection or remove dead infected tissue. Of course, it is necessary to find the focus. In surgery this is commonly abdominal; diagnosis is discussed on page 37.
- Respiratory and cardiovascular support may be required in the intensive care setting.

The therapeutic role of antibodies, both monoclonal and polyclonal, directed against endotoxins is currently being evaluated as an adjunct in the treatment of massive sepsis.

METABOLIC AND IMMUNOLOGICAL DISORDERS CAUSING SHOCK

ADRENOCORTICAL INSUFFICIENCY

This syndrome is rare, but perhaps not as rare as it used to be. De novo it may occur during the course of severe acute sepsis (e.g. the Friderichsen–Waterhouse syndrome in relation to meningococcal septicaemia) or after a severe head injury, but it is more common to encounter it after steroid drugs have been administered which suppress endogenous cortical activity by depressing ACTH production. Thus, it may be seen when surgery is called for in a patient with ulcerative colitis or rheumatoid arthritis.

Adernocortical suppression subsequent to steroid therapy may last up to 2 years, gradually declining in severity, but most instances of acute insufficiency occur within 18 months or take place while the patient is on a maintenance dose but is exposed to additional stress – an operation or infection. The clinical features are non-specific; the diagnosis is made only by a healthy sense of suspicion and the therapeutic trial of a large (200 mg) intravenous dose of hydrocortisone.

INSULIN-INDUCED HYPOGLYCAEMIA

This occurs usually in young, 'brittle', insulin-dependent diabetics when the optimal ratio of circulating insulin to available glucose is exceeded. Mental confusion, profuse sweating and hypotension are rapidly followed by coma. In the surgical context, this form of shock may be seen in a diabetic patient in the postoperative period or any patient receiving parenteral nutrition and insulin supplements. Treatment is an intravenous bolus injection of 50% glucose, having simultaneously taken a blood sample for glucose analysis to confirm the diagnosis.

ANAPHYLACTIC SHOCK

This is the consequence of the release of vasoactive amines by mast cells following repeat exposure to an antigen. The common type of antigen is a drug, and penicillin and its derivatives are often implicated. An urticarial rash is quickly followed by the development of laryngeal oedema and stridor, compounded by severe bronchospasm. Treatment with intravenous adrenaline should precede the use of an antihistamine and is repeated until effective. Tracheostomy is rarely necessary.

FURTHER READING

Glauser M P, Heumann D, Baumgartner J D, Cohen J 1994 Pathogenesis and potential strategies for prevention and treatment of septic shock: an update. Clinical Infections Disease 18 (suppl 2): S205–S216

Parrillo J E (moderator) 1990 Septic shock in humans. Annals of Internal Medicine 113: 227–242

Wilmore D W, Smith R J, O'Dwyer S T, Jacobs D O, Ziegler T R, Wang X D 1988 The gut: a central organ after surgical stress. Surgery 104: 917–923

Surgical infections
John Turnidge

OVERVIEW

Despite major advances in diagnosis and antimicrobial agents, infection still provides a major challenge to the surgeon. This chapter covers all types of bacterial, viral, fungal, and other clinical infections that may be the cause of the initial presentation or may complicate a surgical patient's stay in hospital. The pathogenesis of acute infections is discussed, including opportunistic infections, specific infections such as *Clostridia*, tuberculosis, syphilis and AIDS, as well as infections at specific sites, especially skin, subcutaneous areas and the hand.

Infection is the invasion of the body by pathogenic microorganisms and the reaction of the tissues to their presence and to the toxins generated by them. *Many surgical infections are caused by bacteria that originate from normal bacterial flora.* Infection occurs when the fine balance between host resistance and the virulence of the infecting pathogen breaks down.

SURGICAL PATHOLOGY

Infections may be either acute or chronic.

ACUTE INFECTIONS

Invasion of the body by a bacterial agent produces an inflammatory response which is variable and depends on the resistance of the host and the infecting organism. This response consists of rapid exudation, similar to that produced in the early stages of any injury, called an acute infection. Once the early phase has taken place the infection may resolve, spread or become chronic.

Natural history

Resolution of an infection is the regression of the exudative phase, without any evidence of tissue damage. Many acute infections are aborted at this stage with or without the use of antibiotics. If an infection does not resolve then it may spread. This spread can take place by one of three routes:

- direct spread with or without local tissue death
- spread by lymphatics
- spread by bloodstream.

Direct spread with local tissue death. Direct spread into involved tissues leads to either local tissue death or further spread along tissue planes. Local tissue death takes place as a consequence of two factors:

- bacterial exotoxins, e.g. *Clostridium perfringens* whose exotoxins may produce muscle necrosis with gas formation
- increased tissue tension.

The inflammatory response creates oedema regardless of the exciting agent. If the space in which the reaction takes place is limited, tension is inevitable. Such anatomically-bounded infection may occur in a variety of situations, such as in the pulp space of the finger, the breast or ischiorectal fossa where the fibrous septa separate fat pads; or inside the skull where the bony cavity limits the expansion of the tissue. Thrombosis of veins by the invading organisms will accelerate this process.

Local death of soft tissue results in two things:

- the production of a solid area of infected dead tissue at a body surface – a slough
- the liquefaction of tissues and the products of infection, particularly neutrophil polymorphs – an abscess.

When these events have taken place, the slough must be first cast off or removed, or the abscess drained before healing will occur by granulation tissue formation, i.e. by secondary intention.

In bone, similar processes occur, but outcomes are influenced by the rigidity of structure which causes early vascular thrombosis or obstruction and bone necrosis. When bone dies, the resulting area of septic necrosis is known as a *sequestrum*, although this term is often reserved for a situation in which the dead bone has separated from the living. Progression of the infection leads to subperiosteal abscess formation, which if undrained points to the skin and results in sinus formation.

Gangrene and its relation to infection. Tissues may die in either the presence or absence of bacteria. Aseptic necrosis is tissue death in the absence of bacteria (e.g. myocardial infarction). In the presence of bacteria, two events may occur – the dead tissue may harbour organisms which have little or no action on it, as occurs in a slough; or there may be *wet gangrene* in which proteolytic enzymes derived from the bacteria break down the tissues. These organisms often tend to spread, so that wet gangrene may be associated with cellulitis in the surrounding tissues. *Dry gangrene* is necrosis with desiccation of tissues.

Direct spread without local tissue death. Direct spread without local tissue death is called cellulitis, which is a spreading invasion of the connective tissue; for instance, infection with *Streptococcus pyogenes*, where the bacterial fibrinolysins (exotoxins) break down the protective wall of fibrin and so allow the spread of the organisms along tissue planes.

Spread by lymphatics. This is characteristic of organisms that cause breakdown of fibrin and thus is commonly seen with streptococcal infections. The walls of the lymphatic vessels become inflamed and are often painful (lymphangitis). Embolisation via lymphatics may also occur – though this mode of spread is more common with chronic infections (e.g. tuberculosis) – the bacteria being trapped in the regional lymph nodes, setting up an inflammatory reaction that results in enlargement with pain (lymphadenitis).

Spread by the bloodstream. Two forms are recognised:

- Bacteraemia – this is the carriage of organisms by the bloodstream without specific symptoms being produced
- Septicaemia – this is the presence of organisms in the blood producing systemic symptoms such as fever and chills.

In either case, organisms may set up a focus of infection at a distant site, so-called metastatic infection.

Clinical features

The common local features of acute infection are those seen with any form of inflammation: redness, swelling, increased local temperature and pain (rubor, tumour, calor, dolor). Fluctuation and pointing mean pus (abscess) formation, but slough is present without either. Moderate to severe persistent pain indicates the presence of tension which on occasions may necessitate decompression even in the absence of pus. The nature of the infecting organism may be recognised from its clinical appearance: *Strep. pyogenes* lesions such as erysipelas (an intradermal infection) or lymphangitis, or *Staph. aureus* infection with local necrosis. Enlarged and tender draining lymph nodes indicate lymphatic spread.

CHRONIC INFECTIONS

Chronic infections may develop either as a consequence of untreated or inadequately treated acute infection, or as a direct result of infection with some specific bacterial pathogens. Histologically, lymphocytic and mononuclear cell infiltration, sometimes with giant cell formation, are the typical findings.

Natural history

These infections are characterised by slow destruction of tissues, often with accompanying scarring. The mechanisms of spread are similar to those seen with acute infections, i.e. direct, with or without tissue necrosis, via the lymphatics or via the bloodstream.

Due to rapid bone necrosis, chronic osteomyelitis will almost invariably follow acute osteomyelitis that is undertreated. In addition to sequestrum (dead bone) formation, new, usually distorted, bone will be laid down – a so-called involucrum.

Clinical features

Chronically discharging sinuses and persistent relatively non-tender lymphadenopathy are common features. In some instances, resolution may occur, only to relapse with the same clinical features weeks, months or years later.

MANAGEMENT OF SURGICAL INFECTION

MICROBIOLOGICAL DIAGNOSIS

Although not mandatory to achieve good clinical results, making a microbiological diagnosis can be helpful in the management of many infections. A knowledge of the causative pathogen(s) can:

- confirm the original suspicion
- reveal unexpected pathogens
- allow modification of therapy to more appropriate antibiotics
- give antibiotic choices should the patient develop side-effects.

For wound infections, swabs of pus or exudate provide the most useful sample. For wounds that are not oozing or open, or in cellulitis where there is no obvious wound, a needle aspirate can often provide a useful result. Deep pus should be aspirated, if necessary under ultrasound or CT scan control. Debrided necrotic tissue provides good samples for culture, but superficial slough does not. In the latter case, secondary colonisation is common, and culture results can be misleading.

Patients with fever, malaise, and especially rigors should be considered as possibly septicaemic, and blood cultures should always be collected in these circumstances prior to the initiation of antibiotics. It is important to remember that fever is often absent in up to one-third of elderly patients who are septicaemic. Thus blood cultures should always be collected on suspicion of septicaemia.

In chronic infections, tissue samples provide the optimum samples for culture as well a giving the opportunity for histopathological examination.

PRINCIPLES OF THERAPY

In the exudative phase, an acute infection may halt and resolve either as a consequence of host resistance or with the aid of antibiotics. These measures may be aided by judicious immobilisation. Resolution is achieved by treating an infection early.

Important features in determining outcome are:

- time of treatment in relation to onset
- host resistance
- the vascularity of the tissues; this permits the development of an appropriate inflammatory response and the ingress of the appropriate agents
- an effective antibiotic.

When treatment has failed in the exudative phase or the patient is not seen until tissue death has taken place, surgical intervention becomes necessary; slough must be removed or pus drained, or both. In infections under tension, it is important to reduce this to prevent further tissue death (e.g. osteomyelitis, pulp space infections or ischiorectal abscess). When drainage has been undertaken, a cavity is left. Free escape of exudate must occur until the cavity has contracted and this may mean drainage for some time.

The defect in structures and function produced by an acute infection may require repair.

CHOICE OF ANTIBIOTICS

The scalpel is the most important 'antibiotic' available to a surgeon. Antibiotics are almost never a substitute for drainage of pus, debridement of necrotic tissue or slough, or the relief of obstruction.

As it is usually not possible to know the exact nature of the organism, and in particular its antibiotic sensitivity, before starting an antibiotic, treatment is begun based on:

- the likely organism(s) in the clinical setting
- the prevalence of resistances in those organisms
- the relevant pharmacology of possible choices
- the presence of allergy or host factors that may modify pharmacology or organisms involved
- the degree of severity, and therefore urgency
- the results of culture and sensitivity tests if available.

For example, in cellulitis after minor trauma, which is

usually caused by either *Strep. pyogenes* or *Staph. aureus*, treatment may be commenced with a β-lactamase-resistant penicillin such as flucloxacillin which will cover both organisms and which is necessary because 90% or more *Staph. aureus* strains from the community produce β-lactamase. Oral therapy will be satisfactory for mild infection. In severe infection where septicaemia may be present and where oral absorption may be unreliable, treatment should be commenced intravenously. If *Strep. pyogenes* alone is isolated from specimens subsequently treatment may be changed to penicillin as these organisms remain susceptible.

Often, particularly in serious infections that threaten the patient or tissue death, it is necessary to use more than one agent. In acute peritonitis where the patient is seriously ill and the source of the infection has yet to be determined, coverage of organisms from bowel flora including enterococci, aerobic Gram-negative bacilli and anaerobes is required. This is best achieved with a combination of ampicillin (or amoxycillin), an aminoglycoside (e.g. gentamicin) and metronidazole administered intravenously.

THERAPEUTIC SUMMARY

- Treat early, aiming for resolution without tissue damage or septicaemia.
- Decompress if necessary on grounds of type of infection and tissue reaction.
  - Immobilise adequately.
  - Remove pus and slough completely.
  - Choose antibiotics to cover the likely pathogens.
  - Promote healing and rehabilitation.

INTRA-ABDOMINAL INFECTIONS

PERITONITIS

Peritonitis is an inflammation of a portion or all of the parietal and visceral surfaces of the abdominal cavity. Primary septicaemia peritonitis caused by the haematogenous spread of a single type of bacterium is rare, being seen mostly in patients with cirrhosis and ascites or nephrosis. Rarely streptococci or pneumococci may cause peritonitis in very young girls or elderly women, presumably having traversed the genital tract because of its high pH at these ages. 'Peritonitis', when used by surgeons today, is taken to mean acute sepsis or aseptic secondary peritonitis and it is this condition that will be described.

Surgical pathology

Local. Regardless of cause there are two immediate local responses: inflammation and ileus. Inflammation of the peritoneal membrane leads to increased transudation of fluid into the abdominal cavity, depleting the extracellular fluid (ECF). After a few hours exudation supervenes, the fluid in the abdominal cavity becoming turbid, containing leucocytes, protein, fibrin, cellular debris and blood. Even when the irritant is initially sterile, bacterial contamination usually supervenes after 12 hours. Bacterial culture may show a mixed culture of aerobic (e.g. *Escherichia coli, Proteus mirabilis*) and anaerobic (e.g. *Bacteroides fragilis*) organisms. Bacteria from oral flora are the rule in perforated peptic ulcers.

In cases of ileus, the gut responds to peritonitis by initial hypermotility, quickly followed by paralytic ileus. Fluid accumulates in the bowel as a consequence of increased secretion and decreased resorption. This further depletes the ECF.

General. The hypovolaemia caused by ECF sequestration results in a diminished cardiac output and reduced perfusion of peripheral tissues. In addition, abdominal distension and pain reduce ventilation and consequently the availability of oxygen. The metabolic rate increases in response to stress, with a corresponding increase in peripheral oxygen demand; thus a shift to anaerobic metabolism ensues with a metabolic acidosis.

Commonest causes of acute peritonitis

These are discussed individually in their appropriate chapters and will only be listed here:

- acute appendicitis
- mesenteric lymphadenitis
- acute cholecystitis
- acute salpingitis
- acute diverticulitis
- perforated peptic ulcer
- acute pancreatitis
- abdominal trauma
- ruptured ectopic pregnancy
- mesenteric vascular occlusion
- gall bladder perforation.

Clinical features

These depend on the precipitating causes.

Symptoms. Abdominal pain, nausea and vomiting are all symptoms of peritonitis.

Signs. These include fever, abdominal tenderness, rebound tenderness and rigidity. Bowel sounds may be hyperactive initially, becoming silent later. Without treatment, there is rapid progress leading to abdominal distension, hypotension and shock with, ultimately, respiratory, renal and cardiac failure.

Laboratory findings

Leucocytosis and haemoconcentration are common laboratory findings. Serum electrolytes vary and the urea concentration may be elevated. There is often a picture of metabolic acidosis with compensatory respiratory alkalosis. Plain X-ray of the abdomen may show distension of both the large and small bowels with fluid levels. Free air may be seen under the diaphragm when perforation of a hollow viscus has occurred.

Differential diagnosis

The differential diagnosis includes:

- General:
  - uraemia produces abdominal distension, especially in the elderly
  - diabetes mellitus often presents as an acute abdomen in children
  - rarely, Henoch–Schönlein purpura, acute intermittent porphyria, lead poisoning and lightning attacks of tabes dorsalis may produce severe enough abdominal pain to lead to laparotomy
- Thoracic:
  - Inferior myocardial infarction
  - Basal pneumonia with diaphragmatic pleurisy
  - Ruptured oesophagus
- Gastrointestinal:
  - Severe gastroenteritis
- Retroperitoneal:
  - renal calculi
  - pyelonephritis
  - osteoarthritis of the vertebrae
  - ruptured abdominal aortic aneurysm
- Pelvic:
  - ruptured ovarian follicle
  - torsion of an ovarian cyst
  - acute degeneration of a uterine fibroid.

Treatment

The initial assessment should concentrate on resuscitation of the patient, finding the cause of the sepsis and assessing the need for operative intervention.

Preoperative

Intravenous therapy. It is imperative that the ECF losses are made good. These are best replaced by Hartmann's or similar solution which has an electrolyte composition similar to plasma.

Central venous pressure monitoring. This is essential in the critically ill and the elderly, where cardiac impairment may be exacerbated by large fluid loads.

Nasogastric suction. This is required to empty the stomach and prevent further vomiting.

Urinary catheter. This allows assessment of urinary flow and fluid replacement.

Antibiotics. These should be commenced as soon as the diagnosis is made and should cover a broad range of pathogens (e.g. ampicillin, gentamicin and metronidazole).

Analgesic. Morphine in small doses should be administered intravenously, preferably as a continuous infusion or as a bolus hourly.

Laboratory investigations. The following should be carried out:

- full blood count
- group and cross-match blood
- serum electrolyte concentration
- serum amylase
- blood gases, especially in the elderly
- ECG also in the elderly.

Operative. The operative management will depend on the cause of the peritonitis. There are, however, some general points to note.

Peritoneal toilet and lavage. All necrotic material and contaminated fluid should be removed. Lavage with saline reduces postoperative complications.

Intestinal decompression. Distended bowel should be

decompressed retrogradely via a nasogastric tube. A nasogastric tube is left in place for postoperative decompression of the stomach, as prolonged ileus is a frequent complication of peritonitis.

Drains. Drains should only be placed for the egress of purulent or necrotic debris or blood.

Wound closure. The deep muscle layers should be closed with monofilament nylon or polypropylene sutures. Delayed primary closure of the subcutaneous layers and skin is prudent.

Postoperative

Intravenous replacement therapy. This is required to maintain intravascular volume and hydration of the patient, monitored by CVP measurement and urinary output. It is continued until it is judged safe for oral intake to be resumed, i.e. by the return of the bowel sounds, passage of flatus or faeces and reduced gastric aspirates.

Nasogastric drainage. This should be done continuously until drainage becomes minimal. At this point the nasogastric tube may be removed or spigoted and fluids cautiously started by mouth.

Antibiotics. Those commenced preoperatively are continued unless cultures at the time of operation show that the causative organism(s) is resistant to them, in which case they are changed to appropriate ones.

Analgesia. Intravenous morphine or pethidine given continuously is the most comfortable and safest way to administer analgesia. If this method is not available, small doses at frequent intervals may be administered intramuscularly or intravenously.

INTRA-ABDOMINAL ABSCESSES

These include liver, residual, pelvic and subphrenic abscesses. Only liver abscesses are considered here. The other three are discussed in Chapter 8.

Liver abscesses

Isolated liver abscesses have a number of different causes:

- *Metastatic infection secondary to bacteraemia or sep-*

ticaemia. Bacteraemia or septicaemia with pyogenic bacteria can localise in the liver and result in single or multiple abscesses. Isolated splenic abscesses usually have the same aetiology. The most common organisms involved are *Staph. aureus* and the *Strep. 'milleri'* group of viridans streptococci.
- *Infection due to* Entamoeba histolytica *(amoebic abscess).* Amoebic liver abscess follows intestinal infection with *E. histolytica*, usually several weeks or months later. In many cases, there has been no history consistent with amoebic dysentery.
- *Secondary to 'portal pyaemia'.* Localised pyogenic intra-abdominal infection can spread via the portal circulation to become established in the liver. As with the original infection, the bacteria responsible are usually mixed aerobic/anaerobic 'faecal' flora.

A radiologically guided diagnostic tap of the abscess sent for microscopy, culture and sensitivity will usually distinguish between these types of abscess. Prior to this procedure, consideration should be given to the possibility of hydatid disease as the cause of the problem if the patient comes from a country where this disease is endemic. Hydatid cysts generally have specific ultrasound and CT scan appearances, including peripheral calcification. Indiscriminate tapping of hydatid cysts can result in peritoneal spillage, with disastrous early and late consequences.

Formal drainage procedures are normally required, except for amoebic abscess which can generally be satisfactorily treated with antibiotic therapy alone.

BILIARY TRACT SEPSIS

ACUTE CHOLECYSTITIS (see also Ch. 26)

Although not primarily a bacterial infection, bacteria may play an important role in the pathogenesis of acute cholecystitis. Gallstones are associated with bacteria in the biliary tract in about one-third of cases. The commonest organisms found in the biliary tract are *E. coli, Klebsiella* spp., *Enterococcus* sp. viridans group streptococci and occasionally anaerobic bacteria. In acute cholecystitis due to obstruction of the cystic duct, these bacteria become trapped, multiply and contribute to the acute inflammatory process. Infection may be severe enough to result in gangrene of the gall bladder due to compromise of the blood supply, or less commonly because the organism involved is *Clostridium perfringens*.

ACUTE CHOLANGITIS (see also Ch. 26)

Acute cholangitis is the constellation of fever, rigors and jaundice with or without right upper quadrant pain. It can follow any cause of acute common bile duct obstruction, most commonly the passage of gallstones, but also obstruction due to tumour or inflammation of the pancreatic head. Endoscopic retrograde cholangiopancreatography (ERCP) may also precipitate this infection in the absence of obstruction, especially if foreign bodies such as stents are inserted.

The key element of acute cholangitis is that it is primarily a septicaemic illness, and thus aggressive medical treatment, including broad-spectrum antibiotics that cover the organisms listed above, as well as early surgical intervention are necessary parts of treatment.

EMPYEMA (THORACIC INFECTION)

An empyema is an acute or chronic suppurative pleural exudate, which may be caused by a multitude of organisms.

Surgical pathology

The initial inflammation of the pleura leads to an exudation of fluid into the pleural cavity. Although the exudate may at first be sterile, if the inflammation was caused by an adjacent lung lesion, it is soon invaded by bacteria. Spread is by:

- direct extension of pneumonia
- lymphatic channels from infections in the lungs, chest wall or diaphragm
- haematogenous route
- direct inoculation by trauma, surgical incision of a lung abscess or via an intercostal catheter
- ruptured thoracic viscera (e.g. oesophagus)
- extension of subdiaphragmatic process (e.g. subphrenic, hepatic or perinephric abscess).

Bacteriology

This depends largely on the source of the infection. The organisms most frequently encountered are:

- *Staph. aureus*, most common in all age groups. Spread is directly from staphylococcal pneumonia or via an intercostal catheter.
- *Strep. pneumoniae*, an occasional complication of pneumococcal pneumonia; it is characterised by thick green pus that becomes loculated early. Later in infection, 'sterile' effusions may occur in pneumococcal pneumonia that can mimic empyema.
- *Bacteroides* spp., seen as a complication in women with pelvic inflammatory disease and in elderly debilitated men. It is also seen in pleural rupture of a subphrenic abscess, when it is often associated with other enteric organisms. It is characterised by massive accumulation of thick, foul-smelling pus that rapidly returns after evacuation.
- *Klebsiella* spp., which principally affect the debilitated, elderly, chronically ill or alcoholic patients. They are also common after surgical procedures in the pleural space.

Complications

These include:

- invasion of the chest wall and osteomyelitis of the ribs or costal cartilages
- bronchopleural and bronchial fistulas; these require urgent closure because of a danger of flooding the opposite lung with pus
- mediastinal abscess
- septicaemia
- metastatic abscess.

Clinical findings

Symptoms. These include chest pain, shortness of breath, weakness and haemoptysis.

Signs. Fever and signs of pleural effusion are usually present.

Special tests. FBE: anaemia and leucocytosis; CXR: there is opacification of part of the pleural space, occasionally with a fluid level (pyopneumothorax) – a pneumonic infiltrate may be seen, though this is often obscured by the empyema.

Treatment

Local. Treatment is either with antibiotics or by drainage of the pleural space. In the case of the former, prompt diagnosis and treatment are essential. Sputum, pleural fluid and blood cultures should be obtained and antibiotic treatment instituted on the basis of clinical findings and Gram-stained smears.

When draining the pleural space, early, closed, underwater seal drainage of the empyema is necessary to avoid chronicity. If the CXR suggests loculation this should be broken down through a limited thoracotomy, with removal of all necrotic material and the resection of a short segment of rib. The empyema cavity is usually isolated from the remaining pleura within a week, the underwater seal becoming unnecessary. The tube can be cut down and slowly withdrawn as the cavity becomes obliterated.

General. As for any patient with a chronic deep collection of pus, anaemia should be corrected with blood transfusion. The patient should be fed with a high-energy, high-protein diet supplemented with vitamins.

CENTRAL NERVOUS SYSTEM INFECTIONS

See Chapter 18 for a discussion on these types of infection.

SKIN AND SOFT TISSUE INFECTIONS

Infection of skin or subcutaneous tissue usually follows major or minor trauma with inoculation of specific pathogens. In some cases, obstruction of glands may trap pathogens, and 'traumatic' cellulitis may have no obvious source. Each form of infection is associated with specific pathogens. As in all types of surgical infection, adequate drainage or debridement of slough or necrotic tissue is essential for adequate resolution.

FURUNCLES AND CARBUNCLES

Furuncles (boils) are infections of hair follicles caused by *Staph. aureus*. Most commonly, the lesions are single, painful and eventually suppurative. Constitutional symptoms are absent. Drainage is the optimal method of treatment but is difficult early in the course of infection. There is no evidence that antibiotics alter the course of simple furuncles significantly, although it is felt that if they are started very soon after onset they may reduce the size and discomfort of the lesion.

Carbuncles are furuncles that have invaded the dermis and caused a multiloculated abscess. They are most common at the back of the neck. Formal extensive drainage with rupture of all loci is essential to effect a cure.

ERYSIPELAS

Skin infection characterised by a painful, bright red, thickened and indurated spreading patch of epidermis is called erysipelas. It is almost invariably due to *Strep. pyogenes* and most commonly occurs on the face or the neck. Penicillin remains the treatment of choice. Surgical intervention is rarely necessary.

INFECTIONS RELATED TO SKIN ULCERS
(see also Chs 36 and 37)

Chronic skin ulcers such as decubitus ulcers, venous ulcers and arterial ulcers are always heavily colonised by bacteria. It is a common error to swab slough and/or exudate from these lesions, grow mixed organisms and presume that this means infection. Removal of slough and devitalised tissue will promote healing. Antibiotics will only select for resistant organisms, which may be a problem later if true infection develops.

Skin ulcers should only be presumed to be infected if there is definite spreading cellulitis surrounding the ulcer or if there are systemic features of infection. In these circumstances, it is usually *Staph. aureus* that is the invader rather than the variety of Gram-negative bacteria that are often cultured from the ulcer itself. Empirical treatment for staphylococcal infection (e.g. flucloxacillin) is the best initial therapy if there is evidence of invasive infection. Exceptions include cellulitis associated with lower limb ulcers in diabetes (see below) and decubitus ulcers, where mixed aerobic/anaerobic 'faecal' flora as well as staphylococci are often found and broad-spectrum antibiotic therapy is required (e.g. a first generation cephalosporin plus metronidazole).

HYDRADENITIS SUPPURATIVA

This is a troublesome recurrent condition of sweat glands that often results in sinus formation and scarring. It is most often seen in the axillae and inguinal regions where apocrine glands are plentiful. It is initiated by blocking of gland ducts, and secondary suppurative infection can result. Mixed infection with staphylococci, Gram-negative bacilli and anaerobes may be seen. Multiple deep-seated abscesses may make antibiotic treatment alone ineffective and surgical drainage is almost always required for infective recurrences. Rarely, complete excision of the affected area is required if there is extensive disease to prevent recurrences.

CELLULITIS

Cellulitis after surgery is considered in Chapter 8. Other causes are discussed here.

After minor trauma

Wound infections and cellulitis that occur in normal hosts after cuts, scratches and abrasions, as well as cellulitis that appears 'spontaneously', are for the most part caused by *Strep. pyogenes* or *Staph. aureus*. Initial optimal therapy is with a β-lactamase-resistant antibiotic such as flucloxacillin which will cover both organisms (combination with penicillin G is unnecessary). Antibiotics should be given intravenously initially if there are systemic signs of infection (suggesting septicaemia). If *Strep. pyogenes* alone is isolated from blood or wound, treatment can be changed to penicillin. Surgical intervention is required when there is necrosis, slough or abscess formation.

After animal bites and scratches

Bites from dogs and cats, and scratches from cats will become infected in about 30% of cases. The organism most frequently responsible is *Pasteurella multocida*, a normal resident of the oropharynx in these pets, although other organisms may also be involved. *Pasteurella* is quite susceptible to penicillin. Infections of this type respond rather slowly to treatment. If there is a chance that important underlying structures may be infected, such as tendon sheaths in the hand, early surgical management is important to avoid complications (see Hand infections, p. 43).

After human 'bites'

Human bites are not common injuries, but they have an almost 100% chance of becoming infected if the skin is breached. The commonest problem is the 'clenched fist' injury where the striking fist hits the teeth of the opponent. If the skin is punctured, mixed aerobic/anaerobic oral flora are inoculated into the tissues and often into or around delicate structures such as tendons and metacarpophalangeal joints. Infections when they develop are very aggressive, and early debridement is mandatory. The situation is exacerbated in true bites due to an element of crushing of the tissues. Antibiotic therapy is indicated even before infection develops and should be designed to cover oral flora organisms. The simplest option is clindamycin which covers the likely pathogens.

After underwater injuries

Injuries occurring underwater are a common summer occurrence. A small proportion can become infected. Infection in these circumstances can be due to staphylococci or streptococci as for other trauma, but occasionally aggressive infections with rapidly spreading cellulitis, gangrene and septicaemia develop. These are caused by unusual Gram-negative bacilli that are found in water, such as *Aeromonas hydrophila* (fresh water) and halophilic *Vibrio* sp. (salt water). If the infection developed within a few hours of the injury, the patient should be immediately hospitalised for possible surgical intervention and broad-spectrum antibiotic treatment such as a third generation cephalosporin.

In diabetes and peripheral vascular disease

Patients with vascular disease of the lower limb, particularly microvascular disease seen with diabetes mellitus, are very prone to infection due to local ulcerations or after minor trauma. In diabetics, the term 'diabetic foot' is often used to describe this syndrome. In contrast to lower limb cellulitis that occurs after minor trauma in normal hosts, where staphylococci and streptococci alone are seen, mixed aerobic/anaerobic flora of the 'faecal' type are more frequently involved, with or without staphylococci. In addition, if the infection is of the indolent type, underlying osteomyelitis should always be suspected. Broad-spectrum combined antibiotic therapy (e.g. flucloxacillin, gentamicin and metronidazole, or a first generation cephalosporin plus metronidazole) should be initiated early, even for minor infection in these types of patients, as cellulitis has a great tendency to cause (wet) gangrene. Any slough or necrotic tissue needs aggressive excision back to healthy tissue to ensure success. Infection may progress in some cases, due to very poor blood supply preventing penetration of antibiotics, and amputation back to better vascularised tissue is required.

GAS GANGRENE (clostridial myonecrosis)

This condition is both a medical and a surgical emergency.

Bacteriology

Gas gangrene is an acute and devastating rapidly spreading infection caused by various gas-forming organisms of the clostridia group in which the predominant one is *C. perfringens (welchii)*, and occasionally *C. septicum, C. oedematiens* and *C. sporogenes.* All are Gram-positive anaerobic bacilli which are inhabitants of soil and the large bowel of humans.

Like *C. tetani*, this group of organisms produces disease by virtue of powerful exotoxins but, unlike *C. tetani*, the effect is predominantly at the wound of entry. These organisms ferment sugars (saccharolytic) and destroy protein (proteolytic) and lipids with the liberation of gas and volatile fatty acids, a mixture of which results in the formation of the characteristic foul-smelling gas.

Gas gangrene-prone wounds

The mere presence of toxigenic species of clostridia in a wound does not necessarily lead to gas gangrene; the physical conditions of the wound and the general virulence of the organism determine the outcome. The anaerobic conditions required for the growth of tetanus organisms also pertain to the gas-forming clostridia. These are particularly prone to grow in deep penetrating wounds which are associated with much tissue damage, ischaemia, haematoma formation and soil or faecal contamination. In current surgical practice, the wounds most at risk are amputations of the lower limb in bedridden diabetic patients.

Surgical pathology

There are dramatic changes at the wound of entry. The organisms proliferate and spread rapidly, aided by the destruction caused by the powerful exotoxins. Spread in the subcutaneous tissues results in the formation of a dry, hot and oedematous cellulitis containing gas bubbles. This is followed by destruction of blood vessels and haemolysis of liberated blood, which causes the area to assume a characteristic brick-red colour. Later, proteolytic organisms destroy muscles (myonecrosis) and liberate further gases, and the tissues assume an olive-green colour, the process eventually spreading to involve other muscle groups (spreading myonecrosis).

Clinical features

The incubation period is short, usually 24–72 hours. The wound is never trivial; it soon becomes unusually painful and swollen, with the development of brick-red and olive-green colour changes and a 'sickly sweet' smelling discharge containing gas bubbles. As the infection progresses, the skin becomes gangrenous and black friable muscle is exposed in the depths of the wound. Palpable crepitus beneath the skin can be elicited and visualised in tissue planes on radiographs.

The patient has marked toxaemia associated with tachycardia and fever. Death may ensue within hours from circulatory failure or extensive gangrene.

Differential diagnosis

The diagnosis should always be made on clinical grounds alone and without delay for bacteriological confirmation. Wound infections due to other gas-forming organisms, such as some anaerobic streptococci, coliforms and *Proteus* organisms, occur more slowly and are not associated with putrefaction or the production of the characteristic discharge.

Management

Prevention. Gas gangrene, unlike tetanus, cannot be prevented by the production of active immunity. Moreover, the effectiveness of passive immunisation with polyvalent antitoxin at the time of wounding has never been proved. Prophylaxis is dependent on two measures: wound debridement and antibiotics.

Wound debridement. Meticulous attention must be paid to all gas gangrene-prone wounds. All dead skin, subcutaneous fat, fascia, muscle, loose bone fragments and foreign bodies must be removed so that the wound becomes macroscopically clean. In the presence of gross and widespread crushing of tissues where heavy contamination has occurred, or when suppuration is already present, the wound must be left open and allowed to heal by secondary intention. However, when the wound appears to be clean and not heavily contaminated, primary closure followed by careful observation is permissible; but if doubt exists about the potential infectivity of the wound, then it should be left open and reassessed about 5 days later, when delayed primary closure may be possible.

Antibiotics. Large and frequent doses of intravenous penicillin G (e.g. 1.2 g 4-hourly for an adult) are given for all gas gangrene-prone wounds.

Curative treatment. Once gas gangrene has been established, the following treatment is started.

The wound. Wide and ruthless debridement is essential, with removal of all dead and doubtfully viable tissues and the laying open of all pockets of pus or potential cavities. When more than one group of muscles of a limb is involved, serious consideration must be given to amputation; it will certainly be indicated if all muscle groups are involved. Whatever is done, the wound must be packed lightly and left open.

Antibiotics. Large and frequent doses of intravenous penicillin G are essential. Additional antibiotics may be required if other bacteria are identified in cultures.

Supportive therapy. This includes:

- correction of shock and peripheral circulatory failure with intravenous therapy
- correction of anaemia with blood transfusion
- correction of metabolic acidosis
- hyperbaric oxygen
- relief of pain with analgesia
- sedation, but only if absolutely necessary.

With the increase in the amount of oxygen available to the tissues, the production of clostridial toxins, particularly the alpha toxin of *C. perfringens*, is inhibited. Intermittent exposure of patients with gas gangrene to oxygen at 3 atm absolute causes dramatic benefit in the first 48 hours of therapy. Patients who are severely toxic with clostridial myonecrosis benefit from 2–2.5 hours of hyperbaric oxygen therapy before debridement, provided it is not associated with any complications such as oxygen convulsions or disorientation. Hyperbaric oxygen together with wound debridement and antibiotics has now become standard practice in centres equipped with hyperbaric chambers.

The overall mortality rate from gas gangrene is about 25% and most deaths are due to late diagnosis, inadequate excision of devitalised tissue and multi-organ failure.

NECROTISING FASCIITIS

Necrotising fasciitis is an invasive infection of fascia due to mixed infection with microaerophilic streptococci or staphylococci, as well as Gram-negative bacilli.

Clinical features

The process begins in a localised area such as a puncture wound or leg ulcer and spreads along relatively ischaemic fascial planes. Vessels penetrating between skin and deeper structures thrombose, leading to skin death. The skin becomes anaesthetic, and crepitus may be present. The patient is febrile and has a tachycardia. Surgical findings are of dull-grey necrotic fasica and subcutaneous tissue which contains thrombosed veins.

Differential diagnosis

The differential diagnosis is between ischaemic and clostridial gangrene.

Management

- Antibiotics – initially, penicillin in large doses parenterally, once material has been taken for smear and culture.
- Thorough debridement – the wound should be left open for secondary closure.
- Restoration of tissue perfusion.
- Correction of the disorders, for example diabetes mellitus.

SYNERGISTIC GANGRENE

This condition was first described by Meleney and is often named after him (Meleney's synergistic gangrene). It is a mixed infection with *Staph. aureus* and microaerophilic non-haemolytic streptococcus.

Clinical features

The condition usually starts around puncture sites or wounds and spreads as a painful increasing area of pale red cellulitis with a purplish central area that finally ulcerates. Involvement of the perineum and scrotum is called Fournier's gangrene.

Management

Management is by radical excision of the ulcerated area with secondary closure and antibiotics. Penicillin plus flucloxacillin should be administered in large doses parenterally until culture results are available.

LYMPHADENITIS

This can be either acute or chronic.

Acute lymphadenitis

Acute lymphadenitis is used to describe acute inflammation of a single or contiguous group of lymph nodes, usually due to infection nearby. The typical features are pain, tenderness and swelling of a discrete collection of nodes. Acute lymphadenitis may accompany wound infection or cellulitis, where its presence suggests that the infection is caused by *Strep. pyogenes*. Occasionally, the node infection is prominent while the nearby soft tissue or wound infection is minimal. Other localised forms of acute lymphadenitis include the bilateral anterior cervical lymphadenitis associated with acute pharyngitis caused by *Strep. pyogenes* and adenoviruses, and the preauricular adenitis of adenoviral conjunctivitis.

Chronic lymphadenitis

Chronic, relatively non-tender, localised lymph node swelling is most often caused by mycobacteria of various types. In young infants, unilateral chronic anterior cervical lymphadenitis is caused by *Mycobacterium scrofulaceum* and comes about through the accidental ingestion of small amounts of soil, the normal habitat of this bacterium. Surgical removal of the affected nodes is sufficient for cure.

In adults, this same condition is most often caused by *M. tuberculosis* and occasionally by *M. bovis*. Medical treatment will usually eradicate this infection, and surgical intervention is required mainly for diagnosis (biopsy) and drainage of any (cold) abscess formation.

Chronic lymphadenitis is also seen with *M. marinum*, which usually follows minor trauma and inoculation of the organism into the subcutaneous tissue when cleaning home aquariums. A local granuloma develops at the site of trauma (fish tank granuloma) and spread occurs to the epitrochlear and sometimes the axillary nodes.

Cat scratch disease is another infection that can result in localised chronic lymphadenopathy. This infection is caused by a recently identified organism, now called *Bartonella henselae*, a fastidious Gram-negative bacterium. This infection has characteristic histopathology and responds, albeit slowly, to treatment with appropriate antibiotics.

OMPHALITIS

This is an infection of the umbilicus. Predisposing factors are:

- in neonates, contamination of the umbilical stump
- in adults, poor hygiene.

It is usually a mixed staphylococcal and streptococcal infection, characterised by redness, heat, swelling, tenderness and pus. There may be cellulitis spreading from the navel. Treatment involves drainage of any pus and systemic antibiotics to prevent possible complications. Complications, usually confined to neonates, include septicaemia, portal pyaemia (bacteraemia) and liver abscess by spreading along the patent umbilical vein, and portal vein thrombosis which may result in portal hypertension.

HAND INFECTIONS

Hand infections are principally soft tissue infections and most of their features have been listed above. However, there are some special features that are largely the result of the special anatomy of the hand. They are also responsible for the loss of many work hours in industry.

ACUTE PARONYCHIA (whitlow)

Infection starts as cellulitis of the nail fold, and within a few hours a subcuticular abscess forms. When this is not controlled, rapid spread follows to involve the entire nail fold, usually in association with subungual extensions (Fig. 6.1).

The nail fold becomes red and swollen; later a subcuticular collection of pus appears with or without subungual extension.

PULP SPACE INFECTION (felon)

Infection is most common in the distal pulp space fol-

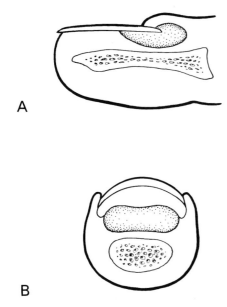

Fig. 6.1 **A. Subungual extension of acute paronychi.**
B. Pulp space infection.

lowing a penetrating injury. An initial phase of cellulitis involving most of the pulp is quickly followed by the collection of pus because of the honeycomb of fibrous bands intersecting the space between phalanx, tendon sheath and the skin (Fig. 6.1). There is rapid necrosis of the pulp tissues and of a varying amount of overlying skin due to the action of necrotising bacterial exotoxins. Untreated, the infection leads to further skin necrosis, and possibly osteomyelitis of the distal phalanx, or suppurative arthritis. In the case of more proximal segments, an important danger is involvement of the tenosynovium which often leads to disastrous effects on flexor tendon function.

Infection of this space is suggested by the onset of throbbing pain following a penetrating injury of the involved segment, in association with a diffusely swollen and very tender pulp. Maximal tenderness overlies the centre of abscess formation. In the early stages the pulp is tense and reddened, but with impending skin necrosis the pulp develops a mauve or blue colour. In an untreated case osteomyelitis or spread to the tendon sheath may result.

WEB SPACE INFECTION

Infection may follow a penetrating injury in the region of the web space and is quite common in manual labourers and hairdressers. Pus collection occurs in the subcuta-

neous compartment of the web beyond the distal palmar crease and is limited on each side by vertical septa of the aponeurosis passing to the intermetacarpal ligaments. Untreated, the infection may spread to involve the deep palmar spaces.

This infection is characterised by the onset of pain and tenderness in the area, together with obvious distension of the web space, usually following a penetrating injury. Considerable swelling of the dorsum of the hand may be associated.

THENAR SPACE INFECTION

This space is bounded in front by the flexor tendons, behind by the fascia covering the transverse head of adductor pollicis, medially by the intermediate palmar septum, and laterally by the fascia covering the muscles of the thenar eminence (Fig. 6.2). True collections in this space are rare, and many which are so called are simply abscesses deep of superficial to the palmar aponeurosis or extensive collections in the first web space. The important features are severe pain and extensive swelling, centred on the thenar eminence and corresponding region of the dorsum of the hand, but without obliteration of the palmar cavity, which distinguishes the infection from one in the middle palmar space. The distension of the thenar space tends to force the thumb into palmar abduction.

MIDPALMAR SPACE INFECTION

This space lies between the medial palmar septum medi-

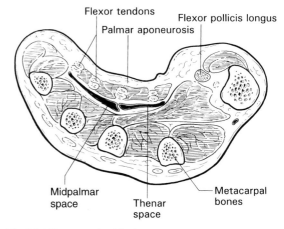

Fig. 6.2 Thenar and midpalmar space.

ally and the intermediate septum laterally and is bounded in front by the flexor tendons and behind by the third, fourth and fifth metacarpal bones and the fascia covering the intervening interossei (Fig. 6.2). Subcutaneous abscesses of the palm may occasionally extend to involve this space.

Characteristic features are swelling and tenderness involving the medial part of the palm, flattening or obliteration of the palmar concavity, and swelling of the dorsum of the hand. The lateral half of the hand is spared.

SUPPURATIVE TENOSYNOVITIS

Although infection of a tendon sheath is uncommon, when it occurs prompt diagnosis is imperative if there is to be any hope of salvaging flexor tendon function. Suppurative tenosynovitis may develop as the result of a penetrating injury, as an extension of one of the aforementioned infections, or following the operative repair of an injury involving the flexor tendon or sheath. The infection is confined to the tendon sheath and, if untreated, it will result in the extensive destruction of the synovial membrane, tendon adhesions and perhaps sequestration of the flexor tendons in advanced infections (Fig. 6.3).

The classical features of a swollen, reddened finger, affecting all segments, with exquisite tenderness along the line of the flexor tendon and excruciating pain on pas-

sive movement, are fairly late signs. If this advanced stage has been reached, even if infection is controlled, considerable tendon dysfunction is likely to result. Pain on passive movement of the fingers is the best early sign of developing tenosynovitis.

NON-SPECIFIC TENOSYNOVITIS

In this category are included infection of the tendon sheath by organisms of low virulence, traumatic tenosynovitis and injuries resulting in haemorrhage within the tendon sheath.

One occasionally encounters patients who have some of the local features of suppurative tenosynovitis, such as pain on finger flexion and localised tenderness along the tendon sheath, but little local swelling, cellulitis or systemic disturbances. These are cases of non-specific tenosynovitis due to trauma of the tenosynovium, as may occur in process workers carrying out long periods of rapid and repetitive hand movements. Suppuration does not occur and recovery takes place fairly quickly with rest of the affected part. A similar condition is De Quervain's disease, which is tenovaginitis of the long extensor of the thumb. There is pain of thumb movement and tenderness over the distal third of the forearm. Most patients recover with rest, but quite a few require incision of the sheath.

MISCELLANEOUS

Traumatic wound infections, infected blisters, boils and furuncles may occur in the hand as elsewhere in the body. Osteomyelitis and septic arthritis also occur, either as a result of one of the above infections or as a primary infection.

PRINCIPLES OF TREATMENT

There are four fundamentals of treatment, as described below.

Drainage

When pus has formed, simple incision suffices to drain unilocular collections in the palm, the web spaces and the proximal segments of the fingers. However, for the honeycombed collection of pus in the pulp space, adequate drainage can only be assured by incision and meticulous debridement of all necrotic tissue. Incisions must be

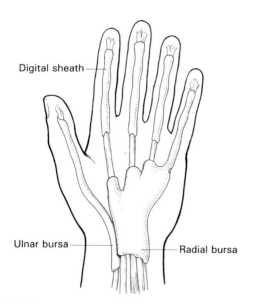

Digital sheath

Ulnar bursa

Radial bursa

Fig. 6.3 Flexor tendon sheaths.

transversely placed parallel to the skin creases, centred over the area of maximal tenderness and swelling; but when there is a draining sinus or area of skin necrosis, this should be included in the incision. In finger collections, any longitudinal extension of the drainage incision must be made in the midlateral axis of the finger to minimise the incidence of longitudinal scar contracture and tenderness.

When local anaesthesia is used, the injection should never be introduced through or in the vicinity of areas of cellulitis. Distal digital pulp infection may be safely drained under a digital block, but infections extending to the arm require a general anaesthetic or an infraclavicular brachial plexus block. There is no place for ethyl chloride freeze anaesthesia in the treatment of hand infections because the duration of anaesthesia produced by this method is too short to allow deliberate removal of necrotic tissue.

Antibiotics

When cellulitis has not progressed to pus formation some early infections can be reversed by the prompt administration of antibiotics. This applies particularly to early paronychia and infections caused by *Strep. pyogenes*, where full suppuration often does not occur.

Antibiotic therapy should begin before surgery, the initial choice usually being empirical, based on the fact that *Staph. aureus* is the most likely pathogen. In this case a penicillinase-resistant penicillin (e.g. flucloxacillin) should be used. If there is suspicion of Gram-negative infection, an aminoglycoside (e.g. gentamicin) should be added. If infection follows a dog bite or cat scratch, *Pasteurella multocida* is the most likely pathogen and penicillin is optimal. After a human bite or tooth damage, clindamycin provides best coverage. At time of drainage, pus should be sent for Gram stain and culture. The initial choice of antibiotic may need revision within 72 hours if the area of cellulitis is extending or pain is not relieved, particularly when the results of culture and sensitivity tests indicate that a more effective antibiotic should be chosen.

Immobilisation

Postoperatively, the area involved and related joints should be immobilised with an appropriate splint and supporting sling. If the infection is severe the patient should be confined to bed with the limb elevated by sus-

pension from a vertical stand. Immobilised joints should be placed in the position of function of slight dorsiflexion of the wrist, with the metacarpophalangeal joint at 90° of flexion and the interphalangeal joint in midposition.

Rehabilitation

Once infection has been controlled and healing is progressing, graduated finger movements are started to minimise stiffness which may result from tendon and joint adhesions. These are always likely complications of hand infections.

FOREIGN BODIES

The presence of a foreign body in the hand must always be considered in hand injuries. The diagnosis may be difficult, the functional consequences if untreated may be significant, and surgical removal can be technically demanding.

The commonest causes of foreign bodies are:

- fragments of glass or metal in lacerations
- penetration by a nail or needle which breaks.

Diagnosis

A foreign body may be present in any puncture wound of the hand. X-rays should always by taken, preferably in two planes, with an opaque marker at the entry site.

Management

Open wounds should be explored and carefully excised until all foreign material is removed. Exploration for a fragment of needle following a puncture wound should be undertaken in an operating theatre with full aseptic conditions, tourniquet control and image intensifier (or X-ray facilities) available.

BONE AND JOINT INFECTIONS

ACUTE OSTEOMYELITIS

Acute osteomyelitis is an abrupt onset infection that can occur in any bone in the body, but it has a propensity for certain bones. It can be initiated by:

- haematogenous spread to a bone
- spread from a nearby wound or soft tissue infection.

Bacteriology

For haematogenously acquired disease, *Staph. aureus* is the commonest pathogen; occasionally streptococci or Gram-negative coliforms may be involved. When the infection is initiated by local spread, the organisms involved are the same as those initially involved in the wound or soft tissue infection.

Surgical pathology

Haematogenous infection attacks different bones at different ages. In infants and children, the metaphysis of a long bone is the commonest site. In adults the vertebrae or sometimes the intervertebral discs are most frequently involved. Local infection can obviously occur at any site, but infection in bones of the foot is one common site seen in association with the 'diabetic foot' (see above).

Clinical features

Localised pain and tenderness in conjunction with fever are the usual features. A young child will stop using the affected limb.

Management

Diagnosis is best made with blood cultures, which are often positive, and nuclear bone scan, which becomes positive earlier than plain X-ray. Appropriate antibiotic treatment is then initiated with the specific attempt to prevent bony necrosis which can occur early in the course of disease and subsequently lead to chronic osteomyelitis. Biopsy of the affected bone to make a bacteriological diagnosis can be considered but should not delay antibiotic treatment. Antibiotic treatment should be given for a minimum of 3–6 weeks.

CHRONIC OSTEOMYELITIS

Chronic osteomyelitis follows delayed or inadequately treated acute osteomyelitis, is associated with prosthetic infections, or can arise de novo with specific pathogens.

Bacteriology

The bacterial causes of chronic osteomyelitis are the same as those of acute osteomyelitis in cases where this is the preceding problem. Coagulase-negative staphylo-cocci are also seen when the cause is a prosthesis, while *M. tuberculosis* can cause infection, especially in the vertebrae, as a single manifestation of tuberculosis.

Surgical pathology

The distinct features of chronic osteomyelitis are bony destruction, bone necrosis (sequestrum) and new bone formation (involucrum). There is often considerable soft tissue involvement around the site.

Clinical features

Localised pain without fever, with or without a discharging sinus, are the hallmarks of this infection. Fever is not seen. Radiological changes in the affected bone are obvious.

Management

Surgical debridement of dead bone is essential unless this would result in major dysfunction. Any surrounding inflammatory tissue or pus should be removed. Unlike acute osteomyelitis, it is important to make a bacteriological diagnosis prior to treatment. This may require aspiration or bone biopsy. Cultures from a discharging sinus can be helpful but are often misleading due to superficial contamination. Blood cultures are usually negative. Antibiotic therapy should be guided by culture results.

PROSTHETIC INFECTIONS

Two forms are recognised: early and late onset.

Bacteriology

Early onset infection results from the inoculation of bacteria at the time of or soon after surgery. Relatively non-pathogenic bacteria are often involved, such as coagulase-negative staphylococci or other skin flora organisms. These bacteria are often resistant to the agent used for antibiotic prophylaxis at the time of insertion. Late onset infection occurs when bacteria causing bacteraemia or septicaemia seed the prosthesis, in a manner similar to that of the pathogenesis of endocarditis. *Staphylococcus aureus* and viridans streptococci are most common in this setting.

Surgical pathology

The features are those of acute or chronic osteomyelitis, depending on the rapidity of onset.

Clinical features

Very early onset infection is usually manifest as wound infection with cellulitis. Drainage of any pus will often reveal tracking of infection down to the prosthesis. With less pathogenic bacteria and late onset infection, symptoms may be delayed, with pain and swelling being the only manifestations. Loosening of the prosthesis may occur and will be seen on X-ray.

Management

If possible, cultures should be obtained by aspiration or surgically. The choice of treatment depends on the likely consequences of removing the prosthesis, which is the only way that cure can be achieved. Antibiotic treatment is based on culture results.

SEPTIC ARTHRITIS

Septic arthritis is acute infection of a joint. Any joint in the body is capable of becoming infected. This can occur either through seeding from a bacteraemia or septicaemia (the commonest), or from local extension of a soft tissue infection or osteomyelitis.

Bacteriology

The agents responsible for septic arthritis are similar to those seen in the same settings as acute osteomyelitis. *Staphylococcus aureus* is most often seen with haematogenous infection, while the bacteriology of contiguously spread infection resembles that infection. In addition, *Neisseria meningitidis, N. gonorrhoeae* and *Haemophilus influenzae* type b can also cause haematogenous infection as part of septicaemic illness.

Surgical pathology

There is rapid purulent effusion into the joint cavity, combined with acute inflammatory changes in the synovium. Adjacent bone may show changes of acute osteomyelitis if this is the source of the infection, or if the infection has had time to progress.

Clinical features

Septic arthritis is manifest as the acute onset of pain, redness, tenderness and swelling in the joint. Signs of effusion may be elicited in large joints. Systemic features such as fever and malaise are common, and are to be expected if the infection is haematogenous. Non-infective acute arthritis can mimic septic arthritis. If a single joint is involved, as is usually the case with septic arthritis, the crystal arthropathies gout and pseudogout must be considered. These diagnoses are confirmed by the finding of their characteristic crystals in aspirated joint fluid.

Management

Joint aspiration should be attempted for diagnosis. Blood cultures should be performed, especially if the joint is not accessible to aspiration. Large numbers of polymorphs are found in aspirated joint fluid, but Gram stain is not always positive. Antibiotic treatment should be initiated early and based on the Gram stain results or tailored to the clinical setting if the Gram stain is unhelpful. Repeated aspiration or operative washout of the effusion can be of assistance in some circumstances.

GENITAL TRACT INFECTIONS

These are discussed in Chapters 34 and 35.

URINARY TRACT INFECTIONS

These are discussed in Chapter 35.

HOSPITAL-ACQUIRED INFECTIONS

These are clinical infections occurring in hospital patients that were not present at the time of admission. They occur in 5–15% of patients admitted to hospital, the incidence being higher in centres that treat the critically ill and do complex surgery, and contribute to an increased morbidity and mortality.

Bacteriology

Gram-negative bacilli and *Staph. aureus* are the commonest causes of hospital-acquired infection. *Staphylococcus aureus* strains with multiple antibiotic resistance (multiresistant *Staph. aureus*, MRSA) are a particular problem in some hospitals. The Gram-negative organisms also have the capacity to develop resistance to many antimicrobial agents in common use, making them difficult to treat satisfactorily.

The main reason for antibiotic-resistant bacteria is the use of antibiotics; by suppressing sensitive organisms, they allow colonisation by resistant organisms, often leading to overt clinical infections. In addition, infections may arise, especially in individuals with impaired host defences, caused by organisms (e.g. *Candida albicans*) not normally regarded as pathogens (opportunistic infections). Transmission is principally through breakdown of asepsis and antisepsis, in particular neglect of handwashing. Thus infection is contracted from contact with hospital staff, either from hands or by respiratory droplets, or via food, water, sinks, contaminated ventilator systems, catheters or respirators.

Common sites of infection

Urinary tract. This accounts for 40% of hospital-acquired infection, secondary to either instrumentation of the urethra, bladder or kidneys or insertion of a urethral catheter.

Pneumonia. Pulmonary infections are a leading cause of death from hospital-acquired infection. Infection with Gram-negative bacilli and *Staph. aureus* both cause a necrotising bronchopneumonia.

Surgical wound infection. Postoperative surgical wound infection can be stratified into clean, contaminated or dirty, according to the type of procedure and the clinical condition being treated. Clean surgery involves incisions only through clean skin; contaminated surgery occurs when the procedure involves a mucosal surface that is normally colonised by bacteria; and dirty surgery occurs when the procedure is carried out when infec-tion is already established or there is gross spillage of intestinal contents during intra-abdominal surgery (see Ch. 8).

Burns. Extensive third degree burns are at high risk of infection. These days *Pseudomonas aeruginosa* is the most frequent organism.

Bloodstream. Intravenous cannulae, especially cannulae used for the infusion of hypertonic nutrient solutions (TPN), are particularly prone to infection and strict asepsis is of paramount importance. With peripheral cannulae, the risk of infection rises with the length of time they are left in a particular site, particularly longer than 72 hours.

Management

Management is by prevention:

- Reduce the risk of patients acquiring infection. The basic principles remain the avoidance of transmission of infection between patients by hospital staff and the identification and correction of potential sources of infection.
- Assume all patients are carrying infectious agents (universal precautions).
- Protect patients by separation of those more susceptible to infection (e.g. patients with burns or depressed immunity).
- Be restrictive with antibiotics. It is obvious that the indiscriminate use of broad-spectrum antibiotics without due consideration to diagnostic possibilities is dangerous and can lead to the emergence of multi-antibiotic resistant organisms. Thus it is essential that antibiotics be used in full dosage only when necessary and only for the length of time required to eliminate the pathogen(s).
- Employ the 'rules of indwelling devices':
  — don't use it unless you have to
  — remove it as soon as possible
  — insert and manage with aseptic technique
  — keep system closed as much as possible.

These rules apply to all indwelling devices such as intravenous cannulae, urethral catheters, endotracheal tubes intercostal drains, etc.

TETANUS

Tetanus is caused by *Clostridium tetani*, an anaerobic spore-forming bacillus that is commonly present in soil and animal faeces.

Surgical pathology

Clostridium tetani is not an invasive organism and does not cause an inflammatory reaction. Instead it colonises wounds and releases a powerful neurotoxin which is transported retrogradely along nerve fibres to the anterior horn cells causing them to be hyperstimulated.

Surgical importance

Tetanus-prone wounds. An understanding of those wounds that are prone to tetanus acquisition is required. The wounds likely to be affected are:

- deep and penetrating, associated with local tissue damage, foreign body implantation or soil contamination
- soil-contaminated, superficial and minor lacerations or abrasions
- crushing injuries of fingers and toes, especially those associated with fractures
- surgical, particularly when a second operation is performed; the operative trauma may activate dormant tetanus spores
- deliberately contaminated raw surfaces, e.g. the umbilicus of a neonate dressed with earth containing spores – a tradition in certain cultures.

In about one-fifth of cases, no obvious source of infection is apparent. Tetanus-prone wounds should be managed according to standard surgical principles, including thorough debridement, and removal of necrotic material and foreign bodies.

Tetanus prophylaxis

Primary. Most individuals have been vaccinated with three doses of tetanus toxoid as a child. Boosters are required every 10 years in order to maintain immunity, but are often neglected, and older individuals can be vulnerable to tetanus for this reason. Each presentation for wound management must be considered an opportunity to boost immunity to tetanus, even if the wound is not tetanus-prone.

Secondary. Passive immunisation with tetanus immunoglobulin must be given to all individuals who have sustained a tetanus-prone wound and whose immune status is unclear, or if boosters were given more than 10 years previously, as well as a tetanus toxoid booster.

MEDICAL INFECTIONS WITH SURGICAL IMPLICATIONS

TUBERCULOSIS

This was once a common surgical disease but is now less common in the Western world.

Bacteriology

Organisms reach the site by inhalation or aspiration rather than by haematogenous spread. Pneumonia is most likely postoperatively following a general anaesthetic or in patients intubated for prolonged periods.

There are two common forms: human (*Mycobacterium tuberculosis*) and bovine (*M. bovis*). The organisms are rods which fail to be visualised on Gram-staining, but stain characteristically with the Ziehl–Neelson (acid-fast) method. Culture, which may take up to 8 weeks to become positive, is the best method of confirming the disease.

Surgical pathology

The effects of tubercle bacilli depend largely on host resistance. A large dose in an undernourished patient may produce a relatively severe subacute infection which is relentless and causes death if untreated. A small dose in a healthy individual with a naturally high level of resistance produces a more chronic infection with which the body may either come into equilibrium or even eliminate.

The lesions produced are granulomas. They destroy the tissue in which they form, leading to the formation of necrotic 'caseous' material and pus (cold abscess), which is 'sterile' on routine culture unless secondary bacterial infection supervenes. Healing is by fibrosis with or without calcification. Common surgical sites are:

- lymph nodes of the neck, mediastinum and abdomen; in the first site, abscesses and sinuses may develop, and any necrotic material should be removed surgically
- serous cavities: joints, pleura, peritoneum, pericardium
- viscera, e.g. terminal ileum, kidneys, ureters and bladder
- bones, especially vertebrae.

Management

All surgical tuberculosis is initially managed conservatively with antituberculous agents unless there is an emergency (e.g. spinal cord compression, intestinal obstruction). Surgery is used to:

- obtain tissue for diagnosis, by either histological examination or culture

- evacuate pus and necrotic tissue
- stabilise or reconstruct
- deal with complications.

ACTINOMYCOSIS

Actinomyces israelii is a branching Gram-positive bacillus which grows anaerobically and microaerophilically. It gains access through a breach in the mucosa of the gastrointestinal tract anywhere from the teeth to the anus but is most common in the neck and right iliac fossa, the latter secondary to appendicitis. It is also found in the vagina and can cause endometritis in association with an intrauterine device.

Surgical pathology

A woody cellulitis is followed by pus formation containing the yellow 'sulphur granules' which are large clumped colonies of bacteria.

Management

Management is usually conservative, with large doses of penicillin over a period of many weeks. Surgical debridement may be required in some cases to hasten recovery or prevent disfigurement.

BLOOD-BORNE VIRUS INFECTIONS

There are three major blood-borne viruses that have implications for surgery: hepatitis B virus, hepatitis C virus, and human immunodeficiency virus (HIV). All have the properties of chronicity, transmission via blood (as well as other mechanisms of transmission), and long-term consequences for the infected individual.

Surgical importance

There are three major surgical issues:

- prevention of transmission between patients
- prevention of acquisition of infection from patients

- prevention of transmission to patients.

Prevention of transmission between patients. Principal strategies here include the need to minimise transfusion use and adequate sterilisation or high-level disinfection of surgical instruments, including fibre-optic endoscopes. Although all donated blood is screened for HIV antibody it is still theoretically possible to transmit the virus very early in infection when the HIV antibody test is negative.

Prevention of acquisition of infection from patients. Surgical staff are at risk because of the volume of body fluids with which they are in contact and the frequent chance of sharps injuries during surgical procedures. Two strategies will assist in reducing this risk. The first is to adopt the policy of 'universal' blood and body fluid precautions, where it is assumed that all patients, regardless of whether they have been screened or not, are treated as potentially carrying blood-borne viruses such as HIV, hepatitis B and hepatitis C viruses. In turn, this requires improving operative technique to minimise the risk of sharps injuries.

Prevention of transmission to patients. In rare instances blood-borne viruses have been transmitted from surgical staff to patients. Individuals who believe they may be at risk of carrying blood-borne viruses should have themselves tested for these agents and exclude themselves from procedures that run the risk of 'reverse' sharps exposure.

FURTHER READING

Adier M W 1993 ABC of AIDS, 3rd edn. BMJ, London
Fry D E 1994 Surgical infections. Little, Brown, Boston
Polk H C 1982 Infection and the surgical patient. Clinical surgery international, vol 4. Churchill Livingstone, Edinburgh
Pollock A 1987 Surgical infections. Edward Arnold, London
Taylor E 1992 Infection in surgical practice. Oxford University Press, Oxford
Watts J Mck, McDonald P J, O'Brien P E et al (eds) 1981 Infection in surgery: basic and clinical aspects. Churchill Livingstone, Edinburgh

7

Wound healing
Jeremy Thompson   David Scott-Coombes

OVERVIEW

The four stages of normal wound healing are described: haemostasis, inflammation, granulation tissue formation and maturation. Most incised wounds heal directly by first intention, but tissue loss and infection may lead to a delayed process of healing by second intention. Infection is one of several factors that inhibit wound healing, others being ischaemia, malnutrition and agents such as irradiation and drugs. Wound complications are considered, notably dehiscence and keloid scar. An understanding of normal and abnormal wound repair should allow the clinician to achieve the best functional and cosmetic results for the patient.

Whether a patient has suffered a wound through trauma or by the hand of a surgeon, all doctors called upon to treat wounds require a basic understanding of the principles of wound healing.

The body has its own repair mechanisms which occur in all organs and tissues. However, the amount of regrowth that occurs following tissue loss varies considerably, from none in the central nervous system to the high capacity for regeneration seen in the liver. Where tissue cannot be regenerated a defect is filled by scar tissue.

Following injury, the management of all wounds should be directed at optimising the conditions that allow speedy healing with the minimum of scarring and maximal function.

This chapter describes the healing and management of wounds to the skin, subcutaneous tissues, muscle and fascia. Injuries to abdominal organs (Ch. 15), bones (Ch. 12) and nervous tissue (Ch. 16) are considered elsewhere.

MECHANISM OF WOUND HEALING

Four stages of wound healing are recognised. These stages are not independent of each other, but merge to form a continuous process of repair. The time course of wound healing is subject to individual variation as well as specific factors that influence wound healing (see below), but a general indication of the timing of these stages is shown in Figure 7.1.

STAGE I: HAEMOSTASIS (first 4 hours)

At the time of injury there is a transient vasoconstriction of arterioles, which is thought to be mediated by a neurogenic reflex. This vasoconstriction lasts seconds to minutes according to the degree of injury. Following injury there is a change in the charge of the damaged collagen, which leads to the immediate activation of the clotting cascade and stimulates platelet aggregation. The platelet and fibrin clot produces a haemostatic plug within hours of injury, and this ensures complete haemostasis.

The surface of this haemostatic plug dehydrates to form a scab, which seals the wound from the external environment. Any excess clot in the deeper layers of the wound has the potential to become infected, and this could delay wound healing.

STAGE II: INFLAMMATION (first 24–48 hours)

Following the transient reflex vasoconstriction, there is a

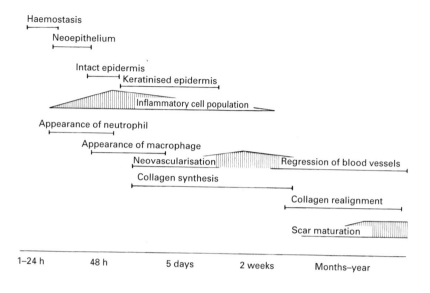

Haemostasis

Neoepithelium

Intact epidermis

Keratinised epidermis

Inflammatory cell population

Appearance of neutrophil

Appearance of macrophage

Neovascularisation   Regression of blood vessels

Collagen synthesis

Collagen realignment

Scar maturation

1–24 h   48 h   5 days   2 weeks   Months–year

Fig. 7.1 Time course for wound healing.

prolonged period of vasodilatation mediated mainly by histamine and serotonin released from platelets and tissue mast cells. This process results in a slower flow of blood in the capillary bed and allows the white blood cells to line up along the vascular endothelium of the capillaries (margination). Intrinsically linked to the clotting cascade is the activation of the complement and kinin systems. Under the influence of a variety of chemotaxins – protein fragments released from injured tissue cells, products of complement (C3a and C5a) and bacteria – the active emigration of white blood cells from the vessels (diapedesis) occurs. In particular, the polymorphonuclear neutrophils migrate into the wound to phagocytose damaged tissue and bacteria, thus combating infection and removing excess blood clot. The increased permeability of the vessels permits the exudation of protein-rich plasma which, together with the neutrophils, constitutes the inflammatory exudate. This fibrin coagulum traps red cells, debris and devitalised tissue and binds the wound edges together.

Clinically the wound is red, warm, painful and oedematous, and frequently normal function is impaired – the classical signs of inflammation (rubor, calor, dolor, tumor and functio laesa).

STAGE III: GRANULATION TISSUE FORMATION (48 hours–5 days)

This stage is heralded by the emergence of the

macrophage as the predominant cell within the injured tissue and by the gradual disappearance of neutrophils. The macrophage has three main functions: (1) a phagocytic role to digest any remaining organisms or necrotic debris; (2) the stimulation of existing endothelial cells to proliferate, migrate and mature as new blood vessels (neovascularisation); and (3) the stimulation of fibroblast proliferation.

Granulation tissue is so called owing to its soft pink granular appearance on the surface of wounds. The characteristic histological appearance is that of a proliferating matrix of fibroblasts and macrophages and new blood vessels (Fig. 7.2). The function of the fibroblast is to synthesise collagen and ground substance. Collagen is first secreted from the fibroblast as immature tropocollagen, which undergoes hydroxylation (vitamin C-dependent) and subsequent cross-linkage to produce a stable polymer. Each collagen molecule is composed of three polypeptide chains (alpha chains) coiled in a left-hand helix. In humans there are five genetically distinct alpha chains, and five types of collagen have been identified. Each type differs in the degree of hydroxylation, glycosylation and the pattern of cross-linking. The collagen usually produced in healing wounds is of the type III variety. Ground substance is an amorphous matrix of connective tissue consisting mainly of mucopolysaccharides.

At the margins on the surface of the wound, basal cells of the epidermis undergo hypertrophy and hyperplasia to

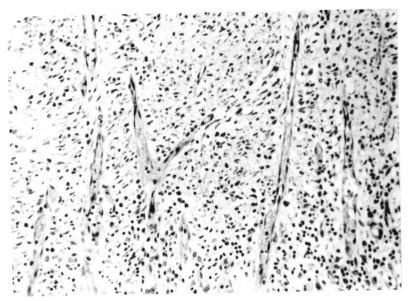

Fig. 7.2 Granulation tissue. New vessels and immature fibroblasts are seen in loose myxoid ground substance (×160, haematoxylin and eosin).

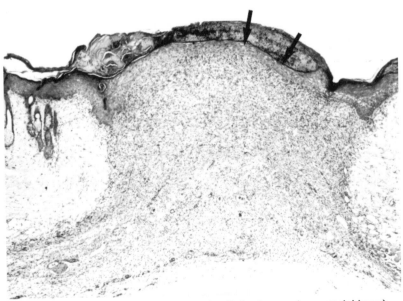

Fig. 7.3 A wound healing by second intention (following previous punch biopsy). The slide shows granulation tissue filling the defect with a regenerated epithelium (arrowed) and residual overlying coagulum (scab) (×45, haematoxylin and eosin).

produce spurs. From these spurs new epithelial cells migrate across the surface of the wound (epiboly), under the scab, and converge by 24–48 hours (Fig. 7.3). At 5 days this new epithelium has undergone surface keratinisation.

In the deeper layers of the wound edges myofibroblasts congregate. These specialised cells contain elements of both muscle cells and fibroblasts, and possess the ability to contract, thus reducing the surface area of the wound (wound contraction).

Clinically the wound remains swollen with a surrounding redness (hyperaemia). The surface of the wound will be sealed off by the scab, or if this has lifted off, the pink granular reflective surface of granulation tissue will be visible. By the end of this stage the wound is less painful unless some complication (e.g. infection) arises.

STAGE IV: MATURATION (5 days–months)

This long process consists of a gradual strengthening, remodelling and realignment of collagen fibres along the lines of tension, together with a steady regression of vascular channels which formed in the early stages of healing but are unnecessary by this stage. This process results in an acellular, avascular, collagenous scar.

Clinically the scar softens and gradually pales from the red/pink colour of a newly epithelialised surface to the whiteness of a mature scar. However, the overall appearance of the scar is dependent upon the age and race of the patient and the anatomical site of the wound.

TYPES OF WOUND HEALING

Although the mechanism for healing is essentially the same in all wounds, we recognise two subdivisions of healing.

Healing by first intention (primary union)

Clean surgical incisions generally heal in this way. There has usually been minimal tissue loss or damage with minimal bacterial contamination. The divided tissue edges are reapproximated (by sutures, clips, tape or glue) without tension.

Healing by second intention (secondary union)

This describes the way wounds with a more extensive defect between the edges undergo healing. Secondary union may arise because of tissue loss or injury (surgical excision or trauma), or the wound edges may be deliberately kept apart because there has been heavy wound contamination (e.g. trauma patients or following laparotomy for faecal peritonitis). There are two problems: wound care is more complicated, and a larger tissue defect needs to be filled. Compared to healing by first intention, there is more fibrin exudation and there may be more necrotic tissue, both of which prolong the

inflammatory stage of healing with a greater production of granulation tissue. In addition, wound contraction, which is minimal in wounds healing by primary union, plays a major role in decreasing the size of the tissue defect when wounds heal by secondary union. The healing process is slower and produces more scar tissue.

WOUND STRENGTH

Most wounds of skin, subcutaneous tissue, muscle, fascia or tendon never regain their pre-injury strength. Figure 7.4 illustrates the time course of establishment of wound strength of the abdominal wall. There is an initial lag phase, but between 2 and 4 weeks there begins a rapid increase in the strength of the wound, which increases to between 70–80% of pre-injury strength by 3 months. Thereafter wound strength reaches a plateau below 100%. Some tissues, however, regain almost full strength much earlier, for example sutured small bowel regains its strength by 10 days.

The development of wound strength is related to the type of collagen produced, the early granulation tissue type III collagen being weaker than the later (maturation stage) type I.

SUTURES

Humans have used artificial ways to close wounds for over 2000 years. Carefully placed sutures will appose the sides of the wound and encourage healing by first intention. In addition the sutures provide support to the wound, which regains 40–70% of its original strength immediately after operation. However, when skin sutures

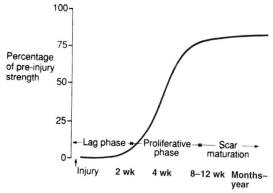

Fig. 7.4 Time course for the development of wound strength following injury.

are removed (usually at 10 days) the wound weakens to only 10% of its pre-injury level.

The disadvantages of sutures are that they provide a route for bacteria to penetrate through to the deeper tissue layers and that they can initiate foreign body reactions. The likelihood of sutures leading to wound complications is determined in part by the mass of suture placed within the wound and also by the innate ability of the suture material to evoke an inflammatory response.

The ideal suture should be strong, non-irritant, biodegradable, cheap and easy to handle. At present no suture satisfies all of these criteria and the surgeon has to choose between suture material that is either inert or absorbable. Non-absorbable sutures maintain the strength of a wound indefinitely, whereas absorbable sutures allow a progressive decline in wound strength such that by the end of 1 month the suture is usually contributing very little to the strength of the wound. However, non-absorbable sutures, in particular braided materials, have the potential to generate a more prolonged foreign body reaction compared with absorbable sutures. The most appropriate suture material is selected on the basis of the need for strength on the one hand and for absorbability on the other. When suturing the skin the final cosmetic appearance is also important.

IMPAIRED WOUND HEALING

Factors that decrease the efficiency of wound healing may be either systemic or local (Table 7.1).

SYSTEMIC

Patients with a poor nutritional status are at risk of poor

Table 7.1 Factors that impair wound healing

Local	Systemic
Infection	Nutritional status – deficiency of vitamins A and C, zinc, manganese, protein
Ischaemia	Steroid therapy
— tension	Anti-cancer chemotherapy
— compartment syndrome	Ionising radiation
— shock	Uraemia
— anaemia	Jaundice
— vascular disease	Malignant disease
Foreign body	Diabetes mellitus
Malignancy	Age

wound healing. Vitamin C is necessary for the synthesis of collagen fibres and low levels can result in scurvy – a disease characterised by poor healing of epithelial lesions. Similarly, zinc is an important cofactor for many enzymes involved in tissue repair. It has been shown that a high-protein diet accelerates the speed of regaining wound tensile strength.

Systemic steroid therapy or antimitotic agents have a major anti-inflammatory action, impair collagen synthesis and enhance its breakdown. Ionising radiation destroys rapidly dividing cells, in particular the newly developing small blood vessels and dermal fibroblasts.

Jaundice delays angiogenesis and impairs fibroblast function, whereas uraemia suppresses connective tissue formation and epithelial repair.

Patients with diabetes mellitus are susceptible to infection and may have poor blood supply to wounds on the extremities of the limbs.

LOCAL

Infection is the most common and most important local factor impairing wound healing. Infection arises from the implantation of bacteria following a breach in the epidermis. Infection prolongs the inflammatory phase of wound healing, retards collagen synthesis and encourages collagen breakdown. The presence of a foreign body, such as a suture, or of necrotic tissue not only prolongs the inflammatory response but also acts as a nidus for infection. Furthermore, the invading organisms compete for the limited oxygen supply with the injured tissues.

Ischaemia of the tissues is the second most common cause for impaired wound healing. Wounds of the face and hands, which have a rich blood supply, generally heal very well. For effective wound healing it is essential for the oxygen demands of the granulation tissue to be met. Ischaemia of the wound can arise in a number of ways, e.g. patients with arterial disease have an impoverished supply of oxygen to the tissues. Local ischaemia of the tissues may arise through increased tissue tension leading to a compressive effect upon the blood vessels. Such an increased tension may arise from sutures being secured too tightly, from a haematoma compressing the vessels or from oedema secondary to infection.

If this swelling occurs in a closed space, the rise in tissue pressure can exceed the blood perfusion pressure leading to a local arrest in the blood flow to the tissues. This is called *compartment syndrome*; left untreated, it leads to necrosis of the muscle and dysfunction of the limb. The common sites for compartment syndrome are the volar compartment of the forearm and the anterior compartment of the leg. Owing to the sensitivity of nerve receptors to anoxia, the patient initially complains of pain apparently out of proportion to the clinical findings, with associated hyperaesthesia in the distribution of the nerves in the compartment. Weakness follows and then paralysis of the compartment musculature. Pain can be elicited by passive stretching of the compartment muscles (e.g. straightening of the fingers in forearm compartment syndrome). An absent distal pulse is not a reliable physical sign as it may be palpable even in the presence of muscle necrosis. The treatment is immediate surgical decompression achieved by performing a fasciotomy of the deep and superficial fascial layers in the compartment. The fasciotomy wound edges are left unsutured.

The presence of a local malignancy, e.g. a squamous carcinoma developing in an ulcer caused by venous hypertension (Marjolin's ulcer), is a rare and sometimes unrecognised cause of impaired wound healing.

MANAGEMENT OF WOUNDS

For any wound the most important priority is to avoid the development of infection. Therefore all wounds should be thoroughly cleaned, necrotic tissue and debris removed (debridement), and haemostasis secured. The decision about whether to close the wound immediately is determined by the degree of wound contamination and tissue loss. Surgical incisions are best managed by primary closure using sutures, clips, tape or tissue glue. Ragged wounds require excision of the skin edges followed by primary closure if this can be achieved without tension. Wounds with abundant crushed or devitalized tissue require more extensive debridement. The wound edges can be left apart for subsequent inspection and if the tissues are viable and clean, then the wound may be closed at 3–5 days (delayed primary closure).

Infected wounds are left open until the infection abates. At that time the wound can either be left to heal (with associated wound contraction) or it may be closed. Closure may be achieved by delayed primary closure when the wound edges can be approximated without tension or by skin grafting onto healthy granulation tissue. Both of these methods reduce wound contraction.

When extensive skin loss occurs, the wound will require skin grafting. This can be performed immediately if the wound is clean (primary grafting) or be delayed if there is infection or extensive devitalised tissue.

HIGH VELOCITY INJURIES

High velocity missiles (>600 m/s) possess enormous kinetic energy which is transferred to the tissues during the missile's passage through the body, resulting in a temporary cavitation of the tissues. The diameter of the cavity may be 30–40 times the diameter of the missile, and these injuries are often complicated by disruption of vessels, bone and nerves, both locally and at a distance from the missile's trajectory (Fig. 7.5). This temporary implosion creates a vacuum which sucks bacteria and foreign material inside the wound as the cavity expands and collapses in a pulsatile manner. Therefore, although the wound may look clean superficially, these wounds should never be closed, as infection and gas gangrene will almost certainly result. As with other heavily contaminated injuries, wounds should be treated aggressively by extensive debridement, preserving as much skin as possible. All high velocity wounds must be left open during the early stages of treatment.

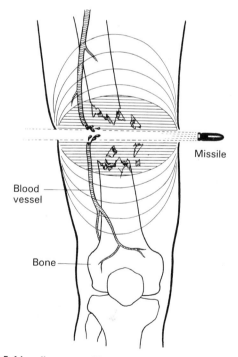

Fig. 7.5 Line diagram to illustrate the implosion cavity ▦ and shock waves ▤ that follow injury with a high velocity missile. A transient cavity is generated by the transfer of kinetic energy from the missile to the tissues, and a permanent cavity may result because of tissue displacement by the missile.

ANTIBIOTICS

Whilst the use of antibiotics is no substitute for appropriate surgical management of the wound, they can help both in preventing wound infection (prophylaxis) and in the management of established infections.

Prophylaxis

Prophylactic antibiotics are only of use if the tissue concentration of antibiotic is in the therapeutic range at the time of operation (contamination). In general there is no place for the use of antibiotics during a clean operation except when the consequences of infection would be catastrophic for the patient, e.g. when prosthetic material is placed within the patient (vascular graft, hip replacement) or in the prevention of gas gangrene following an amputation for peripheral vascular disease. There is no doubt that the prophylactic administration of antibiotics has reduced the wound sepsis rate in operations that could result in tissue contamination with endogenous bacteria (e.g. operations on the gastrointestinal tract). In either situation the surgeon should choose an antibiotic regimen with a specific action against the likely pathogen(s).

Therapeutic use

In established wound infections, the surgeon must ensure that there is adequate drainage of pus and that the tissues are not under tension. The wound should be opened widely and to a depth that maximises free drainage of pus and allows for easy cleaning and dressing. The wound should be dressed regularly according to the rate of production of pus.

If there is surrounding cellulitis and/or the patient is systemically unwell, the surgeon may decide to prescribe an appropriate antibiotic regimen based upon the bacteria isolated and their antibiotic sensitivities.

COMPLICATIONS OF WOUND HEALING

INFECTION

Infection of the wound is the most common complication and the most important cause of impaired wound healing (see previous section). A wound infection will usually present as a cellulitis in the early stages but can progress to form an abscess. The bacteria responsible for wound infections are either endogenous, e.g. anaerobes from the patient's gastrointestinal tract, or exogenous, e.g. *Staphylococcus aureus* from the surgeon's nose.

Wounds of warfare are at high risk of developing infection, in particular gas gangrene, although this can also occur in other injuries. Gas gangrene is caused by *Clostridium perfringens* whose spores reside in soil. This anaerobic gas-producing infection can result in widespread necrosis of muscle and subcutaneous tissues. Clinically the wound is oedematous and discharges a foul smelling brown-coloured pus. Crepitus can be palpated and an X-ray will reveal gas under the skin. The treatment is high-dose penicillin, radical debridement, antitoxin and hyperbaric oxygen.

DEHISCENCE

If an abdominal wound fails to heal, its edges may burst apart allowing loops of intestine to protrude through the wound (dehiscence). In addition to the systemic and local predisposing factors (especially wound infection) to impaired wound healing, poor surgical technique can also lead to dehiscence. This may arise because suture knots become undone, sutures break, the placement of the sutures in the tissues was wrong or the choice of suture material was inappropriate.

Wound dehiscence usually occurs around the 10th postoperative day, often following exertion of the abdominal musculature (e.g. by coughing). The treatment of this dramatic event is to reassure the alarmed patient and proceed to resuture the wound under general anaesthetic.

In abdominal wounds where part or all of the deeper layers give way but the skin heals intact, an incisional hernia results. This may develop either in the early postoperative period or months or even years after operation.

FIBROSIS

Occasionally the healing process itself can lead to problems. Examples of this include intra-abdominal adhesions between viscera, tendon adhesions to the wound, anastomotic strictures and cirrhosis of the liver. In these cases fibrous tissue is formed where it did not previously exist, and this results in impaired function. It is thought that this process occurs as a result of a more intense and prolonged duration of the inflammatory stage of healing.

OVERHEALING

Hypertrophic and keloid scars are further examples of abnormal healing which are seen easily by the naked eye. A hypertrophic scar develops soon after injury, is confined to the wound and usually subsides over time. They favour flexor surfaces and are common over the shoulder joint. Keloid scars may not develop for several months, but they rarely subside and often progress. Keloids overgrow the boundaries of the injury and are prone to develop on the ear lobes and the pre-sternal skin. In contrast to hypertrophic scars, the magnitude of a keloid scar is not proportional to the magnitude of the injury. Keloids recur after surgical excision, but this may be prevented by preoperative radiotherapy or intradermal steroid injections.

FURTHER READING

Hunt T K 1988 Physiology of wound healing. In: Clowes G H A (ed) Trauma, sepsis and shock; the physiological basis of therapy. Marcel Dekker, New York, p 443–472
Lynch S E, Colvin R B, Antoniades H N 1989 Growth factors in wound healing. Journal of Clinical Investigation 84: 640–649
Westaby S (ed) 1985 Wound care. William Heinemann Medical Books, London

8 Preoperative and postoperative care

Robin Williamson

OVERVIEW

Preoperative care starts with a proper evaluation of the patient by history, clinical examination and appropriate investigation. Selection of the patient for operation requires a careful assessment of the risk–benefit ratio, bearing in mind the surgical condition itself and any intercurrent disease. It is often advisable to cover the operation with prophylactic measures against infection and venous thromboembolism, in particular. General postoperative care is discussed together with the common postoperative complications, both general and local.

Surgery is not just a technical exercise. It includes the total care of the surgical patient, i.e. those patients with conditions that can be improved or even cured by means of a surgical operation. Often (although not always) the operation is the centrepiece of surgical treatment, but however skilfully performed, operations are pointless or even harmful if the indications are inappropriate, the preparation is slapdash and the aftercare is inadequate. There is little comfort in the adage 'it was a good operation but the patient died'. This chapter considers the preoperative assessment of the patient and postoperative care, including the prevention and management of common complications. The management of the patient within the operating theatre is covered by textbooks of operative surgery.

PREOPERATIVE ASSESSMENT

SELECTING THE PATIENT

In conditions such as uncontrolled bleeding, a curable cancer, an abscess, or a displaced fracture, the need for operation is so strong that only the most unfit of patients should be denied this chance for the relief of suffering and/or the prevention of death. In other conditions such as hiatus hernia, a cosmetic defect of the skin, haemorrhoids or an arthritic joint, the indications may be less clear-cut and the potential benefits of surgical treatment must be set against the risks, pain and disability that might result. The failure of conservative treatment, the likelihood of a successful operation and the patient's own wishes must be taken into account. Good clinical judgment is based upon common sense, experience and compassion. It includes the ability to refer the patient to a colleague in the same hospital or to a specialist centre if this is clearly in the patient's best interests. It also requires a decision to be made on the extent of operation and the method of anaesthesia, where genuine choices exist.

DETERMINING THE FITNESS FOR OPERATION

The skill lies in assessing the patient's chance of surviving a general anaesthetic and the trauma of a major surgical procedure and avoiding major complications. The assessment starts with a detailed history, looking for important intercurrent disease, followed by a full physical examination. Routine investigations in patients undergoing all but the most trivial operations include haemoglobin, blood grouping and chest X-ray plus ECG (electrocardiography) in older patients or smokers, and urea and electrolytes if intravenous fluids are likely to be needed. Pulmonary function tests are advisable in those with respiratory disease and a clotting screen in those

Table 8.1	ASA physical status scale (simplified)
Category	**Description**
Class 1	Healthy individual with no physical or mental disturbance.
Class 2	Mild to moderate systemic disease not necessarily related to the condition requiring operation (e.g. hypertension)
Class 3	Severe systemic disease (e.g. uncontrolled diabetes)
Class 4	Incapacitating systemic disease (e.g. heart failure)
Class 5	Moribund – operation only performed as a last resort (e.g. for bleeding)
ASA = American Society of Anesthesiologists.	

with any predisposition to bleed (e.g. jaundice). Risk assessment in patients with cardiac, respiratory or renal disease may require the opinion of a specialist physician as well as a preoperative visit by the anaesthetist. Physical status can then be classified according to the ASA scale (Table 8.1).

Certain *risk factors* must be taken into account in determining fitness for operation.

Age. Although elderly patients have reduced cardiac, respiratory and renal reserves, their 'biological age' (i.e. general health status) is more important than their exact chronological age. In general, older people withstand surgery well but may not tolerate serious complications. They are sensitive to fluid overload and narcotic drugs, and they are at greater risk of deep vein thrombosis and mental confusion.

Obesity. This increases the technical difficulties of operation plus the risk of wound infection, chest infection and deep vein thrombosis. Advice to lose weight before an elective operation must be balanced against the severity of the patient's symptoms during that time.

Cigarette smoking. All heavy smokers will have some degree of chronic bronchitis and are therefore at much greater risk of postoperative chest complications. Nicotine and carbon monoxide have adverse effects on the heart, lungs and immune system. Smokers should be strongly advised to abstain for at least 1 month before an elective operation. All patients with pre-existing respiratory disease are likely to benefit from preoperative physiotherapy, and antibiotics and bronchodilators may also be indicated.

Cardiac disease. Ischaemic heart disease is prevalent among older patients. Operations should be avoided within 3–6 months of a myocardial infarct if possible. Specialist advice should be sought in patients with arrhythmias (including those with a pacemaker) or cardiac failure. The anaesthetist must be informed about drug therapy in those with hypertension or other cardiovascular disease. Hypertension that is newly discovered on preoperative assessment should be investigated before proceeding to operation, if time allows. Patients with valvular disease of the heart need antibiotic prophylaxis against endocarditis; penicillin, amoxycillin and eyrthromycin are suitable drugs.

Anaemia. Mild anaemia (haemoglobin >10g/dl) is better corrected during the operation than by an immediate preoperative transfusion. If blood transfusion is needed, it is best performed at least 5 days before operation to allow the circulation to stabilise. Rapid transfusion in older patients should be monitored by central venous pressure measurement, and diuretics may be required to reduce sudden circulatory overload.

Diabetes. Present in about 1% of the population, this condition may be picked up by preoperative urine testing and should be investigated by means of a glucose tolerance test. Insulin-dependent diabetics should be converted to a soluble insulin regime before operation. Insulin should be stopped for at least 4 hours before operation, and an intravenous infusion is set up with 5% glucose. Postoperative insulin is delivered by pump infusion with frequent measurement of blood glucose levels. Dehydration must be avoided. It is easy to miss hypoglycaemic coma in a sedated postoperative patient.

Renal insufficiency. Blood levels or urea and creatinine are relatively insensitive markers of preoperative renal function. Creatinine clearance is a simple measure of glomerular filtration rate (GFR) and is devised from the following equation, using a single blood level and the volume of urine (V) collected over a measured period of time (usually 24 hours):

$$GFR = \frac{urinary\ creatinine\ concentration}{plasma\ creatinine\ concentration} \times V$$

Hyperkalaemia and anaemia are potential problems in patients with renal impairment. In all patients undergoing major surgery, an hourly output of at least 40 ml urine should be sought by judicious use of intravenous fluids and, if necessary, diuretics.

Jaundice. The preoperative preparation of jaundiced patients is considered in Chapter 27 (p. 282). In those with prolonged or profound obstructive jaundice (serum bilirubin >200 µmol/L), preoperative biliary decompression may be advisable.

Drug therapy. Patients on corticosteroids will require the drug to be continued by the intravenous route (e.g. hydrocortisone sodium succinate 100 mg 6-hourly) until they are able to take tablets again. Contraceptive pills that include oestrogen are associated with an increased risk of deep vein thrombosis and should be stopped 1 month before a major operation. Certain psychotropic drugs, notably antidepressants, should be discontinued before operation if possible. Antihypertensive medication must be discussed with the anaesthetist.

PERIOPERATIVE PROPHYLAXIS

PROPHYLACTIC ANTIBIOTICS

The risk of sepsis is high enough to justify the use of prophylactic antibiotics in two different types of operation:

- operations on a contaminated organ system, e.g. gastric, biliary or colorectal surgery, appendicectomy
- operations that involve inserting prosthetic material, e.g. vascular grafts, artificial hips, heart valves.

The choice of antibiotics should reflect the likely pathogen, e.g. metronidazole alone in appendicectomy or in combination with a cephalosporin or aminoglycoside in colectomy. Either a single dose or up to three doses are given intravenously, starting when the patient goes to the operating theatre. Antibiotics are no substitute for good surgical technique, however, especially the avoidance of haematoma formation.

THROMBOPROPHYLAXIS

There is a risk of deep vein thrombosis (DVT) and fatal pulmonary embolus after all but the most minor operations, but this risk reflects several factors: age, obesity, duration, extent and type of operation, period of postoperative bed rest, presence of malignant disease, use of contraceptive pill, cardiac failure, past history of DVT or

pulmonary embolus. Precautionary measures against thromboembolism include:

- graduated compression stockings, which are simpler than any of the following:
- external pneumatic compression using an inflatable device applied to each leg
- low molecular weight dextran
- subcutaneous heparin: 5000 u given by s.c. injection starting 2 hours before operation (or treatments that confine the patient to bed) and continuing 8- or 12-hourly until the patient is ambulant
- intravenous heparin by low-dose infusion in those at especial risk.

A combination of compression stockings and subcutaneous heparin is popular in many areas of surgery; low molecular weight heparins may confer an increased benefit (see Ch. 37). Anticoagulants are contraindicated in neurosurgery because of the risk of intracranial bleeding, but should be given in hip replacement surgery, where manipulation of the joint causes severe distortion of the femoral vein.

SPECIFIC MEASURES

Upper gastrointestinal surgery

In patients with intestinal obstruction or pyloric stenosis, a nasogastric tube should be inserted before operation to empty the upper gastrointestinal tract. Following most operations on the oesophagus, stomach, small bowel, bile duct, pancreas or spleen, nasogastric intubation is used until bowel sounds return and the volume of aspirate falls below the oral intake of fluids.

Colorectal surgery

Some form of bowel preparation is important to reduce infection and anastomotic leakage. Mechanical cleansing involves switching to a low residue diet and the use of bowel cleansing solutions given by mouth (e.g. Klean-Prep, Picolax) or enemas from below. Some surgeons give neomycin and/or metronidazole by mouth to reduce the colonic bacterial count, but others rely on intravenous antibiotics (see above).

Obstructive jaundice

Steps should be taken to counter dehydration and avoid

renal failure (chiefly by intravenous fluid replacement), prevent sepsis (prophylactic antibiotics) and reverse any coagulopathy (giving intramuscular vitamin K to normalise prothrombin time).

Splenectomy

The spleen plays an important immunological role in producing opsonins to assist phagocytosis of encapsulated bacteria. Asplenic patients are at slight risk of overwhelming postsplenectomy sepsis, particularly children receiving splenectomy for blood dyscrasias. All splenectomised patients should be vaccinated against pneumococcus, meningococcus and *Haemophilius influenzae* type B 2–4 weeks before operation, if possible. Children may also be given oral penicillin for 2 years, but compliance is poor.

Malnutrition

Malnourished patients, for example those with oesophagogastric cancer, may have difficulties with the healing of wounds and anastomoses. Serum albumin can be used as a rough index of nutritional status. The normal value is 35–45 g/L, and a value below 30 g indicates moderate malnutrition. Profoundly malnourished patients may require 10–14 days of preoperative nutritional support, either parenteral or enteral according to circumstances, using a central venous catheter or a fine-bore nasogastric tube. In less severe cases a feeding jejunostomy tube may be inserted at operation for postoperative alimentation.

PREPARATION FOR THE OPERATING THEATRE

The following measures should be taken.

Signed consent. It is the duty of the operating surgeon or his deputy to explain to the patient the purpose of the operation and its potential risks. This explanation should be given without frightening the patient, but all questions should be answered honestly. Both the patient (or their representative) and the doctor need to sign the relevant form.

Skin cleansing. Before elective operations the patient should take a bath or a shower. It is customary to shave the relevant area. Topical antiseptic solutions are used to prepare the skin in theatre before the incision is made.

Patient identification. An identity bracelet is applied. Rings and dentures are removed. The side of operation (e.g. nephrectomy, hernia repair) should be clearly marked on the skin.

Fasting. The patient should eat or drink nothing for 4–6 hours before the operation to empty the stomach and prevent the risk of vomiting and inhaling the contents during induction of anaesthesia.

Catheterisation. The patient is asked to empty the bladder before the premedication is given. Urethral catheterisation is carried out after induction of anaesthesia in all pelvic operations and in major operations where accurate measurement of urine output is needed.

Premedication. The drugs should be prescribed on the advice of the anaesthetist. The objective is to relieve the patient's anxiety.

POSTOPERATIVE CARE

Following a relatively minor and uncomplicated procedure the patient can safely be returned to the surgical ward. After a major operation the patient requires more vigilant observation in a recovery area or high dependency unit, where experienced nurses are available and there is immediate access to emergency equipment and an anaesthetist. Patients who cannot be extubated should be transferred immediately to an intensive therapy unit for continuing ventilator support. Written postoperative instructions must be given regarding drug prescriptions, fluid requirements and the management of drains and tubes. Particular attention must be paid to the following.

Oxygenation. This is simply measured by the use of a pulse oximeter. Oxygen by mask will usually correct moderate degrees of hypoxia, but if oxygenation fails to improve, arterial blood gas analysis should be performed. If necessary, the patient must be re-intubated and ventilated.

Pain control (see also Ch. 2). Most methods of postoperative analgesia rely on the administration of opiate drugs, generally by the intramuscular, intravenous or epidural route. Patient-controlled analgesia (PCA) implies the delivery of a drug bolus (within preset limits) when the patient presses a button to activate the machine. Injection of long-acting anaesthetic into the wound and the use of fentanyl skin patches are other useful techniques for pain relief.

Drain and tubes. Surgical drains are generally removed once the volume of effluent diminishes towards zero. Urethral catheters are removed when the patient is stable and able to get out of bed. Nasogastric tubes are removed once bowel sounds return, flatus is passed and/or the volume of aspirate diminishes. After thoracotomy, intercostal drains are clamped when the air leak ceases and are then removed if the lung remains inflated.

Fluid balance. Fluid and electrolyte replacement should be judged according to the measured losses, the patient's general circulatory status, the urine output and the daily measurement of serum urea and electrolyte levels in those dependent upon an intravenous drip. The standard intravenous fluid requirement for an adult patient is 3 L/day, of which 1 L should ordinarily be normal (isotonic) saline and 2 L should be 5% dextrose. Potassium supplements are added provided that urine output is adequate. The first response to a falling urine output or blood pressure should usually be the rapid infusion of a 'fluid challenge' (500 ml).

POSTOPERATIVE COMPLICATIONS: GENERAL

All operations are associated with a risk of complications, which may be conveniently classified as general and local. General complications are those that follow any operation, irrespective of its site. Local complications are those related to a particular type of operation (these are discussed on p. 67).

POSTOPERATIVE PYREXIA

A minor elevation of temperature within a few hours of a major operation is a common event and may reflect the trauma of the surgical procedure and the general anaesthetic and/or the effect of any blood transfusion. Thereafter, the most frequent cause of fever within the first 2–3 days of operation is chest infection.

Pyrexia developing between 3 and 10 days after operation may still be due to respiratory infection, but other causes to consider are wound infection, deep sepsis at the site of operation, urinary infection, deep vein thrombosis and phlebitis caused by an intravenous 'drip'. High fever (to 39°C or above) accompanied by rigors suggests septi-

caemia; blood cultures should be obtained and broad-spectrum antibiotics should be started. One potential source of septicaemia is a central venous line placed for venous pressure monitoring or parenteral nutrition. A swinging fever and a raised white cell count may suggest sepsis within or deep to the surgical wound (see below).

RESPIRATORY PROBLEMS

Pulmonary collapse and consolidation

Several factors predispose to incomplete expansion of the lungs, i.e. atelectasis: the pain from a laparotomy incision (especially upper abdominal) or thoractomy incision, the sedation caused by postoperative analgesia and the viscid tracheobronchial secretions of a cigarette smoker. Air entry is reduced on examination of the chest, and there may be added sounds (râles) or even bronchial breathing if the collapsed lung undergoes consolidation. Treatment is by vigorous and frequent physiotherapy, giving the patient adequate analgesia to cooperate with the physiotherapist. Antibiotics will be needed if fever persists, indicating bronchopneumonia.

Pleural effusion

Effusions developing within the first few days of operation usually follow basal collapse/consolidation of the lung or congestive cardiac failure (especially if bilateral). Effusions developing at 7–10 days may be due to pulmonary embolism or a subphrenic abscess ('sympathetic' effusion). Small effusions (<500 ml) may be left alone to reabsorb if they do not interfere with respiration. Alternatively, pleural aspiration is performed either in the ward, using a two-way syringe to avoid pneumothorax, or under ultrasound guidance. The pleural fluid should be sent for bacteriological culture. Blood-stained effusions suggest pulmonary embolism.

Pneumothorax

This generally arises from pleural puncture during insertion of a central venous line, and a chest X-ray should always be performed after this procedure. Pneumothorax can also follow rupture of an emphysematous bulla in a patient on positive-pressure ventilation, in which case there is a rapid fall in oxygen saturation. Treatment is by inserting an intercostal drain under a water seal.

Aspiration of vomit

This occurs when an unconscious patient vomits with an unprotected airway, typically during induction of anaesthesia. Muscle relaxants abolish the protective reflex that closes the larynx by apposition of the vocal cords and the flap action of the epiglottis. Patients weakened by systemic illness and those with cord paralysis (e.g. following thyroidectomy) are also at risk. Minor degrees of aspiration lead to pneumonia. Massive aspiration causes severe lung injury as gastric acid provokes an intense pneumonitis.

Prevention. This entails:

- keeping the stomach empty in conditions such as acute gastric dilatation or intestinal obstruction
- protecting the airway with a cuffed endotracheal tube or tracheostomy in unconscious patients
- using cricoid pressure to compress the oesophagus during 'crash' induction of anaesthesia.

Treatment of aspiration entails:

- bronchoscopy and bronchial lavage
- respiratory support
- drugs, including antibiotics, bronchodilators and corticosteroids.

Adult respiratory distress syndrome (ARDS)

There is severe lung injury leading to hypoxia and progressive respiratory failure. Systemic sepsis is the main culprit, but shock, trauma, drugs and aspiration of gastric contents may also play a part. There is oedema and consolidation of the lungs, producing diffuse fluffy shadowing on a chest X-ray. The pathophysiology is unclear, but endotoxin-activated leucocytes are thought to be deposited in the pulmonary capillaries, releasing oxygen-derived free radicals, cytokines and other chemical mediators.

Treatment. This is by:

- control of infection by antibiotics and surgical drainage of any pus
- respiratory support with positive end-expiratory pressure (PEEP)
- pharmacological agents such as prostacyclin or antioxidants.

The mortality rate of ARDS is approximately 50%.

Respiratory failure

This is defined as having occurred when the arterial oxygen tension (P_aO_2) falls below 8.0 kPa (60 mmHg).

Causes. These include:

- general anaesthesia and major surgery
- acute chest disease including thoracic trauma
- neurological disease including head injuries
- systemic sepsis leading to ARDS.

Pain, inadequate respiratory drive (e.g. due to opiates), abdominal distension and failure to clear bronchial secretions can all lead to progressive hypoventilation. The classical sequence of collapse–consolidation–infection leads to a right-to-left shunt of the pulmonary blood flow, thereby contributing to hypoxia.

Diagnosis

Clinical. Fatigue, confusion, cyanosis, tachypnoea, laboured breathing.

Arterial blood gases. Low PO_2, low PCO_2, respiratory alkalosis.

Treatment. The procedure is as follows:

1. clear the airway by physiotherapy, tracheal suction or bronchoscopy
2. give oxygen by mask
3. relieve any contributing factors – see above
4. ventilatory support may be needed.

In order to provide ventilatory support, the patient is sedated, an endotracheal tube is passed and intermittent positive-pressure respiration (IPPR) is established. The need for prolonged IPPR is the commonest indication for *tracheostomy* nowadays, but this operation is sometimes required for acute upper airways obstruction or following radical head and neck surgery. Tracheostomy may be performed by an open operation: the trachea is approached through a transverse cervical skin incision, with displacement or division of the thyroid isthmus, and an upside-down U-shaped incision is made through the second, third and fourth tracheal rings. Percutaneous tracheostomy using a needle/guidewire technique is now performed on patients in the intensive therapy unit.

VENOUS THROMBOEMBOLISM.

Prophylactic measures (see p. 62) reduce but do not abolish the risk of deep vein thrombosis and pulmonary embolism. These conditions are described in Chapter 37.

RETENTION OF URINE

Postoperative pain, sedative drugs and intravenous fluid administration may combine to cause acute retention of urine. Even if a urethral catheter has been used during the perioperative period, the patient may be unable to void satisfactorily or at all once the catheter is removed. This problem is discussed in Chapter 35 ('acute micturition difficulty', p. 353).

ACUTE RENAL FAILURE

Patients may develop pre-renal failure because of a hypotensive episode during or after the operation. Hypoperfusion of the kidney may be aggravated by hypoxia, sepsis and nephrotoxic drugs (e.g. gentamicin). Urine output falls, and there is a rise in serum potassium, urea and creatinine. Unless the condition is reversed, acute tubular necrosis will develop. Urethral catheterisation is needed for an accurate measurement of hourly urine output, and a CVP line is required to measure circulating blood volume. Biochemical status is checked by frequent estimations of serum urea and electrolytes, and urine osmolality gives an index of renal function.

Treatment

Treatment can be summarised as follows:

- Restoration of an adequate circulating blood volume without overhydration.
- Diuretics such as frusemide or mannitol in the early stages to provoke the secretion of urine. Diuretics should be stopped if the patient remains oliguric. Low-dose dopamine may increase renal blood flow.
- Measures to reduce hyperkalaemia, e.g. intravenous glucose and insulin or cation exchange resins.
- Renal support by peritoneal dialysis, haemofiltration or haemodialysis. Recovery from acute tubular necrosis can be anticipated in survivors after 2–4 weeks. The patient will then enter a polyuric phase in which fluid and electrolyte balance require further careful monitoring.

POSTOPERATIVE MENTAL DISTURBANCES

Since operations are stressful events, it is not surprising that sometimes mental disturbances follow. They are of three kinds:

- Predominantly psychological responses to changed circumstances, e.g. knowledge of cancer, an amputation or a stoma. These are usually characterised by depression and/or denial, which delays convalescence. Do not forget that malnutrition, lack of family support and an uncertain future can contribute to distress.
- Associated with systemic disturbances – hypoxia and bacterial toxaemia are the commonest. Delirium is the most obvious feature. It follows that in a delirious patient after operation, a physical cause must be sought.
- Withdrawal of psychotropic agents, e.g. delirium tremens from alcohol and 'cold turkey' (acute anxiety, vasomotor disturbances) from opiates.

BED SORES

These are wholly preventable but still occur in the elderly, the obese and the immobile, particularly when insufficient nursing care is given. The proximate aetiological factors are:

- prolonged pressure on a single point – buttock, sacrum, greater trochanter – which causes ischaemia
- shearing of the skin on the deep fascia, which tears subcutaneous blood vessels and produces an ischaemic lesion.

In the case of the latter, there is sloughing of the skin and subcutaneous fat and, unless the causes are corrected, deep penetration down to bone occurs. There is often secondary infection with burrowing abscesses and a mixed bacterial growth.

Sores are prevented by ensuring constant movement so that pressure is not applied to a single place; by care in turning the patient; and by rigorous skin hygiene. If they occur, they are managed in the same way. Most are small and will heal provided that the patient is able to mount a normal wound healing response. Large ulcers may require skilled repair by a plastic surgeon.

FAECAL IMPACTION

Inability to evacuate the bowel after an operation is the consequence of:

- inadequate preoperative preparation
- weakness and sedative drugs
- a bulky hard stool.

The condition is usually seen in the elderly and bedridden but can occasionally occur in those who are frightened to defaecate, e.g. after surgical procedures on the anal verge. The presenting feature may be 'spurious' diarrhoea, which is the trickling down of liquid faeces through channels in an impacted solid collection in the rectum. Whenever diarrhoea or persistent constipation occurs in postoperative patients, a rectal examination is essential.

Unless the condition responds to conservative measures (suppositories or wash-outs), manual evacuation under sedation is usually required.

PSEUDOMEMBRANOUS ENTEROCOLITIS

This is an uncommon complication which may follow the use of antibiotics, with the development of a fulminating bowel infection. It is usually due to resistant staphylococci or clostridia, particularly *Clostridium difficile*.

Surgical pathology

There is partial destruction of the bowel mucosa resulting in inadequate fluid resorption and therefore dehydration. Casts may be passed, along with blood and mucus in the stool.

Clinical features

The diarrhoea usually appears 3–4 days after operation with associated abdominal distension, hypotension and shock because of both extracellular fluid depletion and toxaemia.

Management

Prevention. Unnecessary use of antibiotics should be avoided, particularly courses prolonged for more than a day or two.

Therapy. This consists of conservative management, including intravenous replacement and supportive therapy, together with nasogastric suction and the use of the appropriate antibiotic. Urgent stool culture should be performed, but unless there is reason to think otherwise, *C. difficile* infection should be assumed; in this instance vancomycin is specific.

PAROTITIS

This is now rare but follows serious illness when the patient is dehydrated and mouth hygiene is deficient. The infected gland swells rapidly and pus forms quickly, adding to the systemic burden of illness.

Treatment is to correct the problems, administer antibiotics and drain the area early if there is any thought that pus is present.

STRESS ULCERS

Acute ulceration of the gastric or duodenal mucosa can occur after major surgery, especially in patients who develop complications and are admitted to the intensive therapy unit. The condition usually presents with upper gastrointestinal haemorrhage. The incidence has declined with the routine use of prophylactic drugs, such as ranitidine, sucralfate or alkalies (see also Ch. 25).

POSTOPERATIVE COMPLICATIONS: LOCAL

Unlike general complications, local complications are those related to a particular type of operation. They reflect surgical expertise and the extent of disease.

POSTOPERATIVE HAEMORRHAGE

Bleeding from the wound or the drains is alarming for both the patient and the surgeon. A steady trickle of blood from the skin can often be stopped by a suture inserted under local anaesthetic. Postoperative bleeding is classified as *reactive* or *secondary*.

Reactive bleeding occurs within 24–36 hours of operation. It is caused by a slipped ligature or dislodgement of a diathermy coagulum as the blood pressure recovers from the operation and the patient coughs, vomits or gets out of bed. Unless local pressure controls the bleeding, re-exploration of the wound is required. Subcutaneous *haematoma* is a common prelude to wound infection (see below), and large haematomas may require operative evacuation.

Secondary bleeding usually occurs 7–10 days after operation as a consequence of deep-seated infection. Re-operation is generally needed after correction of hypo-volaemic shock.

WOUND INFECTION

This is the commonest complication in surgery. However, the incidence varies from less than 1% (hernia and clean orthopaedic operations) to 20–30% in colonic surgery when this is unattended by suitable precautions.

Predisposing factors

Preoperative. Infection at or near the site of the intended surgical wound may occur with:

- skin infections – particularly those due to staphylococci from nasal, throat or hand reservoirs
- wound contamination by infection from a diseased or perforated viscus, such as may occur in perforated ulcer or appendicitis
- susceptible patients – particularly where malnutrition, hypoproteinaemia, avitaminosis, diabetes, carcinomatosis and prolonged steroid administration are present.

Operative. These include:

- airborne infection from the theatre environment or the surgical and nursing staff, where the organism is usually a staphylococcus. Although the incidence of this problem is now low, it is of great importance in relation to prosthetic implants.
- contact infection from theatre staff, instruments, fluids (skin preparations, irrigating fluids) and dressings.
- inadequate surgical technique – particularly when there is haematoma formation, incomplete obliteration of dead space, muscle sutures that are excessively tight, or soiling of the wound by bowel contents.
- operations on heavily contaminated areas, e.g. large bowel, or lower limbs of bedridden diabetic patients.

Postoperative. These include:

- continuation of preoperative factors
- self-infection of the wound, particularly with staphylococci from the skin or nose, streptococci from the

throat, or coliform organisms from the faeces (all of these are uncommon)
- cross-infection from the ward environment (surgical and nursing staff and patients) by airborne or contact routes. This is particularly common in the presence of drainage tubes.

Multiresistant staphylococci (MRSA) are now an endemic feature of the surgical environment. They are not necessarily dangerous but can produce troublesome sepsis. Their control requires ward closures and epidemiological measures.

Bacteriology

Many wound infections are caused by a mixture of organisms.

Staphylococci. In the past these have been the commonest organisms; often the coagulase-positive, penicillin-resistant staphylococci carried by the nose, face and hands of patients and attending staff can be incriminated.

Coliform organisms. *Escherichia coli, Proteus* and *Pseudomonas* normally inhabit the bowel, and they are usually the predominant organisms in wound infections after operations on the intestinal tract. Currently they are the most frequent causes of wound infection.

Haemolytic streptococci. Beta-haemolytic streptococci, which are harboured in the nasopharynx in about 5% of the population, can result in wound infection by airborne or contact routes. Although this type of infection is uncommon in general surgical practice, it can be an important cause of free graft failure in plastic surgery.

Anaerobic organisms. Specific infections with clostridia (tetanus and gas gangrene) are discussed in Chapter 6. *Bacteroides* infection is now known to be common following operations on the large bowel (including the appendix), and these organisms may complicate vaginal and middle ear infections as part of a mixed picture.

Clinical features

The onset is usually within 7 days of operation. Symptoms include malaise, anorexia and pain or discomfort at the operation site, and there are signs of local redness, tenderness, swelling, cellulitis, discharge or frank abscess formation, as well as elevated temperature and pulse rate.

Treatment

Prevention of wound infection is aided by preoperative correction of any general problem and bowel cleansing before elective operation on the large bowel. Perioperative antibiotics (beginning before operation) are indicated in the following instances:

- when it is known or suspected that a contaminated or infected operative field will be entered (e.g. an inflamed appendix, operations that involve opening the biliary or alimentary tract)
- when a prosthesis (e.g. arterial, cardiac, orthopaedic) is being inserted
- when there is known valvular heart disease (risk of subacute bacterial endocarditis)
- in debilitated patients and those on steroids
- in accidental wounds when there is any appreciable contamination.

A sterile technique is important – for instruments, skin preparation and drapes – and the wound should be excluded via plastic drapes, particularly when an infected abdomen is opened or when the bowel is to be entered.

Meticulous wound excision and toilet and wash-out of contaminated wounds are also important, and care must be taken in closing the wound, avoiding strangulating muscle sutures, haematoma formation and dead spaces. Wound drains and topical antibiotics should be used before complete closure when contamination has occurred. Sepsis occurs predominantly in the subcutaneous tissue: if a contaminated wound is left open for 3 days and then closed (delayed primary closure), infection is much less likely.

Postoperative wound dressings should be disturbed as infrequently as possible except when they become moist with discharge or exudate.

Therapy. Organisms should be isolated whenever possible, using appropriate aerobic and anaerobic culture. Systemic antibiotics, specific to the infecting organism, are administered when cellulitis or septicaemia is present. When pus is present drainage is essential. Drainage is performed by removing a skin stitch when a suture abscess is present, or by removing all stitches and opening up the wound for a larger collection (which is commonly needed).

All wounds are then allowed to granulate and heal by second intention. Wounds should not be tightly packed.

RESIDUAL ABSCESS

After any operation, sepsis may ensue deep to the wound, but this is commonest in the abdomen and especially if the gut is opened. Further, after operation for sepsis, a focus may persist. In both cases a residual abscess can form.

Predisposing factors

These include:

- inadequate drainage of an abscess cavity
- infection of a haematoma
- persistence of infective sources, e.g. in abdominal surgery the incomplete amputation of an appendix stump; in orthopaedics the presence of dead bone (a sequestrum); in any procedure a foreign body
- failure to carry out adequate treatment (e.g. complete peritoneal toilet in peritonitis or thorough debridement in soft tissue trauma).

General features of residual abscesses

At a varying interval of 2–7 days, but occasionally much later, there are systemic features of sepsis: fever, malaise and a raised leucocyte count and erythrocyte sedimentation rate (ESR). Occasionally, organisms escaping into the circulation may give rise to rigors and, in severe cases, septicaemia may complicate the local condition.

Locally, in accessible sites, there are the physical signs of inflammation – tenderness, heat, redness and swelling. Residual abscesses that lie deep to wounds will usually 'point' to the surface via the wound, but others will have to be formally drained.

Principles of management

Particularly in the abdomen, residual abscess may be difficult to detect (see below), but localisation is the first step in management. Adequate antibiotic therapy should be given, based on either culture or 'best guess'. Drainage should be undertaken when spreading sepsis has been contained.

Sometimes an abscess will discharge spontaneously (see 'pelvic abscess' below), but most will require surgical drainage by either of:

- open operation
- percutaneous techniques in which, under ultrasonographic or CT guidance, a catheter–cannula combination is passed into the cavity, which is either emptied and the tube withdrawn or continuously drained until its walls collapse together.

Abdominal residual abscesses

Abdominal residual abscesses still occur with distressing frequency. In the classic sites – pelvic and subphrenic – they can usually be diagnosed by conventional means (see below), but low-grade persistent sepsis hidden away in the abdomen (e.g. between loops of bowel) may pose much greater difficulty. Modern techniques – ultrasonography, CT scan and labelled leucocytes that can be detected by scintiscanning – are helping to make the diagnosis earlier and to permit precise localisation. There is still an occasional indication for a laparotomy when sepsis is almost certainly present but cannot be precisely located.

PELVIC ABSCESS

Pelvic abscess usually follows an operation for generalised peritonitis – perforated appendicitis, perforated ulcer, or perforated diverticultis. It can be the primary presentation of acute pelvic appendicitis or pelvic inflammatory disease. The organisms involved are usually enteric, *Bacteroides* being of importance.

Clinical features

Urgency of defaecation and mucous diarrhoea are clinical features. Blood may appear with pus if the abscess ruptures into the bowel. Abdominal examination may show either nothing or slight lower abdominal distension from coils of bowel lying in the abscess wall. On rectal examination there is a tender boggy mass, which in the female may also be palpable on vaginal examination.

Treatment

This depends on the maturity of the abscess cavity.

Pointing. This is evidenced by fixation of the abscess, usually to the rectal wall, which becomes thickened and oedematous, and indicates that drainage through the rectum is required. Occasionally the abscess may point into the vagina or anterior abdominal wall and require incision and drainage at these sites.

Not pointing. As long as the patient's general condition remains satisfactory, conservative treatment is indicated. This includes the use of broad-spectrum antibiotics and the maintenance of nutrition. Low-grade intestinal obstruction may arise from adhesions between loops of bowel and the wall of the abscess cavity and may require gastric suction. The abscess may point and discharge, or resolve. Occasionally, deterioration will occur in the absence of localisation of the abscess; then laparotomy and drainage will be indicated.

SUBPHRENIC ABSCESS

The subphrenic spaces are potential spaces only; they become real when distended by pus or fluid. Subphrenic abscess formation is a relatively uncommon sequel of any laparotomy, but can particularly follow operations on upper abdominal viscera such as the liver and spleen.

Surgical anatomy

Terminology and classifications are confusing. In practical terms there are only right and left subphrenic spaces, plus the subhepatic space on the right.

Cause and surgical pathology

Most subphrenic collections follow peritoneal contamination from either gastrointestinal operations or episodes of peritonitis associated with perforation of a hollow viscus. The condition starts as a cellulitis. It is said to occur partly because the subphrenic spaces are in direct communication with the paracolic gutters to which pus gravitates and partly because, once there is air beneath the diaphragm, the liver when it descends acts as a piston, sucking infected material upwards to the subphrenic space. An abscess develops and there is contiguous inflammation of the diaphragm and pleura, so leading to a 'sympathetic' pleural effusion. Gas often forms in the abscess cavity. If untreated, the abscess may rupture into the general peritoneal cavity or into the chest. The latter situation may be associated with empyema, pyopneumothorax, bronchopleural fistula, suppurative pericarditis or mediastinal abscess formation.

Clinical features

A subphrenic abscess can be notoriously difficult to diagnose. It is therefore important to remember that such a complication can occur, especially when conditions favourable to its formation are present.

Symptoms. In the more acute cases the features of a precipitating peritonitis may merge into those of a rapidly collecting abscess with continued pyrexia and general toxaemia. In delayed cases, the onset of suspicious symptoms may occur many days after apparent recovery from the predisposing condition. Later development is probably more likely to occur after intensive antibiotic therapy has been given for the original condition.

Anorexia and nausea are usual. Pain or ache beneath or over the lower ribs should always raise suspicion; rarely there is shoulder pain. Hiccoughs are common.

Signs. The patient may look unwell, pale or even wasted. The classical 'swinging' temperature is present in only 50% of cases, and in about 10% there is no elevation of temperature at all. Tachycardia is usual. Local tenderness beneath the rib margin may be present, but redness and a palpable lump are very late to develop.

In the chest, the classical sequence of percussion changes from above downwards of resonance (normal lung), dullness (pleural effusion), resonance (gas above abscess) and dullness (abscess) is rarely, if ever, detected. However, signs of consolidation or of pleural effusion may be present.

Special tests. As with any abscess the white cell count is raised. Ultrasound scan is probably the simplest and most accurate test, and needle aspiration/drainage of the collection can be performed at the same time. CT scan and labelled leucocyte scan can help if uncertainty persists. Chest X-ray may show a pleural effusion or pulmonary consolidation.

Older tests such as screening the diaphragm and barium meal are seldom needed nowadays.

Treatment

Percutaneous catheter drainage is successful in most subphrenic abscesses and should be attempted before resorting to open operation. A large cavity or one containing viscid pus may require formal surgical evacuation with placement of a wide-bore tube drain. An anterior subcostal incision is usually appropriate, and the procedure should be 'covered' with broad-spectrum antibiotics.

When the diagnosis is not quite certain, continued observation is essential. Rarely the patient's condition fails to improve; then either a diagnostic aspiration or a laparotomy may prove helpful in localising the abscess.

WOUND DISRUPTION

Wounds break down because they are:

- septic
- inadequately closed
- pulled apart by distractive forces
- made in patients who cannot mount a normal healing response.

The common wound disruption in general surgery is burst abdomen, the incidence of which remains at about 1% of all abdominal operations; the mortality rate is about 10%. In that the causes are almost entirely technical, these figures are too high. A common error is to sew up the muscle layer too tightly, merely rendering the tissue ischaemic and causing the wound to give way. Apart from technical and general factors, the common reason for an abdominal disruption is a paroxysmal rise in intra-abdominal pressure from coughing or straining.

Surgical pathology

There are three types of burst abdomen.

Superficial and revealed. This occurs at about 10 days when the skin sutures are removed. There is separation of the skin and subcutaneous layers only, which is most often the result of wound haematoma or infection.

Deep and concealed. This occurs gradually, with separation of all layers of the abdominal wall with the exception of the skin. If not recognised while the patient is in hospital, an incisional hernia always develops at a later date. Most often this type of dehiscence results from a combination of faulty technique and faulty healing.

Complete and revealed. This occurs at about the tenth day, gradually or suddenly, with the protrusion of a knuckle or loop of bowel or a portion of the omentum through a wound which is completely disrupted in the whole or part of its length.

Clinical features

Symptoms. There may be no warning of an impending wound dehiscence. Alternatively, there may be nausea, fever, and local pain or discomfort. Occasionally the patient describes a 'tearing' or 'ripping' sensation in the wound after a bout of coughing or straining.

Signs. These include serosanguineous or thin purulent discharge from the wound; and bowel or omentum protruding through the wound spontaneously or after removal of skin sutures.

Treatment

Superficial and revealed. Evacuate the blood clot and treat wound infection if present. Allow the wound to granulate and heal by secondary intention.

Deep and concealed. If recognised while in hospital by presence of a 'tell-tale' serosanguineous discharge or the appearance of a knuckle of bowel after removal of a few skin sutures, then urgent operation is required. If not recognised and the skin heals, then the subsequent incisional hernia is dealt with on its merits.

Complete and revealed. Cover the exposed bowel loops with a moist pack and sedate the patient while preparing for re-operation. Resuture with closely applied interrupted non-absorbable sutures passing through all layers of the anterior abdominal wall deep to the skin. The skin is best left unsutured. Any attempt to suture each layer separately is of no value, as the tissues are friable and oedematous.

ENTERIC FISTULA

This is any communication between the gastrointestinal tract and the body surface.

Predisposing factors

- A disrupted intestinal anastomosis because of poor technique, avascularity or the persistence of some original disorder at the site of anastomosis (Crohn's disease, carcinoma, tuberculosis)

- Intestinal obstruction distal to the site of anastomosis
- Fistulating diseases such as Crohn's disease and diverticulitis
- Injury to the bowel or its blood supply at operation or subsequently, e.g. by a rigid intraperitoneal drainage tube.

Clinical features

Either spontaneously or at a varying time postoperatively, there are features of systemic sepsis followed by the development of inflammation on the abdominal wall or in relation to a wound. Initially, pus may be discharged but this is rapidly followed by intestinal content, the quantity of which varies according to the site of the fistula.

Clinically fistulas are classified into:

- high output (>500 ml/day)
- low output (<500 ml/day).

A high output fistula occurs predominantly in the upper gastrointestinal tract, where even a fistula in the distal ileum may produce many hundreds of millilitres of fluid a day. A low output fistula generally stems from the large intestine or from an incomplete defect in the small intestine (without distal obstruction).

The local effects of a fistula are variable. A duodenal fistula containing bile and pancreatic enzymes will cause rapid digestion and secondary septic infection of the abdominal wall. Fistulae are not uncommonly multiple, whatever their cause.

The general effects are loss of water and electrolytes (extracellular fluid volume deficiency) and malnutrition. Nutritional failure is the consequence of both lack of normal absorption, even if the patient can eat, and the increased catabolic rate associated with severe local sepsis.

Management

Prevention. Clearly it is essential to avoid the predisposing factors, in particular poor surgical technique.

Treatment. Many fistulae will close spontaneously unless there is distal obstruction of the bowel, mucocutaneous union, or a persistently infective focus. Meanwhile the patient must be supported. Local treatment is directed at protecting the skin around the fistula from digestion. Fluid and electrolyte loss is corrected. With a high output fistula, parenteral nutrition is instituted with the aim of restoring or maintaining the serum albumin level above 30 g/L (see Ch. 4). If any of the factors that prevent closure are present, operation will be required once the fluid and electrolyte loss, malnutrition and sepsis have been corrected.

WOUND SINUS

A sinus is a track lined by granulation tissue which opens on to the skin.

Predisposing factors

In all cases there is persistent infection caused by:

- inadequately drained abscess
- residual dead tissue
- foreign material such as a ligature or swab
- chronic underlying disease such as tuberculosis, Crohn's disease or malignancy.

Clinical features

A sinus is evident by persistent discharge of material, other than gut content, from a wound beyond 1 month after operation.

Management

Prevention. This is by adequate drainage of an abscess so that healing takes place from its base, and by removal of foreign bodies and avoidance of non-absorbable sutures in infected wounds.

Treatment. The sinus is explored and any foreign material is removed. An abscess cavity with an inadequately draining sinus must be opened widely so that it may heal from the base.

FURTHER READING

Clarke J R 1989 Decision making in surgical practice. World Journal of Surgery 13: 245–251

Classen D C, Scott Evans R, Pestotnik S L, Horn S D, Menlove R L, Burke J P 1992 The timing of prophylactic administration of antibiotics and the risk of surgical-wound infection. New England Journal of Medicine 326: 281–286

Cuschieri A 1995 Preoperative, operative and postoperative care. In: Cuschieri A, Giles G R, Moossa A R (eds) Essential surgical practice, 3rd edn. Butterworth-Heinemann, Oxford, p 372–398

Diamond T, Rowlands B J 1995 Preoperative assessment. In: O'Higgins N J, Chisholm G D, Williamson R C N (eds) Surgical management, 2nd edn. Butterworth-Heinemann, Oxford, p 1–14

Jorgensen L N, Wille-Jorgensen P, Hauch O 1993 Prophylaxis of postoperative thromboembolism with low molecular weight heparins. British Journal of Surgery 80: 689–704

Kirk R M 1994 Choose well, cut well, get well. In: Kirk R M (ed) General surgical operations. Churchill Livingstone, Edinburgh, p 1–11

Pettigrew R A, Hill G L 1986 Indicators of surgical risks and clinical judgement. British Journal of Surgery 73: 47–51

9

Minimally invasive techniques in surgery

Jeremy Thompson

OVERVIEW

The last 8 years have witnessed a technical revolution in surgery. Many operations that used to be performed through a single long incision can now be done through multiple tiny incisions by means of video endoscopy. Minimal access techniques reduce the degree of surgical trauma, and this usually results in a quicker recovery, but they have their own potential complications. Access can be obtained either via anatomical (endoluminal) routes, e.g. in gastrointestinal or genitourinary endoscopy, or via non-anatomical routes, e.g. by entering a body cavity at laparoscopy, thoracoscopy or arthroscopy. Careful evaluation against traditional methods is needed in this rapidly evolving field.

INTRODUCTION

Minimally invasive surgery may be used to describe many techniques throughout the range of surgical specialties, although the term has been applied particularly to operations using video endoscopic equipment. Their common feature is a reduction in the trauma of surgical access. In many cases, the actual surgical procedure is the same as or similar to that performed using more traditional or open operations.

For many years, minimally invasive techniques have been used for the diagnosis and treatment of gastrointestinal, urinary, respiratory, gynaecological and joint disease, and the range of operations performed continues to expand. In some specialties, minimally invasive procedures are performed mainly by radiologists (e.g. vascular surgery) or physicians (e.g. cardiology). More recently, minimally invasive techniques have been extended with the creation of artificial 'body cavities' such as pre- and retroperitoneal, mediastinal and subfascial endoscopy.

The development of video endoscopes, whereby the image can be displayed on monitors for the surgeon and assistants, has greatly facilitated therapeutic endoscopic procedures. The parallel development of a wide range of instrumentation for minimally invasive surgery has also increased the scope of procedures that can be performed. At present, a large number of procedures, covering all branches of surgical practice, are being undertaken using minimally invasive methods.

This chapter aims to give an overview of minimally invasive techniques and to discuss their advantages and disadvantages within the context of modern surgical practice. Individual procedures are not described in detail, although many are discussed elsewhere in this book.

ADVANTAGES AND DISADVANTAGES OF MINIMALLY INVASIVE SURGERY

Whilst some of the advantages and disadvantages of minimally invasive procedures are specific to the individual procedure, many are common and these are summarised in Table 9.1.

Many studies have shown reduced postoperative pain following the use of minimally invasive techniques. This is to be expected as most postoperative pain comes from the wound. Minimising the length of surgical incision reduces postoperative pain, particularly when the wounds are sited close to the thorax and are thus subject-

Table 9.1 Common advantages and disadvantages of minimally invasive surgery

Advantages	Disadvantages
Reduced postoperative pain	Longer operations
Shorter hospital stay	Expensive equipment
Improved cosmetic result	Loss of tactile sensation
Shorter convalescence	Loss of 3-D vision
Improved operative visualisation	Poorer visualisation (some sites)
Better teaching	Complications of access techniques
Reduced wound complications	Training problems
Reduced adhesion formation	Difficulties with specimen retrieval
Reduced risk of viral transmission	Possible increased wound metastasis

ed to stress on respiration. Studies comparing laparoscopic with open cholecystectomy have shown improved respiratory function in the postoperative period, almost certainly as a consequence of reduced pain on breathing. Other physiological measures of benefit from the use of minimally invasive techniques have been demonstrated, such as a reduction in the acute phase and inflammatory responses to operation. Reductions in postoperative stay and a more rapid return to work following successful minimally invasive procedures have been clearly documented when compared with traditional open operation.

The cosmetic result of minimally invasive techniques is better than that of traditional operation. Although wound complications such as infection, haematoma and herniation occur with both methods, they are encountered less frequently with minimally invasive procedures. Reduced exposure of the viscera may limit the trauma of handling and minimise cooling and drying of visceral surfaces. These factors help to reduce the development of postoperative adhesions.

Minimally invasive techniques use access routes that are too small to permit the passage of a surgical hand. The resultant loss of tactile sensation is disadvantageous and may compromise assessment of tumour localisation, fixity or extent of spread (e.g. colonic carcinoma). There are additional concerns about the possible increased risk of wound (port site) tumour implantation after laparoscopic cancer surgery. Endoscopic ultrasound probes have been developed and help to overcome some of the problems related to loss of tactile sensation. They are useful for preoperative assessment of the liver, bile ducts,

pancreas and retroperitoneum. Minimally invasive procedures limit the risk of injury to the surgeon and other staff and thus reduce the risk of viral transmission to and from patients.

Whereas open operations permit three-dimensional vision, standard endoscopic imaging is two-dimensional and results in reduced distance perception, with associated loss of surgical dexterity at first. Although attempts to develop three-dimensional video endoscopy have been made, at present they remain unimpressive. Surgeons use other visual clues for judging distance and most rapidly learn endoscopic operating skills. Undoubtedly endoscopic techniques can provide better visualisation of the operative field at many sites, particularly when a magnified video-endoscopic view is obtained. However, for some areas, visualisation is difficult (e.g. the lesser sac, small bowel examination) using minimal access techniques, and superior or much more rapid imaging is obtained at open operation.

Because small incisions are used, removal of intact surgical specimens (e.g. gall bladder, spleen, kidney) may not be possible without extension of one incision. This is usually performed low in the abdomen to reduce postoperative pain and improve cosmesis. Some specimens may be passed per rectum (colonic resections) or vagina (hysterectomy). Others are cut into small pieces (morcellated), although this is contraindicated when formal histological staging of tumours is required.

Video endoscopy provides good opportunities for teaching, either within the operating theatre itself or at a distance by transmission to a lecture room. Surgical trainees and other theatre staff obtain good views of the surgical field, a situation which contrasts markedly with the restricted visualisation of many open operations to all apart from the operating surgeon (Fig. 9.1). However, the widespread and rapid adoption of some minimally invasive procedures (e.g. laparoscopic cholecystectomy) has had training implications for career surgeons and their trainees. Minimally invasive techniques require new operative skills, and the 'learning curve' for some may be flat. The relatively high bile duct injury rate during the development of laparoscopic cholecystectomy services was probably a reflection of inadequate training. Conversely, many trainees are now inexperienced in open operation techniques, which may pose problems when conversion to open operation is required during a difficult minimally invasive procedure. All patients should be warned that conversion to open operation may be necessary.

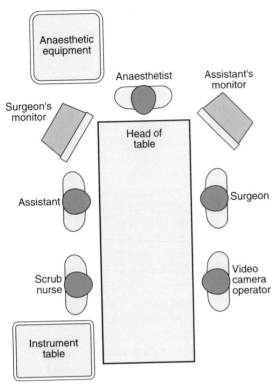

Fig. 9.1 One theatre layout for laparoscopic cholecystectomy. Note that both surgeon and assistants have a clear view of the video monitors.

Table 9.2   Access routes for minimally invasive procedures
Anatomical routes
Gastrointestinal
Genitourinary
Gynaecological
Respiratory
Non-anatomical routes
Radiological (percutaneous)
● ultrasound/CT/MR guided biopsy/drainage
● angiographic
— arterial
— venous
— cardiac
● cholangiography
Transcoelomic
● laparoscopy
● thoracoscopy
Arthroscopic
Artificial cavities
● pre/retroperitoneal
● subfascial

ACCESS METHODS FOR MINIMALLY INVASIVE SURGERY

A large variety of access methods are currently being used for different types of minimally invasive procedure (Table 9.2). The different routes of access in common use and an indication of the range of procedures being undertaken are briefly described here.

ANATOMICAL (ENDOLUMINAL) ROUTES

These techniques use natural orifices to gain access to internal organs. Rigid or flexible endoscopes are used with air or fluid installation to permit mucosal visualisation.

Gastrointestinal endoscopy

For many years, rigid endoscopes have been used for examination of the oesophagus and the rectosigmoid. The introduction of flexible fibre-optic endoscopes allowed good quality routine imaging of the stomach, duodenum, colon and terminal ileum to be obtained. These fibre-optic instruments are being replaced by video endoscopes which can now be used to extend throughout the whole length of the gastrointestinal tract. While initially used for diagnostic purposes, these flexible endoscopes can now permit a wide range of therapeutic procedures. Upper gastrointestinal endoscopy has become the first choice procedure for most upper gastrointestinal symptoms, permitting not only diagnosis but also biopsy and in many cases definitive therapy. Operating proctoscopes have been developed which allow an increased range of per-anal procedures for rectal polyps and cancers. The therapeutic procedures commonly undertaken are listed in Table 9.3.

Genitourinary endoscopy

Rigid and, more recently, flexible endoscopic examination of the urethra and bladder have been widely used for many years. These endoscopes provide the standard route of access for diagnosis and therapy for most urological conditions affecting the urethra, prostate and bladder (see Ch. 35). Endoscopic examination of the ureter is also possible for removal of stones or biopsy of suspicious lesions. A percutaneous approach to the renal pelvis using dilatation of a radiologically established tract to permit access with an endoscope has been used extensively in some centres for the treatment of stones in

Table 9.3 Common procedures in therapeutic gastrointestinal endoscopy

Procedure	Uses
Gastroscopy	Intubation/ablation of malignant strictures (especially oesophagus) Dilatation of benign strictures (especially oesophagus) Dilatation for achalasia Sclerotherapy/banding of varices Injection/diathermy/heater probe therapy for bleeding ulcers Polypectomy Gastrostomy insertion Removal of foreign bodies
Colonoscopy/proctoscopy	Polypectomy Diathermy/laser coagulation of angioplastic mucosal blood vessels Dilatation of colonic strictures Ablation of malignant colonic strictures Excision of early rectal cancers
ERCP (endoscopic retrograde cholangiopancreatography)	Sphincterotomy (major or minor papilla) Sphincteroplasty (balloon dilatation) Removal of stones from bile (or pancreatic) duct – Dormia basket, balloon Lithotripsy for ductal stones (mechanical, electrohydraulic, laser or ultrasound) Stenting (plastic or expanding metal) for bile (or pancreatic) ductal strictures (especially malignant) Dilatation of bile (or pancreatic) ductal strictures (especially benign)

the pelvicalyceal system. However, extracorporeal shock wave lithotripsy (ESWL) is now more frequently used to shatter such stones with ultrasound, allowing their passage through the ureter, which is usually temporarily stented to avoid ureteric colic.

Gynaecological endoscopy

Colposcopic examination of the vagina and uterine cervix has been used for many years for the diagnosis and treatment of local disease. Over the last few years, hysteroscopic examination of the uterine cavity has also been established and is now the preferred procedure for the assessment of endometrial disease. It is used to treat a wide variety of conditions including endometrial resec-

tion for menorrhagia, the removal of endometrial polyps and fibroids.

Respiratory endoscopy

Bronchoscopic examination of the respiratory tract remains an important diagnostic tool. Flexible bronchoscopy carried out under local anaesthetic has now replaced traditional rigid bronchoscopy under general anaesthetic. Bronchoscopy is used therapeutically for removal of foreign bodies and retained sputum.

NON-ANATOMICAL ROUTES

Many minimally invasive surgical procedures use non-anatomical access routes. These require an incision through the skin and underlying structures to gain access to an organ or tissue, or to a natural or artificial body cavity which is filled with gas or fluid so that minimally invasive therapy can be performed.

Radiological (percutaneous)

These techniques rely on indirect imaging of the target organs or tissues using X-ray screening or computed tomography (CT), magnetic resonance (MR) or ultrasound scanning. Most procedures are performed by interventional radiologists, although physicians and surgeons also use these imaging techniques. Percutaneous needle biopsy or aspirational cytology of abnormal organs or tissues is frequently used to establish diagnosis (e.g. biopsy of liver metastases or a lung or breast lesion). Collections of fluid (e.g. abscesses) can be aspirated or drained under direct imaging. Percutaneous cannulation of arteries or veins permits contrast imaging of blood vessels (angiography) and occlusion of bleeding points or tumour blood supply (embolisation). Thrombus can be dispersed by intravascular infusion of thrombolytic agents. Arterial or venous stenoses may be dilated (e.g. percutaneous coronary angioplasty) or stented. Percutaneous transhepatic cholangiography (PTC) permits biliary imaging and stenting of biliary strictures.

Transcoelomic access

These techniques include laparoscopy (endoscopic examination of the abdomen and/or pelvis) and thoracoscopy. Many of the most recent advances in minimally invasive surgery have occurred using these techniques.

While both of these methods have been in use for years, they were largely limited to diagnostic endoscopy (including biopsy) and minor therapeutic procedures such as female sterilisation. With advances in instrument design and the development of video endoscopy, a large variety of therapeutic laparoscopic and thoracoscopic procedures are now being performed (Tables 9.4 and 9.5). Not all of these are widely used and many remain to be formally evaluated by randomised comparison with traditional operations.

Arthroscopic access

Arthroscopy of the knee, shoulder and other joints is increasingly used in diagnosis and therapy (e.g. removal of loose bodies, meniscectomy). The knee joint is particularly accessible for an endoscopic approach.

Artificially created body cavities

It is possible to create an artificial body cavity by insufflation of gas within a tissue plane. This may be performed pre-peritoneally to approach the inguinal or femoral canal or retroperitoneally for access to the kidney, great vessels and other retroperitoneal structures. Subfascial endoscopy allows ligation or clipping of venous perforators. Most of these techniques are currently in the stage of development.

COMPLICATIONS OF MINIMALLY INVASIVE SURGERY AND THEIR PREVENTION

Many minimally invasive procedures are performed under local anaesthetic with intravenous sedation, and respiratory depression leading to hypoxaemia or even respiratory arrest is a serious potential complication. All such patients should be monitored with pulse oximetry, and oversedation should be carefully avoided particularly in the elderly and those with existing respiratory disease.

Some of the complications of minimally invasive procedures are specific to the operation performed, whereas others represent a common hazard of the access techniques used. For example, a trocar injury to the bowel may occur during any laparoscopic procedure, whereas a bile duct injury is specific to cholecystectomy. Whilst the incidence of specific complications may have increased for some operations, e.g. ureteric injury in laparoscopic colorectal operations or bile duct injury in laparoscopic cholecystectomy, these complications also occur at open operation. The complications that relate to those methods used for minimal access will now be considered (Table 9.6).

ANATOMICAL (ENDOLUMINAL) ROUTES

Perforation of the gastrointestinal or genitourinary tract may allow spillage of luminal contents, bleeding and infection. Peritonitis following intra-abdominal perforation or mediastinitis or pelvic sepsis following extraperitoneal perforation may rapidly lead to life-threatening sepsis. Bleeding can occur following therapeutic endoscopy, e.g. colonic polypectomy or endoscopic sphincterotomy for the removal of bile duct stones. Infection may be introduced into the gastrointestinal, biliary, pancreatic or genitouri-

Table 9.4 Some laparoscopic operations

Diagnostic
Tumour staging (e.g. pancreas, stomach)
Biopsy of liver lesions
Investigation of ascites
Investigation of acute abdominal pain
Assessment of abdominal trauma

Therapeutic	
Cholecystectomy	Gastrojejunostomy
Appendicectomy	Small bowel resection
Inguinal hernia repair	Splenectomy
Exploration of the common	Nephrectomy
bile duct	Hepatectomy
Repair of perforated peptic ulcer	Pelvic lymph node
Fundoplication of stomach	dissection
Highly selective vagotomy	Ureteric surgery
Cardiomyotomy	Surgery for ectopic
Colonic resection	pregnancy
Abdominoperineal excision of	Hysterectomy
rectum	Varicocele surgery
Rectopexy	Excision of maldescended
Colostomy	testes
Ileostomy	Divisum of adhesions
	Cholecystojejunostomy

Table 9.5 Some thorocoscopic operations

Cervical sympathectomy
Oesophagectomy
Cardiomyotomy
Lobectomy
Pneumonectomy
Lung biopsy
Splanchnicectomy

Table 9.6   Complications of minimal access

Route	Complication
Anatomical (endoluminal) routes	Perforation
	Bleeding
	Infection
Non-anatomical routes	Vascular injury
	Visceral perforation
	Insufflation problems
	Carbon dioxide absorption
	Diathermy/laser injury
	Trocar wound
	complications

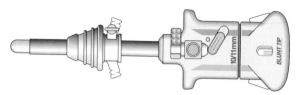

Fig. 9.2 Blunt (Hasson) trocar which is inserted using an open 'cut-down' technique. This method reduces the risk of visceral or vascular injury and is as quick as the closed technique using an insufflation needle and sharp trocar.

nary tract by inadequate cleaning or exogenous contamination of instruments. Both genitourinary endoscopy and endoscopic retrograde cholangiopancreatography (ERCP) may lead to bacteraemia by instrumentation of, or injection into, an infected tract.

NON-ANATOMICAL ROUTES

Insertion of a trocar or needle into a body cavity or other structure may lead to vascular or visceral injury. Perforation of the bowel, bladder or stomach may occur during percutaneous or laparoscopic procedures. Injury to solid organs such as the liver or spleen and to major blood vessels results in bleeding. Damage to the retroperitoneal vessels, particularly the aorta and iliac vessels, is a rare but well-recognised and frequently fatal complication of laparoscopy. Most, if not all, of these laparoscopy trocar or needle puncture injuries can be avoided by use of the open technique for placement of the first trocar (Hasson technique, Fig. 9.2). Carbon dioxide insufflation of the peritoneal cavity leads to absorption through the peritoneal membrane with a rise in the blood carbon dioxide concentrations, which may pose problems in patients with severe respiratory disease. The intra-abdominal pressure is raised during laparoscopic procedures (to approximately 14 mmHg) and this may impede venous return to the heart, particularly if associated with a head-up, foot-down position on the operating table. These factors may predispose to the development of deep vein thrombosis and pulmonary embolus. Insufflation using a needle may occur in the wrong place, leading to pre-peritoneal or intra-omental insufflation. Diathermy or laser injuries can occur during therapeutic endoscopy and care must be taken to ensure that the instru-

ments are kept within the field of view at all times. Trocar wound complications include bleeding and herniation. All large trocar wounds should be sutured, and blood vessels should be avoided at the time of trocar insertion.

CONTRAINDICATIONS

Most contraindications to minimally invasive surgery are relative and they are in many cases similar to those for open operation. Patients with intestinal obstruction, multiple previous abdominal operations, advanced pregnancy or severe respiratory disease may represent contraindications to laparoscopic surgery.

CONCLUSIONS

Minimally invasive techniques have revolutionised the treatment of many surgical procedures. Although they have disadvantages, their introduction has usually benefited patients and often reduced overall health care costs. All new techniques require careful evaluation, preferably by randomised comparison with established methods. Minimally invasive procedures will continue to encroach onto the remainder of traditional surgical procedures.

FURTHER READING

Berci G, Cuschieri A (eds) 1997 Bile ducts and bile duct stones. W B Saunders, London

Büchler M W et al (eds) 1996 Five years of laparoscopic cholecystectomy: a reappraisal. In: Progress in Surgery, vol 22. Karger, Basel

Paterson-Brown S, Garden J 1994 Principles and practice of surgical laparoscopy. W B Saunders, London

Toouli J, Gossot D, Hunter J G 1996 Endosurgery. Churchill Livingstone, New York

10 Principles of surgical oncology

James Shaw

OVERVIEW

The surgeon has a major role in the prevention, diagnosis and surgical management of patients with cancer. In addition, surgeons with a specific interest in oncology tend to be involved in the insertion of devices to facilitate the administration of chemotherapy by medical oncologists, as well as having some involvement in performing clinical trials in patients with cancer.

In this chapter, the various roles of the surgeon in the management of the oncology patient are discussed. In addition, principles of surgical management of cancer are outlined. This applies to both potentially curative surgery and palliative surgery. Furthermore, mention is made of molecular biology and gene studies in patients with cancer and the use of the multimodality approach to manage the cancer patient.

Table 10.1 The role of the surgeon in cancer care

- Diagnosis
- Staging and prognosis
- Surgical resection and reconstruction
- Insertion of catheters and other implantable devices
- Follow-up
- Surgical resection of metastases in selected patients
- Evaluation of new treatment modalities
- Education and research

The surgeon has a major role in the management of most patients with cancer and should not be seen as a mere technician. He has an important role to play in all aspects of patient care including prevention, diagnosis, surgery for cure or palliation and reconstructive surgery. In addition, surgery has a complementary role with other treatment modalities and in follow-up care (Table 10.1).

PREVENTION

Surgery may be required in the treatment of a variety of precancerous conditions. Familial polyposis of the colon is an inherited disease resulting in widespread adenomatosis of the large bowel. If untreated, this disorder progresses to one or more carcinomas of the large bowel. As a result, patients with multiple polyposis and/or those bearing the polyposis gene should undergo prophylactic colectomy prior to the development of malignancy – preferably before the age of 25 years. In addition, the development of mucosal proctectomy, ileal pouch formation and anal anastomosis has allowed many of these patients to avoid a permanent ileostomy (see Ch. 31).

Other examples of precancerous diseases requiring prevention and/or early operation include leukoplakia of the oral cavity mucosa, carcinoma-in-situ of the cervix, and some endocrine abnormalities such as the multiple endocrine neoplastic syndromes. Patients with multiple endocrine neoplasia (MEN) types IIA and IIB have a high risk of developing medullary cancer of the thyroid gland and may require total thyroidectomy. Kindred of these patients may be screened by assessing basal calcitonin levels and the response to pentagastrin stimulation. In addition, recent genetic studies have identified the gene responsible for these syndromes. As a result at risk patients/kindred can now be detected/screened by the presence of the 'ret proto-oncogene' (Table 10.4).

A further example of cancer prevention is the performance of prophylactic bilateral mastectomy (and reconstruction) in women with a strong family history of breast cancer. This is always a difficult issue that requires careful assessment and counselling in a multimodality setting, but for some histological types of breast cancer in some clinical settings prophylactic surgery may be appropriate.

DIAGNOSIS AND STAGING

With few exceptions, cancer diagnosis is based on histological or cytological interpretation of tissue obtained by surgical, radiological or endoscopic methods. The biopsy procedure may simply be a percutaneous fine needle aspiration or endoscopic biopsy; however, in some patients an open surgical biopsy may be required. This open biopsy may range from the excision of a small fragment of superficial tumour to laparotomy, thoracotomy or craniotomy in order that sufficient tissue may be obtained for pathological clarification.

In some clinical settings, excisional biopsy may be preferred to incisional biopsy. Removing the lesion completely (excision) ensures an adequate amount of tissue for examination and has the added advantages of minimising the risk of disseminating the tumour, abolishing the problem of sampling error and, should the lesion prove benign, avoiding the need for further operation. The initial diagnosis of cutaneous melanoma is one example. In contrast, incisional biopsy may be more appropriate in some settings when an excisional biopsy would compromise margins of clearance during a definitive resection. Limb sarcomata and breast cancers often fall into this latter category.

The need to establish the diagnosis and stage of recurrent disease (local recurrence or the presence of metastases) is a common problem. In each circumstance, the simplest and safest technique available should be chosen in order to clarify the situation thereby allowing the use of other therapies for treating the disease recurrence. In order to facilitate this process, surgeons must possess some knowledge of the indications, contraindications and relative merits of the various imaging procedures, e.g. scintillation scanning, ultrasound, computerised tomography (CT) scanning and magnetic resonance imaging (MRI), as well as the more recent modalities of immunoscintigraphy and position emission tomography (PET) scanning.

The oncology surgeon may also be called on to provide staging information. Staging laparotomy was frequently employed in the past to determine more accurately the extent of Hodgkin's lymphoma. Although the stage of disease was often changed by the surgery, the treatment and outcome were not changed enough to justify the morbidity of the procedure. As a result, over the last decade this technique has largely been replaced with more sophisticated radiological methods.

However, staging dissection of regional lymph nodes has a major role in the therapeutic planning of a variety of other cancers. For example, squamous cell cancer of the tongue is frequently associated with occult regional disease in neck nodes. As a result, a staging suprahyoid (limited) neck dissection may be appropriate in addition to partial glossectomy in order to clarify the stage of disease and thereby change the treatment approach and hopefully the outcome. A more common situation is the use of axillary dissection, in patients with clinically node negative breast cancer (clinically clear axillae), in order to stage the disease histologically. This information is especially helpful in pre-menopausal patients as it is used to determine the appropriateness of adjuvant chemotherapy.

Finally, the oncology surgeon may be asked to diagnose non-malignant conditions in cancer patients who are immunocompromised as a consequence of their disease or its treatment. For example, thoracotomy and open lung biopsy may be required to diagnose the causative agent of an opportunistic lung infection.

CURATIVE SURGERY

Many cancers can be cured by surgical removal of the primary disease process. Failure to cure the cancer may be due to a number of factors:

- The primary lesion may have already produced distant metastases prior to surgical extirpation (excision).
- The cancer may be multifocal or multicentric.
- Clinical and/or radiological means are unable to detect micrometastases.
- There was inadequate removal of the cancer and/or the regional lymph nodes.

At present, little can be done by the surgeon to overcome the problem of macroscopic or microscopic metastases, although radiological techniques capable of detecting this problem continue to improve. In those organs where a cancer may be multicentric or multifocal (e.g. ductal carcinoma-in-situ of the breast (DCIS) or papillary cancer of the thyroid), the surgeon must be aware of that possibility and utilise this knowledge of tumour biology in deciding the extent of the resection.

The view that many cancers may be cured by surgical excision is based on the concept that at some time in its development the tumour would have been localised enough to have been completely surgically encircled both locally and regionally. There is evidence to support this hypothesis in some cancers such as colon carcinoma.

To accomplish an adequate cancer operation, it is important that the lines of resection (margins) are far enough from the edges of the tumour to allow for sufficient normal tissue to be included with the lesion. Frequently, cancer may present with microscopic invasion of adjacent tissue or submucosal spread that is not detectable macroscopically. Under those circumstances, a wider margin of apparently normal tissue must be taken around the tumour. In some settings, multiple frozen sections of the margins may be required to clarify that clearance is adequate. This is especially true in surgery for head and neck cancer, where negative margins are critical in determining outcome, and oesophageal cancer, where submucosal spread is common.

Adequate margins of clearance vary for individual tumours, but positive margins (histological presence of tumour cells) are usually associated with an unacceptably high rate of local recurrence (Table 10.2).

Minimal manipulation of the cancer during dissection is an historic principle of cancer surgery that is based on the theory/fact that tumour cells are frequently dislodged into the vasculature during surgery and that this *may* lead to the seeding of metastatic deposits. As a result, *whenever possible*, the arterial supply leading to, and the venous drainage from, the tumour should be interrupted early in the course of the dissection and as far away from the primary lesion as possible. Although theoretically appealing, the scientific credibility of early vascular ligation is questionable. On the one hand, the 'no-touch' isolation technique of early vascular ligation of the mesenteric vessels before dissection – advocated by Rupert Turnbull for colon cancer – indicated that the cure rate could be improved. On the other hand, early ligation of the internal jugular vein, as in a classical radical neck dissection, or not at all, as in a modified neck dissection, appears to have little effect on outcome.

Adequate removal of a primary tumour is intended to include those tissues adjacent to the lesion that contain lymphatic vessels and nodes. In addition, the primary lesion and the adjacent soft tissues should be removed *en bloc* (as a block of tissue) to prevent mechanical spillage and seeding of tumour cells by surgical transection of the cancer or its associated lymphatic channels.

Another dilemma faced when performing major curative resections for cancer is to adequately excise sufficient tissue while at the same time providing for tissue reconstruction for restoring function and achieving an acceptable cosmetic result, especially in head and neck surgery.

In the past, tissue from the subcutaneous chest wall (deltopectoral flap) was used for reconstruction. However, recent improvements in microvascular surgery and the use of large myocutaneous flaps (especially those based on the pectoralis major muscle) provide tissue to reconstruct large anatomic defects in this region. Composite free flaps such as vascularised fibula and associated soft tissue have revolutionised the reconstruction of the resected mandible.

Breast reconstruction after mastectomy with rectus abdominis myocutaneous flaps or the preservation of anal continence following rectal excision using a gracilis muscle sling are two further examples of newer reconstructive surgical techniques.

PALLIATIVE SURGERY

The term 'palliation' implies relief of symptoms or impending symptoms, as well as prevention of complications or potential complications, without altering the progress of the primary disease process. The emphasis is on quality, rather than duration, of life, and a major goal is to provide time away from hospital. The operative mortality and morbidity of a palliative procedure must be minimal or the above goals are unlikely to be met and the

Table 10.2 Acceptable minimal margins of resection

Type of cancer	Minimal margin
Melanoma <1 mm thick	1 cm
Melanoma 1–2 mm thick	2 cm
Melanoma >2 mm thick	3 cm*
Rectal cancer distal margin	>1 cm*
Breast cancer	Few mm*†
In situ breast cancer	1 cm
Colon cancer	>5 cm*
Oesophageal cancer	>5 cm
Soft tissue sarcoma	Few cm

*Staging and/or therapeutic node dissection may also be appropriate.
†Providing adjuvant radiation is to be employed.

maxim 'primum non nocere' ('above all, do no harm') is highly relevant.

Operations are frequently required to relieve a whole host of symptoms and complications resulting from uncontrolled/uncontrollable malignant disease. These vary from correcting an intestinal obstruction due to metastatic tumour; to the excision of a fungating cancer of the breast; to a biliary bypass or a biliary stent procedure to relieve jaundice, and associated itch and cholangitis.

DEBULKING SURGERY

In the past, the concept of 'cytoreduction' and 'relief of tumour burden' by surgical excision was advocated for a variety of tumours. Present-day evidence suggests that it may have a role in the management of patients with ovarian carcinoma, islet cell cancer, testicular carcinoma or Burkitt's lymphoma of the abdomen. However, debulking surgery must always be employed with caution and this is especially true when performing palliative surgery.

ACCESS DEVICES, INFUSION AND PERFUSION THERAPY

A variety of surgical techniques have been developed to assist in the safe delivery of chemotherapy. The direct administration of chemotherapeutic agents into peripheral veins is associated with a high incidence of phlebitis and other complications. As a result, a variety of catheters and related implantable devices have been developed to avoid this problem by providing central venous access with the catheter tip sitting in a large vein with a high flow rate, e.g. the superior vena cava. The catheter is used for both blood sampling and infusion of chemotherapy. The major complication, however, is catheter sepsis. Catheters are tunnelled to reduce infection and may either exit from the skin or be connected to an implantable subcutaneous reservoir which can be accessed as a long-term 'port'.

Other examples of where implantable devices and procedures are used in the oncology patient include limb perfusion of malignant melanomas through surgically placed catheters; perfusion of the liver with surgically placed intravascular catheters; and perfusion of the liver with surgically implanted subcutaneous pumps which are subsequently loaded with chemotherapy. Limb perfusion or infusion chemotherapy in the patient with melanoma and extensive 'in-transit disease' is a well established and effective technique. However, liver perfusion for primary or secondary liver tumours has not been shown to improve survival.

SURGICAL EXCISION OF METASTASES

A highly selected group of patients are known to benefit from surgical removal of metastatic deposits. Examples include pulmonary metastasis from osteosarcoma, some other sarcomata, and testicular tumours. The key principle is that if a single site of metastatic disease can be resected with a low mortality and morbidity, then there may be a survival benefit for the patient. Occasionally, a solitary brain metastasis can be considered for resection if there is no evidence of spread to other sites outside the brain. Resection of melanoma cerebral metastases combined with adjuvant radiation therapy has been shown to yield superior results to the use of radiation alone.

As a general rule, surgery for metastatic disease should be reserved for those patients presenting with a solitary metastasis, preferably where a considerable period of time has elapsed since the resection of the primary lesion. The patient must be well enough to tolerate the operative procedure, and most importantly, the primary lesion must be controlled. If the primary lesion is not controlled then this is an absolute contraindication to resection of metastatic disease.

MULTIMODALITY MANAGEMENT OF CANCER

Over the past 20 years, the treatment of cancer has changed from being single modality (i.e. surgery, radiation or chemotherapy alone) to multimodality (i.e. a combination of treatments and regimens). As a result, multimodality meetings of a variety of specialists are frequently employed to allow discussion and thereby to outline optimal plans of management. In general terms, the groups comprise radiologists, pathologists, surgeons, medical oncologists, radiation oncologists and palliative care physicians. In some clinical settings, nurse specialists, speech pathologists, dietitians, physiotherapists and other health professionals may also be included.

The expected outcome for many different tumours has been dramatically improved with the use of a multimodality, rather than a single modality, approach (Table 10.3).

Table 10.3   Role of multimodality treatment

Tumour	Role for surgery	Adjuvant radiation	Adjuvant chemotherapy
Rectal cancer	Established	↓ Local recurrence	?↓ Liver metastases
Squamous cell carcinoma of the head and neck	Established	↓ Local recurrence	??
Breast cancer	Established but now more conservative	↓ Local recurrence	Established in node positive pre-menopausal women
Melanoma	Established; now more conservative	?↓ Local recurrence	No effective agent
Soft tissue sarcomas	Established; less use of amputation	↓ Local recurrence	Established in children, but adults ??

Table 10.4   Molecular biology and surgical oncology

Tumour	Marker	Significance
Medullary cancer thyroid	*ret* proto-oncogene	Marker of familial disposition to the disease
Familial breast cancer	c-*erb* – B-2 oncogenes	Experimental; may detect kindred at risk
Familial bowel cancer	APC oncogene	Detect kindred with familial adenomatous polyposis
Breast cancer overall	*p51* oncogene	Prognostic predictor of outcome
Gastric cancer	c-*erb* B	Prognostic predictor
Colon cancer	DCC	Chromosome defect in 70% of colorectal cancer patients
Cervical cancer	c-*myc*	Denotes poor prognosis
Soft tissue sarcoma	*p53* mutation	Increased risk of disease

WHAT IS A SURGICAL ONCOLOGIST?

Many cancers can be resected safely and adequately by an appropriate surgeon who is competently trained in his specialty. For example, a neurosurgeon can resect a brain tumour; a general surgeon, a colorectal cancer; a urologist, a carcinoma of the kidney; and a cardiothoracic surgeon, a carcinoma of the lung. Thus, surgical oncology is not truly a specialty, but is a *subspecialty* of several disciplines. However, the surgeon who develops a major interest in cancer treatment within his specialty must develop an expertise in all aspects of cancer care, including diagnosis and staging, as well as the use of other modalities of treatment. The surgeon should be able to provide expert advice in many areas in which the average surgeon is not so well versed. The resection of major soft tissue sarcomata, major lymph node dissections and the use of infusion and perfusion techniques often fall within the province of the oncology surgeon who is part of a team of experts in other disciplines of cancer treatment.

Where possible, oncology surgeons should also be involved with therapeutic advances and clinical trials. In addition, they should be involved with cancer education and research.

MOLECULAR BIOLOGY AND SURGICAL ONCOLOGY

A working knowledge of molecular biology is now important for the oncology surgeon. Oncogenes and genetic markers have been identified to aid in the diagnosis and management of a variety of neoplastic disorders. This expanding field of research is beyond the scope of this book; however, some examples are shown in Table 10.4.

FURTHER READING

Casciato D A, Lowitz B B 1995 Manual of clinical oncology, 3rd edn. Little, Brown, Boston

McArdle C S 1990 Surgical oncology: current concepts and practice. Butterworths, London

Moffat F L, Ketcham A S 1994 Surgery for malignant neoplasia. The evaluation of oncology surgery. In: McKenna R J, Murphy S P (eds) Cancer surgery. J B Lippincott, Philadelphia

Moossa A R 1991 Principles and complications of surgical therapy. In: Moossa R L et al (eds) Comprehensive textbook of oncology, 2nd edn. Williams and Wilkins, Baltimore, p 429–439

Poston G J, Winstanley J H R 1996 Principles of surgery and malignant disease. In: Taylor I, Karran S J (eds) Surgical principles. Arnold, London, p 61–75

Rosenberg S A 1984 The organisation of surgical oncology in university departments of surgery. Surgery 95: 632–634

Organ transplantation
Michael Nicholson

OVERVIEW

Organ transplantation has been one of the most dramatic developments in 20th century medicine. Kidney transplantation is widely regarded as the best treatment for end-stage renal failure, and excellent graft survival rates are being achieved around the world. Liver and heart transplants have also become routine procedures with very high success rates. Whole organ pancreas transplantation is finding an increasing role in the treatment of diabetics with end-stage renal failure; transplantation of isolated islets of Langerhans has proved less successful. The results of combined heart–lung and single lung transplant procedures are improving rapidly. Small bowel transplantation has been attempted but many problems still remain. Improvements in immunosuppression underpin these striking advances.

Immunological rejection has been the major obstacle to successful organ transplantation. Considerable advances have been made in immunosuppressive therapy, and this has been the main reason for an improvement in results. The drugs being used are still not sufficiently specific, and the morbidity of long-term immunosuppression needs to be reduced. Currently the major problems are a lack of suitable organ donors and the process known as chronic rejection, which accounts for most late graft failures. This chapter emphasises renal transplantation, but many of the principles involved apply to the other transplantable organs.

ORGAN DONATION

There are two sources of transplant organs: cadaveric and living donors.

CADAVERIC DONORS

Cadaveric organs are most commonly used, but because of a fall in the death rate from both intracerebral haemorrhage and road traffic accidents, there is a shortage of suitable cadaveric donors. This has led to a progressive increase in the kidney transplant waiting list in many countries, including the UK and Ireland (Fig. 11.1).

Donors can be of any age up to 70 years, but for heart and liver transplantation the upper age limit is normally set at 50–60 years. Malignancy (except primary tumours of the central nervous system which never metastasise), HIV or hepatitis B infection and systemic bacterial infection, including tuberculosis, are contraindications to organ donation.

Patients suffering brain stem death whilst being maintained on a ventilator in an intensive care unit should be considered as potential donors. The family should be approached to ask for permission to remove suitable organs. The concept of brain stem death allows organ retrieval from heart-beating donors, which reduces damage to the organs before removal.

Brain stem death criteria

Death can be defined as an irreversible loss of the capacity for consciousness combined with an irreversible loss

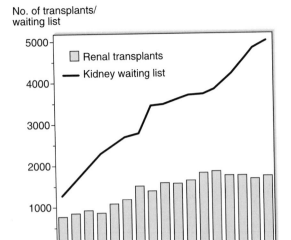

No. of transplants/waiting list

Fig. 11.1 UK and Ireland cadaveric kidney transplants and transplant waiting list 1978–1994.

neys for transplantation. Corneas and long bones can be removed up to 24 hours after death and then stored in tissue banks for subsequent transplantation.

Careful preoperative management of the donor helps to keep the various organs in good condition before removal. Intravenous fluids are given to maintain a good urine output, and inotropic drugs may be needed to support the blood pressure. The organ retrieval operation is carried out under sterile conditions in a fully equipped operating theatre. The key principle is to avoid warm ischaemia by rapid in situ organ cooling. This process is achieved by isolating the vascular supply of the organs and flushing them with cold preservation fluid as soon as the blood flow has been interrupted. This manoeuvre washes out the blood (preventing thrombosis), rapidly cools the organ (reducing metabolic rate and oxygen requirement) and fills the organ with preservation fluid. The composition of preservation fluid is similar to intracellular fluid to prevent ion fluxes across cell membranes. Transplant organs are stored in crushed ice for transport to the recipient hospital.

of the capacity to breathe (and hence to sustain a heartbeat). These two functions are subserved by the brain stem, and 'brain stem death' is a concept accepted by most countries throughout the world. Brain stem death can be diagnosed by a series of simple tests. The patient must first meet strict preconditions, i.e. be comatose and maintained on a ventilator, and have a known cause of irremediable structural brain injury (confirmed on a CT brain scan). Hypothermia, drugs and metabolic or endocrine disturbances that could account for coma must be excluded. The inability to ventilate spontaneously is demonstrated by disconnection from the ventilator for 5–10 minutes following pre-oxygenation to prevent hypoxia. The $P_a\text{CO}_2$ must rise above 6.65 kPa (50 mmHg) during the test. The diagnosis of brain stem death is completed by demonstrating the absence of the following brain stem reflexes:

- pupillary reflex
- corneal reflex
- vestibulo-ocular (caloric) reflex
- response to painful stimulus in the trigeminal nerve territory
- gag reflex.

Cadaveric organ retrieval operations

As far as possible, multi-organ donation is performed, with removal of the heart, lungs, liver, pancreas and kid-

LIVE DONATION

Healthy individuals with normal renal function may donate one of their kidneys for transplantation. The donor is usually a highly motivated parent or sibling. The mortality rate associated with donor nephrectomy is approximately 1 in 2000 operations, and it has been shown that there are few long-term health risks for the donor. Donor nephrectomy is most commonly performed through a loin incision. The recipient is operated on synchronously so that the kidney is transplanted and revascularised within an hour or so of removal from the donor. The renal ischaemic damage in this situation is minimal.

It has recently been shown that the results of living unrelated kidney transplantation from spousal donors are as good as or even better than cadaveric transplants. This is the case despite poor HLA matching, and it is thought to be related to the very short ischaemic times associated with living donor transplantation. Segments of liver and pancreas have also been successfully used for transplantation, but the risks to the donor are considerably higher in these procedures.

SELECTING THE TRANSPLANT RECIPIENT

The names of potential recipients are held on local and

national waiting lists. A number of factors are taken into consideration when choosing a recipient for a particular organ. There must be ABO blood group compatibility between donor and recipient. For kidneys, the tissue type is also taken into consideration and the best matched recipient is usually offered the transplant. The heart, lungs and liver remain viable for shorter periods during cold storage and must be transplanted quickly. This requirement does not usually leave enough time to perform tissue typing before transplantation.

TISSUE TYPING AND MATCHING

All nucleated human cells express a number of surface glycoproteins which are recognised by the immune system as 'self' antigens. As these were first identified on white blood cells, they are known as human leucocyte antigens (HLA). The genes that code for HLA are grouped together on chromosome 6 in a region called the major histocompatibility complex (MHC). The genetic material is arranged in a number of loci of which A, B and DR are the most important. The human MHC is a highly polymorphic region, i.e. many alternative genes (alleles) may exist at each locus. Currently, over 20 A, nearly 50 B and 16 DR locus alleles have been found in humans. Each individual has two alleles at each locus and has a virtually unique combination of HLA. The genetic differences between donor and recipient constitute the major factor underlying immunological graft rejection. Following transplantation, a recipient will mount an immune response to any mismatched donor HLA. This process can be counteracted by optimising the donor–recipient HLA matching and by modifying the immune response with immunosuppressive drugs.

Tissue typing

The determination of the HLA antigens in individuals (or tissue typing) can conveniently be carried out using lymphocytes from the peripheral blood (recipients) or the lymph nodes and spleen (donors). The method used is a complement-dependent cytotoxicity (CDC) assay. Sera containing specific anti-HLA antibodies along with complement are added to the lymphocytes to be typed. The specific antisera were originally obtained from pregnant women who have produced antibodies to mismatched fetal HLA of paternal origin. If antibody is bound and complement fixed, the lymphocytes will be lysed and these dead cells can be identified under the microscope.

The combination of specific antibodies causing cell death defines the tissue type. More modern molecular biological techniques using DNA are now replacing the traditional CDC method.

Cytotoxic cross-match

Potential transplant recipients may have pre-formed anti-HLA antibodies to mismatched donor antigens. These antibodies result from sensitisation to foreign HLA following blood transfusions, pregnancies or previous transplants. The cytotoxic cross-match is designed to detect anti-HLA antibodies in the recipient and must be performed before transplantation in order to avoid hyperacute rejection and immediate thrombosis of the transplanted organ. The test is effectively a preoperative 'transplant in a test tube' and is carried out in a similar way to tissue typing. In a positive cross-match, donor lymphocytes are lysed by recipient serum, and this would contraindicate a transplant between that particular donor and recipient. Some patients have developed antibodies to many different HLA antigens and these highly sensitised individuals are very difficult to transplant.

TRANSPLANT IMMUNOLOGY

Following transplantation, foreign antigens in the graft are recognised by the host immune system. This process is mediated by circulating leucocytes (macrophages and lymphocytes) which migrate into the transplant through the microvascular endothelium. Macrophages in the graft process foreign HLA antigens and present them to recipient donor helper T lymphocytes. This mechanism activates the helper cells, which then secrete a number of important cytokines, including interleukin-2 (IL-2), which stimulates the production of a clone of cytolytic T cells from their precursors. Cytolytic T cells are responsible for the process of acute cellular rejection. An understanding of this process has been used to develop drugs that modulate the immune response, and this is the major factor responsible for the excellent long-term graft survival rates being achieved for most transplant organs.

IMMUNOSUPPRESSION

The mainstay of modern immunosuppression has been cyclosporin. It is usual to give this drug in combination with either steroids (dual therapy) or steroids and azathioprine (triple therapy). The aim of such combinations is to reduce the dosage and hence the side-effects of each agent.

Cyclosporin

This polypeptide is derived from a soil fungus and acts by blocking transcription of the IL-2 gene in T helper lymphocytes. This process prevents the maturation of precursor cytolytic T cells into fully armed cytolytic cells. The main side-effect of cyclosporin is nephrotoxicity mediated by intense glomerular afferent arteriolar vasoconstriction. Blood levels are used to adjust the dose of drug to avoid toxicity.

Corticosteroids (prednisolone)

These drugs cause a non-specific immunosuppression. Their mechanism of action includes preventing transcription of the IL-1 and IL-6 genes. Steroid side-effects have in the past been responsible for a good deal of post-transplant morbidity. Lower doses are now being used as a result. Side-effects include Cushingoid appearance, hypertension, diabetes, peptic ulceration and avascular necrosis of the femoral head.

Azathioprine

This drug is non-specific, acting as a purine analogue which prevents the proliferation of rapidly dividing cells including lymphocytes. The main side-effect is bone marrow suppression (especially neutropenia).

FK506

This is a new immunosuppressive agent derived from a fungal metabolite. Its actions and side-effects are similar to cyclosporin, but it is 100 times more potent in vitro.

General side-effects of immunosuppressive drugs

The art of post-transplant management is to strike the correct level of immunosuppression in individual patients. Over-immunosuppression runs the risk of promoting infection or malignancy, and under-immunosuppression will lead to acute rejection. The dosage of immunosuppressive drugs is reduced gradually following transplantation, but a low dose must be continued indefinitely.

All types of infections are more common in transplant patients, but those organisms eliminated by T lymphocytes are especially likely to cause opportunistic infections. These include viral (cytomegalovirus), protozoal (pneumocystis pneumonia) and fungal (*Candida*) infections. The same spectrum of infections is seen in AIDS patients.

The higher prevalence of certain malignant diseases is thought to be due to a loss of the capacity for immune surveillance. The commonest tumours are squamous cell carcinomas of the skin. Malignant lymphomas (usually non-Hodgkin's) also occur with a much higher frequency in transplant patients compared to the general population.

KIDNEY TRANSPLANTATION

INDICATIONS AND CONTRAINDICATIONS

Most causes of end-stage renal failure requiring dialysis are indications for renal transplantation. These conditions include chronic glomerulonephritis and pyelonephritis, hypertensive and diabetic nephropathies, polycystic kidneys and chronic urinary tract obstruction. The results of kidney transplantation are not as good at the extremes of age, especially in children under 5 years and adults over 70 years. Transplantation subjects the patient not only to the usual risks of surgery and anaesthesia but also to the risks associated with long-term immunosuppression. Potential recipients should therefore have no major cardiorespiratory disease and no contraindication to immunosuppression such as systemic sepsis or malignancy.

THE KIDNEY TRANSPLANT OPERATION

The transplanted kidney is placed extraperitoneally in either iliac fossa. The donor renal vein is anastomosed end-to-side to the recipient external iliac vein, and the renal artery is anastomosed either end-to-side to the external iliac artery or end-to-end to the stump of the divided internal iliac artery. The operation is completed by anastomosing the ureter to the bladder using a technique that creates an anti-reflux mechanism. This manoeuvre can be performed either by opening the bladder and tunnelling the ureter submucosally (Leadbetter–Politano technique) or by a simple extravesical onlay method (Gregoir–Lich). The ureteric anastomosis may be protected by a double-J ureteric stent, which is removed cystoscopically once the anastomosis has healed.

POSTOPERATIVE COURSE OF A KIDNEY TRANSPLANT

Following revascularisation, an immediate diuresis occurs in all living donor kidneys and in approximately 70% of cadaveric kidneys. In the remaining 30%, urine is not produced and dialysis support is required until the kidney recovers. This delayed graft function results from acute tubular necrosis secondary to pre-transplant renal ischaemia and is seen most commonly in kidneys that have been stored on ice for long periods (a cold ischaemic time > 24 hours).

Accurate fluid balance must be maintained. Urine output is measured hourly and is replaced by a combination of 0.9% saline and 5% dextrose. Renal function is assessed by daily serum creatinine measurements.

Acute rejection

This is the major problem in the first 3 months after renal transplantation. Hyperacute rejection, which is antibody-mediated, occurs immediately following revascularisation if the recipient has preformed antibodies to mismatched donor HLA antigens. This possibility is avoided by performing a pre-transplant cytotoxic cross-match. Acute cellular rejection mediated by lymphocytes is more common, occurring in up to 50% of transplants in the first 3 months. The usual presentation is with fever, general malaise, graft pain/tenderness and a fall in urine output associated with a rise in serum creatinine. Many of these features are less prominent in patients treated with cyclosporin, and a clinical diagnosis of acute rejection should be confirmed by a needle core biopsy. Biopsy is performed under real-time ultrasound control, which allows the needle to be accurately introduced into the renal cortex. Histological examination reveals a mononuclear cell infiltrate (lymphocytes and macrophages) within the interstitium and the tubules ('tubulitis').

Treatment. Acute cellular rejection is initially treated by a course of high-dose intravenous methylprednisolone (0.5 g i.v. daily for 3–5 days). Steroid-resistant and severe rejection episodes are treated with anti-T lymphocyte antibody preparations. These may be either monoclonal (OKT3) or polyclonal (antithymocyte globulin) antibodies raised against human T-cells.

Chronic rejection

This is the commonest cause of late graft loss following renal transplantation. Clinically it is characterised by a slowly progressive and irreversible decline in renal function associated with proteinuria and hypertension. These changes usually begin after the first 3 or 6 months post-transplant. The histopathology of chronic rejection is dominated by vascular changes (neointimal proliferation), interstitial fibrosis, glomerulosclerosis and tubular atrophy. So far, no effective treatment has been found.

Complications of renal transplantation

Vascular complications are usually related to technical errors. Venous or arterial thrombosis occur early in 2–6% of patients, and graft loss is the usual outcome. Renal artery stenosis occurs later in up to 10%. Urological complications are related to devascularisation of the ureteric blood supply at the time of organ retrieval. This process may present early as a urine leak from the ureter or later as ischaemic ureteric stenosis and obstruction.

Results of kidney transplantation

These are dependent upon many factors, but ischaemic times and the degree of HLA matching are perhaps the most important. The best results are seen with HLA identical siblings, in whom the 1-year graft survival is over 95%. Kidneys from HLA non-identical siblings or between parents and their children have 1-year graft survival figures in the region of 90%. Cadaveric kidneys would be expected to yield an 80% graft survival at 1 year and 60% at 5 years.

LIVER TRANSPLANTATION

INDICATIONS

Chronic liver disease complicated by life-threatening conditions (e.g. variceal haemorrhage) and decompensated chronic liver failure (ascites, chronic encephalopathy, coagulopathy) are the main indications. Suitable conditions include non-alcoholic cirrhosis (e.g. primary biliary cirrhosis, chronic active hepatitis and Budd–Chiari syndrome) and alcoholic cirrhosis. Transplantation of patients with hepatitis B and malignant lesions is more controversial. Liver transplantation is also the best treatment for acute fulminant hepatic failure, e.g. as a result of paracetamol poisoning.

OPERATION

The diseased liver is removed and replaced by the transplant organ (orthotopic grafting). The recipient hepatectomy can be a very difficult procedure as a result of portal hypertension and intra-abdominal varices. Anaesthetic management during the anhepatic phase is also fraught with difficulty because of marked changes in fluid and electrolyte balance, glucose metabolism and the coagulation system. The five anastomoses required to transplant a liver are performed in the following order:

1. suprahepatic vena cava
2. infrahepatic vena cava
3. portal vein
4. hepatic artery
5. bile duct.

The biliary system may be reconstructed either by direct anastomosis of donor and recipient bile ducts or by suturing the bile duct to a Roux-en-Y loop of jejunum (choledochojejunostomy). The safe cold preservation time for livers was initially limited to 8 hours, but this has now been extended to 24 hours by the use of University of Wisconsin (UW) solution.

Complications

Postoperative thrombosis may occur and is more common in the hepatic artery than the portal vein. Biliary complications are the Achilles heel of liver transplantation. Bile leaks present early and can cause severe sepsis and death. Biliary strictures due to ischaemia present later with the features of ascending cholangitis. They may be treated by endoscopic dilatation and stenting or by revisional surgery.

Results

These are heavily influenced by the indication for transplantation and the general condition of the patient at the time of transplantation. The best results are seen in young recipients with non-malignant liver disease (e.g. primary biliary cirrhosis). The overall 1- and 5-year graft survival rates are 75% and 70%, respectively.

PANCREAS TRANSPLANTATION

INDICATIONS/RATIONALE

The ideal role of pancreas transplantation would be to prevent the development of secondary complications in insulin-dependent but non-uraemic diabetics. However, long-term treatment with insulin is much safer than long-term immunosuppression, and so at the present time the main indication for pancreas transplantation is insulin dependent diabetes mellitus causing end-stage renal failure. The best treatment for these patients is a kidney transplant, and as this will obligate long-term immunosuppression, it is reasonable to consider performing a pancreas transplant at the same time. A simultaneous pancreas/kidney transplant (SPK) will render the patient independent of both dialysis and insulin, and the normalisation of glucose metabolism should also prevent the recurrence of diabetic nephropathy in the renal transplant.

OPERATIONS

The most usual procedure is to perform SPK transplantation (Fig. 11.2). The main problem is to deal with the proteolytic enzyme-rich exocrine secretion of the pancreas, which is liable to cause autodigestion of the surrounding tissues. The most successful method of avoiding this is to perform whole organ pancreas transplantation with urinary drainage of the exocrine secretions. The donor pancreas is removed with a segment of duodenum. The arterial system is reconstructed using a donor iliac artery 'Y' graft anastomosed to the splenic and superior mesenteric arteries of the pancreas. This new arterial system is anastomosed to the recipient external iliac artery, and the portal vein is anastomosed to the

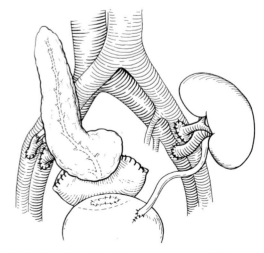

Fig. 11.2 Completed simultaneous pancreas–kidney transplant with bladder drainage technique.

external iliac vein. Finally, the duodenal segment is anastomosed to the recipient bladder using a staple gun. The use of the bladder drainage technique enables the measurement of urinary amylase levels – a fall indicates early acute rejection. Preservation times of 24–30 hours are possible if the UW solution is used.

Complications

SPK remains a difficult procedure with a high rate of graft rejection and infectious complications. With the bladder drainage method, urinary tract infections, haematuria and duodenal segment leaks can all occur.

Results

These have steadily improved. One-year graft survival rates of 75% are achieved by experienced units.

Islet cell transplantation

This is a more logical treatment as it removes all the complications associated with the exocrine portion of the pancreas. Islets are obtained by digesting the pancreas using collagenase and can then be injected into the portal vein to seed in the liver. Unfortunately there have been few clinical successes throughout the world, and the procedure remains experimental. The main problem has been variation in the efficacy of individual batches of collagenase leading to poor islet yields. Islets appear to be strongly immunogenic, and rejection has also been a major problem.

CARDIAC TRANSPLANTATION

INDICATIONS

End-stage heart disease caused by coronary artery disease or idiopathic cardiomyopathy is the main indication.

OPERATION

The safe cold ischaemic time for a heart is only 4 hours. Therefore, only ABO blood group compatibility is used to match donor and recipient. The recipient heart is removed at the mid-atrial level, and the aorta and pulmonary artery are cut just distal to their valves. This technique leaves intact the parts of the right and left atria receiving the vena cavae and pulmonary veins. The donor atria are anastomosed to the recipent atria, and the pulmonary arteries and aorta are then anastomosed end-to-end.

Immunosuppression and rejection

Immunosuppression is with cyclosporin, steroids and azathioprine. Rejection is difficult to diagnose clinically, so regular endomyocardial biopsies are performed using small biopsy forceps introduced via a central vein.

Results

The best centres are achieving 1- and 5-year graft survival rates nearing 80% and 60% respectively.

COMBINED HEART–LUNG TRANSPLANTS

These are being performed for irreversible pulmonary disease causing cardiac failure. The operation involves anastomosis of the donor and recipient right atria, the trachea and the aorta.

FUTURE PROSPECTS

Much of the morbidity of transplantation results from the side-effects of immunosuppression. Nevertheless, our understanding of transplant immunology is increasing. In time, it may be possible to induce a state of immune tolerance in transplant recipients, and this would allow the level of immunosuppression to be greatly reduced or even stopped.

In the future it may also be possible to transplant organs from one species to another (xenotransplantation). This is not yet possible because humans have pre-existing xenoreactive antibodies which mediate hyperacute rejection of xenotransplants. Activation of complement is central to this process, and attempts are currently being made to genetically engineer pigs so that their endothelial cells express the human genes that code for complement inhibitors. Transplantation using such transgenic pig organs is a possibility in the future.

FURTHER READING

Allen R D M, Chapman J R 1994 A manual of renal transplantation. Edward Arnold, London

Kahan B D (ed) 1994 Horizons in organ transplantation. Surgical Clinics of North America 74(5)

Primrose J N, Giles G R 1995 Surgical immunology and organ transplantation. In: Cuschieri A, Giles G R, Moossa A R (eds) Essential surgical practice, 3rd edn. Butterworth-Heinemann, Oxford, p 125–137

Trauma

12 General management of injuries and fractures

Don Howie

OVERVIEW

A systematic approach to the initial assessment, resuscitation and definitive care of the trauma patient will ensure the best outcome. This chapter provides a basis for such an approach and also covers extremity trauma, including fractures, spinal injuries, pelvic fractures and associated injuries.

GENERAL MANAGEMENT OF SEVERE TRAUMA

Approximately half the deaths following motor vehicle accidents, which are the commonest cause of multiple injuries, occur at or about the time of the accident and few of these patients can be salvaged. This data emphasises the importance of community education and preventive programmes.

A further one-third of deaths occur within a few hours and many of these deaths might be prevented by efficient resuscitation programmes. The remainder of deaths commonly occur in the weeks following the injury, as a result of brain death, infection or multiple organ failure. To decrease mortality and morbidity following major trauma there is a need for all those personnel involved in treatment to have an adequate understanding of the initial assessment and resuscitation of the multi-injured patient.

The American College of Surgeons initiated a nationwide education programme – ATLS (advanced trauma and life support) – in 1979 to promote a systematic approach to trauma management. The ATLS programme has also been adopted in the UK, and in Australia it has been modified and called EMST (early management of severe trauma).

The first part of this chapter on initial assessment and management of extremity trauma follows the outline of the ATLS programme.

INITIAL ASSESSMENT

The injured patient must be evaluated rapidly and thoroughly and resuscitation begun at the same time. The patient's vital functions must be assessed quickly and efficiently. An adequate patient history and account of the incident is mandatory.

The initial assessment is divided into five phases:

- *Primary survey* – assessment and treatment of ABCs
  — airway and cervical spine control
  — breathing and ventilation
  — circulation with haemorrhage control
  — disability: brief neurological evaluation
  — exposure and environmental control – completely undress the patient and prevent hypothermia.
- *Resuscitation*
  — shock management – intravenous lines and volume replacement
  — management of life-threatening problems identified in the primary survey is continued
  — electrocardiograph monitoring and placement of nasogastric and urinary catheters.
- *Secondary survey* – total evaluation of the patient from head to toe ('tubes and fingers in every orifice')
  — head, skull and face

— neck and cervical spine
— chest
— abdomen
— perineum and rectum
— extremities – fractures and dislocations
— back
— neurological examination (Glasgow Coma Scale)
— appropriate X-rays, laboratory tests, and special studies.

- *Definitive care* – after identifying the patient's injuries, managing life-threatening problems and obtaining special studies, definitive care begins.
- *Transfer* – if the patient's injuries exceed the institution's immediate treatment capabilities, the process of transferring the patient is initiated as soon as the need is identified. The transfer process should not, however, interrupt the resuscitation process.

PRIMARY SURVEY

Airway and cervical spine

The upper airway should be assessed to ascertain patency. Initial procedures to establish a patent airway include clearing the airway of foreign bodies and the chin lift or jaw thrust manoeuvre. Oesophageal airway, intubation or surgical cricothyroidotomy may be necessary. *Assume a cervical spine fracture in any patient with multisystem trauma*; hence, the patient's head and neck should not be hyperextended or hyperflexed, but cervical spine immobilisation should be maintained with a collar.

Breathing and ventilation

The patient's chest should be exposed to adequately assess rate and depth of respiration. Administer high concentrations of oxygen. When significant cardiovascular, respiratory or neurological instability exists, ventilation should be accomplished with a bag-valve device connected to a mask or endotracheal tube. Three traumatic conditions that most often compromise ventilation are tension pneumothorax, open pneumothorax or flail chest with pulmonary contusion.

Circulation and haemorrhage control

Blood volume and cardiac output. Hypotension following injury must be assumed to be hypovolaemic in origin until proved otherwise. Rapid and accurate assessment of the injured patient's haemodynamic status is therefore essential. Three elements of observation yield key information: status of consciousness, skin colour and pulse.

Bleeding. External, exsanguinating haemorrhage should be identified and controlled. Rapid blood loss is managed by direct pressure on the wound. Occult haemorrhage can account for major blood loss, and should be suspected but dealt with during definitive management.

Disability: brief neurological evaluation

A rapid neurological evaluation is performed at the end of the primary survey. This neurological evaluation establishes the patient's level of consciousness and pupillary size and reaction.

The AVPU method describes the patient's level of consciousness:

- A – alert
- V – responds to vocal stimuli
- P – responds to painful stimuli
- U – unresponsive.

Changes in the patient's neurological condition may indicate intracranial pathology or decreased oxygenation and perfusion of the central nervous system.

Exposure and environment control

The patient should be completely undressed to facilitate thorough examination and assessment, being aware of the environment and keeping the patient warm with a space blanket.

RESUSCITATION

Shock management

Supplemental oxygen therapy is instituted for all trauma patients. A minimum of two large-bore peripheral intravenous catheters should be established. When initiating intravenous lines, blood should be drawn for blood group and cross-match and for baseline haematology and biochemistry.

Vigorous intravenous fluid therapy should be initiated with Hartmann's solution and later colloid. If hypovolaemia persists after infusion of 2–3 L of Hartmann's and colloid, blood transfusion is required. Type-specific blood may be used whilst full cross-match proceeds. If type-specific blood is unavailable, uncross-matched O-negative blood should be used.

When a shock-like state persists despite adequate fluid and resuscitation, and facilities for operation are not immediately available, then the MAST (military anti-shock trousers) suit may be applied, inflated and used in conjunction with continued intravenous fluid resuscitation.

Continuing management

Airway maintenance, cardiopulmonary resuscitation and other life-saving modalities for patient care should be initiated when the problem is identified, rather than after the primary survey.

Monitoring

Adequate resuscitation is best assessed by the quantitative improvement of certain physiological parameters – ventilatory rate, pulse, blood pressure, pulse pressure, arterial blood gases and urinary output – rather than by the qualitative assessment that is done in the primary survey. Actual values should be obtained as soon as is practical after completing the primary survey. Careful ECG monitoring of all patients is required.

The placement of urinary and nasogastric catheters should now be considered. The contraindication for urinary catheterisation is suspected urethral trauma – blood at the urethral meatus, scrotal haematoma or a high-riding prostate on rectal examination. The contraindication for nasogastric catheterisation is a suspected cribriform plate fracture, which is common with facial injuries.

SECONDARY SURVEY

Head and face

The secondary survey begins with evaluation of the head and face and identification of all related and significant injuries. The eyes should be re-evaluated for pupillary size and examined in detail; contact lenses should be removed. Patients with midfacial fractures may have a fracture of the cribriform plate.

Cervical spine and neck

The airway should be maintained and bleeding stopped. Examination of the neck includes both visual inspection and palpation. A lateral radiograph of all the cervical spine should be performed, including all seven cervical vertebrae. A 'swimmer's' view may be necessary. The absence of a neurological deficit, pain or tenderness does not rule out injury to the cervical spine. Such an injury should be presumed present until adequate radiological examination is performed, and even then, if clinical suspicion persists, the cervical spine should be immobilised until injury is definitely excluded.

Chest

A complete evaluation of the chest wall requires inspection and palpation of the entire chest cage, feeling each rib and clavicles individually. Evaluation of the internal structures is done with the stethoscope followed by an erect X-ray of the chest. Decreased breath sounds may be the only indication of a tension pneumothorax, and this is treated by needle thorocentesis followed by intercostal catheter.

Abdomen

Initial examination, close observation and frequent re-evaluation of the abdomen are important in the management of blunt abdominal trauma. Peritoneal lavage may be indicated.

Perineum and rectum

Inspect for lacerations, blood at the urethral meatus or scrotal haematoma. A rectal examination is an essential part of the secondary survey. Specifically, one should assess for the presence of blood within the bowel lumen, a high-riding prostate (indicating a pelvic fracture), the integrity of the rectal wall, and the quality of the sphincter tone.

Extremities

Inspect for deformity and haematoma, and palpate for tenderness, crepitation and abnormal movement. Stress the pelvis. Reduce grossly displaced fractures or dislocations by traction. Splint fractures, relieve pain, and give tetanus immunisation and antibiotics as indicated. In addition, all peripheral pulses should be assessed and their presence or absence documented, along with neurological findings.

Back

Thoracic and lumbar spinal fractures must be considered based on physical findings and mechanism of injury. Log roll to examine for swelling, bruising, tenderness, deformity and penetrating trauma.

Neurological

A comprehensive neurological examination includes not only motor and sensory evaluation of the extremities, but also re-evaluation of the patient's level of consciousness and pupils. The Glasgow Coma Scale is evaluated at this stage.

Any evidence of paralysis or paresis suggests major injury to the spinal column or peripheral nervous system. Immobilisation of the entire patient must be established.

Acute extradural and subdural haematomas, depressed skull fractures and other intracranial injuries should be treated in consultation with a neurosurgeon. Changes in intracranial status may be associated with alterations in the level of consciousness. Oxygenation and perfusion of the brain and the adequacy of ventilation should be reassessed. If these parameters are unchanged, intracranial surgical intervention may be indicated.

DEFINITIVE CARE

The definitive care of each injury will be discussed in other chapters.

TRANSFER

Interhospital triage criteria take into account the patient's physiological status, obvious anatomical injury, mechanism of injury, concurrent diseases, and factors that may alter the patient's prognosis. Emergency department and surgical personnel should use these criteria to determine if the patient requires transfer.

RE-EVALUATE THE PATIENT

The trauma patient should be re-evaluated continuously so that any new signs and symptoms are not overlooked.

RECORDS AND LEGAL CONSIDERATIONS

Precise records are essential to evaluate the patient's needs and clinical status and are helpful for medicolegal reporting. Consent is sought before treatment for obvious reasons. In life-threatening emergencies, the necessary treatment should be given first and formal consent obtained later.

The remainder of this chapter deals with extremity trauma, fractures, joint injuries, spine and spinal cord injuries, and pelvic fractures and perineal injuries.

For details of assessment and management of other specific injuries, see Chapters 13 (brain), 14 (chest), 15 (abdomen), 16 (nerve and vessels) and 17 (burns).

EXTREMITY TRAUMA

Patients with apparently isolated extremity trauma should be managed and assessed in the same manner as multisystem trauma patients.

A primary survey and resuscitation are undertaken. During this assessment the extremities receive little specific attention except for direct control of bleeding, which may include maintaining traction and application of direct pressure. During the secondary survey, the emphasis is on perfusion, alignment and neurovascular injuries. Definitive care involves restoration of perfusion, wound care, restoration of alignment and immobilisation by splints or traction.

EXTREMITY ASSESSMENT

The quality of care administered by pre-hospital (ambulance officers) and emergency department personnel can significantly affect the recovery and ultimate rehabilitation of any patient with extremity trauma.

History

The following information can be obtained from the patient, relatives or bystanders at the accident scene and must be obtained from pre-hospital care personnel. This should be documented and included as part of the patient's medical record.

Mechanisms of injury. If the situation is a motor vehicle accident, this includes the position of the patient in the vehicle; whether the seat belts were fastened and what type they were; whether the patient was ejected; and whether the windscreen or the dashboard was damaged.

Other important information concerning the mechanism of injury includes whether the patient was a pedestrian, fell from a significant height, was injured as a result of fire, smoke and/or an explosion, was injured in an industrial work place, or sustained a crushing injury.

Environment. Important factors are prolonged patient exposure to temperature extremes, near-drowning complications, contaminating factors such as dirt, animal faeces or fresh water, and whether the patient's clothing was torn or intact.

Predisposing factors. These include ingestion of alcohol and/or drugs, emotional problems or illnesses, underlying medical illnesses and previous injuries, especially to the same extremity.

Findings at the accident site. These include the position in which the patient was found, bleeding at the scene, bone or fracture ends exposed, obvious deformity or discoloration, and spontaneous movement of extremities.

Pre-hospital observations and care. These include changes in the limb's function, perfusion or neurological state, spontaneous reduction of fractures or dislocation, dressings and splints applied, extrication procedures and any delays incurred.

Physical examination

The patient must be completely undressed. Always compare an injured extremity with the uninjured extremity. Carry out the following:

- *Look* – examine for colour and perfusion, angulation or shortening, swelling, discoloration and bruising, muscle spasm and wounds.
- *Feel* – examine for sensation, tenderness, crepitation, pulse, capillary filling and warmth.
- *Move* – assess active range of motion. Cautiously examine passive range of motion. Neither an extremity with an obvious fracture or dislocation nor an extremity that the patient refuses to move actively should be moved passively.

Fracture assessment

Fractures are either closed or open (compound).
Any obvious or suspected fracture near a wound should be assumed to be an open fracture. Open fractures are classified by the extent and complexity of the wound, the degree of contamination and the configuration of the fracture as seen on X-rays.

Extremity injuries associated with potentially life-threatening complications. These are crush injuries of the abdomen and pelvis, major pelvic fracture, complete or incomplete traumatic amputations, and massive open long bone fractures with ragged, dirty wounds.

Limb-threatening injuries. These include vascular injuries proximal to the knee or elbow, with or without fractures, crush injuries to an extremity, compartment syndromes, dislocations of the knee or hip, fractures about the elbow or knee, fractures with vascular or nerve injury, and open fractures.

Associated injuries. Certain musculoskeletal injuries are often associated with a second injury that may not be immediately apparent. A history of the injury, clinical suspicion and a full clinical and adequate radiographic examination are important. They include falls onto the hand with wrist, forearm, elbow, arm or shoulder injuries; falls from heights with calcaneal, ankle, tibial, femoral and spinal fractures, femur fracture and hip dislocation, and pelvic fracture with visceral injury.

Occult fractures. These may be easily overlooked in the multiply injured patient and include the following: in cases of head injury, cervical spine fractures and dislocations, particularly C6 and C7; fractures and dislocations of the shoulder girdle; non-displaced fractures of the forearm, femur or pelvis; and complex dislocations of the wrist.

Dislocation and fracture–dislocation assessment

Allowing a major joint to remain dislocated for a protracted period of time can result in accentuated traction injury to the nerve, kinking of vessels with irreversible muscle damage due to vascular compromise, and pressure necrosis of soft tissue and skin. Prolonged delay in reduction of a dislocated hip increases the chances of aseptic necrosis of the femoral head.

All dislocations are painful injuries and pain cannot be relieved until the dislocation is reduced.

Blood loss assessment

Closed extremity injuries may produce enough blood loss to cause hypovolaemic shock – fractures of the pelvis and closed fractures of the femur in particular. Moreover, blood loss from open fractures is far greater than estimated.

Assessment of neurovascular bundle injury

This is discussed in Chapter 16.

Compartment syndrome

Whenever interstitial tissue pressure rises above that of the capillary bed, local ischaemia of nerve and muscle occurs. Permanent paralysis and/or necrosis may result in the form of Volkmann's ischaemic contracture or frank gangrene.

Compartment syndromes usually develop over a period of several hours. They may be initiated by crush injuries, closed or open fractures, prolonged compression of an extremity in a comatose patient, or after restoration of blood flow to a previously ischaemic extremity.

The signs and symptoms of compartment syndrome are as follows: pain greater than that expected from the injury and typically increased by passively stretching involved muscles; decreased sensation of nerves within the involved compartment; tense swelling of the involved region; and weakness or paralysis of involved muscles. Distal pulses and capillary filling do not reliably exclude compartment syndromes. Intracompartmental pressure measurement may help.

Amputation

Amputation is a catastrophic extremity injury. The patient may be a candidate for reimplantation. The amputated part should be rapidly transported with the patient, cleansed of any gross dirt or debris, wrapped in a towel moistened with sterile saline, placed in a sterile, sealed plastic bag, and transported in an insulated cooling chest with crushed ice and water. Do not allow the amputated part to freeze.

EXTREMITY TRAUMA MANAGEMENT

Life-threatening problems, i.e. airway, breathing and circulation, are managed first. After these emergencies are controlled, attention can be directed at the specific extremity injury, usually in the definitive care phase. Patients with extremity injuries are potential candidates for operation and must not receive anything by mouth.

Fractures

If the fracture is open, remove gross contamination and cover the wound with a sterile dressing. Align the fracture and splint the extremity. Initiate appropriate antibiotic coverage and administer tetanus prophylaxis. Open fractures should be definitively treated within 6–8 hours.

Any fracture or suspected fracture must be immobilised to control pain and prevent further injury. Severely angulated fractures should be aligned.

Distal pulses, skin colour, temperature and neurological status are assessed before and after aligning. Gentle traction, as an adjunct to splinting and to facilitate alignment, is beneficial when immobilising long bone fractures. If possible, the splints should extend one joint above and below the fracture site. X-rays, including arteriograms, should not be obtained until the extremity is dressed and splinted.

Joint injuries

Management of dislocations and fracture dislocations has a high priority. Prompt orthopaedic consultation should be obtained for all dislocations and fractures. All dislocations should be reduced as rapidly as possible to prevent or decrease vessel, nerve and skin damage. Immobilise the bones above and below the joint.

Open wounds

Open wounds are best covered with dry, sterile dressings before definitive management. Bleeding is controlled by direct pressure dressings.

Compartment syndrome

When symptoms or suspicion of a compartment syndrome are present, all potentially constricting materials, i.e. circumferential dressings, casts, etc., must be released down to skin over their full length. If symptoms do not respond rapidly with external decompression, prompt fasciotomy will probably be required.

Crush syndrome

The key to management is effective resuscitation, early release of compartment syndrome, maintenance of high urine flow in the presence of myoglobinuria to prevent renal impairment, and early debridement of non-viable tissue.

Antibiotics

Broad-spectrum antibiotics, directed toward the most likely contaminant, should be administered intravenously as soon after the injury as possible, but proper surgical care is the mainstay of wound care. Cultures should be obtained routinely at the time of wound debridement.

Pain control

Care should be exercised in the use of analgesics. Immobilisation of fractures is the safest and most effective method of pain control. If administered, analgesics should be given intravenously. Intramuscular analgesics should not be administered during the initial assessment and treatment phases. If a painful procedure must be carried out, small amounts of analgesics or relaxant, carefully monitored, may be necessary. A 50:50 mixture of oxygen and nitrous oxide (Entonox) may be used during long-distance transfers.

Increasing pain after adequate immobilisation raises the possibility of ischaemic injury or compartment syndrome.

Tetanus immunisation

Tetanus immunisation depends upon the patient's previous immunisation status and the tetanus-prone nature of the wound (see Ch. 15).

Immobilisation techniques

The hand should be splinted temporarily in an anatomical position, achieved by gently immobilising the hand over a large gauze roll. The forearm and wrist are splinted in a flexed position. The arm is immobilised by splinting to the body or by simple application of a sling or binder; circumferential bandages can have a tourniquet effect. The extremity must be monitored frequently for vascular compromise. All splints must be padded over bony prominences. All jewellery, including rings, bracelets, etc., must be removed before splinting.

Femoral fractures are best splinted with traction splints. Traction splints may be used for ipsilateral femoral and tibial fractures. Excessive traction should be avoided. Tibia fractures are best immobilised with a padded board splint or aluminium gutter splint. Ankle fractures may be immobilised with a pillow splint or padded board splint.

SUMMARY

Life-threatening situations must be properly assessed and managed before attention is directed to the injured extremity. Early alignment of fracture and dislocations and proper splinting techniques can prevent serious complications and late sequelae of extremity trauma.

In the multiply injured patient with extremity trauma, operative fixation of fractures within the first 24 hours may reduce mortality and morbidity. It is essential to obtain orthopaedic consultation early in the patient's management.

FRACTURES

CLASSIFICATION

Fractures are classified as either *closed or open*, otherwise known as compound, and 'open' implies a fracture associated with an open wound.

Fractures may be either simple (two fragments) or comminuted (multiple fragments). Fractures are described by the line of the fracture (transverse, oblique, spiral, incomplete, greenstick in children); by their special type (compression/crush, intra-articular, growth plate/physeal, pathological, stress); by the degree of displacement and tilt/angulation; and by their association with joints in fracture dislocations.

THE HEALING OF FRACTURES

Normal healing requires:

- apposition of bony ends without other tissue in between
- adequate blood supply
- relative immobility of the bone ends
- freedom from infection

The normal sequence of healing is as follows:

1. At the time of injury, haemorrhage occurs and a haematoma forms around the fracture site (0–4 days).

2. Granulation tissue forms in the haematoma and osteogenic cells are mobilised (4–14 days).

3. Provisional callus is laid down, forming a bridge between the bone ends (14 days onward).

4. Progressive remodelling of the provisional callus occurs over several months leaving the fracture united by compact bone.

SURGICAL MANAGEMENT OF THE OPEN FRACTURE

The patient is given a general or regional anaesthetic. An uninflated tourniquet is normally applied unless it creates problems in the assessment or definitive fracture treatment; thus massive haemorrhage can be controlled. The wound and limb are cleansed with an aqueous antiseptic and the wound covered with sterile dressings.

Wound excision (debridement)

The various structures are dealt with as follows.

Skin. A minimum of skin should be excised, and dead skin is removed. The wound must be extended if exposure of the deeper tissues is inadequate.

Muscle and fascia. Division of tight deep fascia may be necessary to improve the circulation to muscle which has been compressed by haematoma and oedema fluid. Necrotic muscle is excised and any foreign material is removed.

Vessels. Small bleeding vessels are cauterised. Major arteries are repaired if they are essential for limb survival.

Nerves. Primary nerve suture is undertaken if an ideal wound can be created; otherwise divided ends are marked with coloured monofilament sutures.

Tendons. Tendons can be repaired if the wound is relatively uncontaminated.

Bone. If there is a compound fracture, completely detached fragments of bone are removed; foreign material is carefully cleaned from the bone ends and the fracture is reduced under direct vision. However, if minimally contaminated, large structural fragments may be retained.

Wound closure

Primary wound closure is contraindicated. The wound is loosely packed with Betadine-soaked dressings.

Immobilisation is essential for soft tissue and bone healing. If the fracture allows, external splintage is used, but external fixation is particularly useful, although internal fixation may be employed. If an encircling plaster is used, it should be split from end to end to enable inevitable swelling to take place without compromising the circulation or a plaster splint should be used.

Delayed primary closure should be employed in all compound fractures with few exceptions. It prevents tension on the wound and resultant further ischaemic necrosis, and allows a second 'clean and look'.

The definitive wound closure is by direct suture, split skin graft, local flap or free vascularised flap, and is usually undertaken at approximately 5 days. If the wound is grossly contaminated or if soft tissue trauma is extreme, further debridement should be undertaken approximately every second or third day following injury. The aim is to maintain a clean wound free of dead tissue. Provided adequate immobilisation is achieved initially, definitive fracture fixation can usefully be delayed until the wound is clean and tissues are viable, at delayed closure.

RADIOGRAPHIC INVESTIGATION OF FRACTURES AND DISLOCATIONS

In most instances plain radiographs will be more than adequate to plan and monitor treatment. The 'rule of two' applies:

- *Two* views are necessary as a fracture or a dislocation may not be seen in a single view.
- *Two* joints, those above and below a fracture, must be included.
- Radiographs on *two* occasions may be necessary as some fractures may not be easily seen until 10 days.
- *Two* limbs may be X-rayed, especially in children in which the presence of uncalcified cartilage or the growth plate may confuse interpretation.

Remember that X-rays are shadows; they do not tell the complete story and they do not show the position of the bones at the time of maximal displacement at injury. Sometimes, computerised tomography for the spine and pelvic fractures and radioisotope scans for stress fractures may be necessary.

PRINCIPLES OF FRACTURE TREATMENT

Treatment of a fracture involves reduction, holding the fracture fragments until they unite, preservation of joint movement and function, and rehabilitation.

Reduction

When a bone is broken, the periosteum is also torn but usually remains intact on one part of the bone as a 'hinge of soft tissue'. By understanding the deforming forces of the injury, the site of this hinge can be worked out and used to maintain reduction.

Fractures can be reduced by traction, manipulation or open reduction. With adequate traction, many fractures will reduce. If not, manipulation is indicated. Initially the deforming force is increased, opening the bone ends on the soft tissue hinge, opposing the fragments and then closing the hinge. When traction and manipulation fail, open reduction is indicated.

Holding the fracture

This can be achieved simply by traction, by splintage with plaster, functional braces or external fixation devices fixed with pins to bone, or by internal fixation with plates, screws or nails. Internal fixation is sometimes the treatment of choice. An example of this is fractured neck of the femur in the elderly, where prolonged traction is accompanied by the problems of recumbency with pressure sores, pneumonia and deep vein thrombosis, and immobilisation in plaster is clearly not appropriate. There are many other strong indications for open reduction and internal fixation.

In the immediate post-reduction period (particularly if the immobilisation includes a circumferential plaster), check repeatedly for circulatory inadequacy distal to the fracture, which is best demonstrated by pain on passive movements of toes or fingers. Measures required to deal with impending ischaemia may vary from splitting a plaster to fasciotomy.

Joint movement and preservation of function

Ideally, joint movement should begin immediately as this maintains range of movement, promotes fracture healing by physiological loading of bone by muscle activity and weight-bearing, and prevents muscle wasting. However, experience has shown that a short period of immobilisation of joints around many fractures is acceptable while the fracture unites, provided function of the rest of the limb is maintained.

Rehabilitation

The surgeon's responsibility does not end with healing of the fracture. Rehabilitation starts from the time of operation. Active physiotherapy maintains muscle tone, improves circulation and reduces oedema and subsequent joint stiffness. It is continued after the fracture has united. Occupational therapy is begun as early as possible.

COMPLICATIONS OF FRACTURES

These fall into two categories: general and local.

General complications

These include shock, fat embolism which produces acute post-traumatic respiratory distress, crush syndrome which threatens renal function, gas gangrene and tetanus, and deep venous thrombosis and pulmonary embolism.

Local complications

Delayed wound healing and infection. This can be largely avoided by delayed primary closure. If infection is suspected, operative drainage, culture and appropriate antibiotic therapy are priorities. Chronic infection, osteomyelitis, may result and may not resolve until the removal of the separated dead fragment of infected bone (sequestrum).

Delayed or non-union. If the fracture is mobile and still healing, albeit slowly, delayed union is present and a change in the treatment plan may be necessary to prevent non-union. Non-union implies that fracture healing has ceased and implies intervention in the form of better reduction and immobilisation, often with internal fixation, bone grafting, improved blood supply and more physiological loading may be necessary.

Malunion. The fracture unites in an unsatisfactory position.

Growth disturbance. As a result of injury to the growth plate (physis) in children, progressive deformity may occur due to asymmetrical growth or shortening due to premature fusion of the physis.

Avascular necrosis. Interruption to blood supply is particularly common in areas of bones which are largely intra-articular; common examples include the head of femur and scaphoid.

Joint stiffness. This may result from immobilisation of a joint, resulting in contracture of the joint capsule and ligaments, and is prone to occur with intra-articular fractures. Musculo-tenderness contracture and adhesion may also cause this. Malunion of intra-articular fractures will also produce lack of joint movement.

Heterotopic ossification. This may affect the joint and muscle at the site of injury. Head-injured patients are particularly prone to this condition.

Nerve and vessel injury. See Chapter 16.

Compartment syndrome. See page 97.

Osteoarthritis. Post-traumatic arthritis may develop rapidly following injury to the articular cartilage or incongruity of a joint following fracture.

JOINT INJURIES

Joint injuries may result in a partial or complete tear of the joint capsule and ligaments, an avulsion of bone at the site of ligament attachment, damage to the articular cartilage and damage to bone beneath the articular cartilage. The result is either that the joint remains congruent or a subluxation results in which the articular surfaces are partially displaced, or that a dislocation occurs in which there is complete displacement of the joint. Recurrent dislocation may occur if the ligaments and joint margins are damaged. Habitual dislocation can be achieved by voluntary muscle contraction.

The definitive treatment of ligament injuries will depend on the extent of the injury, the patient's requirements and the known natural history of the condition. Treatment may range from no immobilisation and early exercises, intermittent splintage or protective braces or splints, to surgical repair and/or reconstruction involving ligament or tendon substitution. The complications of joint injuries include nerve and vessel injuries, recurrent instability, avascular necrosis of bone, heterotopic ossification, joint stiffness and osteoarthritis.

SPINE AND SPINAL CORD INJURIES

ASSESSMENT OF SUSPECTED SPINAL INJURY

Any patient sustaining a high speed injury, an injury above the clavicle, or head injury resulting in an unconscious state should be suspected of having an associated cervical spine injury.

History

The history of mechanism of injury, of paralysis immediately post-injury, or deterioration of the patient's sensori-motor status is important.

A conscious patient with paralysis is usually able to identify pain at the site of injury, because loss of sensation is below this level. If the patient is unconscious, and the injury is due to a fall or a vehicular accident, the chance of a cervical spine injury is 5–10%.

Examination

Examination of any suspected case of spinal injury must be carried out with the patient in a neutral position and without any movement of the patient's spine.

The patient is carefully examined for motor strength and weakness, sensory disturbances, reflex changes and autonomic dysfunction. Autonomic dysfunction is identified by lack of bladder and rectal control, and priapism. Preservation of sensation in the sacral region may be the only sign that the spinal cord lesion is incomplete.

Clinical findings that suggest a cervical cord injury include flaccid areflexia, especially with flaccid rectal sphincter, diaphragmatic breathing, ability to flex but not extend the elbow, grimaces of pain above but not below the clavicle, hypotension with bradycardia especially without hypovolaemia, and priapism which is an uncommon but characteristic sign.

Vertebral injuries are usually associated with local tenderness and less often with palpable deformity, swelling and bruising. Muscle spasm limiting movement and head tilt is an important sign. If the patient does not have head control or trunk control then one should suspect an unstable cervical or thoracolumbar spine injury, respectively.

Penetrating injuries, usually from a gunshot, require urgent attention.

Radiographs

Radiographs should be examined for:

- anteroposterior diameter of the spinal canal
- contour and alignment of the spine with particular reference to widening of the interspinous gap and rotational malalignment
- displacement of bone fragments into the spinal canal
- fractures of the vertebral bodies or posterior elements
- soft tissue swelling.

The whole of the cervical spine to C7–T1 must be visualised. A swimmer's view may be required. Definitive radiographs are necessary. Flexion/extension views may be dangerous and should only be carried out under specialist supervision. A CT scan or myelogram will demonstrate spinal encroachment.

IMMEDIATE TREATMENT OF SUSPECTED SPINAL INJURY

The following procedure should be followed:

1. Attend to life-threatening injuries, avoiding any movement of the spinal column.

2. Establish and maintain proper immobilisation of the patient until vertebral fractures or spinal cord injuries have been ruled out.

3. Insert i.v. line and urinary catheter. Maintain respiratory function if necessary.

4. Obtain lateral cervical spine X-rays as soon as life-threatening injuries are controlled. Later, definitive X-rays will be necessary in suspected cases.

5. Documentation of the patient's history and physical examination are of paramount importance to establish a baseline for any changes in the patient's neurological status (i.e. ascertaining progress or deterioration of an incomplete lesion).

6. Obtain consultation with a spinal surgeon.

7. Transfer patient with unstable vertebral fractures or spinal cord injury to a spinal injuries unit.

SPECIAL FEATURES OF SPINAL INJURIES

Neurogenic shock

The term neurogenic shock is generally used to describe the hypotension and bradycardia associated with cervical or high thoracic spinal cord injury resulting in impairment of the descending sympathetic pathways. The blood pressure can often be restored by elevating the legs to promote blood return to the heart. Atropine can be used to counteract the bradycardia.

Spinal shock

Spinal shock refers to the neurological condition shortly after spinal cord injury. The 'shock' of the injured cord causes a conduction defect and may make it appear completely functionless, even though all areas are not permanently destroyed. This produces flaccidity and loss of reflexes instead of the expected spasticity, hyperactive reflexes and Babinski signs. Days to weeks later, spinal shock disappears and, in areas where no function has returned, spasticity supersedes the flaccid state.

Respiratory paralysis

Hypoventilation due to paralysis of the intercostal muscles will result from an injury involving the lower cervical or the upper thoracic spinal cord. If the upper or the middle cervical spinal cord is injured, the diaphragm will also be paralysed.

Mechanism of spinal injury

Spinal fractures most commonly occur as a result of flexion injury in which one vertebral body is driven against another to produce a compression injury. At the same time there is often rotation, fracturing the facet joints and so allowing dislocation with or without damage to the spinal cord. Less commonly, and nearly always in the cervical spine, an extension fracture or fracture dislocation may occur. Axial loading, lateral bending and distraction may also occur.

Stability of the spine

It is important to determine whether the injury is stable or unstable. Patients who have an unstable injury may not be paralysed but may become so. When interpreting radiographs, the spine can usefully be divided into two columns: an anterior column consisting of the vertebral bodies, intervertebral discs and the longitudinal ligaments; and a posterior column consisting of the posterior body elements and ligaments.

However, instability due to major ligament injury may not be obvious initially and treatment is based on clinical suspicion.

Stable injuries include transverse process fractures, isolated spinous process fractures and anterior compression fractures. If there is an injury to both columns or if there is rotational or translational malalignment, the spine is unstable. Unstable injuries include fracture dislocations of the cervical, thoracic or lumbar spine, some burst fractures, and fractures of the atlas and axis.

Treatment of the spinal column injury

Stable vertebral column injuries such as compression fractures of a single lumbar vertebra are treated by initial bed rest followed by rapid mobilisation. There is no place for immobilisation in a plaster jacket, as used to be practised.

The patient with a spinal cord injury, an unstable fracture or a fracture dislocation requires highly specialised treatment and should be transferred to a spinal injuries unit. In the cervical spine, treatment is usually traction initially, and in the lumbar spine immobilisation on a spinal bed. Operative reduction and internal fixation offer considerable advantages in appropriate cases and may be required as a matter of some urgency.

Spinal cord recovery

In cases of mild damage, recovery of function occurs after 24 or 48 hours. If there is permanent damage to the cord, recovery of function is delayed. No recovery after 48 hours is a poor prognostic sign.

Neurological lesions may be partial or complete. With partial lesions, recovery produces a spastic paralysis with extensor plantar responses and variable return of sensation. With a complete lesion there is spastic paralysis which occasionally is associated with a mass flexor reflex. This is massive flexor response to minimal stimulation.

The bladder

The paralysis of spinal shock produces an atonic neurogenic bladder and retention of urine. With recovery, if the level of the lesion is above the level of S2, spinal innervation to and from the bladder is intact and an automatic bladder results, which empties every 2–4 hours.

Below S2, there is no sensation and no reflex arcs,

except the intramural bladder reflexes are intact. The result is an autonomous bladder which would tend to dribble spontaneously were not bladder training undertaken.

Autonomic hyperreflexia

It is important to recognise this potential medical emergency in patients with high spinal cord injuries. A stimulus such as a distended bladder, severe spastic bladder, faecal impaction, skin abrasion or urological procedure indicates a reflex action of the autonomic nervous system precipitating a hypertensive episode that requires immediate treatment. Clinical features include sweating above the level of the injury, goose bumps, flushing, pounding headache and elevated blood pressure.

DEFINITIVE TREATMENT OF SPINAL INJURIES AND SPINAL CORD INJURIES

The major aims of treatment of patients with spinal cord injuries are to prevent complications and to preserve function. Patients are best treated in, or transferred to, a spinal injuries unit. Specifically, treatment consists of:

- obtaining and maintaining reduction of displaced fracture/dislocations
- prevention of pressure sores
- prevention of urinary infection through intermittent catheterisation of the bladder
- prevention of constipation by the use of enemas
- physiotherapy to prevent hypostatic pneumonia and mobilisation of joints to prevent contractures
- rehabilitation and return to the community.

PELVIC FRACTURES AND PERINEAL INJURIES

Of all bony injuries, pelvic fractures are the most likely to be the combined concern of orthopaedic and other surgeons. Pelvic fractures occur in the most severe form as the result of crushing injuries, when they assume particular importance because of the likelihood of associated damage to the bladder and urethra and other organs.

CLINICAL FEATURES

Pelvic fracture

There is tenderness at the site of impact or fracture and

tenderness on springing the pelvis. There is also severe pain and inability to stand when pelvic ring disruption is present.

Shock, which is often marked when there is pelvic ring disruption, is due to pelvic bleeding, especially if associated visceral injuries are present.

Congenital injuries

Intraperitoneal rupture of the bladder, extraperitoneal rupture of the bladder, or rupture of membranous urethra causes suprapubic or abdominal pain, inability or failure to pass urine, and blood at the urinary meatus. Rectal examination is mandatory.

Lumbosacral plexus and sciatic nerve injury

Anaesthesia and weakness of part of the leg occur, particularly in association with vertical sheer type of pelvic ring disruption.

SPECIAL TESTS

These include:

- plain X-ray of the pelvis, including inlet and outlet views
- cysto-urethrogram if bladder or urethral rupture is suspected
- intravenous pyelogram to exclude rectal trauma as the cause of haematuria.

CLASSIFICATION OF PELVIC FRACTURES

These can be classified into one of three categories, as described below.

Stable

These include fractures that are not disrupting the pelvic ring, i.e. avulsion fractures, isolated iliac wing fractures and isolated pubic ramus fractures. Treatment is symptomatic and little or no bed rest is necessary.

Minimally displaced fractures involving the pelvic ring also fall into this category.

Rotationally unstable, vertically stable

This designation includes often book fractures and lateral compression fractures, both contralateral and ipsilateral.

Open book injury with pubic diastasis greater than 2.5 cm should be closed using a pelvic sling, an anterior external fixation frame or internal fixation.

Lateral compression fractures – unless grossly displaced or causing either visceral injury or impingement, or shortening of the leg greater than 1.5 cm – usually require symptomatic treatment and bed rest. If grossly displaced or associated with severe pelvic bleeding then reduction and anterior internal or external fixation are indicated. 'Four post' bilateral pubic rami fractures from lateral or anterior compression are treated similarly, but associated urethral tears are not uncommon.

Rotationally and vertically unstable

These vertical shear injuries require reduction by skeletal traction, but are often best treated by open reduction and internal fixation posteriorly and anterior fixation.

TREATMENT OF PELVIC FRACTURES

Treatment is by:

- Intial assessment and resuscitation.
- Correction of shock. This may include urgent closure of 'open book' fractures of the pelvis by a binder or an anterior external fixation frame, and skeletal traction on a vertically displaced pelvic injury. This tamponades severe pelvic bleeding.
- Urinary catheterisation. An ascending urethrogram is mandatory prior to catheterisation if there is blood at the meatus or suspicion of urethral rupture. If this injury is suspected or confirmed, the bladder is best decompressed by a suprapubic catheterisation.

ACETABULAR FRACTURES

Pelvic fractures should not be confused with fractures of the acetabulum. Acetabulum fractures are associated with central, posterior or anterior hip dislocations and are treated according to the principles of managing any intra-articular fracture. Often, open reduction and internal fixation are indicated. Posterior and anterior hip dislocations require urgent reduction; the reduction must be stable and concentric.

FURTHER READING

American College of Surgeons 1997 Advanced trauma and life support: program for doctors. Course manual, 6th edn.

Apley A G, Solomon L 1987 Apley's system of orthopaedics and fractures, 6th edn. Butterworths, London

Dandy D J 1987 Essential orthopaedics and trauma. Churchill Livingstone, Edinburgh

Duckworth T 1995 Lecture notes on orthopaedics and fractures, 3rd edn. Blackwell Science, Oxford

Grundy D, Swain A 1996 ABC of spinal cord injury, 3rd edn. BMJ Publishing, London

Huckstep R L 1986 A simple guide to trauma, 4th edn. Churchill Livingstone, Edinburgh

Robertson C, Redmond A D 1994 The management of major trauma, 2nd edn. Oxford University Press, Oxford

Skinner D, Driscoll P, Earlam R 1996 ABC of major trauma, 2nd edn. BMJ Publishing, London

Brain injuries
Graeme Brazenor

OVERVIEW

Injury to the brain, often called head injury, from blunt or penetrating mechanisms, is the commonest cause of death and morbidity in all forms of trauma. This chapter describes the mechanisms of primary brain injury and of how other factors can cause secondary brain injury. The clinical features of raised intracranial pressure and the assessment of the unconscious patient using the Glasgow Coma Chart are covered, with investigations and treatment.

Brain injury is caused by the transfer of energy. This commonly occurs in accidents in motor vehicles, industry, sport and in the home.

Brain injury is of two types: primary and secondary. Primary brain injury is that which occurs whilst energy is being transferred to or from the brain. For example, when a cricketer is struck on the head by the ball, primary brain damage can occur only during the collision.

Secondary brain injury is that which occurs after energy transfer is complete. For example, unbeknown to the cricketer, the impact of the ball has fractured his squamous temporal bone and torn the underlying middle meningeal artery. An extradural haematoma begins to collect between dura mater and skull, even as he picks himself up and staggers from the field. Half an hour later he is discovered in the dressing room unconscious, decerebrate and breathing stertorously. Despite being rushed to a neurosurgical unit where the haematoma is evacuated, he remains decerebrate and never leaves hospital, due to secondary brain injury caused by the haematoma.

MECHANISMS OF PRIMARY BRAIN INJURY

There are five well-recognised mechanisms by which primary brain injury is produced:

- acceleration of the brain
- direct disruption in open head injury
- contusion
- contre-coup
- compression.

Acceleration of the brain

Energy imparted to the brain causing its acceleration or deceleration is the primary mode of injury in most closed or blunt head injuries. These are defined as injuries in which the injuring agent does not penetrate the skull and meninges.

When the head (and hence the brain) is accelerated as in Figure 13.1, or decelerated as in Figure 13.2, the brain dissipates the energy imparted to it by internal movements and gyrations. At low energies these gyrations cause only temporary disruption of function (e.g. amnesia for the event, or perhaps brief loss of consciousness), but at higher energies they may cause disruption of neurons or even tearing of the brain substance. The brain may also be lacerated or contused where it strikes dural structures such as the falx cerebri, or bony ridges on the floor of the anterior and middle cranial fossae.

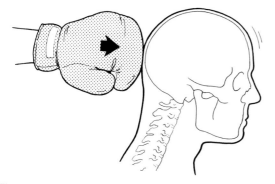

Fig. 13.1 Closed head injury: acceleration of the brain.

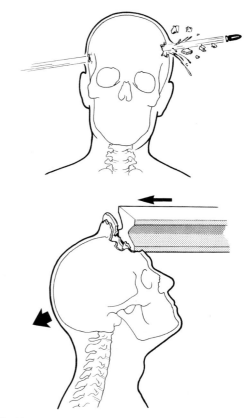

Fig. 13.3 Open head injuries.

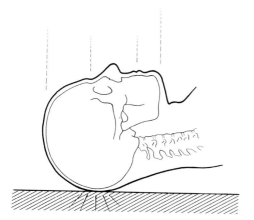

Fig. 13.2 Closed head injury: deceleration of the brain.

Direct disruption in open head injury

An open head injury is defined as one in which the injuring agent penetrates the skull and meninges, as seen in Figure 13.3. When the agent actually traverses brain, as in the two examples shown, primary injury occurs by direct disruption.

The severity of the functional impairment resulting from such an injury depends upon the extent of disruption, as well as on the function of the injured part of the brain.

Note that the direct disruptive effect of a wounding agent is often not its most injurious aspect. In injuries like those shown, the magnitude of the energy transfer is often what determines the patient's prognosis. Thus in a low-velocity missile wound, most of the injury will be due to direct disruption, but with a high-velocity projectile the shock wave spreading outward from its passage will destroy the entire brain in microseconds.

Contusion

Contusion or bruising may occur when the brain strikes bony or dural structures during gyrations of its surface, as described above; or it may occur beneath the skull at the site of impact, due to localised inbending of the skull at the moment of collision (Fig. 13.4). As for direct disruption, the severity of the functional impairment following such an injury will depend upon the extent of the contusion as well as on the function of the injured part of the brain.

Contre-coup

When the brain is accelerated there is an instantaneous positive force generated immediately beneath the site of collision. Because of the physics of acceleration of gelatinous bodies, there is at the same time an instantaneous negative pressure generated in the opposite pole(s) of the brain (Fig. 13.5). Some authorities estimate this as at least -2 or -3 atmospheres (-200 or -300 kPa), and it

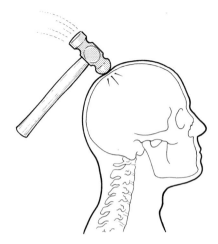

Fig. 13.4 Localised contusion injury.

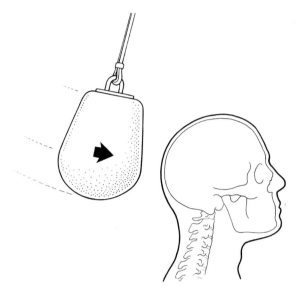

is frequently sufficient to disrupt brain and blood vessels at that point, leading to pulping and haemorrhage opposite to where the blow was delivered. Such a lesion is termed a contre-coup lesion, meaning 'opposite the blow'.

Figure 13.6 shows one cut from a CT scan of a patient who has suffered a blow to the right occipitoparietal region, with a consequent contre-coup lesion of the opposite frontal lobe.

Compression

Compression of the head is an uncommon injury; examples include when the patient's head is stamped upon by an assailant, or when the head is trapped beneath a car which falls off its jack. Such patients not infrequently incur cranial nerve palsies, but injury to the brain is rare, as no momentum is transferred to the cerebrum.

SURGICAL ANATOMY RELEVANT TO RAISED INTRACRANIAL PRESSURE

Figure 13.7 shows a coronal section through the head, demonstrating compartments above and below the tentorium cerebelli, with the midbrain occupying the tentorial hiatus. Figure 13.8 shows the same section in a patient with an extradural haematoma. Note that the plastic brain is herniating: from left to right beneath the falx cerebri, from the supratentorial to the infratentorial compartment, and from right to left across the tentorial hiatus. Figure 13.9 shows a patient with diffuse swelling of the

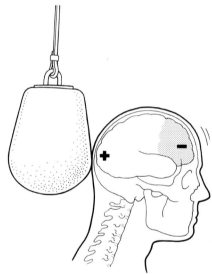

Fig. 13.5 Mechanism of contre-coup injury. In this case, the injury is to the frontal lobes: +, positive pressure in leading pole(s) of the brain; −, negative pressure in trailing pole(s) of the brain.

brain after a severe acceleration injury, in whom symmetrical cephalocaudal herniation of the brain is occurring.

It is these herniations of brain matter which lead to secondary brain injury, when caused by an intracranial haematoma or brain swelling. The aim of head injury care is to anticipate and prevent such herniations or, at worst, to detect them in the extremely early stages so that they may be reversed.

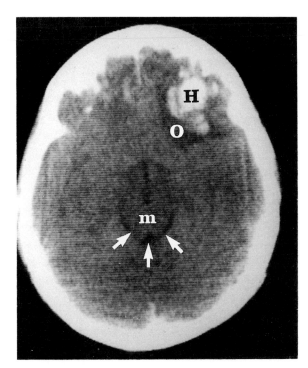

Fig. 13.6 CT scan of brain after impact in right occipitoparietal region. H, haematoma in the left frontal lobe due to the contre-coup phenomenon; o, oedema surrounding the haematoma; m, midbrain; ↑, cisterna ambiens.

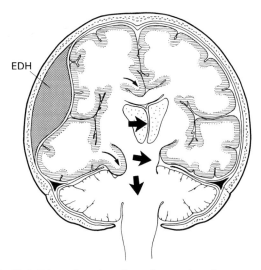

Fig. 13.8 Coronal section of a patient undergoing herniations of brain (indicated by arrows) due to supratentorial extradural haematoma (EDH).

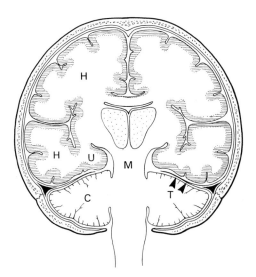

Fig. 13.7 Coronal section through brain stem. T, tentorium cerebelli; H, cerebral hemisphere; U, uncus of temporal lobe; M, midbrain (mesencephalon); C, cerebellar hemisphere.

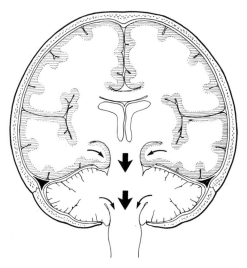

Fig. 13.9 Coronal section of a patient undergoing pure rostrocaudal herniation ('coning') of the brain and brain stem due to diffuse brain swelling after severe acceleration injury.

Note, in Figure 13.8, how the medial aspect of the temporal lobe (the uncus) can be forced down into the tentorial hiatus beside the mesencephalon, thus impinging upon the ipsilateral third nerve to produce a dilating pupil, fixed to light, on that side. Until the advent of the Glasgow Coma Chart (see below) the dilating pupil, fixed to light, was the best yardstick of the patient deteriorating due to raised intracranial pressure. However, it should now be possible in most cases to detect clinical signs of rising intracranial pressure and brain herniation before these processes have progressed to the late stage of dilatation of one or both pupils.

GLASGOW COMA CHART

In 1974 Teasdale and Jennett published the Glasgow Coma Scale. Thus came into being the first useful attempt at quantifying the conscious states of patients. The strength of the chart is that, if the observations are made and recorded in a strictly standardised way, the chart is an extremely sensitive and reliable method for detecting deterioration in conscious state. Measures can thus be taken to reverse the pathological processes threatening the patient's life before permanent neurological injury occurs.

Figure 13.10 shows the 'best response' section of a patient's Glasgow Coma Chart. Observations are taken in three categories: eye opening, best verbal response and best motor response. Observations taken at the same time are recorded in a single vertical column, with the time of the observation at the top. In the first and third categories, an 'X' means that both sides of the body respond in the same way. If this is not found to be the case, an 'R' and an 'L' are recorded on separate lines to indicate the responses of the separate body sides.

EYE OPENING

The minimum stimulus required to elicit eye opening is determined. The patient's eyes may already be open (*spontaneous*); they may open in response to the observer saying the patient's *name*; or they may open in response to a standard *painful* stimulus. Failing that, *none* is recorded.

BEST VERBAL RESPONSE

Following completion of eye-opening observations, the observer presents a standard verbal stimulus to the patient by saying clearly: 'Mr . . . , do you know where you are?' The patient may give an *orientated* response, he may be *confused* as to where he is, he may deliver an answer which is *inappropriate* to the question, the response may be *incomprehensible*, or there may be *no* response at all.

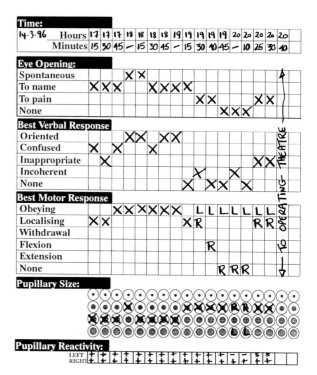

Fig. 13.10 Glasgow Coma Chart of a patient following assault, sustaining a left extradural haematoma (EDH). First deterioration occurred at 19.15 hours, and complete hemiparesis at 19.45 hours. Improvement occurred with intravenous mannitol and intubation with hyperventilation at 20.25 hours. The EDH was confirmed with urgent CT scan followed by immediate craniotomy with evacuation of the haematoma.

BEST MOTOR RESPONSE

Only the arms are tested in this coma chart, as they are better windows on cerebral function than are the lower limbs. The best response of each arm should be recorded separately if they are found to be different.

The patient is first asked to squeeze the observer's fingers with both hands. This will determine if one or both limbs are *obeying*. Failure of a limb to obey will result in the application of a standard painful stimulus to the sternum; if a limb is brought up to where the stimulus is being applied, it is classified as *localising*. If a limb fails to obey or localise, then a standard painful stimulus is applied to the limb itself and the observer records whether the limb undergoes an apparently coordinated *withdrawal*, just spastic *flexion*, decerebrate *extension* or no movement at all.

The exact protocol for taking the observations varies from hospital to hospital, especially in the particular painful stimuli used. The principle of paramount importance, however, is that the observations must be taken in exactly the same way by everyone within the same institution.

Figure 13.10 is a Glasgow Coma Chart recorded on a man who presented to the emergency department after being assaulted. He had a large scalp haematoma in the left parietal region and a fracture on skull X-ray running from the site of impact down to the left external auditory meatus. As can be seen from the figure, when admitted to the emergency department at 17.15 hours the patient was eye opening to name, confused and localising with both upper limbs. Forty-five minutes later he was normal, with eyes open spontaneously, fully orientated and obeying with both hands. At 19.15 hours, however, the first deterioration was noted: he was eye opening only to pain, had no verbal response and was localising bilaterally. By the time another nurse was summoned to check the observations the patient was again obeying with the left upper limb, but the best motor response of the right continued to deteriorate over the next 20 minutes. During this time a resident medical officer was called, who assessed the patient and diagnosed rising intracranial pressure and progressing brain herniation, most probably due to a left-sided extradural haematoma. The resident inserted an intravenous line and administered 20% mannitol in a dose of 1 g mannitol/kg body weight, infused over 20 minutes. In addition he paged the duty anaesthetics registrar to intubate the patient, notified the CT scanning facility and the on-call neurosurgeon of the patient's impending emergency CT scan, and inserted a urinary catheter.

Whilst the resident was attending to all of these tasks, the patient became completely hemiparetic (between 19.45 and 20.10 on the chart) and finally dilated the left pupil. Fortunately the mannitol was being infused by this time and the patient's condition began to improve dramatically at 20.25, at the time he was being loaded into the CT scanner, having been intubated and ventilated to a P_{CO_2} of 30–35 mmHg. CT scan revealed the left temporal extradural haematoma, and the patient was taken straight from the CT scanner to the operating theatre. Craniotomy was rapidly performed over the precise location required. The extradural haematoma was completely evacuated and absolute haemostasis obtained; the bone flap was replaced and the patient was returned to the ward. Ten days later the patient was discharged from hospital apparently neurologically unscathed.

The Glasgow Coma Scale can also be scored, and the

Table 13.1	Method of scoring Glasgow coma responses	
	Response	Score
Eye opening	Spontaneous	4
	To name	3
	To pain	2
	None	1
Best verbal response	Orientated	5
	Confused	4
	Inappropriate	3
	Incomprehensible	2
	None	1
Best motor response	Obeying	6
	Localising	5
	Withdrawal	4
	Abnormal flexion	3
	Extension	2
	None	1

numbers subjected to mathematical analysis. Table 13.1 shows the scoring system.

From Table 13.1 it can be seen that a patient who opens his eyes to pain, has an incomprehensible verbal response and extends his limbs to pain will accrue a Glasgow Coma Score of 6 points out of the maximum possible score of 15. It is a curious feature of this system of scoring that a dead person scores 3 points, rather than zero as one might have expected.

MECHANISMS OF SECONDARY BRAIN INJURY

If there were no causes of secondary brain injury after trauma it would not be necessary to admit patients to acute hospitals after head injury, no matter how severe. We hospitalise head-injured patients in an attempt to prevent secondary brain injury. The major causes of secondary brain injury are as follows.

BRAIN SWELLING

The CT scan has shown that the brain may swell within minutes of an injury, and this is usually not oedema as used to be thought. Rather, it would appear to be dilatation of the microcirculation of the brain, so that it fills with blood within the vascular system, like a sail filling with wind (Fig. 13.11). In severe cases this can occur within 10 minutes of a severe injury, and it may last for up to 2 weeks.

This phenomenon is the single most frequent cause of

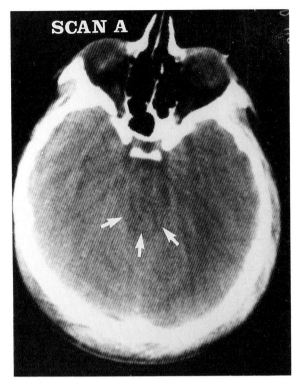
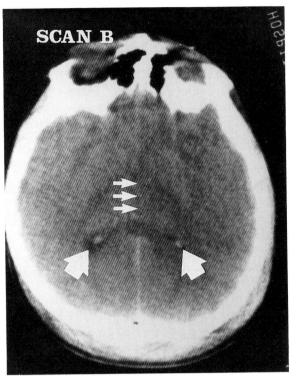

Fig. 13.11 CT scan of brain following severe acceleration injury. Scan A. Note the complete absence of cisterna ambiens around the pontomesencephalic junction. Arrows indicate where it should be seen (cf. normal cistern in Fig. 13.6). **Scan B.** Note the compression of the cerebral ventricles: third ventricle (indicated by ⇉) and atria of lateral ventricle (↑).

life-threatening rise in intracranial pressure after head trauma, and it outnumbers all of the other causes. Treatment is discussed on page 117.

BRAIN OEDEMA

Brain oedema does occur after injury, but it is usually focal. For example, swelling confined to one lobe of the brain on CT scan is most likely to be oedema, secondary either to local contusion or to the contre-coup phenomenon from a blow to the opposite side of the brain.

INTRACRANIAL HAEMATOMA

Haematomata occurring within the cranium after trauma are of three common types: extradural, subdural (acute and chronic) and intra-axial.

Extradural

This haematoma (Fig. 13.12) is common. It is particular-

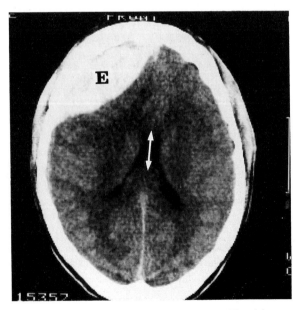

Fig. 13.12 CT scan showing brain compressed by right frontal extradural haematoma (E). Septum pellucidum is indicated (⟷) to show displacement of midline structures.

ly common in young males, perhaps because they move at high velocity and incur skull fractures. It is rare in the elderly, perhaps because the dura mater is more firmly attached to the inner table of the skull.

The extradural haematoma generally occurs beneath the site of a skull fracture, and the patient, like the cricketer described earlier, may experience an early interval of comparatively normal conscious state (the 'lucid interval') before continued accumulation of the haematoma causes brain herniation and loss of consciousness.

Acute subdural

This haematoma (Fig. 13.13) is seen in three sorts of patients. It is seen in infants, where movement of the mobile skull bones can rupture veins crossing the subdural space from the brain to dural venous sinuses. It is seen in the elderly, in whom atrophy of the brain renders it mobile within the skull, so that small traumas may easily result in the tearing of subdural veins.

Lastly, adolescents and young adults suffering massive acceleration injury to the head may sustain such severe gyrations of their brain that the cortical surface is breached and haemorrhage occurs into the subdural space through tears in the arachnoid.

The subdural haematoma is generally thought to carry a less favourable prognosis than the extradural haematoma, probably because in the young adult group of patients subdural haematoma implies greater energy transfer to the brain.

Chronic subdural

These haematomata (Fig. 13.14) occur when the body walls off a small acute haematoma (which may be subclinical) by a membrane of fibrous tissue and proliferating capillaries. Studies have shown these membranes to

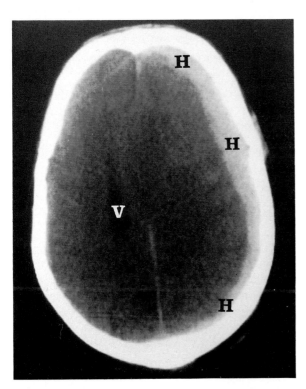

Fig. 13.13 **CT scan showing brain compressed by a large subdural haematoma (H) extending over the entire surface of the left cerebral hemisphere.** V, body of right lateral ventricle. The left lateral ventricle has been compressed out of existence.

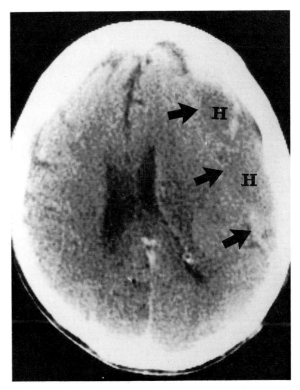

Fig. 13.14 **CT of brain scan showing chronic subdural haematoma (H) over the anterior half of the left cerebral hemisphere.** The brain/haematoma interface is indicated by arrows. Note that the haematoma has almost the same radiological density as brain, because it now consists of a liquid mixture of blood and high-protein fluid. Note also the shift in midline structures.

have a high fibrinolytic activity associated with the pro-liferating capillaries. It is likely that as a consequence there are small microhaemorrhages into the liquid collection from time to time, maintaining or sometimes increasing its size. Patients may present with chronic subdural haematomas as early as 10 days after a major injury, in which case the haematoma contains liquid dark blood. Alternatively presentation may be months or even years after the last significant trauma, in which case the chronic collection may contain straw-coloured fluid with high protein concentration. Presentation is usually with increasing headache and/or deterioration in neurological function.

Intra-axial

These haematomata are produced by the gyrations of a brain exposed to severe acceleration. With small energies the haemorrhages may be pinpoint (petechial), but with greater energies larger blood vessels are ruptured and such patients may incur very large intracerebral haematomata. Common sites for these are the thalamus, basal ganglia (Fig. 13.15), subcortical white matter and sometimes in the brain stem or cerebellum. Intra-axial haematomata have an even worse prognosis than do subdural haematomata because the association with significant energy transfer to the brain is high.

HYPERCARBIA

In most head injuries the blood vessels supplying the brain retain at least a degree of responsiveness to arterial P_{CO_2}. Accordingly, if the arterial P_{CO_2} is allowed to rise for any reason (for example, if the patient also has pulmonary injuries, or if he is oversedated) then there is a general cerebral vasodilatation, the brain fills with even more blood within its vascular system, and intracranial pressure may approach mean arterial pressure.

It is quite possible that patients with only minor or moderate injuries can enter a positive feedback cycle consisting of depressed conscious state leading to hypoventilation and rising P_{CO_2}; consequent cerebral vasodilatation and further rise in intracranial pressure; further depression of conscious state leading to further rise in P_{CO_2}, etc. This is the most likely explanation for patients whose conscious state deteriorates whilst they are under observation but in whom no haematoma is found.

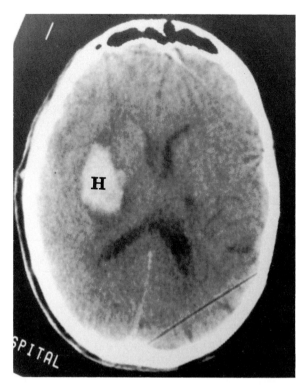

Fig. 13.15 CT scan of brain following severe acceleration injury. An intra-axial haematoma (H) is shown in the right basal ganglia region with shift of the midline structures.

HYPOXIA

There is good evidence to show that the brain injured by trauma is less able to tolerate hypoxia than is the normal brain. Thus it is of paramount importance to try to avoid hypoxia in the brain-injured patient.

HYPOTENSION

The injured brain is also intolerant of hypotension just as it is intolerant of hypoxia. It is therefore mandatory to preserve normotension in the patient with a significant head injury.

INFECTION

The brain and meninges are at risk of infection in the following situations:

- When there is persistent CSF leakage. This usually means either that the tegmen tympani has been fractured, as part of a fracture of the petrous bone (allowing CSF to leak into the middle ear and down the eustachian tube), or that the floor of the anterior cranial fossa has been fractured (e.g. in association with a middle third facial fracture), allowing CSF to leak directly into the nose.

- When there is a compound (usually depressed) skull fracture, with hair or other foreign material driven into the wound.
- When there is a penetrating missile wound, with devitalised brain tissue, fragments of bone and missile along the track within the brain.

In all of these situations surgery is usually necessary to prevent meningitis or infection of the brain itself (cerebritis).

HYDROCEPHALUS

Significant acceleration injuries frequently lead to liberation of blood into the cerebrospinal fluid. Such haemorrhage may be sufficient to occlude CSF pathways over the surface of the brain, with consequent damming up of CSF and dilatation of the cerebral ventricles (hydrocephalus). This condition, if it occurs, is usually seen at a week or 10 days after injury (Fig. 13.16).

VENOUS OBSTRUCTION

It is possible to impair the return of blood from the brain via the internal jugular veins by pressure on these veins in the neck. Thus extreme neck positions should be avoided during nursing and, if the patient has a tracheostomy, the tapes passed around the neck should not be tied too tightly.

CEREBRAL ARTERIAL SPASM

In head injuries in which significant amounts of blood enter the subarachnoid cisterns at the base of the brain, the toxic effects of haemoglobin breakdown products may result in spasm of the arteries in the bloody subarachnoid fluid. As most of these arteries supply the brain, severe spasm may result in ischaemia and even infarction.

Cerebral arterial spasm is rarely a problem in the first 72 hours after trauma, but may then become an important potential cause of secondary brain injury. Treatment is by intravenous volume loading, artificial elevation of the blood pressure or (if a large amount of subarachnoid

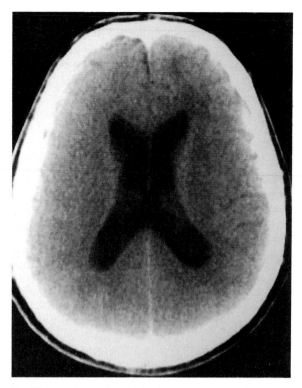

Fig. 13.16 CT scan showing hydrocephalic dilatation of the bodies of the lateral ventricles following trauma, with liberation of blood into the cerebrospinal fluid. Note that there are virtually no sulci visible over the brain surface, indicating compression of the brain by the dilating ventricles and/or blood in the CSF rendering it isodense with brain.

blood is noted on the first post-trauma CT scan) prophylactic use of nimodipine, one of the calcium channel blocking drugs.

CLINICAL COURSE

Concussion is a disturbance in memory and/or conscious state which occurs after transfer of energy to the brain.

The least degree of concussion is seen in the boxer who receives a heavy blow during a bout, staggers but does not fall down, and fights poorly for the rest of that round before recovering in the next. Subsequently he cannot remember anything about that particular round and he cannot remember the blow being delivered. Such a man has amnesia for a brief period before and after the concussive collision, but did not actually lose consciousness. If he were interrogated immediately after such a blow, his conscious state would be found to be impaired.

A more significant impact, such as someone falling heavily on to the back of the head on the pavement, may lead to a minute or two of unconsciousness, an inability to remember the actual collision with the pavement (although there may be memory of falling), and amnesia for the first 5–10 minutes after the collision. Amnesia for the period leading up to the collision is termed retrograde amnesia, whereas amnesia for the period after the event is called post-traumatic amnesia. In almost all cases, retrograde amnesia involves a shorter period than does the post-traumatic amnesia. The lengths of both periods of amnesia are proportional to the acceleration experienced by the brain.

The time-course of recovery of conscious state after the brain has been accelerated to a sufficient degree to cause loss of consciousness is portrayed in Figure 13.17. The patient's conscious state progressively lightens through successive stages until consciousness is fully regained. The time taken to regain consciousness fully is proportional to the acceleration energy imparted to the brain. This is shown in curves 1, 2 and 3, which portray recovery after small, moderate and major energy transfers, respectively. Once the energy of collision exceeds a certain value, complete recovery is no longer possible and the patient is left with permanent impairment of conscious state or intellect (curve 4).

During the observation of patients recovering from concussive brain injuries, the patient who ceases to improve or the patient who improves and then deteriorates (curve 5) must be re-examined and re-investigated as a matter of extreme urgency since they are clearly at risk of further secondary brain injury occurring by one or other mechanism. The detection of such patients is the role of head injury observations.

MANAGEMENT

FIRST AID

The most important first aid measure in head injury patients is the securing of an unobstructed airway. The patient should be placed in the full lateral unconscious position, with due regard to the fact that he may also have a cervical spine injury. Wounds to the scalp or underlying tissues which are actively bleeding should be covered by a sterile dressing held on by winding a crepe bandage around the head. If possible, the Glasgow coma observations, pupillary sizes and reactions, and the time at which the observations were taken should be recorded and sent on with the patient.

In all other ways the first aid of the head-injured patient is the same as that of any other.

ASSESSMENT IN THE EMERGENCY ROOM

History

If possible, the nature of the injury should be ascertained, with special reference to the energy of the collision, the time of the accident and the trend of the patient's conscious state.

Examination

After ensuring that the patient has an unobstructed airway, the examining clinician should then assess the vital signs, including blood pressure, pulse, respiration rate, body temperature (if palpably abnormal) and the pupillary sizes and reactivity to light. Following this, a rapid but thorough examination of the whole body for signs of injury should be carried out. This initial rapid examination should include the taking of the first set of Glasgow coma observations for comparison with repeat observations in a few minutes' time. At this stage the examining clinician must attend to any problems which immediately threaten life. Priority will be given to airway obstruction,

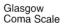
Glasgow
Coma Scale

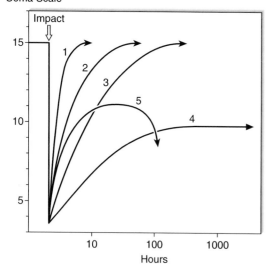

Fig. 13.17 Recovery of conscious state following acceleration injuries of increasing energy (curves 1, 2, 3 and 4). For an explanation of curve 5, see the text.

tension pneumothorax, uncontrolled haemorrhage and similar conditions, as discussed in Chapter 14.

After assessing all body systems for injury and ensuring the patient's immediate survival, the neurological injury may now be fully assessed. First the Glasgow coma observations are repeated and compared with the initial set. Any patient who is thereby shown to be deteriorating will need to be managed with the utmost rapidity. In general, any patient who has lost consciousness or who still does not attain a Glasgow Coma Score of 15 should be subjected to a CT scan of the cranium, with an urgency proportional to their rate of deterioration and inversely proportional to the total Glasgow Coma Score.

The neurological examination of the unconscious patient should be organised and recorded under the same headings as a full neurological examination in any patient, namely:

- conscious state/mental state
- cranial nerves
- motor system: tone, power and reflexes
- sensory system
- coordination.

Of these, only coordination cannot be properly examined in the unconscious patient.

MANAGEMENT OF RAISED INTRACRANIAL PRESSURE

When Glasgow coma observations and/or intracranial pressure monitoring reveal rising intracranial pressure with the risk of cerebral herniations, it is imperative to deal with any surgical intracranial lesion.

All acute haematomata causing raised intracranial pressure, whether extradural, subdural or intra-axial, are managed by craniotomy and evacuation under direct vision. Particularly in the case of subdural haematomata, the craniotomy often has to be quite large, as subdural haematomata frequently spread over the entire surface of the brain on that side (Fig. 13.13). In the case of extradural haematoma, craniotomy is necessary because it is essential to stop all bleeding from dural vessels prior to closing the wound. It should be understood that almost all acute haematomata, in whatever compartment, are clotted and extremely tenacious. They cannot be removed via burr holes.

Burr hole exploration is to locate acute intracranial haematoma. This operation is now performed only where CT scan is unavailable, or sometimes when the patient's deterioration is very rapid, such that the surgeon decides that the extra time taken to obtain a CT scan would be fatal to the patient. Most neurosurgeons now believe that the extra 10–20 minutes taken to obtain a CT scan, particularly with the patient protected by intubation, hyperventilation and intravenous diuretic administration, save much more time than is lost. The operating room can be setting up whilst the scan is proceeding; the whole head does not have to be shaved and prepared and draped, as it must if a haematoma is to be hunted by burr holes; and a craniotomy, perfectly sited with respect to the haematoma, can be immediately raised without the necessity for exploratory burr holes. In addition, the CT scan has taught us that of all people deteriorating whilst under neurological observation, many do not have an intracranial haematoma but have brain swelling (Fig. 13.11) or focal brain oedema.

Treatment of a patient with raised intracranial pressure in the absence of a surgically remediable lesion requires the following measures, in order of precedence:

1. Establish normal blood gases if possible, with arterial P_{CO_2} 30–40 mmHg and P_{O_2} 70 mmHg or more. Hyperventilation to levels less than 30 mmHg may be injurious in the presence of raised intracranial pressure, in so far as it may add a further reduction in cerebral blood flow (due to hypocarbic cerebral vasospasm) to a cerebral circulation already compromised by raised intracranial pressure. Furthermore, hyperventilation loses any effect that it may have on intracranial pressure after a few hours, whereupon the artificially low level of P_{CO_2} has to be maintained for some time, lest intracranial pressure rise during the relative hypercarbic state induced as the CO_2 levels are allowed to return to normal.

2. Nurse the patient with slight elevation of the head to facilitate venous drainage from the brain.

3. Keep serum osmolality between 290 and 310 mmol/L. This involves caution in the use of crystalloid infusions in the resuscitation of the patient. Where intracranial pressure is critical, diuretics such as frusemide and/or mannitol may be used periodically to maintain the plasma osmolality in the upper part of the recommended range.

4. Normotension should be preserved, preventing systemic hypertension in excess of 100 mmHg diastolic or 200 mmHg systolic. Whether or not measures should be taken to control hypertension even more strictly is a difficult question as, in the presence of raised intracranial pressure, the brain may require elevated levels of blood pressure in order to perfuse.

5. Where all other measures fail, a patient may be pharmacologically paralysed and intubated, purely for the control of intracranial pressure.

6. Where intubation and paralysis fail, bolus administration of thiopentone may result in control of rising intracranial pressure.

7. Where bolus thiopentone fails, deep barbiturate coma may be induced to the level of the phenomenon of 'burst suppression' on the EEG, or to a plasma level of 2.5–3.5 mg/100 ml (pentobarbitone).

8. If all else fails in the presence of diffuse brain swelling and uncontrolled intracranial hypertension, wide bilateral craniotomies may be raised and the dura stroked gently with a sharp scalpel in order to allow it to bulge smoothly out on either side. The skin is sutured and the bone flaps are kept sterile in a deep freeze. On occasions such heroic measures have led to the survival of patients in good condition.

FURTHER MANAGEMENT

Allowed home

Patients are allowed home after 4 hours of observations if they are fully conscious; oriented in time, place and circumstances; have no skull fracture; and have lost consciousness for less than 10 minutes. Ideally they should be discharged to the care of a relative or friend, and warned to return immediately in the event of severe headache, vomiting, confusion or drowsiness. Arrangements should be made for their review in an outpatient clinic or by their local doctor in the next day or two.

Admitted to the ward

Criteria for admission to a hospital ward will vary somewhat from place to place, but in general a patient will probably be admitted if he has any of the following:

- a skull fracture
- loss of consciousness for more than 10 minutes
- if he is still not fully oriented in time, place and circumstances, 2 hours after impact
- any abnormal neurological sign
- any abnormality on cranial CT scan.

Sent for urgent cranial CT scan

A CT scan should be carried out as part of urgent management and in the following circumstances:

- skull fracture seen on skull X-ray
- a patient not fully oriented in time, place and circumstances, 2 hours after impact
- loss of consciousness for 10 minutes or more
- failure of Glasgow coma observations to improve
- deterioration in Glasgow coma observations.

Transfer to a neurosurgical unit

As a general guide, any patient who has not improved to a Glasgow Coma Score of 10 or more at 4 hours after injury should probably be transferred to a hospital having a neurosurgical unit. Similarly, any patient whose Glasgow Coma Score is not clearly improving over a 4 hour period, and certainly any patient whose Glasgow Coma Score is deteriorating, should prompt a telephone communication with a neurosurgeon at the very least, if not transfer of the patient to a neurosurgical unit.

Indications for urgent operation

These include:

- raised intracranial pressure due to an intracranial haematoma
- depressed skull fracture
- a compound wound with certain or possible contamination
- requirement for a monitor of intracranial pressure.

Indications for the insertion of intracranial pressure monitoring devices in head-injured patients vary from unit to unit, but the following would be generally accepted indications:

- any patient who requires intubation and paralysis or sedation for control of respiratory status, where conscious state was not normal at the time of intubation
- any patient showing a significant non-surgical mass lesion on CT scan, e.g. focal cerebral oedema, a significant intra-axial haematoma not amenable to easy removal, or diffuse brain swelling
- any patient whose Glasgow coma observations are deteriorating, who has no surgically remediable lesion on CT scan.

Indications for later operation

These may include:

- persistent CSF leak beyond 24 hours after injury
- hydrocephalus – where this occurs and is persistent it should be shunted
- chronic subdural haematoma or hygroma in the presence of impaired mental state or other neurological signs.

Subdural hygroma is a collection of straw-coloured fluid with greater concentration of protein than is found in CSF. It is likely that the hygroma arises by sequestration of cerebrospinal fluid in the subdural space, having issued through a tear in the arachnoid. Although exerting little mass effect, such collections can lead to a persistently disturbed mental state, particularly in an elderly patient. They are easily evacuated by burr holes.

CARE OF THE UNCONSCIOUS PATIENT

In addition to all of the foregoing measures, care must be taken to ensure the patient's adequate nutrition, hydration (without lowering the plasma osmolality) and skin care. In particular, the patient's position must be changed at a minimum 2-hourly and pillows used to protect the skin over bony prominences. Regular skin massage together with the application of lotions to prevent alterations in skin hydration are valuable measures. Care of the urinary tract demands condom drainage or catheterisation of the male unconscious patient and catheterisation of the female. Strict asepsis must attend these procedures and the urine must be regularly checked for infection. Pulmonary care is of utmost importance in patients with disturbed conscious state. Those who have tracheostomies or are intubated must have regular gentle and skilfully applied aspiration of secretions from the tracheobronchial tree and regular controlled hyperinflation of the lungs to prevent alveolar atelectasis. Patients who are not intubated should receive regular chest percussion or vibration in the lateral position, at least 4-hourly. In such cases the upper airway must be preserved either by nursing the patient in the full (lateral) unconscious position or else by the use of an oropharyngeal airway.

REHABILITATION

Almost all head-injured patients who have been unconscious for more than 6 hours or whose post-traumatic amnesia extends for more than 48 hours will need, at the very least, to undergo neuropsychological assessment before being allowed to return to their occupations.

Patients who are clearly neurologically impaired following their head injury, together with many of those who are not but who show impairment on neuropsychological testing, will require formal rehabilitation of one sort or another. It is of no use to apply sophisticated intensive care and neurosurgical techniques to salvaging patients after head injury if the task is not to be completed by providing the fullest rehabilitation possible.

POST-TRAUMATIC EPILEPSY

Epilepsy is a state of intermittent disruption of neurological function due to abnormal electrical discharge within the brain. Patients with post-traumatic epilepsy may experience generalised or partial seizures. Most severe are the generalised 'grand mal' convulsions, with loss of consciousness, incontinence of bowel and bladder and the very real possibility of injury to the patient or others. Partial seizures may involve localised focal motor activity (such as the twitching of a digit or part of a limb), sensory seizures or a period in which normal activities are suspended and 'automatic' activities occur, as in complex partial epilepsy.

The incidence of epilepsy after non-missile head injuries is approximately 5% of all cases. After missile injuries the incidence is much greater and approximates 30–40%.

The highest incidence of post-traumatic epilepsy is found in patients who have one or more of the following factors:

- early epilepsy (from 24 hours after trauma until the end of the first week)
- intracranial haematoma
- penetrating missile injury.

Certain other factors are associated with an increased risk of epilepsy, and these 'secondary' factors (of which any two add up to the significance of one of the above three) include:

- dural penetration
- depressed skull fracture
- intracranial infection
- focal neurological signs
- post-traumatic amnesia exceeding 24 hours.

BRAIN DEATH

This is discussed in Chapter 11.

FURTHER READING

Ashpole R, Hardy D, Klein J 1996 Guidelines for the management of head injuries. Haigh and Hochland, Cheshire

Bullock R, Teasdale G 1996 Head injuries. In: Skinner D, Driscoll P, Earlam R (eds) ABC of major trauma. BMJ publishing, London

Currie D G 1983 The management of head injuries. Oxford handbooks in emergency medicine 5. Oxford University Press, Oxford

Lang D 1995 Management of head injury. In: Johnson C D, Taylor I (eds) Recent advances in surgery 17. Churchill Livingstone, Edinburgh

Wilkins R W, Rengachary S S (eds) 1985 Neurosurgery. McGraw-Hill, Boston, p 1531–1688

14 Chest injuries
Peter Smith

OVERVIEW

Chest trauma, whether blunt or penetrating, is quite a common cause of preventable death. Fractures of the ribs and sternum are often associated with injury to the underlying lung and less often with injury to the heart, great vessels or diaphragm. Tension pneumothorax requires urgent insertion of an intercostal drain. Haemothorax can generally be treated with simple drainage, but thoracotomy is required for persistent bleeding. Mechanical ventilation may be needed if there is a flail chest or associated head injury.

Trauma to the chest is a common occurrence, particularly after road traffic accidents, and it may be associated with potentially lethal pulmonary and cardiovascular injuries.

GENERAL CLASSIFICATION

Chest injuries are broadly classified as follows:

- open injuries – from gunshot, knife or other projectile
- closed injuries – from blunt trauma such as steering wheel, crush, deceleration (e.g. aircraft crashes with restraints in position), blast.

SURGICAL PATHOPHYSIOLOGY

EFFECTS OF INJURY TO THE LUNG

Puncture of the lung from without, either by a weapon or by a broken rib, allows air to escape into the pleural cavity. Any of the following may take place:

Subcutaneous emphysema. If the lung puncture seals there will be a variable degree of collapse and pneumothorax with or without the presence of blood, but provided the other lung is healthy there is not much respiratory embarrassment. If the parietal pleura does not seal then air from the pneumothorax will escape subcutaneously (subcutaneous emphysema) and a continued leak from the lung may result in emphysema stretching from neck to groins.

Tension pneumothorax. If the wound in the parietal pleura seals but air continues to escape, then tension inside the pleural space rises – *tension pneumothorax* (Fig. 14.1). The lung collapses and the encroaching air displaces the mediastinum to the opposite side. Two effects follow:

   — the contralateral lung is compressed so that it becomes less and less effective in gas exchange

   — the inferior vena cava is angled in relation to the diaphragmatic opening, so interfering with venous return.

'Sucking' pneumothorax. A large wound in the chest wall (rare in civilian practice) produces a 'sucking' pneumothorax. On inspiration, air is drawn into the chest, so displacing the lung and mediastinum; on expiration the reverse happens. Air may pass from one lung to the other on inspiration, thus making ventilation even less effective.

Contusion of the lung – usually in severe blunt trauma. The lung is literally bruised and does not function until the haematoma has resolved.

DAMAGE TO THE CHEST WALL

Chest wall trauma is common, occurring in approximately 40% of all torso injuries.

An isolated rib fracture rarely causes much disturbance except in the elderly or frail. A row of fractures more severely embarrasses respiration because of the

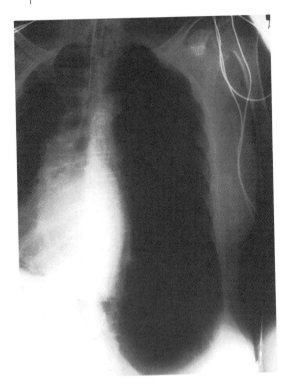

Fig. 14.1 Chest X-ray of a left tension pneumothorax. The heart is displaced into the right hemithorax.

pain caused and also because there may be contusion of both chest wall and underlying lung.

If a number of ribs are broken in *two* places, this creates a *flail segment* which moves independently of the chest wall – inwards on inspiration and outwards on expiration, i.e. *paradoxical* movement. The underlying lung does not expand; furthermore, the work of breathing is increased.

Fracture of the clavicle is common and very painful but is usually not a cause of major injury.

Up to 10% of all thoracic injuries are associated with a fracture of the sternum. Other serious intrathoracic injury is often seen in these patients.

CARDIAC AND LARGE-VESSEL INJURY
See page 125.

RUPTURE OF THE OESOPHAGUS
See page 125.

RUPTURE OF THE DIAPHRAGM
See page 126.

CLINICAL FEATURES

Chest trauma often occurs in association with major trauma in other areas of the body, particularly of the head and within the abdomen. It is extremely important not to assess the chest in isolation.

SYMPTOMS

Symptoms of chest injury include:

- Pain from the presence of chest wall bruising or rib fractures.
- Dyspnoea as a consequence of hypoxia and the shallow breathing caused by pain. Gasping respiration is characteristic of tension pneumothorax and must be regarded as a herald of impending doom.
- Cough and haemoptysis – due to tracheobronchial injury, lacerated lung with or without a haemothorax or to pulmonary haematoma.

SIGNS OF CHEST INJURY

Hypotension. This occurs as a result of blood loss, mediastinal shift or cardiac tamponade (see p. 125).

Chest wall trauma. This will be evidenced by bruising, a sucking wound of the chest wall, paradoxical chest wall movement or pain on 'springing' the chest wall when rib fractures are present.

Surgical emphysema. This produces a crackling sensation beneath the examining fingers.

Tracheal deviation is associated with displacement of the apex beat if there is pulmonary collapse (e.g. pneumothorax) or intrapleural collection (e.g. haemothorax). A tension pneumothorax will displace the trachea away from the affected side.

Elevated jugular venous pressure. This occurs with cardiac tamponade.

Lung fields. Hyper-resonance indicates pneumothorax, and diminished or absent breath sounds indicate haemothorax, pneumothorax or pulmonary collapse.

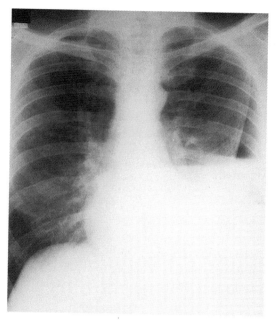

Fig. 14.2 Chest X-ray of a left haemopneumothorax after blunt chest trauma.

SPECIAL TESTS

Chest X-ray

Chest X-ray should always be taken erect unless the patient's condition totally precludes this (which is very rare). Supine X-rays provide limited information. X-ray can demonstrate fractured ribs, pneumothorax, haemothorax (Fig. 14.2), ruptured diaphragm (sometimes), lung contusion and atelectasis. Injuries to the aorta and its major branches are associated with haemorrhage and widening of the upper mediastinal shadow, while a haemopericardium shows up as an enlarged heart shadow.

Other tests

The following tests are of somewhat lesser urgency but are of potential importance in the light of the clinical and chest X-ray findings.

Electrocardiogram. This should be used in blunt injury to the anterior chest wall, particularly a fractured sternum.

Computed tomography (CT scan). This can be useful to demonstrate intrathoracic anatomy, particularly vascular anatomy. In addition, in the stable patient with a sharp instrument or bullet in situ, CT can define the relationship of the foreign body to major anatomical structures.

Aortography. This is useful in violent deceleration injuries or if there is unexplained hypotension or widening of the mediastinal shadow on chest X-ray.

Magnetic resonance imaging (MRI). This form of imaging can be used to define the anatomy of the mediastinum and hemithoraces, and is particularly useful to define the integrity of the aorta.

Estimation of blood gas tensions. Regular estimation of arterial oxygen and carbon dioxide partial pressures is essential in estimating the degree of respiratory insufficiency, particularly in those patients with paradoxical respiration and flail chest wall segments.

MANAGEMENT

URGENT RESPIRATORY MANAGEMENT

1. Clear airway, including removal of dentures, blood and pharyngotracheal secretions.
2. Relieve a tension pneumothorax at once, initially with a wide-bore needle then with a chest drain. A drain is also urgently indicated when it is thought there may be appreciable unilateral or bilateral pneumothorax or haemopneumothorax.
3. Temporarily close a sucking chest wound by any feasible means – pack, large sutures, occlusive dressing.
4. Put up an intravenous line and replace blood volume loss as necessary.
5. Operate. Very occasionally, and particularly in gunshot wounds, bleeding continues into the chest in spite of a chest drain and re-expansion of the lung. A thoracotomy is then required. Laparotomy may be needed for associated intra-abdominal injuries. Be extremely wary of removing a sharp instrument from the chest wall in an emergency situation, e.g. a knife protruding through the ribs. It is usually safer to remove the weapon in the operating theatre.
6. Assess whether the patient can support his own respiration. Inadequate movement may occur:
   — in flail chest
   — in severe head injury

— from pain in multiple fractures
— when there is pre-existing lung disease.

If there is any doubt and if the Po_2 is less then 7.3–7.9 kPa (55–60 mmHg) and/or the Pco_2 is greater than 6.6 kPa (50 mmHg), intubate and ventilate the patient until full assessment is possible.

SUBSEQUENT MANAGEMENT

Pain relief

This can be achieved by:

- continuous intravenous opiate or a patient-controlled analgesic (PCA) system
- local infiltration of long-acting local anaesthetic (for rib fractures)
- epidural opiate.

Of these the first is probably the easiest and most effective.

Physiotherapy

Vigorous physiotherapy is required, aided by nasopharyngeal suction to avoid retained secretions. Bronchoscopy may occasionally be necessary.

Antibiotics

Opinions are divided about prophylactic use. Pneumococcal and *Haemophilus* infection may complicate chest injuries. A broad-spectrum antibiotic should be prescribed prophylactically.

Other

In mild to moderate chest injuries, the above may be all that is required. However, there is often a tendency to deteriorate over the first 24–72 hours, and laboured breathing and adverse changes in blood gas tensions are indications for assisted ventilation.

In open wounds, particularly contaminated trauma wounds, consider tetanus prophylaxis.

There is no indication for tracheostomy in the early management of chest injuries unless there is associated upper airways obstruction. If assisted respiration has to be prolonged into a second week, then consideration should be given to performing a tracheostomy.

SPECIFIC INJURIES

ISOLATED FRACTURED RIBS

This is the commonest injury to the thoracic cage. Though usually trivial in themselves, because of the associated pain on breathing, fractured ribs may cause poor ventilation, sputum retention, atelectasis and pneumonia, particularly in the elderly.

Treatment

Treatment is by:

- relief of pain – see above
- physiotherapy and encouragement to cough
- prophylactic antibiotics – rib fractures often occur in elderly people whose lung function is already compromised, e.g. chronic bronchitis and emphysema.

FLAIL CHEST

The treatment depends on the severity.

Mild to moderate

This is characterised by a small flail segment with respiratory movements maintained. Treatment is by:

- adequate analgesia
- adequate sedation
- prophylactic antibiotics
- posturing and physiotherapy
- intranasal oxygen
- respirator with mouthpiece.

Severe

In severe cases of flail chest, intermittent positive pressure respiration is required for at least 10 days in addition to the simple measures above. The flail segment may rarely require surgical fixation.

PNEUMOTHORAX AND HAEMOTHORAX

Treatment of pneumothorax

Small pneumothorax (i.e. not inhibiting respiratory activity) does not require any treatment unless a general anaesthetic or intermittent positive pressure respiration is indicated for some other purpose.

Large pneumothorax (i.e. large enough to inhibit respiratory activity) requires the insertion of an intercostal drain. Ideally the drain should be in the fifth intercostal space in the mid-axillary line. An alternative site of drain insertion is the second intercostal space anteriorly in the mid-clavicular line.

For a discussion of *tension* pneumothorax, see page 121.

Treatment of haemothorax

Except in some penetrating wounds, bleeding is usually mild and of low pressure. Chest drainage and lung re-expansion are all that is necessary.

Continued bleeding of 300–500 ml/hour requires thoracotomy. It is important to note the trend in the quantity of bleeding. Increasing blood loss over the first hours after trauma increases the likelihood of the need for thoracotomy.

Very occasionally a large haemothorax clots and then has to be evacuated surgically.

BRONCHIAL RUPTURE

A rare injury, bronchial rupture is to be suspected with:

- mediastinal emphysema
- failure of lung expansion with adequate drainage of a pneumothorax or haemopneumothorax
- bloodstained sputum often associated with recurrent paroxysmal coughing
- development of tension pneumothorax.

Confirmation is by bronchoscopy. Treatment is by thoracotomy and repair.

LUNG CONTUSION AND LACERATION

Areas of bruised lung can usually be left to resolve, although respiratory support may be required while this is taking place. Lacerations are nearly always associated with penetrating injury and rarely require specific treatment.

RUPTURED OESOPHAGUS

Traumatic rupture of the oesophagus is rare, but it may follow penetrating or crush injury. The oesophagus may also be torn from within by an oesophagoscope or a swallowed sharp instrument. Finally, non-traumatic rupture occurs in violent vomiting.

When rupture is due to a crushing injury, there is generally a longitudinal tear sometimes associated with a tear in the posterior wall of the trachea, which allows a tracheo-oesophageal fistula to develop.

When rupture is due to oesophagoscopy, the tear is often near the level of the cricoid cartilage. It results from crushing of the posterior wall of the oesophagus between the instrument and the cervical spine, particularly when the spine is osteoarthritic.

Clinical features

Ruptured oesophagus presents with mediastinal emphysema and mediastinitis; when suspected the diagnosis is made on oesophagoscopy and X-ray with oral water-soluble contrast media (Gastrografin).

Treatment

This is by:

- early thoracotomy and repair
- intravenous replacement therapy or feeding jejunostomy
- respiratory support.

CARDIAC TRAUMA

Crushing, deceleration and blast injuries can cause haemopericardium, cardiac contusion and laceration, cardiac rupture, pericardial rupture and injuries to the interatrial septum, interventricular septum and the valvular mechanisms. Myocardial infarction can occur following both blunt and sharp chest trauma.

The symptoms and signs of cardiac tamponade (i.e. inability of the chambers to fill) are a low arterial pressure, a high venous pressure and pulsus paradoxus with an enlarged cardiac silhouette on chest X-ray.

Electrocardiography may show non-specific changes, QRS anomalies, various arrhythmias or the signs of myocardial infarction.

Echocardiography, both transthoracic and trans-oesophageal, is extremely useful in the diagnosis of pericardial effusions and in the assessment of cardiac valves and ventricular function.

It should always be remembered that the patient's heart may have been abnormal before trauma occurred, e.g. with coronary artery or valve disease.

Treatment

In the presence of tamponade, thoracotomy is indicated.

RUPTURED THORACIC AORTA

Rupture occurs typically just distal to the origin of the left subclavian artery and usually follows a deceleration injury. Most injuries are fatal. If the patient survives, it is because a wall of mediastinal pleura and aortic adventitia has contained a pulsating haematoma.

If the patient reaches hospital alive, the diagnosis should be suspected if chest X-ray illustrates a widening of the upper mediastinum and tracheal displacement. An aortogram by way of the right brachial artery will then reveal the defect.

Usually the flow of blood is not impeded, but occasionally aortic obstruction occurs with a 'coarctation-like effect' – proximal hypertension, distal hypotension and occasionally anuria and paraplegia.

Treatment

This consists of left thoracotomy and suture or prosthetic replacement utilising left heart bypass.

In a small number of survivors the injury goes undetected, and a false aneurysm is discovered months or years later on routine chest X-ray or because it begins to expand. Operative repair is recommended.

RUPTURED THORACIC DUCT

This is a very rare complication which may result from a severe crushing injury or hyperextension to the spine.

Dyspnoea develops due to chylothorax (usually right-sided). The diagnosis is established on paracentesis, when white milky fluid is aspirated containing fat droplets, cholesterol, lymphocytes and having a high protein content.

Treatment

Treatment is by frequent aspiration or intercostal drain and suction.

If conservative methods fail, thoracotomy is indicated with ligature of the thoracic duct between the cisterna chyli and the site of injury.

RUPTURED DIAPHRAGM

This may follow a penetrating, crushing or deceleration injury. Most ruptures occur in the left hemidiaphragm and most are centrally situated. Herniation of stomach, spleen, omentum and small bowel may occur through the defect, and often these structures are themselves traumatised by the injurious forces applied.

There are two phases of the condition:

- Immediate consequences of rupture
  — shock
  — pain
  — blood loss
  — haemoperitoneum or haemothorax
- Effects of migration of abdominal viscera into chest
  — displacement of pulmonary, cardiac and mediastinal contents
  — abdominal visceral obstruction or perforation.

There are five signs of a ruptured diaphragm, none of which is particularly reliable:

- diminished chest excursion
- impaired chest wall resonance
- absence of retraction of the intercostal spaces on diaphragmatic movement
- adventitious gastrointestinal sounds in the chest
- cardiac displacement.

Treatment

This includes:

- laparotomy or thoracotomy, or both
- reduction of abdominal contents
- repair of diaphragmatic rupture
- drainage of pleural cavity.

Beware of placing a chest drain into air-filled bowel in the left chest after thoracic trauma.

FURTHER READING

Akins C W et al 1981 Acute traumatic rupture of the thoracic aorta: a ten year experience. Annals of Thoracic Surgery 31: 305–309

Craven K D, Oppenheimer L, Wood L D H 1979 Effects of confusion and flail chest on pulmonary perfusion and oxygen exchange. Journal of Applied Physics 47: 729–737

Deslauriers J et al 1982 Diagnosis and long term follow up of major bronchial disruptions due to non penetrating trauma. Annals of Thoracic Surgery 33: 32–39

Shields T W 1994 General thoracic surgery, 4th edn. Lea and Febiger, London

Sugg W L 1968 Penetrating wounds of the heart. Journal of Thoracic and Cardiovascular Surgery 56: 531–545

15 Abdominal injuries

Robin Williamson

OVERVIEW

Virtually any abdominal organ can be injured either by a penetrating wound or by blunt trauma of sufficient severity. Injuries to solid organs, notably the spleen, liver and mesentery, lead to intraperitoneal bleeding, which may be of sufficient severity to require urgent resuscitation and laparotomy. Injuries to hollow organs, notably the small intestine and colon, present with progressive peritonitis over the next few hours. Injuries to the retroperitoneal organs vary in their behaviour; many renal injuries can be managed conservatively, whereas ruptured pancreas generally requires operative intervention. Injuries to the pelvic organs, notably the rectum, bladder and urethra, also require individual management.

Trauma is the leading cause of death in young adults. In civilian practice, 75% of abdominal trauma follows non-penetrating injuries, except in some communities with a tradition of using the hand gun and the knife to settle differences. Sometimes a force considered trivial may cause serious visceral damage. Even with an acute awareness of such a possibility, the diagnosis or elimination of intra-abdominal trauma can be extremely difficult, especially in the presence of a multiplicity of associated injuries.

CLASSIFICATION

Abdominal injuries can be classified into:

- non-penetrating (closed) injuries
- penetrating injuries.

SURGICAL PATHOLOGY

NON-PENETRATING INJURIES

In general the extent of damage depends on the speed, direction and size of the force applied.

Abdominal wall

Contusions are common. Haematoma of the rectus sheath may occur with rupture of an epigastric vessel as the result of direct violence or sudden contraction of the rectus abdominis muscle.

Intra-abdominal contents

Solid organs. The liver, spleen and kidneys are commonly affected by closed abdominal trauma because they are relatively fixed, large and comparatively exposed.

Haemorrhage is the outstanding feature and, when severe, hypovolaemic shock will occur. The common sources of a traumatic haemoperitoneum are shown in Figure 15.1.

Hollow organs. The intestine is relatively mobile and able to move away from the path of a blow. It is therefore less likely to be damaged than solid organs, except at areas of relative fixation such as the duodenum, duodenojejunal flexure, caecum, ascending colon and colonic flexures.

When the body undergoes acute deceleration, for example in a road traffic accident, the abdominal contents will continue to move forward. This process may tear the mesentery of the small or large bowel.

Peritonitis is the outstanding feature of hollow organ

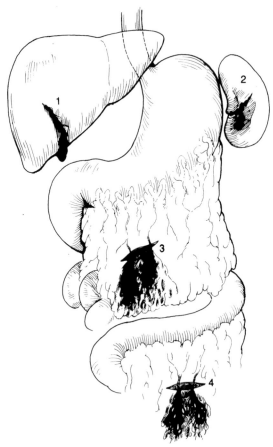

Fig. 15.1 Common sources of a traumatic haemoperitoneum. 1, ruptured liver; 2, ruptured spleen; 3, laceration in greater omentum; 4, laceration in small bowel mesentery. There may also be bleeding from a renal or pancreatic injury or a fractured pelvis (following blunt trauma).

rupture and is due to bowel contents spilling out from tears, crushes or bursting defects in the bowel. Bursting injuries are uncommon but may be seen in shipwrecked sailors as the result of underwater blasts from exploding depth charges during major conflicts.

The mortality rate from hollow organ injuries is higher than that associated with injuries of solid organs because of the increased risk of infection. This risk is greatest with colonic trauma.

PENETRATING INJURIES

The major effects depend on a combination of haemorrhage and shock when solid organs or major vessels are

involved, and peritonitis and infection when bowel is perforated.

When a missile traverses soft tissue, the following may occur:

- Low-velocity missile (a stab or a missile up to 200 m/s) – structures traversed are lacerated.
- Very high velocity missile (over 200 and up to 1000 m/s) – the missile accelerates the medium through which it passes and moves it away from the path with such force that it continues to move once the missile has passed. As a result 'temporary cavitation' occurs, which causes severe and widespread bruising, with tearing, stretching and rupture of nearby viscera.

CLINICAL FEATURES

HISTORY OF VIOLENCE

Road traffic accidents, falls, assaults and sporting injuries are the commonest reasons for blunt abdominal trauma. Compulsory wearing of seat belts and motorcycle crash helmets has reduced the number and severity of injuries.

PREDISPOSING FACTORS

Adhesions and a flaccid abdominal wall (in the unsuspecting or drugged) may increase the risk of intra-abdominal trauma.

PRESENTATION

There are two groups of patients: those in whom the diagnosis is certain and those in whom it is uncertain.

Diagnosis certain

When there is haemorrhage from a solid organ or a major vessel or peritonitis as the result of a perforated viscus, then little diagnostic acumen is necessary and operation is imperative. The outstanding features include:

- acute and persistent abdominal pain
- marked abdominal tenderness, rebound tenderness and rigidity indicating peritonitis owing to blood, bile or bowel contents
- systemic evidence of continued internal haemorrhage despite resuscitation

- shoulder tip pain owing to diaphragmatic irritation from blood or bowel contents.

(Abdominal distension is a late sign and indicates paralytic ileus due to peritonitis or a large retroperitoneal haematoma.)

Diagnosis uncertain

Abdominal signs may be masked at first by shock, associated injuries, unconsciousness or analgesics. Upper abdominal signs may, on the other hand, be exaggerated by the presence of fractured ribs. In all these circumstances the diagnosis should be confirmed or refuted by peritoneal lavage. After urinary catheterisation, 500 ml of saline is run into the abdominal cavity through a subumbilical peritoneal dialysis catheter and then allowed to drain back under gravity into the i.v. container (Fig. 15.2).

Return may be:

- crystal clear – no intraperitoneal injury
- blood or gut content – laparotomy essential
- slightly bloodstained – 10% chance of injury; re-analyse the clinical picture.

Other special tests

These include:

- Plain erect X-ray of the chest to show pneumoperitoneum from rupture of a hollow organ, and abdominal X-ray to show fluid levels indicating paralytic ileus.
- Ultrasound and/or CT scanning in liver, spleen and kidney trauma. Ultrasound is cheaper and can be performed at the bedside (using a portable machine in a shocked patient), but the appearances on CT scan may be easier for the clinician to interpret (Fig. 15.3)
- Selective angiography in selected cases may prove to be of great value, particularly when trauma to the liver or renal vessels is suspected.

TREATMENT

Treatment depends on the classification of the injury.

NON-PENETRATING INJURIES

If the diagnosis is *certain*, treatment involves resuscitation and operation.

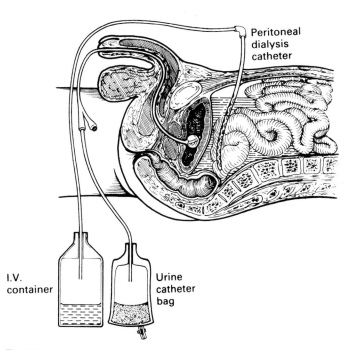

Fig. 15.2 Peritoneal lavage in blunt trauma. Note that a urinary catheter has been passed to empty the bladder and protect it from injury by the peritoneal dialysis catheter.

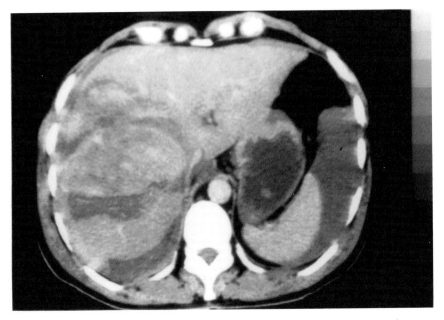

Fig. 15.3 CT scan showing traumatic rupture of the right liver in a young man who was injured in a motorcycle accident. Emergency right hepatectomy was required to control the bleeding.

If, in spite of CT scan or peritoneal lavage, the diagnosis is *uncertain*, then close and continuous observation is essential. This regimen must include:

- frequent recordings of pulse, blood pressure, temperature and respiratory rate
- frequent examination of the abdomen
- avoidance of analgesics such as morphine, pethidine or omnopon (papaveretum).

Features on observation that suggest the presence of intra-abdominal trauma include:

- persistent abdominal tenderness
- persistent abdominal guarding or rigidity
- persistent elevation of pulse and temperature
- progressive loss of bowel sounds
- development of paralytic ileus.

The decision to operate in the difficult case must be made on strong suspicion alone in the absence of frank signs, and after careful and repeated observation. However, integrity or otherwise of the liver and spleen on scanning will assist clinical judgment, while serial scans allow progress to be monitored.

Laparoscopy can be valuable in an equivocal case.

Any haemoperitoneum is washed out and the source of haemorrhage is identified. Active bleeding requires laparotomy, but if bleeding has ceased then consevative management can be continued. The integrity of the bowel can be checked and it may be possible to oversew a simple traumatic perforation.

PENETRATING INJURIES

In low-velocity injury (stabs) penetration of the peritoneum may not mean visceral damage. Absolute indications for operation are:

- visceral or omental prolapse
- continued bleeding – particularly dark venous blood, which probably comes from a portal radicle
- discharge of intestinal contents from the wound
- signs of spreading peritonitis
- shock (in the absence of other major injuries to the body).

All these features being absent, it is reasonable to observe the patient, making frequent abdominal examinations. Only about a quarter of stab wounds managed this way require exploration.

In high-velocity injury, exploration is mandatory. The principles of operation are as follows:

- thorough laparotomy with assessment and treatment of all injuries encountered
- wounds of entry (and exit, if present) must be excised and left open in the first instance.

SPECIAL CONSIDERATIONS

RUPTURED SPLEEN

This accounts for about 50% of visceral injuries following closed abdominal trauma. A diseased spleen (e.g. in malaria or leukaemia) is more likely to rupture than a healthy one.

About 25% of patients with splenic trauma remain well for days or even weeks before frank rupture occurs. In these cases a subcapsular haematoma probably forms and gradually increases in size before breaking through the capsule into the peritoneal cavity.

Clinical features

History of violence. This is often the cause in a crush injury to the left lower chest.

Evidence of internal haemorrhage. This is provided by:

- signs of hypovolaemia – pallor, restlessness, tachycardia, hypotension
- signs of peritoneal irritation – abdominal pain, shoulder pain, guarding and rigidity
- signs of ileus – distension, absent bowel sounds
- signs of fluid – shifting dullness (rare).

Special tests

A plain X-ray of the chest and abdomen should be carried out to exclude haemothorax, fractured ribs or a ruptured hollow organ. Kehr's sign is reliable if positive – elevation of the foot of the bed causes pain to be experienced in the left shoulder.

Ultrasound scans are useful for showing subcapsular or adjacent haematomas when trauma to the liver, spleen or kidney is suspected. Actual disruption of the organ may be seen in severe cases.

CT scan can demonstrate these changes with even greater clarity, but it is more expensive and more difficult to arrange in a shocked patient.

Treatment

Treatment is by resuscitation with intravenous fluids and blood. Expectant treatment should be provided in favourable cases, i.e. in a stable patient with a low blood transfusion requirement (not >2 units) and where there is no evidence of organ disruption on scanning.

Urgent laparotomy and usually splenectomy are required. Preservation of some or all of the spleen is now commonly practised, particularly in the child where there is a real risk of overwhelming postsplenectomy sepsis with pneumococci and other encapsulated organisms. New compounds such as fibrillary collagen are more effective haemostatics and may be associated with effective cessation of bleeding in superficial tears. If splenectomy is carried out below the age of 20, antipneumococcal vaccination is mandatory.

If the spleen cannot be preserved in situ, then slices may be implanted in the greater omentum in the hope of regeneration.

RUPTURED LIVER

Liver injury may follow both open and closed trauma. In open injury the wound may be a simple stab which does not produce much damage, or a high-velocity wound which tears and disrupts the liver substance. In closed injury the damage varies from a simple capsular tear to gross irregular splitting throughout the whole organ. In some cases large fragments of liver may be completely devitalised.

The effects on the patient vary according to the amount of haemorrhage and the amount of bile leakage.

Clinical features

History of violence. This should be considered, particularly in crush injuries to the right lower chest.

Evidence of internal haemorrhage. Signs are the same as these in a ruptured spleen, but maximum pain, tenderness and rigidity are found on the right side of the abdomen.

Special tests

Plain X-ray of the chest and abdomen is performed to exclude haemothorax, fractured ribs or a ruptured hollow organ. CT or ultrasound may show a filling defect (Fig. 15.3).

Hepatic angiography is of considerable value in experienced hands, particularly when major liver trauma is suspected and the patient is not in shock.

Embolisation of the hepatic artery may sometimes help to control bleeding.

Treatment

In cases of *suspected minor liver trauma*, continuous and close observation is required if the patient is rapidly recovering from shock, and abdominal signs are well localised or progressively improving. When minor liver trauma is found at operation, small lacerations may be sutured, packed or covered with omentum or the falciform ligament.

However, in cases of *suspected major liver trauma*, when shock persists despite repeated blood transfusion or when abdominal signs progressively worsen, laparotomy is an urgent requirement.

If severe liver trauma is present, the first essential is to control haemorrhage. Deep 'through-and-through sutures' or packing of deep liver lacerations may be unsatisfactory because a bleeding cavity is left within. Occlusion of the inferior vena cava above and below the liver together with compression of the portal vein and hepatic artery in the porta hepatis may be required through an extended incision.

With haemorrhage controlled and after blood replacement has been achieved, the second essential is resection of non-viable liver fragments. This may require a partial or complete hepatic lobectomy. Deep lacerations of the liver that involve the hepatic veins or inferior vena cava are very difficult to manage and carry a high mortality rate. Unless an experienced hepatobiliary surgeon is available, the liver should be packed; the patient is then stabilised and transferred to a specialist centre.

Occasionally *haemobilia* complicates liver trauma, usually a stab wound. It is manifested by right upper abdominal pain, gastrointestinal haemorrhage and transient jaundice. Selective hepatic arteriography may demonstrate the bleeding intrahepatic artery, and treatment is by embolisation or ligation of the feeding artery.

RUPTURED PANCREAS

This may follow closed abdominal trauma when the pancreas is compressed against the vertebral column, and in its extreme form complete transection of the pancreas may occur. Damage may also occur with penetrating injuries, which usually involve other organs as well. Varying degrees of pancreatitis are liable to occur with oedema, haemorrhage, necrosis, infection and later pseudocyst formation.

Clinical features

There are two common methods of presentation.

Solid organ rupture. This may occur with shock, severe abdominal pain, internal haemorrhage, spreading peritonitis and abdominal distension. The serum amylase is generally raised.

Pseudocyst formation. This develops at a variable period after the injury. The patient recovers but gradually develops an upper abdominal mass, which may take weeks or even months to become obvious.

Treatment

Treatment is by:

- laparotomy after resuscitation – remove necrotic pancreas, secure haemostasis and drain the lesser sac
- pseudocyst drainage.

RUPTURED INTESTINE

Perforation of the *small bowel* is treated by simple closure. The one possible exception is rupture of the duodenum. There are two special points about this injury:

- It is usually retroperitoneal, so that it can be difficult to diagnose; severe retroperitoneal cellulitis can develop before a laparotomy is done.
- A closed injury is the consequence of severe blunt trauma and thus there may be extensive bruising of the duodenal wall.

Both these facts make for a high complication rate from simple closure. It is usually recommended that the duodenum is patched with an adjacent loop of small bowel, but some surgeons exclude the duodenum by dividing it close to the pylorus and closing the ends, restoring continuity with a gastroenterostomy.

Injuries of the *large bowel* are more difficult to treat. Civilian injury from knives or blunt trauma is now usually managed by primary closure. Left-sided injury is either exteriorised or repaired and exteriorised. Military injuries by high-velocity missiles call for extensive resection and end colostomy, as does close-range shotgun injury. The rectum can be injured either by a gunshot wound to the pelvis or by insertion of a foreign body. Suture repair may be required with or without diverting colostomy, depending upon the site of injury and the extent of contamination.

RUPTURED KIDNEY

Trauma to the kidney may follow a heavy fall or a blow or crushing injury to the abdomen or loin. As a result there may ensue a subcapsular haematoma, parenchymal contusion, parenchymal rupture, complete split of the kidney or an avulsion of the kidney from its vascular pedicle.

Clinical features

There is usually a history of violence associated with:

- pain, bruising or swelling in the loin
- haematuria
- ureteric colic due to passage of clots.

Special tests

Intravenous urogram should be carried out (once the patient has recovered from shock) to assess renal function, to determine the presence or absence of extravasation and to demonstrate the presence of a normal opposite kidney.

In selected cases renal arteriogram may be of great value in determining the nature and extent of renal trauma. It may permit selective external ligation, conservative resection or embolisation of a bleeding vessel.

A CT scan with contrast can be used as an alternative to arteriography.

Treatment

Conservative management. This is indicated when the clinical features and radiographic evidence indicate minor trauma, when there is no loin swelling and when haematuria subsides rapidly.

The patient is kept in bed until all symptoms and signs have abated.

A careful follow-up is necessary and should include X-ray examination to detect complications which may develop later, such as infection, hydronephrosis, calculus formation or hypertension.

Operation. This will be indicated if there is:

- rapid deterioration with continuing shock despite transfusions
- continuous massive haematuria
- expanding loin swelling
- increasing pain, tenderness and rigidity, suggesting haemoperitoneum.

At operation, partial or total nephrectomy will usually be indicated. Rarely do the circumstances permit suture of lacerations with conservation of the kidney.

RUPTURED BLADDER AND URETHRA

Intrapelvic rupture of the bladder typically follows a kick to the abdomen when the victim is inebriated and has a full bladder. There is abdominal distension and inability to pass urine. The diagnosis is confirmed by urethral catheterisation and cystography. The defect is repaired at laparotomy, and the catheter is left in situ.

Either extraperitoneal rupture of the bladder or intrapelvic rupture of the posterior urethra can complicate displaced fractures of the pelvis. The diagnosis should be suspected if there is blood at the external urethral meatus and the patient is unable to void. Urethral catheterisation should be avoided because of the risk of converting a partial into a complete urethral tear. Retrograde urethrography should be performed to assess the damage. If the urethra is intact, then a catheter can be passed and the decision to repair the bladder depends upon the extent of the injury. Partial rupture of the urethra is managed by suprapubic catheterisation alone; complete rupture may be suitable for repair by an experienced urologist. In either case, there is a risk of subsequent urethral stricture.

FURTHER READING

Chisholm G D 1991 Urological trauma. In: O'Higgins N J, Chisholm G D, Williamson R C N (eds) Surgical management, 2nd edn. Butterworth-Heinemann, Oxford, p 279–286

Demetriades D, Rabinowitz B 1987 Indications for operation in abdominal stab wounds. A prospective study of 651 patients. Annals of Surgery 205: 129–132

Hernando H C, Alle K M, Chen J, Davis I, Klein S R 1994 Triage by laparoscopy in patients with penetrating abdominal trauma. British Journal of Surgery 81: 384–385

Hollands M J, Little J M 1990 The role of hepatic resection in the management of blunt liver trauma. World Journal of Surgery 14: 478–482

Hoyt D B, Moossa A R 1995 Abdominal injuries. In: Cuschieri A, Giles G R, Moossa A R (eds) Essential surgical practice, 3rd edn. Butterworth-Heinemann, Oxford, p 531–544

Schweizer W, Böhlen L, Dennison A, Blumgart L H 1992 Prospective study in adults of splenic preservation after traumatic rupture. British Journal of Surgery 92: 1330–1333

Nerve and vessel injuries
Don Howie

OVERVIEW

Because of their close proximity to bones and joints, nerves and vessels are often vulnerable to injury, when trauma causes long bone fractures or dislocations. This chapter provides guidelines for classification, assessment and the treatment of nerve, vein and arterial injuries.

Blunt or penetrating injuries to limbs may involve damage to peripheral nerves and blood vessels. Such damage should always be suspected, especially in the presence of a fracture.

NERVE INJURIES

CLASSIFICATION

Nerve injuries may occur with open wounds, fractures or as a result of crushing or traction of the nerve.

Three stages of nerve injury are recognised:

- *neuropraxia* – the axons are intact but their ability to conduct has been lost, usually because of mild pressure or stretching
- *axonotmesis* – there is destruction or division of the axons in an intact neural sheath, a more severe injury
- *neurotmesis* – this is complete division of the whole nerve sheath due to transection or tearing. Initially it may not be possible to distinguish between these three types of injury on clinical examination.

ASSESSMENT

History

It is important to elucidate the mechanism and circumstances of the injury. Tidy injuries caused by broken glass or household utensils will frequently be associated with damage to deeper structures. Adequate tetanus prophylaxis (p. 250) should be assured for tetanus-prone wounds such as those occurring outside the home and with soil contamination. It is important to note the time from accident to examination, from the point of view of administering a general anaesthetic and also because prolonged periods of delay in treatment may influence the degree of closure carried out, primarily in certain untidy wounds.

The patient's occupation should especially be noted, for this may influence the choice of operation.

Examination

Nerve injuries are frequently missed during the initial examination, often because the possibility of division is not considered or the patient does not properly comprehend the instructions given by the examiner.

Tests of motor and sensory function are performed and where possible compared with the other side. To assess motor function, it is simplest to place the patient's joint in the position of maximal contraction of the muscle to be tested and ask the patient to 'hold it there' against pressure exerted by the examiner. Pin-prick is the only reliable test of sensation. Remember that the patient will try to convince the examiner (and so herself) that her sensation is normal. In all penetrating wounds where nerves are at risk, it must be assumed that the nerve is divided until proved otherwise, usually by direct vision at operative exploration.

Specific nerve injuries

Median nerve. This is most often damaged at the wrist, possibly following a self-inflicted wound, because at the distal transverse crease the nerve is quite superficial. It can also be damaged at the elbow by a supracondylar fracture of the humerus. The motor function of the median nerve is tested by assessing the ability of the thenar muscles to maintain the thumb abducted.

Ulnar nerve. This is susceptible on the medial aspect of the elbow, at the wrist and in the palm affecting the deep branch following penetrating wounds. A reliable test, especially for distal injuries, is the ability to maintain abduction of the little finger or adduction of the thumb as in Froment's test. This is elicited by asking the patient to grip a card in the cleft between index and thumb. In an ulnar nerve palsy, this can only be done by flexing the interphalangeal joint of the thumb, because of loss of thumb adduction. Integrity of the proximal nerve can be assessed at the same time by palpating the flexor carpi ulnaris tendon on ulnar deviation of the wrist.

Radian nerve. This is most commonly damaged by a fracture in the upper arm as it runs around the radial groove of the humerus. The accompanying wrist drop and loss of extension of the thumb are characteristic. Lacerations in the forearm may cut the superficial, sensory branch of the radial nerve, which gives rise to a deficit on the dorsum of the web space between the thumb and index finger.

Brachial plexus injuries. In birth trauma there are two main lesions: Erb's palsy and Klumpke's palsy.

In *Erb's palsy*, the head is distracted from the shoulder, stretching the upper part of the plexus, causing a lesion at the upper trunk (C5 and C6). The external rotators of the shoulder, flexors of the elbow and extensors of the wrist are paralysed. The arm is held in internal rotation, extension and flexion of the wrist – the 'waiter's tip' position. There are sensory changes in the C5 and C6 dermatomes.

Klumpke's palsy is the result of forced abduction of the arm, disrupting the first thoracic root. The small muscles of the hand are paralysed and the sympathetic supply to the pupil, which runs with T1, is affected, producing Horner's syndrome.

In adult trauma these injuries are caused by high-velocity impact and stretch injuries such as motorcycle accidents, usually producing a C5/6 lesion or, when more severe, involving the whole plexus. Local pressure in the axilla from a crutch or back of a chair may produce a Klumpke palsy.

Spinal injuries. See page 101.

Sciatic nerve. This may be damaged by fractures of the pelvis or dislocation of the hip. It is also at risk from injections into the buttock and during operations on the hip. The common peroneal nerve is the major component of the sciatic nerve and foot-drop is the hallmark of any sciatic nerve lesion, with sensory changes on the sole of the foot.

The common peroneal nerve itself is vulnerable as it winds around the neck of the fibula. The clinical signs may be the same as for a high sciatic nerve lesion, as only very severe injuries of the proximal sciatic nerve result in hamstring paralysis.

Femoral nerve. Injury is uncommon, but the usual cause is a penetrating injury of the groin. Paralysis of the quadriceps is produced, which can be missed clinically because the patient soon learns to lift the leg without flexing the knee by internally rotating the hip and using the tensor fascia lata to raise the leg.

Causalgia. Any incomplete nerve injury, particularly lower limb injury, can be followed by episodes of severe, burning pain which is very resistant to treatment. This is causalgia, the cause of which is unknown.

PRINCIPLES OF TREATMENT

Divided nerves should be repaired as soon as possible. There is no advantage in delayed primary or secondary repair. The only circumstances in which secondary repair is advised is when there is a dirty wound in which skin closure is not possible.

Complete divisions must be repaired with an avascular field, adequate exposure of the nerve ends and magnification during repair.

The ends must be trimmed with a sharp blade until normal funiculi are identified, and then the nerve ends are precisely apposed while matching up corresponding funiculi with fine material. The related joints must be immobilised in such a position that all tension is taken off the repair.

Where there is a loss of nerve substance, this may be overcome to a certain extent by mobilisation of nerve ends and posturing of related joints.

If the nerve ends still cannot be apposed easily, nerve grafting must be carried out. This is usually done using three or four equal lengths of suitable nerve, such as sural nerve, interposed loosely between the cut ends and again anastomosed with fine sutures under magnification.

Nerve injuries repaired by suture are completely immobilised for 4 weeks, and then graduated mobilisation is begun.

VESSEL INJURIES

A vascular injury may be readily apparent with obvious ischaemia or haemorrhage; however, severe arterial damage, such as an intimal tear, may be present with few initial symptoms or signs. Prompt diagnosis is vital to achieve satisfactory results. In any injury, vessel damage must be suspected until proved otherwise. In civilian trauma, vessel injuries are most likely to occur in young males involved in motor car accidents, whereas gunshot and stab wounds account for only a small number of cases outside the USA and some other violent communities.

ASSESSMENT AND EARLY MANAGEMENT OF VASCULAR IMPAIRMENT

The aim of management is to identify vascular injuries before critical ischaemia develops. Signs suggestive of a vascular injury are:

- bleeding
- expanding haematoma
- bruit
- abnormal pulses
- impaired distal circulation
- decreased sensation
- increasing pain.

Phases of vascular injury

Three phases of vascular injury may be present.

Possible vascular injury. Some vascular injuries, such

as arterial intimal tears, may not be immediately apparent. Capillary refill may be normal and the distal pulses may be minimally changed. These injuries may be difficult to identify in the first hour, particularly if there is no obvious bleeding and perfusion of the extremity appears adequate. Reassessment must be done frequently, particularly in the presence of fractures/dislocations with a high incidence of vascular impairment, especially those about the knee and elbow.

Suspected vascular injury. Vascular injuries associated with impaired circulation represent an immediate or potential threat to limb viability and must be recognised and managed promptly. In the patient who is haemodynamically stable, pulse discrepancies, pallor, paraesthesia, hypoaesthesia and/or any abnormality of motor function suggest possible impairment of blood flow.

With all cases of suspected vascular injury in the presence of fracture or dislocation, the doctor should check the immobilisation device, assess the fracture alignment, reassess distal perfusion, consider a compartment syndrome and obtain surgical consultation.

If a traction device has been applied to an injured extremity with vascular impairment, the status of the traction must be assessed and any necessary adjustments made. Failure to fully align a long bone fracture with insufficient traction, or stretching an extremity through excessive traction can result in vascular impairment. If a circular dressing, splint or cast has been applied, assess for constriction. Release the device if there is any suspicion of it being too tight. If any of these abnormalities, particularly any change in pulse, persists after aligning and immobilising the extremity, a careful investigation for possible vascular injury should be undertaken.

When an arterial injury is suspected, Doppler pressure studies are useful but arteriography may be necessary. The angiogram should not be done until the patient's condition is stabilised and the injury extremity evaluated, dressed and splinted. For some patients with obvious and complete arterial occlusion, prompt surgical consultation is mandatory, and surgical exploration may be considered without waiting for an arteriogram.

Obvious vascular insufficiency. The classical picture of late, complete extremity ischaemia – pain, pallor, pulselessness, paraesthesia and paralysis – indicates profound ischaemia. This late manifestation of severe ischaemia indicates a surgical emergency, with little time remaining to salvage the extremity.

CLASSIFICATION

Contusions or crush injuries

These are probably the most common cause of vessel damage, as they are associated with fractures and dislocations, the brachial and popliteal arteries being most susceptible. External transmural compression of the artery produces a circumferential intimal tear, creating a 'valve' of infolded intima, with the formation of an intra-luminal thrombus and an intramural haematoma.

Incisions and lacerations

These are usually caused by glass or sharp objects and may or may not produce overt haemorrhage. A completely divided vessel may retract and constrict, with little bleeding, but a small lateral laceration may bleed profusely.

Perforations

High-velocity missiles or sharp objects may perforate a vessel without external evidence of injury. The subsequent development of shock or pulsating haematoma reveals the injury.

Puncture wounds

Percutaneous puncture of peripheral arteries (in hospital for either arteriography or blood gas analysis) may result in a pulsating haematoma (false aneurysm).

Chemical injury

Inadvertent intra-arterial injection of thiopentone or other agents will cause severe pain and intense vasospasm. A superficial ulnar artery at the elbow, a not uncommon anomaly, is often involved.

Ruptured thoracic aorta

This is discussed on page 125.

CLINICAL MANIFESTATIONS

Haemorrhage

External pulsating arterial bleeding or a persistent ooze of dark venous blood is obvious, but concealed haemorrhage may present as either shock or an expanding haematoma.

Ischaemia

The clinical signs of acute ischaemia are a pale, cool, extremity with decreased sensation and movement and absent pedal pulses. The palpation of pedal pulses is subjective and can be inaccurate at the best of times but especially in the presence of systemic hypotension. A normal ankle/brachial Doppler pressure index excludes a significant arterial lesion. An abnormal Doppler index or clear signs of ischaemia are an indication for either arteriography or exploration, depending on the urgency of other injuries and the severity of ischaemia.

False aneurysm

A false aneurysm may be formed by the outer layer of an encapsulated haematoma, following bleeding from a side hole in the artery. Proximal flow is not usually disrupted. An expansile and pulsating mass is palpable over the artery. At an early stage there is an expanding haematoma rather than a pulsating aneurysm.

Arteriovenous fistula

This may be acute, following synchronous laceration or ligation of artery and vena comitantes, or delayed, when infected arterial haematomata erode into adjacent veins. A continuous thrill and murmur are usually present.

Venous injury and obstruction

Prominent distal veins and peripheral induration and oedema may indicate venous compression or obstruction.

PRINCIPLES OF TREATMENT

Severe associated injuries are common and should be treated appropriately. Arteriography is seldom required and may delay prompt treatment.

Haemorrhage

External bleeding is best controlled by continuous pressure or packing. Tourniquets and the blind application of artery clips should be avoided.

Operative repair of arterial injuries

The feasibility of repair is determined by the magnitude of the wound. For extensive wounds with gross contamination, as seen in military casualties, proximal arterial ligation and amputation may be life-saving.

The majority of civilian vascular injuries are, however, repairable, as contamination and tissue damage are often minimal. The following principles therefore apply. The artery is exposed by an ample incision in the long axis of the vessel, above and below the level of the injury. Proximal and distal control is achieved using slings and then vascular clamps, and intravenous heparin is given to prevent distal thrombosis.

The injured area of the artery is dissected free and repaired according to the injury:

- Simple laceration is repaired by suture, and when it is longitudinal a vein patch is incorporated to reduce the narrowing of the artery.
- Partial or complete disruption may be repaired by sutures, but more commonly contusion and retraction of the artery necessitate excision and reconstruction with interposed autogenous vein graft. The use of a prosthetic graft in trauma is avoided because of an increased risk of infection and thrombosis.
- In the case of an intimal tear, the segment of artery involved is excised and repaired by either end-to-end anastomosis or interposed vein graft.
- Arterial spasm alone is rarely responsible for vascular occlusion except after chemical injury; then intra-arterial heparin and reserpine are infused.

Fasciotomy distal to a vascular reconstruction to free swollen, ischaemic muscle compressed within fascial compartments should always be performed. Wherever possible, fractures are stabilised by rigid internal or external fixation *before* arterial reconstruction to avoid distraction forces on the repair.

Operative repair of venous injury

The need for concurrent venous and arterial reconstruction is uncertain, as the results following venous ligation alone are comparable. It would seem logical, however, to repair a damaged major venous drainage of a revascularised limb. Venous reconstruction is mandatory during microsurgical repair of severed digits or limbs. The principles of venous repair are similar to those for arteries; however, thrombosis is a more common problem and intravenous heparin is continued postoperatively.

FURTHER READING

Hallett J W, Brewster D C, Darling R C 1995 Handbook of patient care in vascular surgery, 3rd edn. Vascular trauma. Little, Brown, Boston, ch 24

Segelov P M 1990 Complications of fractures and dislocations. Chapman and Hall, London

Sunderland S 1978 Nerve and nerve injuries. Churchill Livingstone, Edinburgh

Burns
John Masterton

OVERVIEW

Thermal injury to the largest organ in the body – the skin – causes major tissue damage and marked physiological effects on other body functions, requiring specific treatment regimens and a team approach. This chapter covers all these issues, emphasising the importance of clinical assessment, initial resuscitation and transfer to a designated burns unit. Definitive treatment is outlined and chemical burns are also discussed.

An extensive burn is one of the most dangerous and devastating of injuries. This equates with the community's perception. There is real fear of pain, disfigurement and death.

In physical terms, a burn involves the transfer of an excessive amount of heat energy to the body. The extent of injury will depend on the temperature, and the scale and period of exposure to the heat source. It will be modified by certain factors:

- the insulating effect and flammability of clothing
- the local blood supply – a good blood supply to an area (e.g. the face) will lessen the effect of the burning agent because a rapid flow of blood acts as a heat exchange mechanism tending to reduce local damage
- the speed with which local external cooling can be applied; good first aid is important.

Cell damage occurs at temperatures at and above 44°C. Rapid cooling of a burn by application of cold in the form of ice or cold water may lessen the injury at the interface of damaged and viable tissue. Diving off a burning boat with clothing on fire is a practical example of this.

PATHOLOGY

When a burn occurs, there is damage or death of cells. The capillary bed of the skin is particularly susceptible. Damaged capillaries leak, leading to loss of water, electrolytes and plasma proteins. The fluid that escapes accumulates in the interstitial space causing oedema which can also be accompanied by blistering or actual surface fluid loss as well as insensible loss. Such losses can amount to a very considerable volume in an extensive burn (defined as one covering more than 10% of total body surface area) and lead to shock if not dealt with by appropriate fluid replacement.

As well as damage to the capillary network, there is damage to or death of cells in the area of a burn. Such an environment is admirable as a culture medium for bacteria which can multiply without interference. Burned tissue is like an ischaemic or gangrenous limb: there is dead material in which bacteria multiply and from where showers of bacteria can invade the rest of the body across the interface of living and dead cells.

An understanding of the simple pathology of a burn as described above should lead to an understanding of the two major areas of initial endeavour in management:

- prevention of shock
- what to do with the burn wound to prevent infection.

Both of these are influenced by:

- the extent of the burn
- the depth of the burn.

EXTENT OF THE BURN

The bigger the burn and the older the patient, the greater is the likelihood of death. Other factors affecting the outcome are:

- how much of the burn is full thickness
- associated respiratory tract injury
- pre-existing problems such as obesity, pulmonary disease and diabetes.

The simplest way to estimate the extent of a burn for adults is by the 'rule of nines' (Fig. 17.1). It should be emphasised that what might appear to be an easy method requires great care. Dirt, clothing and poor light can all prevent an accurate assessment. Early estimates done hurriedly tend to be inaccurate. Review and reassessment are essential. In children, the 'rule of nines' figures are a little inaccurate, in that the area of an infant's or a young child's head is comparatively greater compared with the rest of the body.

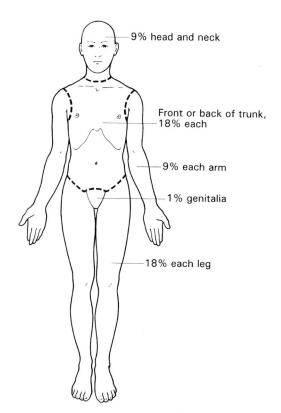

9% head and neck

Front or back of trunk, 18% each

9% each arm

1% genitalia

18% each leg

Fig. 17.1 'Rule of nines' for estimating burn extent as a percentage of total body surface area.

DEPTH OF THE BURN

When examining a burned area, the question the clinician wants to answer, as does the patient, is whether the area is going to recover. Is it partial thickness skin damage or is the area going to require grafting because the full thickness of the skin is damaged?

Skin consists of epidermis and dermis, including hair follicles and sweat glands (Fig. 17.2). A partial thickness burn ranges from one that spares some epidermis and all the dermis to one where there is involvement of all epithelial elements apart from some dermis from which re-epithelialisation can occur. Re-epithelialisation occurs best from surviving elements of epidermis, but if this is destroyed, it can occur from hair follicles and sweat glands. Provided infection does not cause further and total destruction of all epithelial tissue, skin grafting will not be necessary except in certain circumstances (see below).

A full thickness burn is one which destroys epidermis and dermis completely. Unless the area is grafted, healing can occur only by growth of scar tissue. A full thickness burn which may extend to involve fat, muscle, tendon, nerve, major vessels and bone is the most dangerous in terms of local restoration of function and risk of infection.

Differentiation of a partial thickness from a full thickness burn clinically is not always easy, even for an experienced clinician. However, certain clinical signs help in mapping out areas of partial and full thickness damage. By doing this, the treatment programme can be planned.

Methods of assessment of burn depth

Inspection. Partial thickness burns are red, often blistered, and have a moist appearance. Full thickness burns can be red, indicating entrapped red cells in damaged capillaries, but more often the surface is pale and parchment-like or has an appearance like marble. Blistering is rare in full thickness burns and, if it has happened, the blisters have usually ruptured and there are tags of loose, dead skin hanging from the surface. In extreme examples, the tissue is charred and cracked. In such instances, there is never any doubt.

Palpation. A partial thickness burn, particularly the most superficial variety, is extremely sensitive to touch. With increasing depth of the burn, there is blunting of sensation. Thus, the presence of pinprick sensation rang-

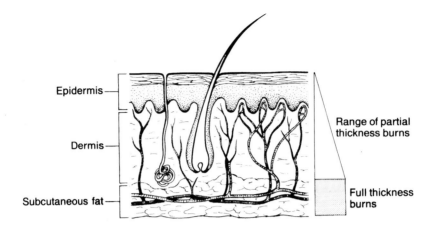

Fig. 17.2 Anatomy of the skin and depth of burns.

ing from hyperaesthesia to hypoaesthesia is indicative of a partial thickness burn. If there is absence of sensation to pinprick, the burn is full thickness: the nerve endings in the dermis have been destroyed. The use of pinprick sensitivity is the most reliable method of differentiating and mapping the extent of partial thickness and full thickness burning. The red colour of partial thickness burns caused by capillary vasodilatation disappears on pressure. The capillaries are emptied and there is blanching. This does not happen with full thickness burns. The partial thickness burn has a resilient, soft feel about it; the coagulated skin of a full thickness burn feels firm, like leather. It is inelastic.

MANAGEMENT

The following discussion addresses the management of burns in adults. While the principles are the same in children, details may be different. This is particularly the case with resuscitation. These differences will not be discussed.

SHOCK

General aspects of the treatment of shock are covered in Chapter 5 and need not be repeated here because the problem of hypovolaemic shock in a burn is not unique. Shock is likely to occur in a burn involving more than 10% of the body surface. The degree of shock is proportional to the total area burned and the depth. The hypovolaemic state is entirely due to loss of water,

electrolytes and plasma proteins from widespread damage to the capillary bed. It is important to realise that losses occur into the interstitial space, into burn blisters and outwards from the burn surface, from which the fluid drips away, as well as due to evaporation. Oedema can be gross. For example, when the face is burned it swells to an inordinate degree, leading to inversion of eyelids and eversion of lips accompanied by a swollen tongue. The latter sometimes leads to partial upper airway obstruction, which is further aggravated by neck swelling. Oedema spreads beyond the burn into undamaged tissue.

A special circumstance may happen in burn shock but can also occur in the crush syndrome. This is the phenomenon of haemoglobinuria and myoglobinuria. Heat destroys red blood cells in burned capillaries and if continued may also damage muscle; perfusion washes the products of muscle and red cell destruction back into the circulation. This material is secreted in the glomerular filtrate and, as it flows down the loop of Henle, it is concentrated in the tubule, where it may cause blockage. Clinically, this possibility is suspected when dark, claret-coloured urine of small volume is produced. This is a warning sign of the imminent risk of anuria.

Management of burn shock

A number of formulae exist which provide a guide to appropriate volume replacement in burn shock. These are helpful but usually depend on an accurate estimate of body weight and the area burned; both of these are not always available with any degree of accuracy and a practical alternative is to re-infuse the patient according to changes that occur in the usual parameters for assessing shock. Thus, it is appropriate to measure pulse rate, blood pressure, central venous pressure, urea and electrolytes, rate of urine output and haemoconcentration by haematocrit or haemoglobin. Arterial blood gas levels and acid/base balance must also be known. In addition, pulse oximetry is an excellent guide to peripheral perfusion. Other and more sophisticated measures may be needed, such as mean arterial pressure via an intra-arterial cannula or pulmonary arterial wedge pressure via a Swan–Ganz cannula.

Guidelines and objectives for fluid replacement. Shock is unlikely in burns covering less than 10% of the body surface. Therefore, intravenous resuscitation is usually unnecessary. In those over 10% of total body surface area (TBSA), certain guidelines should be followed, as described below.

Burns of 10–20% TBSA, usually require an intravenous infusion and may require urethral catheterisation, particularly in elderly people who are more susceptible to changes in fluid dynamics. There are circumstances where a burn of just over 10% in a very fit adult may not require either intravenous infusion or urethral catheterisation. The clinician must judge each case on its merits.

Burns of between 20% and 30% TBSA require both an intravenous infusion and urethral catheterisation and it may be necessary to use a central venous cannula. The latter may be required even in smaller burns because the arms are burned. Nevertheless, an intravenous line can be inserted through burn tissue if necessary either by puncture or by cut-down. Leg veins should be avoided at all costs because of the risk of early thrombophlebitis. If one is used, it should be discontinued as soon as possible.

In *burns of greater than 30% TBSA*, insertion of a central venous line is mandatory in order to measure central venous pressure and possibly provide access for adjuvant parenteral nutrition later. However, the latter should be avoided if the patient can eat adequately or tolerate enteral feeding.

The objectives of treatment of shock should be to maintain:

- a pulse rate of less than 120 beats/min
- a systolic blood pressure at or above 120 mmHg
- a steady central venous pressure at between 5 and 8 cmH$_2$O.
- a urine flow rate of between 50 and 100 ml/h.; in a

burn of 50% this may mean infusion rates of the order of 1 L or more per 2 hours in the first 24 hours.

The fluids to be used are a balanced or physiological salt solution (e.g. Hartmann's solution) and a plasma expander, preferably plasma itself or its equivalent or one of the synthetic plasma expanders. It is customary for blood banks now to supply human colloid as a derivative of plasma, generally in the form of 5% albumin. This varies in different countries. In burns of less than 20%, plasma may not be required but in excess of this it is appropriate and practical to replace what may be quite substantial plasma losses to maintain intravascular osmotic pressure. The infusion is administered by giving crystalloid, alternating with colloid in equal volumes. Usually, maximum volume infusion rates are reached in the first 24 hours, after which the full picture of burn oedema will have developed and the situation will have become more stable except that there will still be a continuing loss of water from the burn surface by both exudation and evaporation. On about the third or fourth day post-burn, oedema begins to lessen. At this time there is, in effect, an infusion of fluid back into the circulation from the interstitial space. When this occurs, the intravenous infusion rate has to be reduced quite abruptly to avoid the risk of overloading which can lead to cardiac embarrassment, particularly in elderly people. Good management requires meticulous care and attention to detail.

Haemoglobinuria or myoglobinuria. This occurs only in the very early post-burn period. The risk of tubular blockage is overcome by inducing a free urine flow at or above 50 ml/h. If this does not occur with a fluid load then it may be necessary to give frusemide intravenously (an initial dose in an adult of 10–20 mg) or mannitol 20% in a bolus dose of 200 ml.

There are quite marked differences in management of shock from one centre to another. Whatever method is used, the aim is to maintain adequate tissue perfusion and the very best guide to this is urine output with, in addition, measurement of pulse oximetry.

Pain relief. Contrary to popular belief, pain, particularly in full thickness burns, is not an overwhelming problem. It may become so later when grafting occurs. However, it is imperative to give effective pain relief with morphine or its equivalent. In big burns, this is best achieved by giving the drug intravenously, and a continuous infusion has much merit. Analgesics should be avoided until effective resuscitation has begun. The subcutaneous route is inappropriate because absorption is unpredictable in shock.

LOCAL MANAGEMENT OF THE BURN WOUND

A tetanus booster should be given to all who have been previously immunised. Active immunisation is begun on anyone not previously immunised. In burns greater than 10% TBSA, particularly if full thickness, immediate passive immunisation with human hyperimmune globulin should be considered in the unimmunised.

Small burns (less than 10% TBSA) can be dressed shortly after admission, because they do not require resuscitation. The wound is cleaned with antiseptic solution and any loose skin tags snipped away. If possible, intact blisters are left, as they protect the extremely painful underlying epidermis. Silver sulphadiazine (SSD) cream or its equivalent is applied to the burn, and gauze dressings and bandages are wrapped around it as appropriate. In certain circumstances, it may be neither practicable nor necessary to use antiseptic cream. For example, the face is sometimes best left alone particularly in less extensive and less severe burns. Small burns (less than 1%) may only require a sterile dressing.

Big burns (greater than 10% TBSA) should be dealt with differently. First, if there are obvious circumferential full thickness areas causing constriction of a limb or the chest, it may be necessary to incise these down to (and including) deep fascia to provide decompression (escharotomy/fasciotomy) and thus prevent underlying muscle damage. Such areas of full thickness burning are insensitive and therefore analgesia is desirable but not essential for the procedure which can be carried out in the emergency department or in the ward. However, more often than not, it is more appropriate to do it in the operating theatre. At the same time, the burn injury can be assessed and thoroughly cleaned and dressed. In other less serious circumstances, the burn wound should simply be covered with a sterile sheet and left alone until resuscitation is underway and shock is controlled or prevented. This usually means a wait of 4–6 hours. Meanwhile, it is essential to keep the patient warm and covered not only with a sterile sheet but also with blankets and if necessary an insulating 'space blanket'.

Prophylactic systemic antibiotics are not recommended at the beginning of therapy, particularly when the patient is likely to be nursed in a clean environment such as most modern hospitals can provide. However, in less ideal circumstances, such as an open ward where staff are unused to burn care and techniques of preventing cross-infection, the patient should be given a course of prophylactic antibiotics for 10 days in the first instance. One of the penicillins is appropriate. Irrespective of whether systemic antibiotics are used, the mainstay of infection control is a vigorous programme of burn wound antisepsis using some form of antiseptic washing, which can include bathing, coupled with the application of an antibacterial cream such as silver sulphadiazine. In most circumstances, a closed dressing technique should be used.

If the burn is entirely partial thickness, there is no need to progress beyond the stage of antisepsis and expectant treatment with baths and dressings until healing occurs. Nevertheless, some partial thickness burns may be dealt with best by the technique of tangential excision and split skin grafting to facilitate more rapid and better quality healing. Tangential excision is where serial slices of the burn are cut away until a healthy bed of bleeding dermis is reached. If there is a full thickness burn, it is expedient to attempt to excise the area of full thickness as soon as possible because such tissue remains a constant hazard for infection. Where extensive areas are involved with a full thickness burn, excision can rarely be done in one stage and a series of theatre visits will be necessary in order to achieve total wound excision and grafting. A conventional plan is to begin a programme of wound excision when the capillary lesion is on the way to recovery. This will mean as soon after the fourth post-burn day as is convenient. It is usually found that around 10–20% of the body surface can be excised and grafted in one session. Excision of areas greater than this can be done but requires experience and care regarding blood loss. It is recommended that grafting is undertaken immediately after burn excision if at all possible. There are many variations and techniques that are advocated and are acceptable. For example, many would now advocate even earlier excision of defined full thickness burns than the fourth postoperative day. Broadly speaking, skin grafting is done using thin split skin autografts taken from whatever unburned or healed areas that are available, but preferably arms, legs or the abdominal wall. Less common areas can even include the scalp. It is customary to mesh donor skin in a meshing machine, thus permitting cover of a larger area as well as enhancing graft take. Meshed skin lessens haematoma formation by allowing any bleeding to take place through the mesh holes. Consequently, the percentage of graft take is higher. Donor skin not used immediately can be stored for up to 2 weeks in an ordinary domestic refrigerator at +4°C. Techniques are available where allograft or xenograft skin can be used as temporary skin cover when there is a shortage of autograft material. More recently, cultured autograft keratinocyte sheets have been used successfully in very extensive burns. Furthermore, a synthetic but biologically compatible dermis will soon be available to be used in conjunction with cultured keratinocyte sheets.

PROBLEMS OF MANAGEMENT IN BURN PATIENTS

Infection

By undertaking a vigorous programme using surface cleaning and topical antibacterial agents, it is possible to guide a patient through a major burn injury without any clinically apparent infection and without any need for systemic antibiotics. Nevertheless, the risks of infection are ever present.

Different environments create different sets of circumstances, and the organisms causing burn wound sepsis vary. In well-run burn units in temperate climates, streptococcal infection has virtually ceased to be a major problem. Characteristically, it occurs when patients are admitted with neglected, infected burns that until then had been treated at home. The organisms seen most frequently are staphylococci and the whole range of Gram-negative bacilli, headed by *Pseudomonas aeruginosa*, *Klebsiella*, *Proteus* and coliforms. The burn wound can become colonised quickly and bacteria can migrate inwards remarkably rapidly from the surface. Infection is suspected when there is fever, tachycardia, metabolic acidosis and there are positive cultures from either the burn or the bloodstream. Hand in hand with burn wound infection, there is often pulmonary infection, and invariably the organisms isolated from sputum are the same as those from the burn. Similarly, organisms cultured from urine are generally the same as from the burn. The need to monitor urine output demands a urethral catheter with the inevitable hazard of infection. Intravenous cannulation sites must be carefully watched for sepsis, and cannulae should be changed and cultured on suspicion. There is a characteristic progression of infection in a big burn. For a number of weeks, all is well and few cultures of the burn produce significant growth. Clinically, there

is no obvious infection. Then, after several visits to the operating room, the chest radiograph begins to cause concern. Blood gas measurements deteriorate, assisted ventilation is necessary and Gram-negative organisms appear in sputum and from wound cultures. This is a dangerous period when, unless the infection can be controlled, the prospect of survival is gloomy. Nevertheless, with the many strategies available in an intensive care unit, patients with the most horrendous infection can and do survive.

Burns scars

Even in the best of circumstances, it is unusual in very extensive burns (> 40% TBSA), where it is necessary to excise and graft large areas, for infection not to occur and for all grafts to take completely the first time. Were that to happen regularly, big burns would not present the major problem they do and the mortality would not be so high. Apart from any risk to life, there is an increased likelihood of development of hypertrophic scars when grafts fail and regrafting has to be done. It should be noted that in certain circumstances even healed partial thickness burns can lead to hypertrophic scars. Such scars are unsightly and, in addition, they can lead to stiffness and disability through scar contracture, particularly when they are crossing joints. Intensive efforts have been made using physiotherapy, splinting and compression bandaging to lessen the effects of contractures and facilitate joint movement. Often, repeated and complex plastic surgical procedures are necessary to improve matters. Much is demanded of the patient and many have emotional problems requiring understanding and support from their families and the whole medical team. The distortion of body image that occurs, not only in a big burn but also in smaller ones affecting the hands and face, can be devastating and long-lasting. The aim of therapy should be to provide the support necessary to overcome or mitigate this. Doctors, nurses, social workers, physiotherapists, occupational therapists, family, friends, clergy, other patients and employers all play a part. Hope and faith in the future have to be maintained.

Chest problems

In the initial accident, there may be burning of the upper or lower respiratory tract. This may result from flames sweeping across the face, fauces, pharynx and larynx, or even extending lower down into the trachea. Apart from flame, hot gases and noxious chemicals can be inhaled. The latter occurs more often now because of the widespread use of plastics in furnishings and in industry. When these become involved in fire, toxic gases can be produced that cause significant alveolar damage when inhaled. Such injuries are more likely when the burning accident is in a confined space. Respiratory tract injuries should always be suspected and looked for by examining the upper air passages. Stridor is an obvious sign that may demand immediate intubation. A chest X-ray immediately after the burning incident is singularly unhelpful. Damage to the lower respiratory tract is less easy to pinpoint clinically and may go hand in hand with pre-existing pulmonary disease or a problem of overinfusion during the shock phase. The early development of a picture of pulmonary oedema is suspicious. Clinical examination, regular follow-up chest X-rays, monitoring of blood gases, adjuvant oxygen therapy, antibiotics for added infection and intubation with assisted respiration are all part of the therapeutic regimen. Steroids are not recommended. Tracheostomy can usually be avoided, provided recovery takes place in 7–10 days. If there is a neck burn leading to compression of the trachea, intubation may be very difficult if left too late and then one is committed to tracheostomy in less than ideal circumstances. Tracheostomy can be done through burn tissue but is best avoided. The technique of percutaneous tracheostomy is preferable to open tracheostomy. Nevertheless, the latter may be necessary where there is gross neck swelling.

Nutrition

Burns of greater than 20% TBSA invariably pose a problem of nutrition and the very lack of adequate nutrition can materially affect the outcome. Energy and nutrients in excess of normal demands are required in order to offset the deficit caused by heat loss, plasma loss and increased metabolic rate. If infection is added, the combined metabolic demands may lead to energy expenditure of the order of 4000–5000 kcal/day (16–20 000 kJ) in an average adult. It frequently happens that the burned patient is too sick, apathetic and physically handicapped because of burns to hands and face to be able to partake of a diet that in any way matches energy needs. Not surprisingly, such patients can and do lose weight. Only by the most vigorous countermeasures can this be prevented. Adequate oral feeding is the ideal but is seldom attained, particularly when the feeding regimen is interrupted by frequent visits to the operating theatre. Consequently, it is necessary to supplement oral food with either liquid tube feeds or intravenous food. The latter can now be given easily and in effective quantities via a central venous cannula. By a combination of oral or tube feeding and intravenous food, patients can and must be adequately nourished. Hopefully, intravenous feeding can be avoided if nutrition is maintained with oral and enteral feeds. In addition, it is essential to recognise that these patients need to have an adequate haemoglobin level at all times. Frequent and ample blood transfusion (sometimes twice a week) is part of the total nutritional package.

Stress ulceration (see Ch. 25)

Upper gastrointestinal bleeding, whilst relatively rare and lessened by anti-ulcer prophylaxis, remains a difficult and serious problem in the big burn victim who is often septic. If major bleeding occurs, requiring transfusion, the mortality is in excess of 30%. The surgeon is faced with a dilemma. Conservative management with continuing anti-ulcer medication is not always effective. Operation may arrest the haemorrhage but impose an insuperable burden on the patient's ability to respond to yet another injury. If the patient is elderly, the problem is close to insurmountable.

THE AFTERMATH

Anyone dealing with a large number of burn victims will be impressed that after they have left hospital there are still many problems. The management of scars has been discussed and remains the principal and most difficult problem long term. There are two others worthy of consideration:

- pruritus
- inappropriate sweating.

For as long as a year or more after burns have healed either spontaneously or by grafting, there is troublesome and almost continuous itching. This can be very disturbing. The victim wakes at night scratching and finds that delicate recently healed surfaces have been damaged and are bleeding. Treatment is not easy. Lanolin and other bland moisturising creams may help, as do antihistamines. A reliable hypnotic may be necessary to provide restful sleep. Only with the passing of time does the matter improve.

In very extensive burns which have been grafted, there has been a loss of large areas of sweat gland activity. Thermoregulation is deranged and in hot weather is difficult to control. Sweat rates from unburned areas are high and, with females in particular, there is anxiety and embarrassment about this. The victims feel they have unacceptable body odour. Reassurance is necessary to allay fears and anxiety over a problem that cannot be completely solved. Nevertheless, with the passage of time it tends to get better.

SCALDS, CHEMICAL BURNS, ELECTRICAL BURNS AND IRRADIATION

These four types of burn require separate brief mention.

SCALDS

Scalds are mainly seen in paediatric practice, among epileptics and in elderly, infirm patients burned in the bath or shower. The lesion is from steam or a brief exposure to hot water. The injury is usually a partial thickness burn and not life-threatening unless it involves very large areas of the body. Treatment is as for other types of burn and it is imperative to appreciate that there is no place for complacency in extensive scalds which can be every bit as serious as other big burns.

CHEMICAL BURNS

These are caused by many different agents. Usually, the clinician first encounters the lesion when it is fully developed and treatment follows conventional lines. As a first aid measure, copious washing in water helps to neutralise any chemical. However, there are a number of chemicals that cause burns that are progressive – phosphorus is one, chromic acid and hydrofluoric acid are others. These should be dealt with by very early excision to prevent extension of the injury into deeper tissues. The effects of hydrofluoric acid can to some extent be lessened by using calcium gluconate as a paste applied to the surface or by injection.

Particular mention must be made of caustic soda (sodium hydroxide) which is used widely in industry and the home. It is arguably the commonest cause of serious chemical burns. Tragically, it is often splashed into the eyes and can cause immediate and permanent blindness or severe conjunctival damage. Immediate prolonged (15 min) irrigation of the eyes with saline should be carried out. However, this may be too late. Prevention of the accident is much more appropriate.

ELECTRICAL BURNS

These are usually caused by alternating current as used in domestic power and in industry. Apart from death from electrocution, electricity by releasing heat energy can cause very severe deep burns. The more resistance to the passage of the current, the greater the injury. There is usually an entry and an exit wound. The possibility of damage to tissues between these two sites must always be considered. Only by early exploration can one establish the full extent of the injury, which may include arterial thrombosis and severe muscle damage. Electrical injury ought to be treated in a specialised burn unit.

RADIATION BURNS

Radiation burns will be encountered only when there is a very occasional problem of patients accidentally being exposed to an excess of local radiation as a therapeutic measure for the treatment of malignant disease. Treatment is essentially one of protection of the area burned and application of antibiotic creams if there is infection. It is not within the scope of this book to discuss the problem of radiation burns in the event of a nuclear accident or war.

PREVENTION

A burn is a preventable illness. High-risk groups can be identified. It affects the young, the socially deprived, the elderly, the ill-educated and alcoholics, particularly those who smoke. Epileptics are a very high-risk group. Public education and appropriate legislation can and have made an impact on the problem.

Finally, there is a group of people beyond our control in terms of prevention – those who see self-destruction by burning as a release from the burdens of life. For these people, there seems to be no solution.

FURTHER READING

Achauer B M 1987 Management of the burned patient. Appleton and Lange, Hemel Hempstead

Cason J S 1981 Treatment of burns. Chapman and Hall, London

Clarke J A 1992 A colour atlas of burn injuries. Chapman and Hall Medical, London

Robertson C, Fenton O 1996 Management of severe burns. In: Skinner D, Driscoll P, Earlam R (eds) ABC of major trauma, 2nd edn. BMJ Publishing, London, p 118–123

Settle J A D 1996 Principles and practice of burns management. Churchill Livingstone, New York

Wardrope J, Smith J A R 1992 The management of wounds and burns. Oxford handbooks in emergency medicine 3. Oxford University Press, Oxford

Head and neck surgery

18 Scalp and intracranial conditions

Graeme Brazenor

OVERVIEW

The scalp provides the cranium and its contents with a tough protective covering of thick skin with a rich blood supply. This chapter discusses, briefly, scalp conditions with more detail given to intracranial disorders, especially the mechanisms for and presentation of raised intracranial pressure, with appropriate investigations. Intracranial haemorrhage, abscess and tumour are discussed in detail.

SCALP

SURGICAL ANATOMY

The scalp is superficial to and freely mobile upon the pericranium (the periosteum of the skull) and consists of four tissue layers:

- *skin*
- *subcutaneous connective tissue* – this makes the scalp stiff and unyielding, and is the layer within which blood vessels ramify
- *aponeurotic layer* or *galea* – to this layer are attached the frontal and occipital muscles
- *loose areolar tissue*.

The arterial blood supply is from terminal branches of the external carotid artery and from the ophthalmic artery, a branch of the internal carotid. Scalp lacerations bleed profusely because the walls of these arteries are tethered by connective tissue of the subcutaneous layer, which reduces arterial spasm and contraction.

Venous drainage is via venae comitantes of the arteries, but drainage of the frontal area occurs via emissary and diploic veins which traverse the skull, communicate with the cavernous sinus and can be paths for the intracranial spread of scalp infection.

COMMON CONDITIONS

Laceration

Minor lacerations of the scalp form a major part of the suturing load of most emergency departments. More extensive wounds may involve an underlying skull fracture or defect of scalp tissues.

When the scalp is struck with a blunt instrument it may incur a laceration with surprisingly sharp edges, because of the 'anvil' effect of the underlying skull. Impacts with flat surfaces often produce stellate lacerations.

Haemorrhage from scalp lacerations may be so profuse as to cause shock even in the absence of any other injury. Treatment involves the following stages.

Stop the bleeding. Digital pressure with the fingertips placed at the edge of the laceration is the best first aid measure until clotting occurs. Avoid attempting to grasp each bleeding artery with artery forceps; instead use a series of forceps, grasping the galea and swinging each forceps back over the wound edge. This manoeuvre controls bleeding by local tamponade.

Closure. Generous sutures picking up all layers will not only control bleeding but will be sufficient for apposition of the skin edges. Elective incisions, by contrast, are closed in two layers: galea first and then skin. Healing is rapid because of the rich blood supply.

Repair of scalp defects. The hair-bearing skin should be shaved well clear of the laceration to prevent hair from contaminating the operative field whilst the wound is being explored and sutured. For large defects with loss of scalp tissue, the scalp is extensively mobilised, deep to the galea, in the areolar layer. Large defects are closed by flaps and split-skin grafting is rarely necessary.

Antibiotics. The rich blood supply restricts the need for antibiotics to circumstances of already established infection. The practice of using prophylactic antibiotics for compound skull fractures (that is, a skull fracture underlying a scalp laceration) has not been supported by prospective clinical trials.

Haematoma

Whether as a result of the obstetrician's forceps (causing cephalohaematoma – a scalp haematoma in the newborn which causes diagnostic uncertainty in that its raised edges and soggy centre falsely suggest a depressed fracture) or because of an unsuspected low doorway, haematomata of the scalp are common. Predictably, the haemorrhage after blunt trauma is within the subcutaneous layer and spread is restricted by the dense connective tissue, producing the characteristic egg shape. Subaponeurotic haematomata may develop after penetrating injuries or neurosurgical procedures, and spread of blood in such cases is limited by the bony attachments of the muscles that attach to the galea, the frontal bone and the occiput. A black eye or ecchymosis of the periorbital skin is therefore a not uncommon sequel to penetrating scalp wounds.

Treatment is conservative in that scalp haematomata resolve quickly because of rich venous and lymphatic drainage.

Infection

Because of a rich blood supply, primary infection of the scalp and scalp wound infection are both uncommon. Spread of infection from underlying osteomyelitis of the skull may present as a subaponeurotic abscess with localised tenderness and pitting oedema, termed Pott's puffy tumour.

When scalp infection does occur, particularly in the frontal region or on the face, retrograde septic thrombophlebitis may cause cerebral abscess or cavernous sinus thrombosis. This is rarely seen in Western societies today.

Tumours

All tumours of the skin (see Ch. 39) may occur on the scalp. Specific scalp tumours are as described below.

Epidermoid (pilar) **cyst** (wen). These are often multiple, arise in the skin layer and may be excised with ease under local anaesthesia. Recurrence at that site or elsewhere on the scalp is not uncommon.

Cock's peculiar tumour. This is an infected and ulcerating epidermoid cyst, which may resemble a squamous cell carcinoma.

Cylindroma (turban tumour). Histologically, a hyaline membrane outlines well-circumscribed masses of basaloid cells. The clinical behaviour is usually benign.

RAISED INTRACRANIAL PRESSURE

The cranium contains three separate elements whose volumes may vary. Because the cranium is wholly rigid and inelastic, the increase of any of the component volumes has the potential to cause a rise in intracranial pressure with compression and deformation of the brain.

INTRACRANIAL VOLUME

The three components of the total intracranial volume are brain, cerebrospinal fluid (CSF) and intracranial blood.

Brain volume

Normal brain volume is approximately 1400 ml, or about 90% of the total intracranial volume. Brain volume may be increased by the presence of a space-occupying lesion within it or by the phenomenon of brain oedema, which is of two types:

- Vasogenic oedema due to the accumulation of excess extracellular fluid, secondary to changes in endothelial permeability. Such changes may be seen in the presence of tumour or abscess.
- Cytotoxic oedema, seen when agents such as hypoxia or cellular toxins result in increase in intracellular sodium and water.

Cerebrospinal fluid volume

There is approximately 75 ml of CSF within the cranium under normal conditions, accounting for 5% of the total intracranial volume. Cerebrospinal fluid is formed in the choroid plexus of the ventricular system of the brain and passes out from the lateral ventricles via the foramina of Monro into the third ventricle, along the aqueduct of Sylvius to the fourth ventricle, then via the foramina of Luschka and the median foramen of Magendie to the cisterna magna and the spinal subarachnoid space. It recirculates through the cisterna ambiens (around the midbrain at the level of the tentorium cerebelli) (see Fig. 13.7) to the subarachnoid space over the cerebral hemispheres and is absorbed by the arachnoidal villi of the superior sagittal sinus into the venous circulation. Obstruction at any point along the course of CSF flow will cause dilatation of the cerebral ventricles (hydrocephalus).

Intracranial blood volume

This, like the CSF volume, approximates 75 ml under normal conditions, or about 5% of the total intracranial volume. Cerebral vasodilatation due to hypercapnia, hypoxia, increased central venous pressure or after trauma (see Ch. 13) may cause a marked increase in brain blood volume. Respiratory obstruction and trauma are therefore potent causes of raised intracranial pressure.

After consideration of the three intracranial compartments, it can be seen that a space-occupying lesion may increase the intracranial pressure by:

• increasing the brain volume, by virtue of its own mass
• altering endothelial permeability, resulting in cerebral oedema
• obstructing CSF flow.

INTRACRANIAL COMPLIANCE

Experimentally, Löfgren discovered that as a sequestrated intracranial volume (such as an expanding rubber balloon) is gradually increased, the intracranial pressure follows a curve like that illustrated in Figure 18.1. Such a curve may be arbitrarily divided into three sections. Phase I represents a phase in which there is little increase in intracranial pressure (ICP), during the early phases of expansion of the balloon. During this phase CSF is being displaced from the head into the spinal subarachnoid space. In phase II, most of the displaceable CSF has left the head and further increase in the sequestrated volume

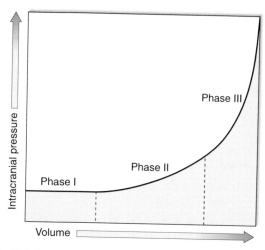

Fig. 18.1 Intracranial pressure vs expansion of a sequestrated intracranial volume.

leads to emptying of veins on the surface of the brain and crossing in the subdural space. In phase III, further increase in the sequestrated volume leads to compression and near occlusion of the veins, impairing egress of venous blood from the brain.

Intracranial compliance is defined at any one point on the pressure volume curve as dV/dP – in other words, the extra volume introduced at that point, divided by the rise in intracranial pressure which it causes. Thus phase I of the curve is the phase of high intracranial compliance, whereas phase III is the phase of lowest, and indeed rapidly diminishing, intracranial compliance.

The clinical application of this curve is most important. A patient with normal intracranial compliance can tolerate a physiological insult such as hypercarbia; intracranial pressure rises, but not to injurious levels. By contrast, a patient already in phase II or phase III of the intracranial pressure–volume curve, subjected to a hypercarbic insult, may experience a further rise in intracranial pressure to injurious or fatal levels. Understanding of this pathophysiology reaches its most critical application in the induction of anaesthesia in patients with raised intracranial pressure. The avoidance of hypercarbia, hypertension or other conditions which might lead to critical rise in intracranial pressure is of paramount importance.

CLINICAL FEATURES OF RAISED INTRACRANIAL PRESSURE

The common clinical features of raised ICP are described here.

Headache

Headache is not caused by raised intracranial pressure per se but by deformation of intracranial blood vessels and dural membranes, which often occurs with conditions that lead to raised intracranial pressure. Typically, such a headache is at its worst in the mornings and is aggravated by coughing, sneezing or stooping.

Vomiting

This also occurs in the mornings and is most common in children with posterior fossa tumours. Typically the patient awakens, vomits and is thereafter able to eat breakfast.

Papilloedema

The optic nerve is an extension of the brain with all its meningeal coverings. Raised CSF pressure in the subarachnoid space around the optic nerve impairs the flow of axoplasm along the axons of retinal neurons as they pass out of the globe through the optic disc. This 'back-up' of axoplasmic material causes swelling of the nerve fibres at the optic disc – papilloedema. In later phases the retinal veins become congested, and haemorrhages may result.

When present, papilloedema is highly suggestive of raised intracranial pressure. Unfortunately, when absent there is no guarantee of normal intracranial pressure.

Cushing response

Rising blood pressure in combination with falling pulse rate signals rising intracranial pressure until proved otherwise. The significance of these changes in the patient's vital signs was first described by Harvey Cushing, a pioneer neurosurgeon.

In fact, the Cushing response (or reflex) probably depends on deformation or ischaemia of the brain stem, rather than on raised intracranial pressure per se.

Decrease in conscious state

Decrease in conscious state, beginning with confusion and progressing through various grades of coma, reflects disruption of the reticular activating system (RAS) which ramifies through the brain stem and thalamus. Thus, it is possible to resect a significant portion of a cerebral hemi-

sphere without impairing the patient's conscious state, but is it not possible to deform or render ischaemic any part of the reticular activating system in the brain stem without disturbance of consciousness.

Figure 13.7 shows a coronal section of brain and brain stem within the skull. Figure 13.8 shows the brain compressed by an extradural haematoma, and in Figure 13.9 there is diffuse brain swelling following significant acceleration of the brain in a blunt head injury. In Figures 13.8 and 13.9, arrows indicate the directions of herniation of the plastic brain, and it is these deformations and herniations which initially impair the function of the RAS and cause permanent injury if allowed to go on untreated.

If the case of pure rostrocaudal migration of the brain and brain stem in Figure 13.9 is considered, a number of (idealised) stages of impairment of the patient's neurological function can be identified. These stages, in sequence, are:

- *Diencephalic stage*. The patient is confused or drowsy and may have bilateral constricted pupils. Occasionally the eyes are downcast and convergent.
- *Mesencephalic stage*. The patient is unconscious, assumes a decerebrate posture, and the pupils become dilated and fixed to light. There may be hyperventilation, termed central ventilatory hyperpnoea.
- *Pontine stage*. The pupils may become constricted down to almost pinpoint size, and no light reaction is discernible. The patient remains decerebrate but the respirations may become irregular in both volume and rhythm. Corneal reflexes are absent.
- *Medullary stage*. The patient may become flaccid during this phase, and the vegetative functions begin to fail. Body temperature may begin to rise rapidly; blood pressure, almost always raised as part of a Cushing response until this point, begins to fall to subnormal levels; and the pulse rate, almost always bradycardic until this point, increases to tachycardic levels. Respiration assumes the cyclical or Cheyne–Stokes pattern and eventually ceases, followed by cardiac arrest.

It must be stressed that these phases are idealised, and often a patient will skip a stage (or stages) or show only some of the signs of a stage. Nevertheless, in a patient undergoing rostrocaudal migration of the brain stem (often termed 'coning'), the succession of stages as above is not infrequently seen. The pathophysiological basis for the stages is thought to be the sequential ischaemia of segments in the brain stem from rostral to caudal, because the vertebrobasilar arterial tree is relatively fixed with respect to the clivus and, as the brain stem moves caudally, the perforating arterial branches entering its substance are occluded.

PRESENTING FEATURES OF INTRACRANIAL MASS LESIONS

Patients with intracranial mass lesions may present with any or all of the following clinical features:

- raised intracranial pressure (with the clinical features described above)
- focal neurological symptoms or signs (e.g. hemiplegia, hemianopia, cranial nerve palsies)
- epilepsy – a transient disturbance of neurological function caused by abnormal electrical discharge within the brain.

Epilepsy is seen usually with lesions involving the cortex of the cerebral hemispheres, and it is uncommon with lesions involving only white matter or brain stem. The most 'epileptogenic' areas of the cerebral hemispheres are the frontal lobes, medial temporal lobes and the areas of motor and sensory cortex anterior and posterior to the central sulcus, respectively.

INVESTIGATIONS

There are now a large number of different ways of investigating the cranium and its contents. The major indications for each are described in this section.

Plain X-rays of skull

These should be performed on everyone who is suspected of having an intracranial lesion or pathology in the bones of the cranium when, for some reason, a CT scan will not be done.

Even in patients who undergo CT scanning or other investigations, skull X-rays are also valuable in two ways:

- for the detection of signs of chronically raised intracranial pressure – these signs include thinning of the cranial vault, expansion of the pituitary fossa and erosion of the clinoid processes
- for the detection of pathology within the bones of the cranium (such as fractures, fibrous dysplasia or bony tumours).

CT scan with intravenous contrast enhancement

The CT scan is a relatively non-injurious procedure and is the investigation of first choice in any patient thought to have an intracranial lesion. The head is scanned both before and after the administration of intravenous contrast in cases where any vascular lesion (such as a tumour, arteriovenous malformation, aneurysm or infarct) is suspected.

Lumbar puncture

This investigation is done either to obtain cerebrospinal fluid for examination or culture, or on some occasions to measure the CSF pressure.

If lumbar puncture is performed in the presence of raised intracranial pressure due to an intracranial mass lesion, the reduction in spinal CSF pressure may lead to rostrocaudal migration of the brain (see above) with abrupt deterioration in the patient's neurological condition. This may occur either during the procedure or in the hour or so thereafter, as CSF leaks out of the spinal puncture into the extradural tissues. When mass lesions are not present, however, lumbar puncture is an important diagnostic procedure, as in suspected meningitis (without abscess); in suspected subarachnoid haemorrhage; in the measurement of CSF pressure in communicating hydrocephalus (i.e. where there is free egress of CSF from the ventricular system to the subarachnoid cisterns); in cases of suspected multiple sclerosis; and, indeed, in all cases of central nervous system disease where diagnosis is unclear and mass lesions appear to be absent.

Angiography

The injection of contrast material into the carotid and/or vertebrobasilar arterial systems is still a very necessary investigation for most vascular intracranial lesions. The advent of digital subtraction angiography (DSA) has vastly improved the images obtained and decreased the amount of intra-arterial contrast medium required.

Magnetic resonance imaging

Magnetic resonance imaging depends on the property of certain atomic nuclei with an odd number of nucleons which tend to align when placed in a strong magnetic field and to precess, at a rate unique for that particular nucleus, around the axis of the field. A pulse of radio waves at the same frequency as the precession can be used to deflect the nuclei to an extent determined by the amplitude and duration of the pulse, and also to synchronise the phase of the precession. On cessation of the pulse, the nuclei emit the absorbed energy as a minute characteristic radiofrequency signal, as they realign in the magnetic field. The scanner receives these radiofrequency signals and compiles them into tomographic images.

No ionising radiation is used and as far as is known this is a totally non-injurious investigation. It is capable of showing demyelinating plaques within the brain, cerebrospinal fluid within the cranium and the spine and, perhaps most significant of all, can be used to show sagittal and parasagittal sections of the neuraxis, which can greatly assist the neurosurgeon in planning and executing operations in the posterior fossa and spine.

Isotope cisternography

In this test, an isotope such as technetium (^{99m}Tc) is labelled onto human serum albumin and introduced into the lumbar subarachnoid space by needle puncture. Scintigraphic scans are taken, following the circulation of the isotope tracer into the subarachnoid cisterns around the base of the brain and (in normals) around the convexities of the brain leading to absorption into the superior sagittal sinus.

In patients with hydrocephalus due to impairment of CSF circulation over the convexities of the brain, isotope commonly enters the cerebral ventricles and fails to circulate from basal cisterns to the superior sagittal sinus. This can be a useful test in a patient in whom CT scan shows an equivocal degree of dilatation of the ventricular system.

Electroencephalography

This involves the recording of electrical activity over the surface of the brain by means of scalp electrodes. The major indication for this test today is when epilepsy is suspected.

Positron emission tomography (PET scanning)

In this mode of scanning, positron-emitting isotopes are generated in a cyclotron and rapidly transported and administered to patients (the rapidity being necessary because of the short half-lives of most positron-emitting isotopes). By incorporating a positron-emitting isotope of carbon in the glucose molecule, for example, a tomographic scan can be obtained showing the pattern of glucose metabolism in the brain. Other isotopes may be used to demonstrate parenchymal blood flow or the distribution of chemical receptors within the brain.

INVESTIGATION OF A PATIENT WITH SUSPECTED INTRACRANIAL MASS LESION

Whether the patient presents with focal neurological symptoms or signs, with epilepsy or with clinical features suggestive of raised intracranial pressure, most clinicians will proceed to a CT scan or magnetic resonance scan as the first investigation. If there are likely to be changes of interest in the bones of the skull (if, for example, the patient presents with a hard lump beneath the scalp) then skull X-rays may also be useful.

The nature of the lesion revealed on the first CT or magnetic resonance scan will determine the other investigations performed. Vascular lesions such as aneurysms and arteriovenous malformations will require some form of angiography, either digital subtraction or magnetic resonance.

Magnetic resonance imaging has risen to prominence dramatically in the past 5 years, because of its ability to show abscesses, demyelinating plaques, arteriovenous malformations and most tumours with a clarity which exceeds that of CT scanning. Further, magnetic resonance scanning is able to project sagittal cuts of the neuraxis, which can be extremely helpful to the neurosurgeon in planning an operative approach.

Isotope cisternography is rarely used now but occasionally is employed to adjudicate on equivocal cases of hydrocephalus. Electroencephalography is used when there is a question of epilepsy.

INTRACRANIAL TUMOURS

All intracranial tumours of any significant size can be considered to be biologically malignant, because if left untreated they may lead to death by causing raised intracranial pressure and brain herniation.

PRIMARY INTRACRANIAL TUMOURS

Primary brain tumours are the second most common cause of cancer-related death in children under 14 years.

In this age group, 70% of tumours are infratentorial (below the tentorium cerebelli) and 30% are supratentorial. In adults the distribution is reversed. In general, primary brain tumours do not metastasise outside the central nervous system.

Primary intracranial tumours may be classified as follows:

- gliomas
- embryonal tumours
- pituitary adenomas
- meningiomas
- schwannomas
- chordomas and other skull base tumours.

Gliomas

Glial cells are the connective tissue of the brain and are of three main types: astrocytes, ependymal cells and oligodendrocytes. Gliomas are the malignant tumours of glial cells. Astrocytomas are the commonest variety, grow diffusely and are poorly encapsulated. They are graded I–IV on the basis of histological differentiation and the presence of haemorrhage and necrosis. The most anaplastic form (grade IV) is termed a glioblastoma multiforme (Fig. 18.2). Astrocytomas graded III or IV are the most malignant tumours of the glioma series, although astrocytomas in the posterior fossa are sometimes less aggressive than those above the tentorium cerebelli. Ependymomas arise from the cells lining the ventricular system and may be spinal or intracranial. The intracranial variety is most common in children, often involving the floor of the fourth ventricle. Oligodendrogliomas often occur in the cerebral hemispheres and are frequently calcified. They can be very slowly progressive indeed, allowing the patient a reasonable quality of life for many years. They may finally convert to the glioblastoma multiforme.

For grade I astrocytomas the 3-year survival is approximately 50%, whereas for glioblastoma it is of the order of 4%. Ependymomas and oligodendrogliomas may exhibit slow growth and a tendency to remain static for long periods, at least initially.

In general, the treatment of advanced gliomas is to obtain a complete resection if possible, but obviously this will depend upon the extent of the tumour and its location at the time of diagnosis. Useful techniques in attempting to obtain a complete macroscopic excision include vision magnification, and ultrasonic disintegration and aspiration of the tumour by means of a hand-held 'wand'. In some

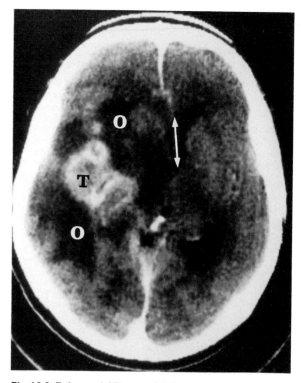

Fig. 18.2 Enhanced CT scan of right temporal glioblastoma multiforme. T, tumour; O, oedema; ←→, septum pellucidum, overlined to indicate shift of midline structures.

cases a surgical laser is used to vapourise the tumour, and in some centres a three-dimensional stereotaxic navigation system is used to enable the surgeon to determine the three-dimensional location of the laser point or of the tip of the ultrasonic wand with respect to the CT or magnetic resonance scan from which they are working.

Deep X-ray therapy has been demonstrated to extend the postsurgery survival times of all grades of gliomas. Megavoltage therapy is therefore almost always given after any attempt to resect an intracranial glioma.

Despite being the commonest single type of brain tumour, gliomas are the least satisfactory to treat. A new technique, photo-irradiation using haematoporphyrin, is used in some centres but has its limitations. When high intensity light of a particular wavelength is shone on the area, the haematoporphyrin exerts a selective cytotoxic effect upon tumour cells.

Embryonal tumours

Neuroblastomas and medulloblastomas of neurectodermal

origin are thought to arise from embryonic 'rests' of neuronal stem cells. They are most common in children but occasionally medulloblastomas may present as late as the fifth decade of life. In children the typical clinical picture of posterior fossa medulloblastoma includes morning headache, vomiting and a staggering gait. Treatment involves excision, irradiation of the neuraxis and chemotherapy. Cure rates of 70% are now attainable.

Pituitary adenomas

Although usually cytologically benign, these tumours may be biologically malignant. They may undergo unrestricted growth, spreading beyond the pituitary fossa either intracranially or into the sphenoidal sinus and nasal passages. Furthermore, they may produce hormones: growth hormone leading to gigantism or acromegaly, ACTH leading to Cushing's syndrome, or prolactin leading to gynaecomastia in the male or infertility and galactorrhoea in the female.

Treatment is by excision – via trans-sphenoidal or transethmoidal approaches if the adenoma is confined to the pituitary fossa, or via subfrontal craniotomy if the tumour has extended intracranially to any significant extent. Radiotherapy and the drug bromocriptine are important adjuncts to surgical therapy for some types of pituitary adenoma – particularly prolactin-producing growths.

Meningiomas

These tumours arise most probably from rests of arachnoidal granulation cells and compress the brain and brain stem from without. They are usually histologically benign. They occur at various characteristic locations within the skull and spine and present with epilepsy or focal neurological signs as a result of slow progressive growth.

Treatment is by surgical excision. They are frequently very vascular tumours and preoperative angiography is often useful in defining the anatomy of major arterial feeders. If the blood supply is shown to be exceptionally profuse, they can be embolised preoperatively by a neuroradiologist. In addition, angiography is useful in defining the patency or otherwise of major venous sinuses nearby, to determine whether these sinuses may be safely resected en passant in the removal of the tumour.

Schwannomas

These are tumours of nerve root sheaths and most commonly affect the vestibular component of the eighth cranial nerve, growing slowly from within the internal auditory meatus to fill the cerebellopontine angle. Patients with so-called *acoustic neuroma* present at first with nerve deafness and tinnitus, and later with cerebellar ataxia, nystagmus, facial weakness and trigeminal distribution numbness.

Schwannomas also affect the fifth nerve, and such patients may present with facial pain and/or disturbance of trigeminal nerve function.

The treatment of schwannomas is excision – which may be difficult – and they rarely recur after complete surgical removal.

Chordomas and other skull base tumours

The chordoma is a locally invasive skull base tumour which arises from notochord remnants. It may occur anywhere along a path from the odontoid process of C2, up along the clivus to the dorsum sellae. It commonly presents with cranial nerve palsies and is a most difficult tumour to eradicate surgically because of its extensive ramifications within the bones of the skull base.

For this and other skull base tumours, the essence of surgical removal is adequate exposure of the bones of the skull base, avoiding the need for hazardous retraction of brain.

SECONDARY TUMOURS OF BRAIN

Intracranial secondaries may be intra- or extra-axial. Extra-axial tumours are almost always based on the dura mater, secondarily compressing the brain. Intra-axial tumours commonly grow at the interface between white and grey matter in the cerebrum or cerebellum. They may also lodge in the brain stem.

The commonest intracranial secondary tumours are carcinomas of lung, breast and kidney and deposits of malignant melanoma. Nevertheless, other tumours can metastasise to the brain and these include other varieties of carcinoma and all of the lymphoproliferative tumours. Prophylactic cranial irradiation has greatly reduced the clinical incidence of intracranial deposits from systemic leukaemia.

The treatment of an isolated single secondary tumour, particularly if it is making the patient ill, is excision followed by irradiation. It makes little sense to attempt primary irradiation of a single secondary tumour (that is, without first excising it), unless the cell type is extremely radioresponsive. Even single secondary tumours in relatively eloquent areas can now be removed by careful surgery without doing further harm to the patient. At the very least the patient gains some months of good quality existence, and in a proportion of cases there is a local cure of that secondary lesion with the help of radiotherapy. In general, the surgical removal of an intracranial secondary tumour is contraindicated by the presence of more than one intracranial lesion and by the presence elsewhere in the body of secondary deposits which are likely to cause the patient's death within months.

INTRACRANIAL ABSCESS

SURGICAL PATHOLOGY

Intracranial abscesses develop as a consequence of spread of infection:

- From adjacent chronic suppuration. This may include otitis media, frontal or ethmoidal sinusitis or osteomyelitis.
- By haematogenous spread. Usually this is from the heart, especially from bacterial endocarditis in association with congenital cyanotic heart disease.

In a proportion of cases the source of infection is never found.

Anatomically, three intracranial planes may be involved:

- extradural – due to osteomyelitis, otitis media or sinusitis
- subdural – due to thrombophlebitis of veins crossing the subdural space, with resultant formation of a subdural abscess or empyema over the convexity of the brain
- intra-axial or parenchymal – involving the brain substance; this is the common 'brain abscess'.

The common causative organisms are streptococci (particularly microaerophilic species), anaerobic Gram-negative bacteria such as *Bacteroides*, and staphylococci, both *Staph. aureus* and *Staph. epidermidis*. Some abscesses contain more than one type of organism, and in general these abscesses are found to have been caused by spread of local infection.

CLINICAL FEATURES

Extradural. See Pott's puffy tumour (p. 150).

Subdural abscess/empyema. These patients are often quite toxic, with pyrexia, disturbed conscious state, signs of raised intracranial pressure and acute-onset epilepsy resistant to pharmacological control.

Intra-axial. This is generally a more subacute presentation, with malaise, headache, irritability and (usually) pyrexia. Finally, neurological signs and raised intracranial pressure supervene. The combination of cyanotic heart disease, pyrexia and neurological signs is highly suggestive of intra-axial brain abscess, secondary to haematogenous seeding from bacterial endocarditis. Fortunately this clinical syndrome is uncommon today.

INVESTIGATIONS

CT scan or magnetic resonance imaging are the investigations of first choice. In almost all cases, CT scan following the injection of intravenous contrast material will show the characteristic 'ring' enhancement of the abscess wall because of increased vascularity. Magnetic resonance scanning will show the abscess cavity, and both modalities will demonstrate the extensive oedema in surrounding brain and the mass effect.

Lumbar puncture should not be done on a patient known to have an intra-axial brain abscess showing significant mass effect on CT scan (see p. 153). It therefore follows that any patient who may have meningitis, but who may also have a brain abscess on clinical grounds, should receive a CT scan before diagnostic lumbar puncture.

TREATMENT

Extradural abscess

Treatment involves excision of the osteomyelitic bone with surgical drainage of the infected compartment and administration of high-dose intravenous antibiotics for a protracted period.

Subdural abscess

This may be drained through multiple burr holes, with irrigation of the subdural space with antibiotics. Catheters may be left in situ to continue intermittent antibiotic irrigation for some days postoperatively. Intravenous antibiotics are essential.

Intra-axial abscess

Aspiration of pus from each individual abscess by means of a brain needle inserted through an appropriately placed burr hole will significantly reduce intracranial pressure. Whilst the brain needle is still in situ, the abscess cavity may be gently irrigated with a dilute solution of antibiotics. One million units of crystalline penicillin and 1 g of kanamycin together in 1 L of sterile Ringer's solution make up a suitable irrigating fluid. An infant-feeding catheter may be left within the cavity of the abscess and brought out through the skin. This allows gentle and strictly aseptic irrigation of the abscess cavity at 6-hourly intervals on a number of occasions, prior to withdrawing the catheter.

In patients in whom there have been one or more abscesses adjacent to the cerebral cortex, the incidence of epilepsy thereafter is very high.

SPONTANEOUS INTRACRANIAL HAEMORRHAGE

Spontaneous intracranial haemorrhages are usually either intra-axial or subarachnoid, and the main causes, in order of frequency, are:

1. arterial hypertension
2. saccular aneurysms
3. congophyllic angiopathy (cerebral vascular amyloid)
4. arteriovenous malformation
5. abnormalities of blood clotting.

INTRA-AXIAL HAEMORRHAGES OF HYPERTENSIVE ORIGIN

Such haemorrhages are a major cause of morbidity and mortality in hypertensive subjects.

Surgical pathology

The commonest anatomical site for haemorrhage is in brain supplied by lenticulostriate perforating branches of the middle cerebral artery, i.e. in the basal ganglia or external capsule of the cerebral hemisphere. Such a haemorrhage is commonly attended by severe headache coming on over seconds or minutes, followed by hemi-paresis and sometimes loss of consciousness. Some hypertensive haemorrhages are seen in the cerebellum, and such patients may become apnoeic due to compression of brain stem structures.

Investigation

The investigation of choice is CT scan, and angiography is frequently done in order to exclude the presence of cerebral aneurysms or an arteriovenous malformation.

Treatment

If the haematoma is causing or threatening to cause brain herniation, and provided the patient is still salvagable, treatment is by craniotomy and evacuation of the haematoma under direct vision. However, patient selection is important. Operation on some very large haemorrhages in the dominant hemisphere is not recommended: if such patients recover, they may have such severe receptive and expressive dysphasic defects that they cannot be rehabilitated and they live out their remaining years in a miserable state. The neurosurgeon should therefore be consulted as to which hypertensive haemorrhages should be operated on.

Control of hypertension is also of paramount importance in the management of such patients, both in the acute stages and during the remaining years of life.

SACCULAR ANEURYSMS

Surgical pathology

These are saccular outpouchings which form on cerebral arteries, usually in relation to the circle of Willis at the base of the brain. Saccular aneurysms almost always occur at vessel bifurcations, and few of them are congenital as was previously thought. Such aneurysms are found in 5–10% of postmortem subjects, and are of two main types:

- Those occurring as the result of a congenital weakness of the cerebral artery wall. This is due to a defect in the media and/or internal elastic lamina. Most aneurysms presenting in the first three or four decades of life are of this type.
- Those occurring due to atherosclerotic degeneration of the cerebral vessel wall. From the fourth decade of life onwards, an increasing proportion of intracranial aneurysms are of this type.

Systemic hypertension increases the likelihood of cerebral aneurysms, but at least half the afflicted patients are not hypertensive.

The commonest sites for aneurysm formation are at the anterior communicating artery, at the first bifurcation of the middle cerebral artery, and at the junction of internal carotid and posterior communicating arteries. They also occur at the basilar artery bifurcation, where the posterior inferior cerebellar artery is given off from the vertebral, and where the ophthalmic artery is given off from the internal carotid.

Clinical features

Aneurysms most commonly present when they rupture, leading to a subarachnoid haemorrhage. They may also present because of increase in size, with compression of neighbouring neurological structures. Finally, and least commonly, they may present due to distal embolisation of platelet aggregates, resulting in stroke or transient ischaemic attacks.

Rupture. When an aneurysm bursts it produces instantaneous onset of headache, often with vomiting and loss of consciousness. The haemorrhaging ceases in most cases after 10 or 20 seconds, when the local subarachnoid pressure approximates diastolic arterial pressure. Symptoms persist for some days, however, including headache, nuchal rigidity, photophobia and malaise. These persistent symptoms reflect chemical meningitis caused by blood in the subarachnoid space.

Enlargement. Aneurysms may enlarge gradually over a long period, or they may undergo relatively rapid enlargement over days. The most common syndrome of an enlarging intracranial aneurysm is an isolated third nerve palsy due to an internal carotid artery aneurysm at the origin of the posterior communicating artery. Carotid –ophthalmic aneurysms may cause progressive visual failure, and large carotid aneurysms in the cavernous sinus may compress third, fourth, fifth and sixth cranial nerves.

Investigations

Lumbar puncture will reveal bloodstained cerebrospinal fluid if the aneurysm has presented with haemorrhage. CT scan will confirm this, showing blood in the basal subarachnoid cisterns. Cerebral angiography is essential

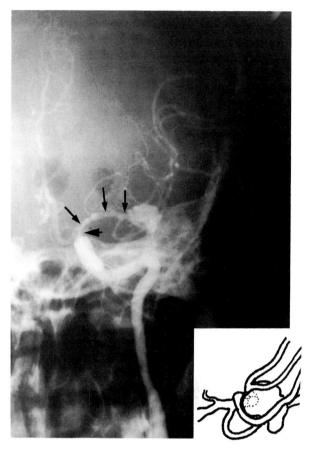

Fig. 18.3 AP projection of left carotid angiogram showing middle cerebral artery aneurysm. Note the spasm of the supraclinoid internal carotid artery (←) and the middle cerebral artery system (↓↓↓). The inset shows a schematic representation of the aneurysm anatomy.

to reveal the number and site(s) of intracranial aneurysms (see Fig. 18.3). It is essential to inject both carotid arteries and both vertebral systems to be sure of detecting all of the patient's aneurysms. About 10–15% of patients have more than one aneurysm.

Treatment

If patients are treated conservatively with bed rest, control of hypertension and general nursing care, the mortality of subarachnoid haemorrhage (even in that relatively select group of patients who reach hospital alive) is in excess of 40%. Many of the survivors of such conservative therapy are neurologically injured. The causes of this high mortality and morbidity are twofold:

● The thrombus which formed in the aneurysm and terminated the original haemorrhage is gradually dissolved by the body's fibrinolytic system, leading to aneurysmal rebleeding, which is often fatal.

● Those cerebral arteries which are encased by blood clot in the subarachnoid space commonly manifest vasospasm, some time during the first 10 days after haemorrhage, as a consequence of the toxic effects of the blood on the arterial wall. Cerebral vasospasm may cause cerebral ischaemia, which commonly progresses to permanent neurological injury or death (Fig. 18.3).

With contemporary operative treatment, case mortality may be reduced at least to 15%. The essentials of achieving low mortality in patients following subarachnoid haemorrhage include operation as early as possible in salvagable cases; skilfully placed craniotomy to facilitate atraumatic access to the circle of Willis without brain retraction; gentle dissection of the aneurysm(s) to minimise vascular spasm and the chance of intraoperative aneurysm rupture; accurate application of one of the numerous technologically sophisticated spring clips now available, to exclude the aneurysm sac from the arterial circulation without occluding the cerebral artery of origin (Fig. 18.4); and assiduous pre- and postoperative monitoring of the patient so that the advent of cerebral ischaemia can be met with prompt and vigorous action.

Occasionally the particular anatomy of an aneurysm will mean that it cannot be clipped, even using one or several of the various geometric forms of spring-loaded clips. Alternative means of dealing with such aneurysms include other surgical techniques on the one hand, or endovascular techniques in the hands of an experienced neuroradiologist, on the other hand. The alternative surgical techniques include proximal ligation, arterial bypass (to the distal vessel of supply) followed by proximal clipping; and wrapping or reinforcement of the sac using plastic, Teflon or other synthetic material. The endovascular neuroradiological technique of choice at present is the insertion of very fine platinum wire coils (named after Guglielmi who invented them) into the aneurysm sac via a very fine, flow-directed angiographic catheter. The platinum coils cause clotting of blood within the sac of the aneurysm and can obliterate it. Even in experienced hands, this technique has an incidence of distal embolus beyond the aneurysm, causing cerebral infarction.

Early craniotomy and clipping of the patient's aneurysm (s), within the first 48 hours after haemorrhage

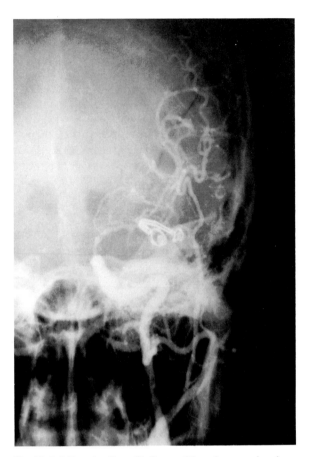

Fig. 18.4 AP projection of left carotid angiogram showing that the middle cerebral artery aneurysm has been exluded from the circulation by two spring clips – one straight and one curved. Note that the supraclinoid internal carotid artery and middle cerebral arterial system are in more severe spasm than in Figure 18.3.

if possible, immediately eliminates the chance of rebleeding. Furthermore, if the patient experiences cerebral ischaemia due to arterial spasm, the fact that the aneurysm has been secured allows application of the only proven treatment for spasm-induced ischaemia: hypertransfusing the patient's intravascular compartment with colloid solutions such as plasma, albumin or blood. This therapy increases cerebral perfusion and can dramatically reverse the symptoms and signs of cerebral ischaemia if action is prompt. Where volume infusion alone is not sufficient to reverse neurological deterioration, sympathomimetic drugs may be used to induce hypertension to 'force-perfuse' the brain. Clearly, such therapy cannot safely be used if the aneurysm remains unclipped.

There are now two important drugs which have been demonstrated to decrease the incidence of death or neurological injury in patients after aneurysmal subarachnoid haemorrhage. The first of these is nimodipine, one of the calcium channel blockers. This is used prophylactically in the hope of preventing cerebral vasospasm, although it may also have other actions (such as free-radical scavenging) which may contribute to its protective effects. The second drug is the 21- aminosteroid tirilazad, which has recently been shown to decrease the incidence of death and neurological injury, particularly in male patients severely affected by the subarachnoid haemorrhage. The exact mechanism of its action remains unclear.

CONGOPHYLLIC CEREBRAL ANGIOPATHY

This is a condition of medium- and small-sized cerebral arteries in the elderly in which amyloid protein accumulates in the media of the arterial wall, rendering it susceptible to rupture, particularly in the presence of hypertension. Such bleeds arise classically in the vicinity of the cortical/white matter interface and may occur anywhere throughout the cerebrum. The incidence of haemorrhages is substantially reduced by satisfactory control of hypertension. In the absence of hypertension control, the patient may experience a number of discrete haemorrhages in different parts of the cerebrum at different times.

ARTERIOVENOUS MALFORMATION (AVM)

Surgical pathology

These lesions are truly congenital and range from microscopic connections between an artery and a vein on the one hand, to huge racemose, convoluted masses of abnormal feeding arteries and arterialised veins which may be as large as a fist on the other.

Clinical features

Arteriovenous malformations commonly present with one of the following:

- haemorrhage, either into the brain substance or into the subarachnoid space
- epilepsy
- progressive or episodic cerebral ischaemia.

Investigation and treatment

The investigations of choice are magnetic resonance imaging (MRI) scan and cerebral angiography.

Surgical treatment is by excision. Using optical magnification and microneurosurgical techniques, the lesion is painstakingly dissected from surrounding brain, during which process feeding vessels are clipped or coagulated with bipolar diathermy, allowing excision of the whole structure. Because of altered vascular reactivity in the brain surrounding large lesions, operative mortality is amongst the highest in neurosurgery, sometimes as high as 10%. As a consequence of this, and bearing in mind that untreated arteriovenous malformations are much more benign in the long term than are cerebral aneurysms, the indications for neurosurgical excision of arteriovenous malformation need to be defined. In general they are:

- significant haemorrhage
- intractable epilepsy
- progressive ischaemia.

An alternative treatment to surgery is embolisation via an arterial catheter in the hands of a neuroradiologist experienced in such procedures. Under X-ray control, measured aliquots of cyanoacrylate glue or silicon spheres are injected into arteries directly feeding the arteriovenous malformation, permanently obliterating sections of its nidus. Embolisation is indicated when there has been significant haemorrhage or progressive ischaemia from an AVM which is inoperable because of its size or location. This procedure, like surgical extirpation, has a significant morbidity and mortality.

Haemorrhage from arteriovenous malformation has a lower mortality than does haemorrhage from aneurysms, probably because less blood is liberated into the subarachnoid space by arteriovenous malformation haemorrhage, with consequently lower risk of cerebral vasospasm. In addition, arteriovenous malformations are less likely to rebleed soon after a first haemorrhage. Epilepsy probably occurs because of progressive gliosis in the surrounding brain following recurrent haemorrhages over the years. Episodic or progressive cerebral ischaemia in surrounding brain was once thought to represent 'steal' of blood into the low-pressure arteries directly supplying the AVM. There is now some evidence to suggest that the ischaemia is due to congestion of veins draining surrounding brain because of the direct arterial input from the AVM.

FURTHER READING

Black P McL, Rossitch E 1995 Neurosurgery. An introductory text. Oxford University Press, Oxford

Jennett B, Lindsay K W 1993 An introduction to neurosurgery, 5th edn. Butterworth-Heinemann, Oxford

Kaye A H 1997 Essential neurosurgery, 2nd edn. Churchill Livingstone, Edinburgh

Head and neck

John Webb

OVERVIEW

Several medical and surgical disciplines are involved in managing head and neck disease. This chapter concentrates on the important lesions to try and ensure that treatable lesions are not missed. Students should aim to achieve a reliable clinical technique, concentrating on specific aspects in the history, visual appreciation and skill in palpation. Anatomical knowledge of lymph node groups is essential, together with a sound understanding of the major salivary glands, their deep relationships and neural connections. Considering both local and general disease, the head and neck is a fascinating and important site for pathology.

Clinicopathological lesions of the neck, face, lip, mouth and tongue constitute an important area in medicine and surgery. A wide range of specialties may be involved in management. For instance, short-lived mouth ulcerations are easily diagnosed and treated by general practitioners, but more complex and protracted lesions require oral medical or surgical expertise. Also, there is a developing move to manage malignancies of this wide region by dedicated multidisciplinary 'head and neck' teams. Hence only common disorders will be discussed in this chapter.

It must be emphasised that the task of general practitioners and 'generally based surgeons' will be to recognise important symptoms and perform competent examinations. For the mouth, examination requires a bright light source, a tongue depressor and gloved bidigital and bimanual examination. For superficial lesions of the skin and mouth, a simple magnifying glass is invalu-able. Perhaps more 'generalists' should acquire skills in indirect laryngopharyngoscopy.

CLASSIFICATION

Head and neck disorders can be classified into:

- congenital disorders
  — cleft lip and palate
  — preauricular sinus
  — tongue tie
- inflammation
  — facial infections
  — glossitis
  — stomatitis
  — ulcers of the tongue
- cysts
  — retention cyst of buccal mucous glands
  — jaw swellings
  — skin cysts of pilosebaceous origin
- carcinoma of the face, lip, tongue and floor of mouth.

CONGENITAL DISORDERS

CLEFT LIP AND PALATE

Cleft lip, cleft palate and combinations of the two are second only to club feet in frequency as congenital anomalies. The incidence of cleft lip varies from 1/600 to 1/1300 live births. Overall, cleft lip and palate each arise in 25%, and in the remaining 50% both are present. Seventy-five per cent of cleft lips are unilateral; they occur eight times more often in Caucasian than in black infants. There is a male dominance in cleft lip (2 > 1) and a female dominance (2 > 1) in cleft palate.

Surgical anatomy

The key to understanding the failure of embryological coalescence that results in cleft deformities is the *incisive foramen*, which lies in the hard palate just behind the incisor teeth. Anterior to the incisive foramen is the *primary palate*, comprising the alveolus and lip. Posterior to this is the *secondary palate*, which is formed by medial growth of two shelves from the maxillary arches, comprising the hard and soft palate. These developments take place from the fourth to the seventh week of intrauterine life.

Classification

Clefts of the lip and palate may be:

- Partial or complete. This depends on whether the primary or secondary palate is involved alone (partial) or both are involved (complete).
- Unilateral or bilateral. Left clefts outnumber both right and bilateral clefts. The most common anomaly is a left complete cleft involving the lip, alveolus and hard and soft palate.

There are three anatomical groups:

- cleft lip and alveolus (cleft of primary palate) – this is usually partial and unilateral with cleft of lip and dimple alveolus
- cleft lip, alveolus and palate (cleft of primary and secondary palate) – the cleft is complete with premaxillary deformity, flattening of the nose and abnormality of the alar cartilage and nasal septum
- cleft of the palate behind the alveolus – the cleft is midline with a bifid uvula.

Predisposing factors

Factors known to be related to an increased incidence of clefts are:

- previous family history – inheritance is polygenic; urogenital and facial defects may affect relatives
- exposure to X-rays, corticosteroids or viral infection (especially rubella) in the first trimester; medication, especially for epilepsy, may be implicated.

Problems of function

Feeding difficulties. Because with a cleft palate the baby cannot suck, breast feeding may be impossible. Special teats, bottles and even an obturator may be required to aid sucking. Cleft lips do not usually present any major problem.

Speech. Consonants cannot be pronounced adequately with a cleft palate, and speech therapy is required after closure.

Dentition. Abnormalities in the growth of teeth occur with alveolar deformity.

Hearing. Secondary oedema of the eustachian tube causes some hearing loss and the child is prone to ear infections, particularly 'glue ear'. Long term ENT care is advisable.

Treatment

Treatment of cleft lip and palate is a long-term process and should involve a team of specialists which includes plastic, oral and ENT surgeons coupled with speech therapy and sometimes psychological counselling. Further surgical procedures may be indicated well into adult life. This congenital abnormality is very distressing to parents; fortunately modern surgical correction is both cosmetically and functionally acceptable in 80–90% of patients.

The aims of reconstruction are to:

- achieve drastic correction of the cleft lip, especially the vermilion border – near perfection is the aim
- correct any associated misshape of the nostrils
- achieve adequate speech and dentition.

The timing of reconstruction depends on the anomaly.

Cleft lip. Use 'rule of tens': weight is greater than 10lb, haemoglobin is at least 10g/dl and baby is over 10 weeks old.

Cleft palate. The repair may need to be staged: the soft palate at 9 months but the hard palate from 10–24 months.

Principles of repair

Cleft lip. There is a wide variety of plastic repairs.

Cleft palate. Bilateral releasing incisions are made in

the roof of the mouth to allow extensive mobilisation of the palatal muscles and thus to achieve midline apposition.

Revision procedures may be required in later years to improve appearance and function, especially for speech defects.

PRE-AURICULAR SINUS AND ACCESSORY AURICLES

These result from imperfect fusion of the tubercles of the first branchial cleft during formation of the pinna. The result is a discharging sinus or a cyst that forms at the root of the helix or on the tragus and is often bilateral. Treatment is difficult and involves complete excision of the sinus tract to prevent infective complications.

'TONGUE TIE'

This congenital variation is a tight frenulum linguae. Although it never results in feeding problems, it does produce other effects. Because the tongue tip is relatively fixed, natural cleansing of the teeth is limited and in speech there is a tendency to lisping.

A commonsense and effective approach is to perform a short operation under general anaesthesia at the age of 3 years. The frenulum is cut transversely well away from the sublingual papillae. The incision is mobilised and sutured longitudinally with absorbable sutures. The results are excellent.

FACIAL SKIN LESIONS

The face, forehead and pinnae are favoured sites for important skin lesions. The effects of chronic ultraviolet exposure and age give rise to scaly areas known as keratoses. These may be multiple and persistent. Some will evolve into squamous carcinomas (epitheliomas). Such damaged skin may also develop small ulcerated neoplasms know as basal cell carcinomas (rodent ulcers). Flat malignant melanomas (lentigos) may appear on the temple or cheek. Apart from the above, the helix of the pinna is affected by a strange persistent ulceration known as chondrodermatitis helicis. The face is a popular site for benign intradermal naevi, subcutaneous lipomas, epidermal cysts and cutaneous horns.

INFLAMMATION

FACIAL INFECTIONS

Though acne vulgaris is by far the most common type of infection of the face, more important are boils and carbuncles, especially those that occur in the 'danger' or 'mask' area of the face. Deep venous communications from the anterior facial vein at the medial canthus via the angular vein to the ophthalmic veins and from the deep facial vein to the pterygoid plexus may result in spread of infection to the cavernous sinus. *Thrombosis of the cavernous sinus* causes localising neurological signs; in the pre-antibiotic era it was fatal.

Treatment includes specific medication for acne, improving skin hygiene and administering broad-spectrum antibiotics when infection of the mask area persists. Abscesses may need to be incised under antibiotic cover.

GLOSSITIS

Acute superficial glossitis

This is caused by minor trauma and scalds or by herpes simplex virus. Treatment is with mouthwashes.

Acute parenchymal glossitis

Typically this follows an insect bite of the tongue and presents with acute pain and swelling. Subcutaneous adrenaline relieves the allergic vasodilatation and 'oral ice' can be helpful. The situation may become a dire emergency as airway obstruction can swiftly ensue. Urgent transfer to an accident department is ideal. Failing that, a medical or paramedical attendant may be forced to establish an airway by cricothyroid large needle puncture, cricothyroidotomy or, in expert hands, tracheostomy. The risk should never be underestimated.

STOMATITIS

Vincent's stomatitis and angina

This uncommon condition is more accurately described as *ulceromembranous stomatitis* and occurs almost exclusively in young adults as a consequence of poor oral hygiene and untreated dental caries. Bacteriologically there is an overgrowth of *Borrelia vincenti*, an anaerobic spirochaete, and *Fusiformis fusiformis*, an anaerobic spindle-shaped Gram-negative bacillus.

Clinical features. General malaise and pyrexia progress to toothache and bleeding gums. The patient has a foul-smelling breath. The gums are inflamed and covered with a yellow-white pseudomembrane, and superficial ulceration. There may be extension elsewhere in the mouth with tender cervical lymphadenopathy. In neglected instances, further spread takes place in the fascial planes of the neck and threatens the airway. Angina infers that the fauces are involved.

Treatment. Mouthwashes with dilute hydrogen peroxide are combined with parenteral penicillin and metronidazole. When the acute phase has settled, oral hygiene is improved and carious teeth are extracted.

Aphthous stomatitis

'Aphthous' is a term used to describe a common non-specific ulceration of the mouth. Three ages of man are inflicted by three different causes. Due to infection from *Candida albicans*, babies in the first few weeks of life may develop monilial stomatitis, with white furry plaques on the mouth, tongue and lips. Treatment is with nystatin drops.

Small, tender aphthous ulcers which affect mainly the tongue but also the buccal mucosa may develop in preschool children. They are self-limiting and heal spontaneously within 10 days. Recurrent ulceration of this type may have an autoimmune basis. Adults may be similarly affected. Local salves with 0.2% aqueous chlorhexidine gluconate, local steroids or chlorine salicylate paste (Bonjela) are popular remedies.

In adult oral ulceration, there are many additional causes. Herpes simplex virus is a member of the human papilloma virus (HPV) or Papova group. HPV-2 affects the mouth and lips, producing tender vesicles, ulcers and scabs. This sequence is commonly recurrent. The virus resides in the trigeminal ganglion and tracks down the nerves to an oronasal skin or mucosal locus. Acute stress, upper respiratory infections, sunlight and acute debility from other causes may precipitate an outbreak. Currently of ominous significance are orogingival infections from the human immunodeficiency virus (HIV), which reduces the CD4 T cell circulating lymphocyte population. The possibility of HIV infection should always be suspected in 'at-risk' patients and otherwise by clinical instinct. Other immune deficiency states can result from drugs or haematological disease (acute lymphocytic leukaemia).

Noma

This full-thickness gangrenous condition of the cheek area may be seen in deprived and debilitated populations. It probably results from symbiotic infection with aerobic and anaerobic organisms. Treatment is by antibiotics and excision of gangrenous areas.

ULCERS OF THE TONGUE

These may be either benign or malignant.

Benign

These include:

- Dental ulcers, caused by sharp teeth or ill-fitting dentures. They occur on the side of the tongue.
- Chronic non-specific ulcers, usually on the tip of the tongue. Such indolent ulcers often heal after excision biopsy.
- Aphthous ulcers.

Local application of choline salicylate paste is the treatment of choice when a specific cause has been excluded. Topical steroids may be useful for recurrent aphthous ulcers.

Epulis. Epulides are chronic swellings related to the gums. There are four main types:

- fibrous epulis which resembles normal gum
- pregnancy epulis which is soft, pink and vascular
- pyogenic granulomas which affect males and non-pregnant women; these are associated with dental caries and tend to bleed spontaneously
- giant cell epulis which is larger than the above, purple in colour and often pedunculated.

All require oral surgery.

All forms of stomatitis and gingivitis tend to be associated with poor general health, inadequate nutrition, lack of vitamins or situations of stress.

It is important to remember that, when a patient is due to undergo a major surgical procedure, a full examination of the mouth and general dental state is obligatory. Dental caries and gingivitis should be dealt with before general anaesthesia and operation. This is particularly relevant for patients with prosthetic heart valves and joint replacements.

Malignant

The majority of these will be epithelial tumours.

CYSTS

RETENTION CYST OF BUCCAL MUCOUS GLAND

Accumulation of fluid in an obstructed mucous gland causes a cystic swelling on the inner aspect of the lip, the gingivolabial sulcus or the cheek.

Treatment is unroofing, which allows the gland to drain or excision.

CYSTS OF THE JAW

A smooth swelling associated with the mandible may be a non-neoplastic dental or dentigerous cyst. A neoplastic cyst is likely to be an adamantinoma. Appropriate X-rays will clarify the situation and the patient should be referred to an oral surgeon.

CARCINOMA OF THE LIP, TONGUE AND FLOOR OF MOUTH

These cancers are less frequent than was formerly the case, largely because of better oral hygiene, a reduction in the incidence of syphilis and reduced local irritation from tobacco. Whereas 50 years ago carcinoma in these regions was 10 times more common in men, the incidence is now equal in both men and women. In the latter, other factors such as iron deficiency anaemia may apply. In the UK, cancer of the tongue accounts for 1% of cancer deaths. In developing countries, orolingual cancers remain a major problem. In the USA, there are 19 000 new cases of oral cancer and 7000 of oropharyngeal cancer annually.

PREDISPOSING FACTORS

Leukoplakia

This simply means a 'white plaque'. It represents increased keratinisation of the superficial cells of the epidermis, which may be a local physiological response to a chronic irritant. The condition is premalignant and the frequency of neoplastic change is about 25%. Frank neoplasia is preceded by dysplasia.

Macroscopically there are two outstanding features:

- a 'cracked white paint' appearance with areas of adherent grey-white plaques of abnormal keratinised epithelium
- a 'raw beef' appearance which represents areas of shed plaque and is sometimes called erythroplakia.

Microscopically the epithelium shows all degrees of cellular atypia ranging from mild dysplasia to carcinoma in situ.

Chronic irritation

This is most important and may result from cigarette smoking, tobacco chewing, alcohol (especially overuse of spirits), chronic dental sepsis with irritation and snuff.

SURGICAL PATHOLOGY

Macroscopic features

These include:

- ulcer – with raised irregular rolled margin and red indurated base
- fissure – chronic in nature with no signs of healing
- protuberant lesion – varying from a small projection beyond the surface to a large 'cauliflower-like' mass.

Microscopic features

Virtually all are keratinising squamous cell carcinomas with typical tongue-like projections of cells into the dermis or beyond. Lesions of the posterior tongue may also be lympho-epithelial or of salivary gland origin.

Spread

Spread is direct, lymphatic or through the blood.

Direct. This may be through the substance of the lip to involve, if untreated, the cheek, gum and alveolus.

Spread may also take place through the substance of the tongue to involve the floor of the mouth, alveolus, tonsillar region and palate. Involvement of the lingual nerve may cause pain to be referred to the ear by way of the auriculotemporal nerve.

Lymphatic. In the case of the lip, only 10% have evidence of spread to the submental or submandibular lymph nodes by 1 year. Drainage is sometimes contralateral.

Spread in the tongue is earlier than with the lip. The tip drains bilaterally to the submental lymph nodes, the posterior third of the tongue drains bilaterally to the upper deep cervical lymph nodes, and the anterior two-thirds drain unilaterally to the submandibular lymph nodes and thence to the deep cervical chain (Figs 19.1 and 19.2).

The submandibular lymph node is normally palpable if the bimanual method is used. However, it is soft and usually less than 1 cm in diameter.

Invasion of a lymph node by tumour cells causes it to become larger and firmer than normal. Later it becomes fixed to surrounding structures.

Blood. This is extremely rare, as local and lymphatic spread and recurrence of disease nearly always occur above the clavicles.

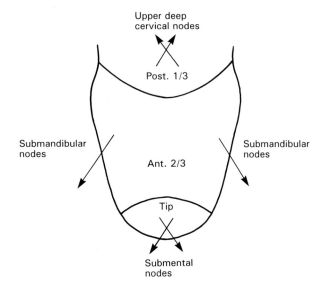

Fig. 19.1 Lymph drainage of the tongue.

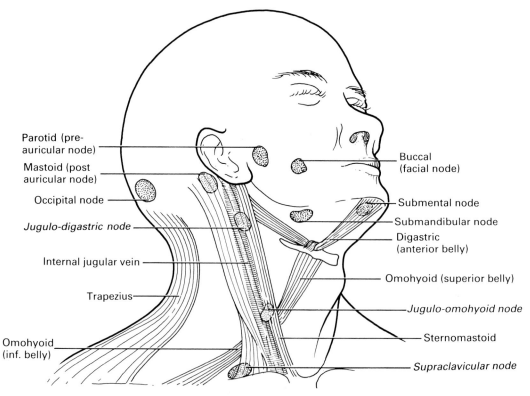

Fig. 19.2 Lymph nodes of the head and neck. Vertical (deep cervical) and outer circular groups of lymph nodes (see p. 70).

DIFFERENTIAL DIAGNOSIS

In the *lip*, this includes:

- benign chronic fissures and ulcers
- benign tumours, e.g. papilloma, haemangioma, lymphangioma, fibroma and accessory salivary gland tumours
- syphilitic chancre, which is rare and usually on the upper lip
- ulceration from HIV infection.

In the *tongue* and *floor of the mouth*, differential diagnosis includes:

- fissures – leukoplakia
- dental ulcers – related to decayed or broken teeth or poorly fitting dentures
- aphthous ulcers – tiny punched-out, white-based painful ulcers surrounded by erythema
- tumours – papilloma, haemangioma, lipoma, rhabdomyoma, mixed salivary origin.

TREATMENT

Prophylaxis

Treatment is by the following procedure:

1. Remove the source of chronic irritation.
2. Allow 2 weeks for the lesion to settle spontaneously and then biopsy suspicious sites.
3. Excise unresolving or suspicious areas of leukoplakia.
4. Stop smoking and alcohol.

Definitive treatment

Surgery, radiotherapy, or a combination, give good results for early cancers. Radiotherapy is best delivered by local implantation of iridium wires.

Early cases. When the primary lesion is small (less than 2–3 cm), without infiltration of surrounding structures, and when any involved lymph nodes are freely mobile, then the following treatment is indicated.

Primary lesions. Surgery or radiotherapy are probably equally effective, but 'tridimensional excision' is probably the treatment of choice. Up to one-third of the tongue can be removed without serious loss of function.

Lymph nodes. If cervical nodes remain enlarged and firm after the primary lesion has been healed for 3 weeks and if infection and postirradiation effects on the nodes have been eliminated by fine needle cytology, then either a suprahyoid or complete neck dissection of the deep cervical lymph nodes is indicated. Usually only unilateral clearance is performed. The prognosis is so poor if bilateral nodes are involved that massive excisional surgery may not be justified.

If cervical nodes are impalpable or clinically normal, then 'prophylactic' excision is unnecessary but careful follow-up is indicated.

Late cases. When there is a tumour greater than 3 cm and/or bony involvement or recurrence after previous treatment and nodes are palpable then treatment is as follows.

Primary lesions. Operation is indicated after a preoperative course of external beam irradiation. It may entail resection and the use of full-thickness skin flaps for a lip lesion or an en bloc removal of half the tongue, mandible and floor of the mouth for a laterally placed tongue lesion. Large defects of the tongue may be repaired with a forehead flap or a quilted split-skin graft to cover defects in the floor of the mouth.

Lymph nodes. If the deep cervical lymph nodes are fixed, operation is contraindicated and radiotherapy is used. If the nodes are still mobile, they may be excised in continuity with the advanced primary lesion. A combined excision of primary tumour and block dissection of the deep cervical nodes, with the removal of part of the intervening body of the mandible, is called a composite excision. It is popularly referred to as a 'commando' operation and is best performed by a team of ENT, plastic and oral surgeons. The patient requires a temporary tracheostomy, intensive postoperative physiotherapy and multidisciplinary care thereafter.

PROGNOSIS

In the lip there is an 80% 5-year cure with surgery or radiotherapy when cervical lymph nodes are not involved.

In the tongue and floor of the mouth, prognosis depends on the following factors:

- Site
  — anterior tumour – 50% survive 5 years
  — posterior tumour – 10% survive 5 years

- Stage
  — early – 60% survive 5 years
  — late – 15% survive 5 years
- Nodes
  — involved – 15% survive 5 years
  — not involved – 60% survive 5 years.

Women have a better prognosis than men.

LYMPHATICS OF HEAD AND NECK

ANATOMY

Lymphatic drainage from carcinoma of the head and neck ultimately reaches the deep cervical chain of lymph nodes, which surround the length of the internal jugular veins from the base of the skull to the root of the neck. Jugular lymph trunks are formed, which empty into the thoracic duct on the left side and the internal jugular or brachiocephalic vein on the right side.

The arrangement of the head and neck lymphatics can be conveniently separated into two groups: vertical and circular.

Vertical group

These are the deep cervical nodes. They are arranged about the internal jugular vein but three of them are named (see Fig. 19.2).

Jugulo-digastric node. This lies below the posterior belly of the digastric muscle as it crosses the internal jugular vein. It is also called the *tonsillar lymph node* and receives lymph drainage from the tonsil.

Jugulo-omohyoid node. This is behind the internal jugular vein where it is crossed by the inferior belly of the omohyoid muscle. All the lymph from the tongue ultimately reaches this node.

Supraclavicular nodes. These extend from the nodes around the inferior part of the internal jugular vein, behind the sternomastoid muscle into the supraclavicular region. The scalene nodes lie in the fat over scalenus anterior.

Circular group

There are three 'circles' of lymphatics, and with few exceptions they drain into the nearest nodes of the vertical group.

Innermost circle. This surrounds the pharynx and trachea and comprises the following nodes:

- retropharyngeal
- paratracheal
- pretracheal.

Inner circle. This is situated in the nasopharynx, is sometimes called Waldeyer's ring and comprises the following:

- tubal tonsils
- nasopharyngeal tonsil (adenoids)
- pharyngeal tonsils
- lingual tonsil.

Strictly speaking these are not lymph nodes but collections of lymphoid tissue.

Outer circle. These superficial glands around the head and jaw comprise the following (Fig. 19.2):

- occipital
- mastoid
- preauricular (parotid)
- buccal (facial)
- submandibular
- submental.

It is essential that students are familiar with these nodal sites.

BLOCK DISSECTION OF DEEP CERVICAL LYMPH NODES

In the slowly growing tumours of the lip and face and the more rapidly growing tumours of the tongue and floor of the mouth, the lymph nodes of the neck should be removed whilst they remain mobile if there is clinical or cytological evidence of nodal metastases. Radiotherapy to nodes greater than 2 cm in diameter is unlikely to be successful.

The operation entails unilateral removal en bloc of the deep cervical lymphatic chain together with the internal jugular vein, sternomastoid, omohyoid and digastric muscles, the submandibular lymph and salivary glands, submental lymph glands, the lower pole of the parotid gland, the deep cervical fascia and cervical nerve plexus. The dissection extends from the midline of the neck up to the mandible, down to the clavicle and back to the anterior border of the trapezius muscle.

Modified block dissection, which removes localised groups of nodes or the total deep chain without sacrifice of the sternomastoid muscle, is favoured for metastatic spread from primary papillary cancer of the thyroid.

Special complications of block dissection

The operation can have the following complications:

- Nerves – damage may occur to the following nerves:
  — glossopharyngeal, vagus, hypoglossal or lingual nerves
  — accessory nerve as it penetrates the sternomastoid
  — phrenic nerve
  — mandibular branch of the facial nerve
  — cervical sympathetics
  — brachial plexus branches.
- Thoracic duct – a chylous (lymphatic) fistula may result.
- Skin flap necrosis.
- Secondary haemorrhage – infection and skin flap necrosis may result in the erosion of the underlying unprotected carotid artery. If a bilateral neck dissection is indicated then the second procedure should be delayed at least 6 weeks and one internal jugular vein preserved.

The surgery of malignancy of the head and neck has been made much more acceptable by primary repairs using *skin flaps* mobilised from the forehead and acromiothoracic region. The principle upon which these flaps are based is simple – they have a large artery and accompanying vein in their base so that they are both well vascularised and drained. Consequently, they can be made relatively long for their width. They are used both for *lining* inside the mouth and pharynx and for *covering* large surface defects. This is very specialised surgery.

NECK SWELLINGS

These derive from a variety of lesions which may be either specific to the region or a local manifestation of systemic disease. This is an important area of clinical diagnosis because errors are easily made.

SURGICAL ANATOMY

The broad and extensive sternomastoid muscles divide the neck into anterior and posterior triangles (Fig. 19.3A). These main triangles are further subdivided by the digastric muscle above and omohyoid below. Above, the digastric separates the submandibular triangle from the carotid triangle. Below, the inferior belly of omohyoid separates the smaller suprascapular or subclavian triangle from the larger occipital triangle. The important parotid region lies between the ascending ramus of the mandible and external auditory meatus with the mastoid process posteriorly (Fig. 19.3B).

The deep or investing layer of cervical fascia splits to envelop the sternomastoid muscles. Turning the head to the side against resistance tenses the fascia and usually helps to clarify whether a palpable swelling is superficial or deep to the fascia. For the purpose of simplicity, the

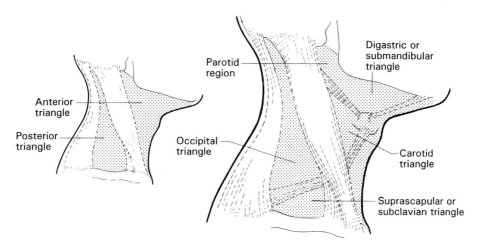

Fig. 19.3 Surgical anatomical subdivisions of the neck.

neck is regarded as extending from the mandible, mastoids and superior nuchal lines above, to the clavicles below.

Swellings that lie superficial to the fascia may not be specific neck lesions.

Swellings superficial to the deep fascia

These include:

- epidermoid (sebaceous) or pilar cysts
- lipomas
- neurofibromas and neurilemmomas
- some lymph nodes.

Swellings beneath the deep fascia

These include midline and lateral swellings.

SURGICAL PATHOLOGY AND GENERAL MANAGEMENT: MIDLINE SWELLINGS

There are from unpaired midline structures (Fig. 19.4):

- thyroglossal cyst
- pharyngeal pouch
- median sublingual dermoid cyst
- subhyoid bursa

- dissecting or plunging ranula
- laryngocele.

Thyroglossal cyst

This is an embryological fault. A cyst may develop anywhere along the thyroglossal tract, which extends from the foramen caecum in the posterior tongue down through the neck in close relation to the hyoid bone and thence to the thyroid isthmus. A sizeable cyst may actually occupy the region of the thyroid isthmus and rarely develop a papillary carcinoma.

Thyroglossal cysts may be infrahyoid or, uncommonly, suprahyoid. They are mostly sited just off the midline but occasionally lie more laterally in the submandibular region. The cyst appears in childhood or early adult life as a rounded tense smooth swelling. The specific diagnostic test is that the cyst elevates with protrusion of the tongue because of attachment to the hyoid bone, which is integral to the tongue musculature. Sometimes it is easier to detect descent of the cyst when the tongue is retracted.

The cysts are lined by squamous, columnar or cuboidal epithelium with islands of thyroid and lymphoid tissue in the wall. They contain clear or mucoid fluid. Because of the lymphoid tissue, thyroglossal cysts are susceptible to acute infection and abscess formation. Infected cysts should be aspirated and not incised. Antibiotic treatment will usually resolve the problem.

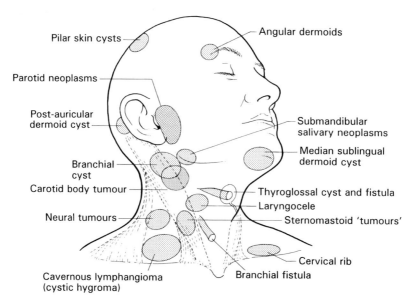

Fig. 19.4 Location of some head and neck swellings.

Inappropriate incision will lead to fistula formation. The surgical treatment is tricky and comprises Sistrunk's operation, which involves excising the cyst, track and 1 cm or so of the central part of the hyoid bone. Careful surgery usually eliminates the chance of recurrence.

Pharyngeal pouch (see also p. 239)

This rare condition represents a pulsion diverticulum resulting from muscular imbalance at an area of weakness in the posterior pharynx between the two components of the inferior constrictor muscle (thyropharyngeus and cricopharyngeus), the dehiscence of Killian. A pouch develops which emerges in the midline but then deviates to the left. It is a thin-walled mucosal sac and may become quite large. Depending on its size, regurgitation or obstruction of the upper oesophagus will ensue.

Treatment is by exploration of the left side of the neck, mobilising the sac, excising or elevating it, and adding cricopharyngeal myotomy.

Median sublingual dermoid cyst

This is also rare but should be suspected when a smooth submental swelling is present. Examination of the mouth will show a sizeable swelling, filling and distorting the sublingual region. The cyst which contains sebaceous-like material is developmental. It lies above the mylohyoid muscle and within the intrinsic muscles of the tongue.

It is excised through a curved submental incision which divides the mylohyoid muscle in the line of its raphe.

Subhyoid bursa

When enlarged, this bursa produces a soft fluctuant swelling below the hyoid bone. It is difficult to distinguish clinically from a thyroglossal cyst.

Dissecting or plunging ranula

This rare condition is usually encountered in childhood. A simple ranula is not uncommon and, being a myxomatous or mucoid degeneration of the sublingual salivary gland, lies laterally in the floor of the mouth. It is a blueish grey almost translucent swelling.

A ranula may enlarge downwards to insinuate itself laterally to the submandibular region or through the

fibres of mylohyoid towards the midline. The surgical treatment is per-oral and is by either excision or deroofing.

Laryngocele

This is a fascinating but uncommon problem. Wind instrument players are said to be subject to it, but persistent coughing from chronic obstructive airways disease is another factor. It shows as a soft variable unilateral or bilateral swelling which arises at the upper part of the thyroid cartilage. It will empty on gentle compression, only to reappear with a Valsalva manoeuvre. Sometimes it mimics a branchial cyst, and surgical excision may be advisable for a thin mucosal cyst which emerges through the thyrohyoid membrane.

SURGICAL PATHOLOGY AND GENERAL MANAGEMENT: LATERAL SWELLINGS

These are from paired lateral structures (Fig. 19.4):

- lymph nodes
- thyroid swellings or goitres
- salivary glands
- branchial cysts
- cervical ribs
- carotid body tumour (chemodectoma)
- cystic hygroma (cavernous lymphangioma)
- sternomastoid tumour
- arteriovenous fistula and cirsoid aneurysms
- soft tissue (muscle, neural or fatty) tumours
- spinal and cervical abscesses, e.g. actinomycosis, pyogenic pharyngomaxillary abscess
- clavicular tumours, primary or secondary.

Lymph nodes

The term lymphadenopathy implies that nodes are enlarged and pathological. Enlargement beyond 2 cm is highly suspicious of malignancy. These important structures give rise to the commonest swellings in the neck. The nodal swelling is usually secondary to either an inflammatory or neoplastic process in the organs drained. Some generalised disease processes may present and/or originate in the cervical nodes, e.g. sarcoidosis, lymphoma or histiocytosis.

Inflammation. In *acute and subacute lymphadenitis*,

superficial lymph nodes may be secondarily infected from skin sepsis such as boils, carbuncles, lesions on the eyelids (meibomian cysts) and insect bites.

The deep nodes tend to be inflamed from dental infections and other sources in the mouth, larynx or nasopharynx (tonsillitis and adenoiditis).

Chronic lymphadenitis is now fairly uncommon in developed countries but may arise rarely from toxoplasmosis (*Toxoplasma gondii*), 'cat-scratch' disease, sarcoidosis and some fungal infections. *Tuberculosis* was once a common cause but is now mainly confined to immigrant populations. The mycobacterium is often atypical and resistant to chemotherapy. The enlarged nodes are part of the primary focus, with the tonsil the source of entry. The jugulodigastric gland is characteristically involved. These nodes are non-tender and become adherent to deep tissues. Caseation may develop, and the node breaks down to form a 'cold abscess'. The pus tends to track through a gap in the deep fascia and form a subcutaneous collection. When such an abscess is drained the offending deep node(s) must be exposed by dividing the deep fascia and then be excised. Tuberculous abscess formation has been described as 'collar stud'. With atypical tuberculous lymphadenitis, several groups of infected adherent nodes require excision. Attachment to the internal jugular and other veins renders dissection difficult.

Neoplasm. Lymphatic metastases from scalp, face, lip, tongue, floor of mouth, tonsil, pharynx, larynx, thyroid, stomach, pancreas, breast and lung may result in hard painless enlarged nodes. Initially the nodes can be mobile but later they become fixed. Of this group two are worthy of particular comment.

'Lateral aberrant thyroid'. This description is inaccurate but it is of historical interest. Papillary thyroid cancer may present as a cystic chronic deep cervical lymphadenopathy. The primary tumour in the thyroid is often small (occult sclerosing carcinoma).

Troisier's sign. This is an enlarged node in the left supraclavicular fossa (Virchow's node) deriving from gastric carcinoma. Other intra-abdominal cancers (pancreas, colon, ovary, testes, oesophagus) and intrathoracic cancers (bronchus, oesophagus) may cause a similar clinical presentation.

Search for the primary lesion. When a neck swelling appears and is proven by fine needle aspiration cytology to be lymphadenopathy, three questions must be considered:

- *Is it part of a local inflammatory process?* Consider:
— tonsillitis
— pharyngitis
— infected skin lesion.
- *Is it part of a generalised lymphoid disease process?* Examine all other nodal sites, particularly the axillae and groins, and palpate for hepatosplenomegaly. If enlargement is present, such conditions as infective mononucleosis, 'cat-scratch' disease and lymphoreticular malignancy may apply.
- *Is it part of a malignant (carcinomatous) process?* Depending on the situation of lymphadenopathy, epithelioma of scalp, face, lips, tongue, floor of mouth, and tumours of the jaw, lung, stomach and breast enter the diagnostic field. Do not forget malignant melanoma. All patients require a detailed intra-oral, general and pelvic examination.

Systemic disease. With generalised lymphadenopathy the following list of diagnoses should be helpful:

- lymphoma – Hodgkin's or non-Hodgkin's
- lymphoid leukaemia
- rubella (German measles)
- infectious mononucleosis (glandular fever)
- sarcoidosis
- chronic skin disease and sepsis (dermatopathic lymphadenopathy)
- cat-scratch disease (a generalised form of this infection can occur)
- tuberculosis
- childhood rheumatoid arthritis (Still's disease)
- adult rheumatoid arthritis (with splenomegaly and leucopenia – Felty's syndrome)
- secondary syphilis
- HIV infection.

Thyroid swellings (generalised goitre, dominant and solitary nodules)

These are discussed in Chapter 20.

Salivary gland swellings

A localised or diffuse swelling in the region of the major salivary glands (parotid, submandibular) can arise from a variety of causes. The term 'salivary gland swelling' is a sensible one. Acute or chronic inflammation, neoplasms, functional and organic obstruction may cause swellings. Mumps is perhaps the most widely known salivary swelling. For the parotid gland, it is important to remember the anatomy and realise that lymph nodes lie in close relation to the salivary tissue; within the gland lie fat, nerves and blood vessels. All of these tissues may develop neoplasms and present as a salivary gland swelling.

Acute salivary swellings. *Acute parotitis* may be viral (mumps), which is common, or bacterial, which is uncommon. Postoperative parotitis is rare but develops in sick, debilitated patients.

By contrast bacterial infection may supervene in a condition known as the 'sicca syndrome', in which an autoimmune process interferes with parotid function and the duct system dilates. Salivary secretion lessens and ascending infection occurs. Also recurrent irritation or actual stenosis of the parotid papilla from ductal tumour induces dilatation of the whole ductal tree. With diminished secretion, bacterial invasion can easily lead to diffuse sepsis or localised abscess. Rehydration, careful mouth toilet, local heat and antibiotics (amoxycillin, flucloxacillin) are the bases of therapy. For duct stenosis, dilatation under a short anaesthetic may be necessary.

Recurrent swelling is often caused by *salivary calculi* and the submandibular gland is affected most often, perhaps because its secretions are more viscid and affected by gravity. By contrast, calculi are uncommon in parotid ducts. Reduction of secretion and mild infection lead on to calculus formation (calcium, phosphate and carbonate stones). After eating or taking stimulating drinks, the ductal stones cause obstruction, so that the gland swells and becomes painful. The pain may be referred to the ventral surface of the tongue. The gland slowly reduces in size thereafter but often remains chronically enlarged. Frank infection and abscess formation may follow if the obstruction is complete.

Bimanual digital palpation may discern a stone in the floor of the mouth or at the hilum of the gland. The superficial and deep parts of the gland are thickened. Plain X-rays including intra-oral views will usually show up the radio-opaque stones. Sialography is rarely indicated for radiolucent stones.

The calculus is removed by intra-oral incision of the duct mostly under a short general anaesthetic by a precise surgical technique. Recurrent calculi or those fixed in the gland hilum ('comma' stones) necessitate excision of the whole submandibular salivary gland. Care must be taken in siting the skin incision for this operation, so as to avoid the mandibular branch of the facial nerve which dips below the angle of the mandible; injury causes an unsightly droop to the corner of the mouth.

Chronic salivary swellings. These may be caused by chronic inflammation and saliva-associated neoplasms.

Chronic inflammation. Any chronic swelling tends to be non-suppurative except where a low-grade infection is associated with major duct dilatation (sialectasis). The *'sicca' syndrome* is probably autoimmune and results in lymphoid infiltration within the parotid gland and fragility of the small (intercalary) ducts. A sialogram reveals multiple areas of small duct dilatation known as 'punctate sialectasis'. Disturbance of parotid function leads to lowered secretion, hence the the term 'sicca' (Latin: dry). Organisms can ascend from the mouth into an affected gland. This condition causes recurrent infective episodes in childhood and variable chronic swelling in adults.

Salivary-associated neoplasms. These may be subdivided into:

- salivary neoplasms proper
- secondary neoplasms
- soft tissue neoplasms
- lymphoreticular neoplasms.

Salivary neoplasms proper are derived from the ductal and acinar tissue and are classified into:

- benign
  — pleomorphic salivary adenoma (mixed tumour)
  — monomorphic adenoma
  — adenolymphoma (papillary cystadenoma lymphomatosum)
- malignant
  — well-differentiated, e.g. muco-epidermoid carcinoma, adenoid cystic carcinoma, acinic carcinoma
  — poorly differentiated or high-grade carcinoma, e.g. squamous and other cell types, malignant change within a pleomorphic adenoma.

A secondary neoplasm is a rare event but clinically simulates a primary neoplasm. Metastases from carcinoma of breast and lung, brain tumours and malignant melanoma are the most likely possibilities.

Soft tissue neoplasms are usually benign and include lipoma and neurilemmoma. Haemangioma is the commonest neoplasm in childhood.

Lymph nodes within the parotid fascia may become enlarged due to Hodgkin's or non-Hodgkin's lymphoma. The disease may arise there primarily or represent a locus of a generalised disease.

Apart from high-grade parotid carcinoma, which tends to be rapidly growing and forms a hard adherent mass which is clearly malignant, the lesions in the above list present as chronic swellings and are clinically indistinguishable from each other. As the pleomorphic adenoma comprises at least 70% of such swellings, it is not unreasonable to assume that all swellings are such. This assumption leads to important clinical mistakes: even skin cysts have been mistaken for parotid neoplasms.

The clinical error in assessing these lesions is around 50%. For this reason some surgeons prefer to make a preoperative diagnosis by careful fine needle aspiration cytology – a technique which can be 90–100% sensitive depending on the lesion. A preoperative diagnosis allows the surgeon to tailor the operation to match the lesion. Otherwise superficial parotidectomy is performed for every operable swelling with an intraoperative reassessment if malignancy appears likely. It is only fair to state that preoperative salivary fine needle biopsy is a controversial issue amongst 'salivary' surgeons.

The *plemorphic salivary adenoma* (mixed tumour) grows slowly and is a firm, elastic, slightly lobulated lesion to feel. It is always essential to look inside the mouth with any salivary examination. Very rarely a parotid tumour may present as a faucial mass. Microscopically the pleomorphic adenoma matches its name. The myoepithelial cell is probably the origin of a tumour which usually shows ductal and stromal elements. The stromal elements contain mucus and cells which resemble or actually are chondrocytes.

The *adenolymphoma* (papillary cystadenoma lymphomatosum), which accounts for 6–8% of parotid tumours, is a fascinating oncological lesion presenting at all ages but especially in middle-aged men who are smokers. It tends to lie superficially in the cervical process of the parotid and often varies in size and consistency. Sometimes it may be soft enough to show fluctuation. The tumour arises from metaplastic (oncocytic) ductal epithelium, which somehow induces a lymphoid response from the host. Cystic change is usually present and even frank necrosis may arise. The lesion is some-times bilateral and may be treated by controlled enucleation with the aid of a facial nerve stimulator to preserve nerve branches.

Well-differentiated carcinoma has a slow clinical progress and on palpation may exactly resemble a pleomorphic adenoma. Superficial parotidectomy at least is required, with sacrifice of facial nerve divisions if invaded. Nerve grafting should be feasible at the time of primary surgery. High-grade or poorly differentiated carcinoma is occasionally operable or may become so after irradiation. The prognosis is sadly very poor unless an early diagnosis is made. Block dissection of cervical nodes is rarely a rewarding addition.

Treatment of salivary gland tumours proper depends on the neoplasm, but *superficial parotidectomy* under controlled hypotension and with a facial nerve stimulator is the commonest operation. The facial nerve is exposed by a precise anatomical approach, and the superficial lobe of the gland is dissected off the nerve divisions. If the neoplasm lies in the deep lobe, operation is far more difficult and less precise. The pes anserinus (i.e. facial nerve and its major branches) is retracted, and the whole deep lobe with tumour is enucleated. It is important to avoid bursting the tumour during removal for fear of local recurrence. Enlarged lymph nodes, soft tissue neoplasms and adenolymphomas can be safely removed by controlled enucleation.

Specific syndromes. It is probably not helpful to maintain terms such as Sjögren's and Mikulicz's disease. The 'sicca syndrome' includes enlargement of the parotid, lacrimal and other salivary glands. Polyarthritis and chronic inflammation of the uveal tract may coexist. Infiltration with both sarcoidosis and lymphoma affect bilateral salivary glands. A form of low-grade non-Hodgkin's lymphoma which affects the gut and salivary glands is known as MESA (myoepithelial sialadenitis) or MALTOMA (mucosal associated lymphoid tumours). In around 90% of cases, fine needle aspiration cytology (FNAC) will clarify the diagnosis.

Branchial cysts

If a branchial cyst includes a deep connection into the nasal or oral pharynx then an embryological basis is likely. Most do not, however, and the cyst probably derives from epithelial inclusions within upper deep cervical lymph nodes.

A branchial cyst has the following characteristics:

- It usually presents in adolescence or young adulthood. One should be careful of making the diagnosis in patients over 40 years of age.
- The swelling lies in the upper neck and protrudes into the anterior triangle.
- It may lie deep to the sternomastoid muscle which partially obscures the cyst.
- Consistency varies but fluctuation may be detected.
- Infection may develop which increases the size and renders the swelling painful.
- The swelling can mimic an enlarged tonsillar lymph node.
- Fine needle aspiration reveals thin pus-like fluid with a characteristic cytology of degenerate squames, lymphocytes, debris and cholesterol crystals.

Surgical excision is advisable. The cyst lies deep to the fascia and is closely related to deep structures. An embryological aberration is a branchial fistula, which shows as a discharging point at the anterior border of the sternomastoid low in the neck. The track passes upwards and runs between the internal and external carotid arteries and then opens into the oro- or nasopharynx.

Sternomastoid tumour

This is a fibrous mass which develops within the sternomastoid muscle and shows soon after birth. It is presumably due to intrauterine or birth trauma. There is often some deformity of the skull, and if it is untreated a 'wry' neck develops. The treatment is entirely dependent on early recognition. Surgical correction is nowadays hardly ever required if the correct physiotherapy is commenced without delay.

Cervical rib

A bony or fibrous extra rib at the seventh cervical level is not uncommon and may be a completely asymptomatic chance finding. Otherwise paraesthesiae related to the first thoracic nerve root may develop. If the subclavian artery is distorted, vascular phenomena in the fingers will be the cardinal feature. Arteriography or Doppler studies are necessary to clarify the symptomatology, but it is occasionally helpful to resect the extra rib and fibrous band.

Cystic hygroma

This is another embryological fault and is more precisely

termed a cavernous lymphangioma. It may be present at birth and of such size and extent in the neck as to require emergency operation to free the airway. Otherwise it is seen in childhood or adolescence as a soft, often transilluminable swelling in the posterior triangle of neck. Excision is not easy as natural structures (nerves and blood vessels) lie virtually within the lesion.

Vascular swellings

Aneurysms, arteriovenous fistulas and other vascular abnormalities are complex. Arteriovenous fistulas may occur in the parotid region where they require a difficult surgical excision.

An entity that comprises dilated small arteries and veins is rarely found to affect the face and scalp and is termed a cirsoid aneurysm.

Carotid body tumour or chemodectoma

This is an uncommon tumour of the chemoreceptors within the carotid body, which develops in middle life as an ovoid, firm, painless lump in the line of the carotid vessels at the upper border of the thyroid cartilage. Delicate palpation may detect expansile pulsation. The differential diagnosis between chemodectoma, carotid aneurysm, metastatic lymphadenopathy and nerve sheath tumours is difficult but critical. The lateral movement on palpation is helpful.

Duplex scanning of the neck vessels is the ideal diagnostic mode, but carotid angiography is also used. The lesion is vascular but can usually be dissected from the main arteries. The most important point is that a vascular surgeon and vascular instruments are available for the operation.

Unusual infections

Actinomycosis, sublingual sepsis (Ludwig's angina) and pharyngomaxillary abscess are all very rare nowadays. Any unusual cervical abscess should be elucidated by CT scanning, coupled with expert surgery and microbiology. The advice of an oral surgeon should be sought.

Unusual tumours

It is very rare to encounter a soft tissue or bony tumour in the neck apart from the ubiquitous lipoma, which can be subcutaneous, subfascial or intramuscular in position.

The possibility of a neural origin (neurilemmoma and neurofibroma) should be remembered. Neurilemmoma may present deeply in the posterior triangle. Here again, CT or MRI scanning is invaluable together with fine needle aspiration cytology (FNAC). Surgical exploration must be planned on such bases. Primary bony lesions of the skull and jaw (histiocytosis and Ewing's tumour) have been known to extend into parotid and submandibular sites.

SPECIAL INVESTIGATIONS

Neck swellings are both a diagnostic paradise and a nightmare, so additional tests can help:

- Endoscopy of the oropharynx, nasopharynx and larynx to identify a cryptic primary squamous carcinoma
- Fibre-optic bronchoscopy and biopsy, to seek carcinoma of the lung
- Fibre-optic oesophagoscopy for postcricoid and oesophageal carcinoma
- Chest X-ray and views of thoracic inlet to identify lung, mediastinal and thyroid disease or a generalised process that may be the cause of metastatic nodes
- Full blood examination, in particular to detect anaemia or a leukaemia
- Mammography if cryptic breast cancer is a possibility
- Fine needle aspiration cytology of a cervical swelling
- Excision biopsy of lymph nodes.

Fine needle aspiration cytology of a cervical swelling is a well-established technique but is not available in all centres. It demands an interested and expert needling surgeon to provide adequate smears and a skilled cytopathologist to read them. The sensitivity of the technique can reach 90–95% for the diagnosis of metastatic nodes, branchial cysts, pleomorphic salivary adenoma and lymphoma. To classify the lymphoma type, excision biopsy is required to allow refined monoclonal studies.

Excision biopsy of lymph nodes should be confined to cases of doubt and lymphoma. Nodes suspected of harbouring secondary carcinoma should not be incised or excised. General anaesthesia and an experienced surgeon are obligatory. In the left scalene node area, the thoracic duct is vulnerable. The node(s) should be excised without undue squashing and sent fresh to the laboratory for lymph node imprints, monoclonal antibodies and routine histopathology. This will hopefully allow precise categorisation and assist the oncologist in deciding the appropriate treatment regimen. The importance of lymph node excision and handling should never be underestimated.

TREATMENT

Excision will usually be indicated for branchial cysts, thyroglossal cyst, pilar and epidermoid cyst,* carotid body tumour, dissecting ranula, sublingual dermoid, laryngocele, salivary tumours and calculi, pharyngeal pouch, cervical rib and lymphangiomas.

FURTHER READING

Edgerton M T, Angel M F, Morgan R F 1991 The mouth, tongue, jaws and salivary glands. In: Sabiston D C, Jr (ed) Textbook of surgery, 14th edn. W B Saunders, Philadelphia, p 1209–1234
Fried M P 1994 The evaluation of a neck mass in an adult patient. In: Morris P J, Malt R A (eds) Oxford textbook of surgery, vol 2. Oxford University Press, New York, p 2215–2220
Routledge R T 1994 Block dissection of the glands of the neck. In: Keen G, Farndon J R (eds) Operative surgery and management, 3rd edn. Butterworth-Heinemann, Oxford, p 369–376
Stell P M, Maran A G D 1988 Head and neck surgery. In: Cuschieri A, Giles G R, Moossa A R (eds) Essential surgical practice, 2nd edn. Wright, London, p 345–371

---

*Most 'sebaceous' cysts derive from the pilosebaceous follicle. Pilar cysts, which are largely confined to the scalp, are histologically distinct from epidermoid cysts.

Breast and Endocrine surgery

20 Thyroid

John Webb

OVERVIEW

The thyroid gland and its disorders dominate the specialty of endocrine surgery. Goitres are common worldwide, affecting 3–5% of the population. They are generally simple or multinodular in type, but the clinician needs to recognise the occasional neoplasm, most of which are malignant. The student must develop a well-rehearsed technique for the clinical assessment of goitres, understanding standard protocols for investigation and watching for minor degrees of hyper- and hypothyroidism.

SURGICAL ANATOMY

The adult thyroid gland weighs between 20 and 30 g and possesses two lobes, the right of which is slightly larger and higher in position than the left. The upper pole is obscured by the attachment of the sternothyroid muscle to the thyroid cartilage (Fig. 20.1) and lies closely applied to the inferior constrictor and cricothyroid muscles. The lower parts of the lobes rest at the side of the trachea and oesophagus. They are joined by an isthmus of gland which lies across the upper four tracheal rings. The pyramidal lobe is a variable tongue of glandular tissue which extends upwards towards the hyoid bone. It is an embryological remnant (Fig. 20.2). It is important to note that the anatomical form of the thyroid gland does vary and that small islands of natural tissue can lie seemingly separate from the main structure.

The gland is composed of lobules and has a definite fine capsule. Surrounding it is the pretracheal fascia and anterior to the thyroid another thin layer known as the infrahyoid fascia. On the deep surface of the thyroid lobe the pretracheal fascia is condensed into a firm and surgically important attachment to the cricoid cartilage and upper trachea (ligament of Berry). Because of this ligament the thyroid elevates with the larynx on swallowing.

Anteriorly lie the strap muscles (sternothyroid and sternohyoid) which are covered by the deep cervical fascia. Superficial to these are the anterior jugular veins covered by platysma and skin.

The parathyroid glands are commonly four in number but vary (Fig. 20.3) from three to six. They are orange-brown in colour and usually surrounded by a small fatty component. Each gland has dimensions of approximately $6 \times 4 \times 2$ mm, weighing around 20 mg. The superior parathyroid glands are the most constant in position and lie on the posterior border of the lobe, on or near a projection known as the nodule of Zuckerkandl, midway between the entry of the inferior thyroid artery and the upper pole. The inferior glands are much more variable and sit somewhere around the lower thyroid pole. They tend to lie posteriorly but may be found on the surface of the pole. Because of embryological migration, the inferior glands can also hide amongst pretracheal lymph nodes within the thymus or thoracic cavity.

BLOOD SUPPLY

The superior thyroid artery arising from the external carotid artery descends in anterior and posterior branches to the superior pole where, in 20% of patients, it is closely related to the external laryngeal nerve from the superior laryngeal branch of the vagus nerve.

The inferior thyroid artery, a branch of the thyrocervical trunk which arises from the first part of the subclavian

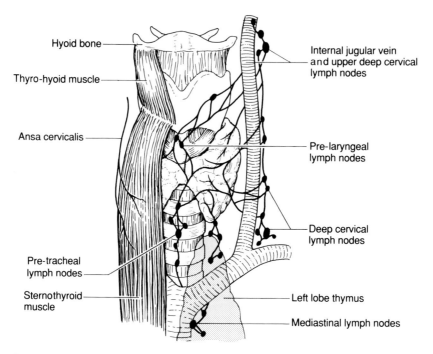

Hyoid bone

Thyro-hyoid muscle

Ansa cervicalis

Pre-tracheal
lymph nodes

Sternothyroid
muscle

Internal jugular vein
and upper deep cervical
lymph nodes

Pre-laryngeal
lymph nodes

Deep cervical
lymph nodes

Left lobe thymus

Mediastinal lymph nodes

Fig. 20.1 Thyroid gland – anterior relations and lymphatic drainage.

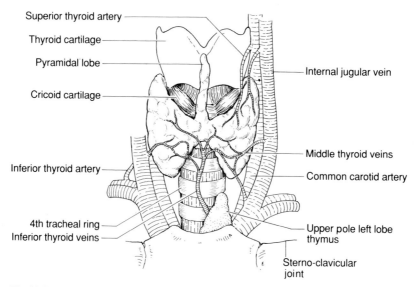

Superior thyroid artery

Thyroid cartilage

Pyramidal lobe

Cricoid cartilage

Inferior thyroid artery

4th tracheal ring
Inferior thyroid veins

Internal jugular vein

Middle thyroid veins

Common carotid artery

Upper pole left lobe
thymus

Sterno-clavicular
joint

Fig. 20.2 Thyroid gland – blood supply. Anterior view with strap muscles removed.

artery, ascends in the neck and arches medially behind the common carotid artery and divides into two main divisions at or near its entry into the lobe. It is a large vessel and varies somewhat in its entry point. Branches from this artery supply both parathyroid glands. The inferior thyroid artery bears an important relationship to the recurrent laryngeal nerve (Fig. 20.4). The nerve may pass anterior or posterior to the arterial divisions, or indeed between them. The relationship on the right side is more complex than on the left. Higher up, where the

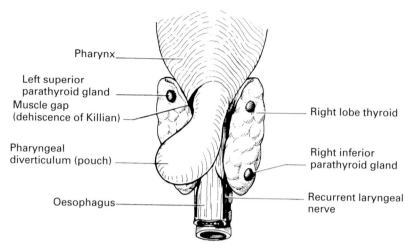

Fig. 20.3 Posterior view of the thyroid gland showing parathyroids and pharyngeal pouch.

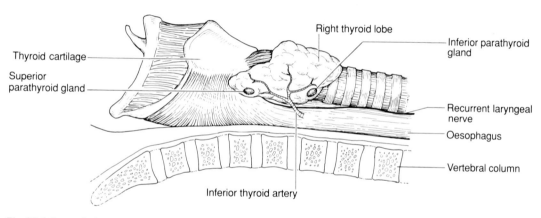

Fig. 20.4 Lateral view of the thyroid gland.

recurrent nerve enters the larynx, a branch of the artery lies closely applied and medial to it.

The thyroidea ima artery is an inconstant and unimportant small vessel which arises from the aorta or brachiocephalic artery and runs into the isthmus.

A variable number of small tracheal arteries enter the deep surface of the thyroid lobe in a paratracheal position.

VENOUS DRAINAGE (Fig. 20.2)

The superior thyroid veins drain into the internal jugular vein. The middle thyroid veins are variable and often multiple. They arise from the surface of the thyroid lobe and, passing over the common carotid artery, drain into the internal jugular vein.

The inferior thyroid veins are very constant and stream from the lower thyroid poles in a pre- and paratracheal position to the brachiocephalic veins. Sometimes they are closely related to an aberrant recurrent laryngeal nerve.

A collection of small veins drain from the deep surface of the strap muscles into the surface of the lateral lobes.

LYMPHATIC DRAINAGE

There is a rich intraglandular network of lymphatics with extensive and widespread drainage from the gland into lymph nodes. On general principles, the vessels follow the arteries, except inferiorly where lymphatics accompany the veins toward mediastinal nodes. The deep cervical chain along its whole length receives lymphatic drainage from the thyroid. Prelaryngeal, pre-isthmic and pretracheal lymph nodes are also present (Fig. 20.1).

PHYSIOLOGY

A basic understanding of thyroid physiology is helpful as it does carry clinical relevance. The biosynthesis of thyroid hormones – thyroxine (T_4) and tri-iodothyronine (T_3) – occurs in three stages within the thyroid follicle:

- iodine trapping
- iodine organification by combination with tyrosine to form inert iodotyrosines
- coupling of iodotyrosines to form active T_4 and T_3.

Release of the hormones involves two further stages:

- hydrolysis of thyroglobulin
- passage of iodotyrosines into the circulation.

The thyroid gland is the sole source of T_4, the hormone in greatest quantity, but not the most active. T_3 is functionally the more important and is produced peripherally by enzymatic conversion from T_4. Both T_4 and T_3 are transported in the blood, bound mainly to thyroid-binding globulin (TBG) and to a lesser extent to thyroid-binding albumin. A small proportion (2%) of T_4 and T_3 is free in the circulation.

Thyroid function is delicately controlled through secretion of thyroid-stimulating hormone (TSH) from the anterior pituitary lobe. Two feedback mechanisms control TSH secretion, central positive and peripheral negative. In the first, the hypothalamus secretes thyroid-releasing hormone (TRH) which exerts a positive feedback on the pituitary, causing release of TSH. The TSH then stimulates the thyroid to synthesise and release thyroid hormones.

In the second, peripheral levels of circulating free T_4 constitute a feedback mechanism on the pituitary TSH secreting capacity. Low circulating levels induce increased TSH secretion (as in Hashimoto's disease), and high circulating levels depress TSH secretion (as in oral thyroxine therapy). T_3 has a minimal effect on TSH secretion, and this physiological property is employed in regimens for radioactive iodine therapy in follicular thyroid cancer.

INVESTIGATION OF THYROID DISORDERS

With some exceptions it is both advisable and rewarding to employ a *standard schedule* of investigations for thyroid disease.

Full blood count/ESR. As some clinical goitres will require operative treatment, a full blood count with ESR or plasma viscosity measurement is obligatory. In cases of viral thyroiditis, the ESR is usually elevated.

T_4 and T_3 levels. Serum T_4 and T_3 levels are standard tests. Nowadays free T_4 and T_3 are measured. An artificial increase in protein binding capacity as in pregnancy or oral contraceptive treatment (oestrogen–progestogen combinations) will increase the serum bound levels.

TSH level. TSH level in peripheral blood is an important and widely used parameter, particularly useful in hypothyroidism when the level is elevated. Serial measurements in the course of T_4 therapy are essential to ensure correct replacement. The TSH level will be fully suppressed in primary, secondary or autonomous thyrotoxicosis apart from a not uncommon mild form of disturbance seen with hyperplastic nodular goitre – T_3 toxicosis. It is important that serum T_3 measurements are requested to diagnose and treat this often obscure clinical problem.

Thyroid antibodies. Thyroid antibodies are measured by radioimmunoassay and are an essential component of the investigation of any form of goitre or possible thyroid disease. Thyroglobulin and microsomal tanned red cell agglutination (TRCA) titres are usually provided, and a level beyond 1/80 is significant. The microsomal TRCA levels are the most sensitive. The levels will be elevated in classical diffuse lymphocytic thyroiditis (Hashimoto's disease), but atypical lymphocytic thyroiditis, which may arise in a pre-existing nodular goitre is more difficult. Primary thyrotoxicosis is associated with elevated antibody levels. In future, serum thyroid peroxidase (TPO) antibodies may be a more sensitive measurement. Thyroglobulin (Tg) antibodies are sometimes used in the management of differentiated thyroid cancer.

IMAGING

Scintillation scan

Three isotopes are used for thyroid scans, as imaged by the gamma camera:

- Technetium. ^{99m}Tc pertechnetate is widely used and

is the isotope of choice for routine thyroid scanning – particularly in young people.

- Iodine (^{131}I) was the first isotope used for thyroid scans. It is more expensive than ^{99m}Tc and requires a higher dose to obtain a useful image. Some centres prefer it for patients over 40 years of age.
- Iodine (^{123}I) is the most efficient imaging agent for the thyroid but its expense rules it out for routine use.

There is considerable difference of opinion regarding the clinical value of scintiscanning. ^{99m}Tc is taken up by the thyroid but is neither organified nor stored. ^{131}I is more reliable as an imager. For the diagnosis of problem goitres in childhood and adolescence, ^{99m}Tc is invaluable, but ^{131}I maintains an essential position for scanning and therapy in well-differentiated thyroid cancer.

The gamma camera technique is one method for thyroid gland representation or mapping after isotopic uptake. Nodules are particularly important and, if large enough, may be outlined on the scan as 'hot', 'warm' or 'cold'. Areas of poor uptake, especially solitary nodules, suggest gross anatomical alteration such as cystic change, thyroiditis or malignancy. 'Cold' solitary nodules demonstrated clinically and on scintiscan bear a risk of malignancy of between 12% and 15%, but the majority will be cysts within an unrecognised nodular goitre.

Ultrasound scan

Real-time ultrasound scanning with a high resolution transducer probe remains the subject of controversy. Ultrasound demonstrates physical characteristics within the thyroid plus even lymph nodes and parathyroids. The technique is sensitive for delineating cysts and demonstrating whether a solitary nodule is solid, cystic or mixed. It may be used to guide precise needle biopsy.

Plain X-ray

Chest and thoracic inlet views are necessary to assess the presence of cardiac failure, pre-existing lung disease, lung metastasis, retrosternal goitre and mediastinal lymphadenopathy. The degree and extent of tracheal deviation or compression is also demonstrated together with the identification of calcification within the thyroid, which may rarely alert the clinician to the presence of thyroid malignancy (papillary or medullary). In complex clinical situations such as recurrent benign or malignant goitres, magnetic resonance imaging (MRI) is invaluable.

Thyroid needle biopsy

This is a controversial subject but the technique is gaining acceptance in many surgical centres. There are two types available:

- large needle (1–2 mm dia.) biopsy, e.g. Vim-Silverman type or 'Tru-Cut'
- fine needle aspiration cytology (FNAC).

Large needle biopsy is inserted under local anaesthetic to obtain a core of tissue for histopathology.

Fine needle aspiration cytology is aspirative as opposed to exfoliative cytology. The procedure is aspiration of the thyroid by a 20 ml syringe attached to a fine needle (21–25 gauge). Tissue sludge, tissue fragments and blood are aspirated and air-dried smears are produced, which are stained by May–Grünwald or 'Diff Quick' staining. Ideally the examination and aspiration are performed by a cytologist who then reads the smears. Diagnostic accuracy can be high and sensitivity rates for defining malignancy can be over 90%. Problems do exist especially in the distinction between benign and malignant follicular lesions, but taken overall, the surgeon is provided with an 80–90% diagnostic certainty before operating.

GOITRE

Terminology

'Goitre' means an enlargement of the thyroid gland which may be diffuse, generally nodular or solitary nodular.

'Toxic' is an abbreviation of the term thyrotoxicosis or hyperthyroidism. 'Non-toxic' is synonymous with a clinically euthyroid goitre. Hashimoto's disease means chronic lymphocytic thyroiditis.

Classification

Goitres are classified as non-toxic, toxic or specific.

Non-toxic goitres. These are:

- diffuse – hyperplastic or colloid
- multinodular
- solitary nodular
- recurrent nodular (following previous surgery).

Toxic goitre. These can be:

- diffuse – primary thyrotoxicosis (Graves' disease) and toxic thyroiditis ('Hashitoxicosis' or self-resolving thyrotoxicosis)
- multinodular – secondary thyrotoxicosis
- solitary nodular – autonomous toxic follicular adenoma.

Specific goitre. This category includes:

- thyroiditis – lymphocytic thyroiditis (Hashimoto), granulomatous thyroiditis (De Quervain)
- neoplasms of thyroid – adenoma carcinoma and lymphoma
- fibrous or ligneous thyroiditis (Riedel) – very rare.

NON-TOXIC GOITRE

Aetiology

Physiological enlargement of the thyroid gland may occur at puberty, pregnancy and the menopause, largely due to hormone changes affecting iodine uptake by the gland.

Pathological goitre may develop as a result of:

- iodine deficiency
- goitrogenic substances
  — dietary
  — drugs
- genetic defects.

A low dietary uptake of iodine (less than 100 μg per day) results in a hyperplastic response in the gland, and this is a major factor in the production of endemic goitres. Iodinisation of salt, bread or margarine is a means of overcoming this common problem.

There is some evidence that goitrogenic substances may be present in turnips, swedes and soya beans. Fluoride excess has been incriminated as a goitrogen in Punjab and calcium excess in Colombia, Cape Province, Burma and West China. In Great Britain, high calcium levels in drinking water may be a cause of endemic goitre. In Himalayan India and elsewhere generally, contaminated drinking water is suspect. All these agents seem to prevent the uptake of iodine and the natural synthesis of thyroxine.

Overtreatment of hyperthyroidisim with blocking drugs (thiouracils, carbimazole) may increase the size of a pre-existing goitre. Lithium salts prescribed for depressive illness may induce goitres. Hypothyroidism and a coexistent goitre may be extant in neonates if the mother has taken antithyroid drugs during pregnancy.

Rarely a goitre develops when there is a genetic defect in the enzyme systems that form thyroxine. Distinct biochemical defects have been described; in general this is known as dyshormonogenesis. Defects include:

- inability to concentrate iodine in the thyroid
- inability to bind iodine organically. This may be severe enough to cause congenital hypothyroidism and goitre. If congenital deafness is associated, it is known as Pendred's syndrome.

Whatever the aetiological cause, the thyroid reacts in a similar manner. If thyroid hormone production is inadequate or if there is an increased demand, the gland enlarges due to hyperplasia and multiplication of follicles in response to increased TSH stimulation. The end result is a hyperplastic goitre which is clinically diffuse. In some circumstances the demand for thyroid hormones eases off, but the gland remains enlarged or increases in size due to increased colloid storage.

For unknown reasons, such a goitre may regress in an irregular fashion. Some areas remain hyperplastic, others colloid; within the latter coalescence and degeneration can form either large colloid nodules or cysts. Fibrosis and calcification may develop within and around these lesions. This change may be gross, producing huge irregular goitres (200–300 g), or remain limited in size, localised and barely progressive. Haemorrhage may occur into cystic areas.

In certain instances (dyshormonogenesis, lithium medication) the goitre remains largely hyperplastic with multiple cellular nodules and cytological changes that closely mimic malignancy.

Clinical features

The common feature of non-toxic goitres is a visibly and palpably enlarged thyroid. *Inspection* is very important. A goitre moves on swallowing unless very large and impacted retrosternally or adherent owing to malignant invasion. Inspection is often the best means of deciding whether a goitre is diffuse or nodular. A glass of water for the patient to sip and swallow is essential. Examine the patient from behind and in front, feeling with both sets of fingers. Solitary nodules are more difficult; it is sometimes helpful to gently deviate the larynx when palpating. Thereby a nodule can be less obscured by the sternomastoid muscle. Varying the degree of flexion of the neck is also helpful.

Treatment

Diffuse goitre. Physiological goitres rarely require treatment. For established diffuse goitres, sodium thyroxine (T_4, 50–100 μg/day) should be given to suppress the TSH level. If clinical resolution becomes evident, the treatment should be continued for up to a year. Thyroidectomy may be required for pressure symptoms or cosmetic detriment.

Multinodular goitre. Multinodular goitre is the commonest goitre encountered by physicians and surgeons. All cases should be properly investigated. There is little doubt that thyroid malignancy (follicular and anaplastic carcinoma) is commoner in endemic areas. With the aid of ultrasound scanning, any uncertain nodule should be sampled by FNAC. For cytological atypia, pressure symptoms, secondary toxic change or cosmetic reasons, subtotal thyroidectomy should be advised. Some surgeons prefer total thyroidectomy for glands above 100 g in weight.

Solitary nodules. On clinical grounds, only 50% of seemingly solitary nodules are truly solitary. The remainder are part of a nodular gland and constitute a dominant nodule. Especially careful investigation is required and should include a scintiscan, ultrasound and FNAC.

If the nodule is solitary, solid, 'hot' or 'warm' (on scintiscan) and cytologically benign, it is a follicular adenoma. Radioactive ^{131}I treatment can be used, but most surgeons settle for total lobectomy with excision of the isthmus, controlling any possible mild toxicity with a beta blocker (e.g. nadolol 40 mg b.d. or t.d.s).

If the nodule is 'cold', one should proceed to FNAC (repeated if necessary). If solid, cytology is critical. It will be benign, malignant or atypical.

If benign or atypical it is probably a follicular adenoma. Total thyroid lobectomy with the isthmus is necessary. Should the paraffin histopathology show carcinoma, a second operation to complete a near-total thyroidectomy is indicated.

If the cells show undoubted malignancy, near-total thyroidectomy is advisable preserving at least two parathyroid glands and minimal protecting thyroid tissue (about 1 g).

Cystic nodules are problematic. Ultrasound is invaluable to clarify the precise physical features. FNAC is performed from more than one site. Provided that the cells are benign, the fluid is not grossly bloodstained and the swelling disappears after aspiration, a conservative policy with thyroxine therapy (50–100 μg/day) is acceptable. If the swelling recurs, lobectomy is wise. If the cells are malignant or suspicious, then total lobectomy with frozen section histopathology (to outline a papillary carcinoma) is necessary. The operation proceeds according to the pathology and size of the tumour.

Recurrent nodular goitre. This difficult disease can usually be prevented by regular thyroxine therapy following subtotal thyroidectomy. However, if a swelling recurs, full and precise investigation is obligatory. The goitre should be subjected to scintiscan and ultrasound; T_4 and T_3 toxicosis must be excluded. An ENT surgeon should be requested to check the larynx for previous recurrent or external laryngeal nerve damage. FNAC is necessary to exclude malignant change, but hyperplastic nodules can yield very atypical cells and this is a practical problem. Operation by an experienced surgeon is usually indicated, and the patient must be warned of risks to both parathyroid and nerve function. A debulking procedure with preservation of important anatomy is the aim.

Retrosternal goitre is particularly taxing. Postoperative thyroid treatment is essential.

TOXIC GOITRE

Aetiology

The causes of hyperthyroidism or thyrotoxicosis are not fully understood, but autoimmune factors are probably involved. Sometimes a psychological upset seems to trigger the onset, such as bereavement, rejection or academic failure.

Surgical pathology

Diffuse toxic goitre (Graves' disease, primary thyrotoxicosis). The gland is enlarged and smooth, the cut surface uniform, reddish and vascular. Microscopically epithelial hyperplasia, increased vascularity and variable lymphocytic infiltration are seen.

Multinodular toxic (secondary toxic) goitre. The goitre has usually been present for many years before hyperthyroidism develops. The gland is irregularly enlarged, and its cut surface reveals many nodules which are solid (cellular) or cystic (colloid-filled). Microscopically, areas of epithelial hyperplasia can be identified.

Toxic solitary nodule. The cut surface shows a single lesion with a thin discrete capsule. The nodule may show cystic change, fibrosis and calcification. Microscopically the features of follicular adenoma are seen.

Toxic Hashimoto's disease. In its classical form the gland is enlarged and very firm, the surface pale and grossly nodular (bosselated). Microscopically the gland is grossly disturbed by lymphoplasmocytic infiltrate and germinal centres. The thyroid follicular cells are stimulated by a high TSH level to cytoplasmic and nuclear enlargement (Hürthle or Askanazy cells).

Clinical features

Diffuse toxic goitre (Graves' disease and toxic Hashimoto's disease). Clinical features include weight loss despite a good appetite, preference for cold environment, sweating, tremor of hands and nervousness. Eye signs may be present. These include lid retraction, protrusion of the eyeball (proptosis) and, in severe cases, oedema of the eyelids and paresis of the extrinsic ocular muscles.

Multinodular goitre and autonomous 'hot' nodule. Hyperthyroidism from these conditions will often differ from the pattern seen in Graves' disease in the following ways:

- onset in middle or later life – Graves' disease affects younger people
- eye signs are minimal or absent
- cardiac arrhythmias (atrial fibrillation) and insidious cardiac failure are common
- there may be pressure signs in the neck; however, weight loss, irritability and gastrointestinal upsets can also occur.

Treatment

The treatment of thyrotoxicosis is urgent and requires careful supervision. There are few disorders in which the choice of treatment has to be so delicately balanced. This choice may be determined by the wishes of the patient, the facilities available and the patient's geographic location. Antithyroid drugs are used to render the patient fit for operation combined with beta-adrenergic blockade.

Antithyroid drugs. Carbimazole is given at a dose of 10–20 mg 8-hourly (depending on the severity), coupled with (paradoxically) sodium thyroxine (100 mg). Once the patient has been rendered euthyroid, both clinically and biochemically (and this takes 1–2 months), the dosage is slowly reduced to a basal level of 5 mg three times a day for 1–2 years. The drug is then gradually withdrawn.

Advantages. The advantages of antithyroid drugs are that they avoid the possibility of operation, which may not appeal to the patient and carries risks if the patient is otherwise unfit, and they avoid the potential hazards of radioactive iodine.

Disadvantages. The relapse rate is high, around 50–60%. Reactions to the drug occur in about 10–15%, of which the most serious are drug rashes and leucopenia; the white blood count should be checked regularly. Resistance to the drug may also occur.

Regular follow-up for 2 years and beyond is essential and this may be unreliable, uneconomic or generally unacceptable to the patient.

Special indications. These include:

- childhood
- mild thyrotoxicosis in adolescents
- recurrence after operation, as an alternative to radioactive iodine
- patients with cardiac features – these require carbimazole in combination with digoxin, diuretics and radioiodine
- pregnancy.

With any form of thyrotoxicosis, complementary treatment with beta-adrenergic receptor antagonists (beta blockers) is invaluable, e.g. propranolol 40 mg 6-hourly or nadolol 80 mg b.d., plus the tranquillizer diazepam 5–10 mg b.d. For secondary thyrotoxicosis, this combination is the ideal therapy and carbimazole should be withheld.

Radioactive iodine (^{131}I)

Advantages. ^{131}I can be simply given as a drink, and it avoids the risks of operation in unfit or unwilling patients and also the risks of long-term antithyroid drug therapy.

Disadvantages. The efficacy of ^{131}I is slow and hypo-thyroidism always develops with time (35–40% after 10 years). Theoretical risks of carcinogenesis mean that for some patients avoidance will be preferred.

Indications. ^{131}I should be used in:

- adults over 40 years of age, particularly women
- recurrent thyrotoxicosis after operation, particularly if there is proven recurrent laryngeal damage, but prefer-ably when no appreciable goitre is present
- severely affected thyrocardiacs.

Operation

Advantages. Operation is rapidly effective and there is a low incidence of recurrence.

Disadvantages. Even in skilled hands it can be a techni-cally difficult procedure. There should be a low rate of permanent hypoparathyroidism (1–2%) and of recurrent or external laryngeal nerve injury.

There are rare complications such as thyrotoxic crisis and postoperative haematoma formation.

Indications. Operation is indicated in the following:

- large toxic goitres – the larger the goitre the poorer the long-term response to carbimazole
- toxic nodular goitre – with preoperative control of any cardiac disease
- intrathoracic goitre, toxic or otherwise
- failure of antithyroid drug treatment
- social, economic and preferential factors when the patient is unable or unwilling to undergo long-term drug therapy and supervision.

Special considerations

Thyrocardiac patients. Once the thyrotoxic and cardiac components are controlled with medication, operation is offered. If cardiac failure is refractory, radioactive iodine is indicated. The worst scenario is where ^{131}I is only par-tially effective and a sizeable goitre is present.

Pregnancy. When the toxicosis is under control, thy-roidectomy is safe in the second trimester. The patient is then able to breastfeed, which is inadvisable if the moth-er is taking antithyroid drugs, as the infant can be affect-ed.

Exophthalmos. This is a problem and may worsen after thyroidectomy, drug therapy or radioiodine. Thyroxine should be given to correct hypothyroidism and reduce TSH levels. Steroids, azathioprine, tarsorrhaphy and orbital decompression are further options. The patient should be under ophthalmological supervision.

SURGICAL MANAGEMENT

Preoperative investigation and control of toxicity

The following should be carried out:

- Plain chest X-ray and thoracic inlet views: to assess tracheal state, calcification in the goitre and any intrathoracic (retrosternal) extension.
- Indirect laryngoscopy to assess vocal cord function is probably wise before all primary operations but not obligatory if the voice is unchanged. For secondary operations it is essential.
- Full blood investigations as previously described.
- Adequate sedation (e.g. with diazepam) to induce a sleeping pulse rate of 60–70/minute.
- Drugs to render the patient euthyroid, e.g.
  — carbimazole or propylthiouracil
  — beta blockers such as propanolol or nadolol
  — lugol's iodine (5% iodide in 10% potassium iodide solution) 0.5 ml (10 drops) t.d.s. in milk is popular with some surgeons to reduce the vascularity of the goitre.
- Complete bed rest under the care of an endocrine physician will control severe cases of thyrotoxicosis. Normally 4–8 weeks of traditional treatment is effec-tive.

Operation

A subtotal thyroidectomy is the standard procedure. Whatever the goitre size (the normal thyroid weighs 20–30 g), a remnant of about 3–4 g is retained on each side (total 6–8 g); this remnant measures about 5 × 1 cm. The external and recurrent laryngeal nerves are pre-served together with the parathyroid glands. With nodu-lar goitre the remnants can be smaller, provided the important structures are preserved, as thyroid supple-mentation will be required in any case.

Postoperative complications: local

Any form of thyroidectomy is associated with an excellent outcome in most cases. However, there are certain potentially dangerous local and special complications.

Haemorrhage. This is rare but can be devastating. It is reactionary and occurs within 12 hours of operation, arising deeply from the cut surface of the thyroid or from vessels. If haemorrhage is allowed to continue, blood will collect beneath the deep fascia and cause venous obstruction and secondary laryngeal congestion with glottic oedema leading to hypoxia and death.

Clinical recognition is crucial. There is tachycardia, tachypnoea, pallor or cyanosis, stridor and agitation. A neck swelling may be obvious. Treatment is urgent: the emergency 'crash-call' team is summoned. Meanwhile in the ward the dressing is taken down, the skin clips or sutures are removed and the strap muscles are separated digitally to evacuate the clot. Urgent return to theatre for general anaesthesia, exploration and adequate haemostasis is obligatory. Transfusion may be necessary. Should the glottis be narrowed, intubation or tracheostomy must follow.

If, on the ward, the respiratory emergency is acute then emergency tracheostomy falls to the most competent attendant. A 'thyroid tray' with skin staple remover, a tracheostomy set and other equipment should sit next to a post-thyroidectomy patient during their hospital stay. Even though no neck swelling is present, any mild stridor or glimmer of respiratory difficulty post-thyroidectomy should warn that the patient must be transferred to the intensive therapy (care) unit (ITU) without delay.

Liquefying haematoma. At around 7–10 days postoperatively, a lump may slowly develop in the neck. This will soften and discharge spontaneously through the wound. Occasionally surgical drainage will hasten resolution.

Wound infection. In patients with chronic obstructive airways disease, disturbance of lymphoid tissue at the root of the neck can release organisms which cause an infected haematoma. Antibiotics and drainage may be necessary.

Unsatisfactory scar. Most thyroidectomy wounds heal well, but hypertrophic and keloid scars do sometimes develop. Careful siting of the incision and precise closure of the platysmal layer may prevent some problems. Once healed, the patient should be encouraged to move the neck normally and soften the scar with skin creams.

Postoperative complications: special

Glottic oedema. Previous recurrent laryngeal nerve injury and over-treatment with antithyroid drugs may induce thickening of the true cords and glottic narrowing.

Tracheal collapse is a rare complication which may develop when the trachea is subject to long-term compression and distortion by a large goitre. Intubation or tracheostomy may be required if any respiratory embarrassment is detected.

Nerve injuries. This is a serious complication of thyroidectomy and may be unilateral or bilateral, transient or permanent. Laryngeal nerves may be damaged.

The recurrent laryngeal nerves. These may be injured from bruising, stretching, ligature or division. Damage is most likely to arise in operations for large multinodular and recurrent goitres when the nerves can be stretched over nodules or obscured by scar tissue. Malignancy may actually invade these nerves. If one nerve is damaged, the vocal cord on that side lies motionless in the mid- or cadaveric position. The voice is slightly hoarse and weak. If both nerves are paralysed, tracheostomy is necessary.

Transient paresis may develop postoperatively. Phonation is lost and the cords sit in single or bilateral cadaveric positions. Recovery takes place within days, weeks or months. Bruising and oedema comprise the presumed mechanism. Even simple endotracheal intubation can give rise to cord paralysis.

Prevention of recurrent nerve damage at operation requires a sound knowledge of the variable relationship of the nerves to the main trunk branches of the inferior thyroid artery and the ligament of Berry.

Exposure of the nerves is also required. Most thyroid surgeons expose the nerves at operation and trace them upwards to the inferior constrictor muscle. Great difficulty arises, however, if the nerve (or a division of it) lies stretched over a thyroid nodule.

A delicate surgical technique is necessary, keeping the nerves moist with normal saline, and there should be meticulous control of haemorrhage. Care should be taken to avoid excessive retraction on thyroid lobes.

Treatment of recurrent nerve damage is as follows. If injury is detected at operation, the recurrent laryngeal nerve is directly sutured with the aid of operating loupes and very fine sutures. Tracheostomy is required for respiratory obstruction.

If injury is detected postoperatively, up to 9 months can be allowed for recovery to ensue. An ENT opinion should be obtained. Late operations for permanent paresis include exploration and resuture of the nerve, arytenoidopexy with permanent lateral position of the cord and Teflon paste injection of the vocal cord(s).

The external laryngeal nerves. These nerves have been neglected in the discussion and practice of thyroidectomy. Injury to them may be a commoner cause of vocal insult after thyroidectomy than recurrent laryngeal nerve damage, which always tends to show good spontaneous recovery due to compensation of the other cord.

The external laryngeal nerves may be injured during dissection and ligation of the superior thyroid pole. Damage leads to marked voice weakness manifested by loss of power and quality. Injury can be avoided by a precise technique in mobilising the superior pole away from the larynx and ligating the vessels as close to the lobe as possible. There is no treatment if damage has occurred.

The cervical sympathetic chain. This is very rarely at risk with a large nodular goitre or papillary carcinoma with many involved deep cervical lymph nodes. A Horner's syndrome (miosis, enophthalmos, partial ptosis and skin sweating loss) may follow but tends to recover spontaneously.

Endocrine changes. These can result in hypoparathyroidism, hypothyroidism, recurrent thyrotoxicosis, progressive exophthalmos and thyroid crisis.

Hypoparathyroidism. This is an important complication which may be transient or permanent and follows excision, bruising or devascularisation of the parathyroid glands. The parathyroids are small (normal, $6 \times 4 \times 2$ mm), fragile and often elusive. For subtotal thyroidectomy, up to 5% of patients suffer mild transient hypoparathyroidism. For total or near total thyroidectomy, between 1% and 15% of patients will suffer permanent effects.

Clinically the patient should be carefully assessed on each postoperative day for symptoms of hypoparathyroidism (paraesthesias, etc.) and neuromuscular irritability (Trousseau's and Chvostek's signs). The serum calcium level should be measured on the fourth or fifth postoperative day unless the patient is tetanic, in which case it is measured at once.

To *prevent* hypoparathyroidism, removal of or damage to parathyroid glands at operation should be avoided. If a gland is found 'lying free', it should be diced into 1 mm fragments and implanted into a sternomastoid muscle. Many surgeons performing total lobectomy or total thyroidectomy prefer to ligate the terminal branches of the inferior thyroid artery and not the main trunk.

The *treatment* of this problem depends on whether it is minor or severe. For minor hypocalcaemia, calcium gluconate tablets 2–8 g daily will usually suffice. If the serum calcium level does not recover quickly, 1–2 μg daily of alfacalcidol (One-alpha vitamin D) is added.

For more severe hypocalcaemia (i.e. tetanic symptoms and signs), 10–20 ml of 10% calcium gluconate is given either by intravenous drip or by slow intravenous injection over 20 minutes. With persistent symptoms it is correct to estimate the serum magnesium and also to institute supplementation with magnesium chloride.

Hypothyroidism. Tiredness, lethargy and weight increase point to hypothyroidism. After subtotal thyroidectomy, 5–10% of patients develop such symptoms. Following operations for nodular goitre and autoimmune thyroiditis, supplementation with T_4 (50–150 μg) should be routine. Following operations for primary thyrotoxicosis, up to 1 year should be allowed for the remnants to recover. Serum estimations of T_4 and TSH should be made every 3–6 months until the patient is stabilised.

Recurrent thyrotoxicosis. On rare occasions it does develop. The diagnosis is confirmed by repeat serum tests and ^{131}I scintiscan. If possible, radioactive iodine is preferred, but a sizeable thyroid remnant will require a repeat operation.

Progressive exophthalmos. The effect of thyroidectomy on exophthalmos is unpredictable. Following surgery it is wise to continue T_4 treatment postoperatively so as to suppress TSH secretion. An ophthalmic surgeon should be involved with all but the most minor cases, as expert surgery may be required (tarsorrhaphy or orbital decompression).

Thyroid crisis. This dire complication was once a great problem and responsible for deaths following thyroidectomy for primary thyrotoxicosis. Nowadays, with adequate control, it should not arise. The problem lies with the mild unrecognised case, usually in secondary thyrotoxicosis with elevated T_3 levels.

Postoperative agitation, tachycardia, tachypnoea, fever and mental disturbance are danger signs. Immediate management includes serum estimation of thyroid hormones and treatment with intravenous beta blockers (propranolol, nadolol) plus sedation with chlorpromazine or diazepam.

SPECIAL CONDITIONS

THYROIDITIS

This term embraces a group of conditions which may be part of an autoimmune process. Excluded is the acute bacterial (pyogenic) thyroiditis, which is a rare condition caused by staphylococcal organisms.

Classsification

Thyroiditis can be classified into:

- chronic lymphocytic thyroiditis (Hashimoto's disease)
- viral or granulomatous thyroiditis (de Quervain's disease)
- Riedel's thyroiditis.

Surgical pathology

Hashimoto's disease (autoimmune thyroiditis, chronic lymphoid or lymphocytic thyroiditis). This process probably results from a perversion of host immunity whereby the body becomes sensitised to thyroglobulin and the microsomal function of the follicular cell. There is infiltration of the thyroid with lymphoid and plasma cells of B cell type, resulting in progressive destruction of the thyroid follicles and colloid. Autoantibodies to thyroglobulin and the cytoplasmic organelle (the microsome) are detectable in the serum. The process varies in severity; a mild degree of thyroiditis causes little alteration of thyroid function and no goitre. Generally the thyroid becomes diffusely enlarged over a 1–2 year period and firm in texture.

Microscopically there are several changes. Follicles become infiltrated with round cells, causing dispersion of colloid. Epithelial changes occur due to TSH stimulation. The follicular epithelium transforms to large cells with eosinophilic cytoplasm. Nuclear pleomorphism develops.

Within the stroma, lymphoplasmacytoid infiltration takes place, which may reach the stage of germinal centres. Histiocytes and Langhans' giant cells are present.

In time the lymphoid reaction diminishes and is replaced by sclerotic fibrous tissue. There are plenty of reactive lymph nodes draining the thyroid.

De Quervain's disease (granulomatous thyroiditis, subacute thyroiditis, giant cell thyroiditis, viral thyroiditis). Although this is an uncommon condition, many cases are unrecognized as the symptoms are so mild. There is circumstantial evidence implicating mumps and other viruses. The patient may complain of malaise, sore throat, painful swallowing and a tender goitre.

Microscopically, gross changes are evident. The follicles are disrupted and filled with histiocytes and degenerate follicular cells. These cells coalesce to become giant entities which are very distinctive.

In the stroma, inflammatory cells (polymorphs and lymphocytes) develop associated with fibroblasts.

Since the disturbance can be so gross, it remains surprising that recovery takes place in the vast majority of cases.

Riedel's thyroiditis (ligneous thyroiditis). This process is very rare, and its exact nature the subject of controversy. Non-Hodgkin's lymphoma must be excluded. A true case will present a very hard fibrotic gland which becomes fixed to surrounding structures.

Clinical features

Hashimoto's disease. There are two clinical types: the classical form where the whole gland is uniformly affected, and the atypical or nodular variant where the goitre appears nodular. Features of the classical form are as follows:

- Women are predominantly affected, especially in middle age.
- There is insidious development of a goitre, which is firm, symmetrical and has a smoothly nodular surface (termed bosselation).
- Mild hyperthyroidism occurs at the onset of disease, which tends to resolve spontaneously.
- Hypothyroidism is the usual sequel in established disease.
- Thyroid function tests reveal a low or low normal T_4 level with elevated TSH readings.

De Quervain's disease. The typical features are:

- usually young or middle-aged women
- abrupt febrile episode with sore throat, malaise and fever
- painful, tender, moderately enlarged thyroid
- investigations show an elevated erythrocyte sedimentation rate or plasma viscosity.

Riedel's thyroiditis. In this situation a dense, hard and fixed thyroid gland will cause pressure symptoms and concern as to the presence of malignancy.

Diagnosis

Fine needle aspiration cytology is useful for every form of thyroiditis. In Hashimoto's disease, the stimulated follicular cells (Askanazy or Hürthle cells) are mixed with lymphocytes and plasma cells. In De Quervain's disease, scattered thyroid cells are mixed with histiocytes, degenerate thyroid macrophages and multinucleate giant cells. In Riedel's thyroiditis a scanty yield of fibrocytes, fibroblasts and scattered thyroid follicular cells is expected. Open biopsy and wedge resection may be indicated to exclude cancer in Riedel's thyroiditis.

Treatment

Hashimoto's disease. Treatment consists of thyroid replacement for life (sodium thyroxine, T_4, 150–250 μg/day). The gland normally recedes to a minimal goitre; should it not do so, subtotal thyroidectomy is advisable.

De Quervain's disease. Once the diagnosis is made, it requires simple analgesia with aspirin and clinical surveillance. Occasionally in severe cases, a short course of oral prednisolone (10–20 mg/day) is beneficial.

Riedel's thyroiditis may produce tracheal compression, necessitating surgical decompression or even tracheostomy.

CARCINOMA OF THE THYROID

Malignancy in the thyroid is rare, but the incidence is slowly increasing.

Classification

These malignancies are:

- papillary
- follicular: micro- and macroinvasive
- anaplastic
- medullary.

Predisposing factors

Pre-existing goitre. There is a positive correlation between endemic goitres of multinodular type and both the follicular and anaplastic types of carcinoma. Perhaps an increased TSH level leads to areas of unstable hyperplasia and stromal proliferation.

Radiation. Exposure to low-dose irradiation in childhood is a proven cause of papillary thyroid cancer. At one time – particularly in the USA – therapeutic irradiation was the fashion and induced many cases. Currently, 'background' irradiation due to nuclear accidents is of great concern.

Genetic. In a small proportion of medullary cancers, multiple endocrine neoplasia is present and genetic abnormality is likely.

Surgical pathology

Papillary carcinoma. This is the commonest type (50–60%). Whilst affecting all ages it is most likely in young adults.

Macroscopically, there are solitary nodules limited by a thick irregular fibrous capsule and cystic spaces with small calcific bodies (psammoma bodies). Lymph node metastatic presentation is common.

Microscopically, there are papillary processes within cystic spaces and some follicular areas. Lamellated psammoma bodies are very characteristic.

Papillary cancer is slow growing but has a propensity to spread via lymphatics within the thyroid to lymph nodes. The primary tumour varies considerably in size. Apart from childhood up to 10 years of age, biologically, papillary cancer differs according to age. Under the age of 40 years in the male and 50 in the female it behaves very favourably.

Follicular carcinoma. This is less common (15–20%) and appears from young adulthood onwards.

Macroscopically, there seems to be a thin capsule, but invasion of neighbourhood structures may be detectable. The cut surface differs from the natural thyroid; it is paler, fleshy and may contain haemorrhagic and cystic areas.

Microscopically, these tumours vary a lot. The well-differentiated microinvasive types are difficult to separate from follicular adenoma. With the macroinvasive type there is invasion through the capsule, and tumour lies within blood vessels.

Follicular carcinoma has a specific tendency to spread via the bloodstream, and the disease may turn up as bony or pulmonary metastases.

Anaplastic carcinoma. In some series this tumour is second in incidence to papillary carcinoma, but in general the proportion is 10–15%. It affects elderly adults, especially women, and is an appalling tumour with few patients surviving beyond 1 year. The tumour grows rapidly and soon becomes fixed to neighbouring structures. Venous obstruction often supervenes. In some cases there is a history of a pre-existing goitre.

Macroscopically, the thyroid is hard, irregular, fixed and vascular. *Microscopically*, there is considerable pleomorphism. Giant, spindle, squamous and Hürthle cell types are seen.

Respiratory obstruction, dysphagia, venous obstruction and nerve pareses indicate a malignant tumour.

Medullary carcinoma. This is a rare tumour (6–8%) that was only properly delineated in 1954. Its biological behaviour is variable. Some tumours grow slowly as a long-standing solitary nodule, but others are far more rapid and present with lymph node, pulmonary and hepatic metastases. Around 40–50% of patients will survive 10 years after treatment. Operation is the only effective treatment; adjuvant chemotherapy and irradiation for metastatic disease are of little avail.

Macroscopically, it is a hard, solid, circumscribed tumour with a greyish, off-white or yellowish surface. Lymph node metastases are especially obvious on macroscopy.

Microscopically, the cells are small, spheroidal, ovoid or spindle in shape and lie in small groups. Stromal fibrosis is present, within which lies amorphous material which stains for amyloid.

The tumour spreads by lymphatics to regional lymph nodes in the neck and mediastinum, while bloodstream spread facilitates metastases in the liver. The tumour is of considerable oncological interest. It is thought to develop from parafollicular or C cells which derive embryologically from neural crest tissue incorporated within the thyroid. These cells produce the hormone calcitonin. Radiology may demonstrate both fine and gross calcification within medullary cancers. The hormone can be used as tumour marker, and high serum levels are detectable in patients with widespread metastases.

A minority (20%) of these tumours are familial and may be associated with parathyroid adenomas and phaeochromocytomas in the MEN (multiple endocrine neoplasia) type II syndrome.

Clinical features

It is important to realise that at least 50% of thyroid cancers present clinically as a 'benign' entity. Hence diagnostic errors and delay in recognition are common.

Carcinoma presents in one of the following ways:

- metastatic lymphadenopathy in the neck, often cystic and usually in one group (papillary carcinoma)
- solitary thyroid nodule (see below)
- as a clinically malignant thyroid, when the gland has enlarged rapidly and is hard and irregular with evidence of direct local spread (oesophagus, trachea, recurrent laryngeal nerve)
- sometimes, distant metastases, an abnormal chest X-ray or destructive bone lesion are the first discovery. For a bony lesion, proven by some form of biopsy as a metastasis, thyroid is one of the possible primary sites.

Solitary thyroid nodules (see also p. 185)

As already stated, half the solitary nodules represent one dominant nodule within a nodular goitre. The incidence of malignancy in truly solitary nodules is around 12–15%, but the figure will rise for solid (ultrasound) and cold (scintiscan) nodules to 25% or even more.

The investigation of a solitary thyroid nodule is particularly important as the risk of malignancy is higher than with multinodularity. Nevertheless a dominant or newly developing nodule within a long-standing nodular goitre deserves equal attention. Some form of preoperative needle biopsy (fine or large) can provide an 80–90% sensitivity rate for defining the presence and type of neoplasia. Otherwise a total lobectomy with frozen or urgent paraffin section is the procedure of choice.

Management of thyroid cancer

In all cases, preoperative tissue diagnosis is of great help to the surgeon.

Papillary. Surgeons differ in their approach, but one acceptable aim is to 'tailor' surgery to the biological state of the patient with tumour. In females under the age of 50 years, provided the tumour is confined to the thyroid, survival with treatment matches that of the standard population. Over the age of 40 (male) and 50 (female) the tumour is unpredictable, but overall a 20% 10-year death rate is likely.

Lymph node spread has paradoxically little effect on survival. Conservative surgery involves total lobectomy on the affected side with further excision of the isthmus, pyramidal lobe and 60% of the grossly unaffected lobe. Radical surgery involves near-total thyroidectomy, which leaves the contralateral thyroid capsule with at least two viable parathyroid glands or 1 g of thyroid tissue, depending on the anatomy. The involved lymph nodes are resected in groups ('node-picking') without resorting to block dissection of the neck. Occasionally the sternum is split and mediastinal nodes are removed with the thymus. The patient's TSH level is thereafter kept suppressed by oral T_4 (150–300 μg/day). Unless the tumour has invaded beyond the thyroid to involve larynx, oesophagus or muscles, adjuvant irradiation and ^{131}I are not widely used. Even multiple lung metastases will disappear on T_4 treatment (thyroid feeding). Surgeons differ as to when to employ conservative or radical surgery and I_{131} therapy, but age, size of tumour (> 3 cm diameter) and local spread are discriminant factors.

Follicular. For micro- or macroinvasive tumours, many surgeons opt for total or near-total thyroidectomy with attempted preservation of parathyroid function. The patient is placed on T_3 supplements while ^{131}I tracing and therapy are undertaken at intervals over a 2–3 year period. After two clear scans, the patient can revert to T_4.

Medullary. Total thyroidectomy with block dissection for involved lymph nodes is the standard surgical approach and is likely to be most rewarding if the tumour is discovered early and confirmed by preoperative FNAC. Adjuvant therapy is largely unhelpful, but radiotherapy is the least disturbing for the patient. Serum *calcitonin* levels are useful tumour markers postoperatively. They also have a distinct place in MEN II families, in whom serial serum levels are carried out. Clinically occult medullary cancers are treatable by prophylactic total thyroidectomy. However, such families are very rare and the sporadic medullary cancer dominates.

Anaplastic. The only real chance of relief is to discover the tumour early when total thyroidectomy is worth an attempt. This involves a high level of suspicion for any goitre and the liberal use of FNAC, especially in elderly women. Mostly the tumour is too advanced for surgical resection and radiotherapy is of little avail.

Lymphoma (non-Hodgkin's). This is an important but uncommon lesion. Some clinicians and pathologists hold the view that many cases derive from Hashimoto's disease – hence the general principle that a residual Hashimoto goitre of any size should be excised. Preoperative diagnosis by FNAC or large needle core biopsy is imperative. If resectable, near-total thyroidectomy may be carried out; if irresectable, then irradiation coupled with chemotherapy can help. Survival rates which exceed those for anaplastic carcinoma (54% at 5 years) are achievable.

FURTHER READING

Dudley N E 1994 The thyroid gland. In: Keen G, Farndon J R (eds) Operative surgery and management, 3rd edn. Butterworth-Heinemann, Oxford, p 333–356

Hall R, Besser M (eds) 1989 Fundamentals of clinical endocrinology, 4th edn. Churchill Livingstone, Edinburgh

Larsen P R, Ingbar S H 1992 The thyroid gland. In: Wilson J D, Foster D W (eds) Williams textbook of endocrinology, 8th edn. W B Saunders, Philadelphia, p 357–487

Lennquist S, Smeds S 1990 The hypermetabolic syndrome: hyperthyroidism. In: Friesen S R, Thompson N W (eds) Surgical endocrinology, clinical syndromes, 2nd edn. J B Lippincott, Philadelphia, p 127–159

Norton J A, Wells S A, Jr 1990 Medullary thyroid carcinoma and multiple endocrine neoplasia. Type 2 syndromes. In: Friesen S R, Thompson N W (eds) Surgical endocrinology, clinical syndromes, 2nd edn. J B Lippincott, Philadelphia, p 359–375

21

Endocrine disorders

Paul Anderson   James Shaw

OVERVIEW

Endocrine disorders may be uncommon but it is important to recognise them early as surgical treatment usually provides cure. This chapter covers the non-thyroid-related disorders of the parathyroid and adrenal glands. Hyperparathyroidism in its primary, secondary and tertiary types is covered in detail, as are Conn's syndrome, Cushing's syndrome and disease and phaeochromocytoma. There is a small section on adrenal incidentalomas. For endocrine tumours of the pancreas, see Chapter 27.

PARATHYROID GLANDS

ANATOMY AND PHYSIOLOGY

The parathyroid glands are typically four in number (15% of patients have more than four), yellow/brown in colour, 'tongue-shaped' and 0.5 cm in size. Their total weight is approximately 120 mg.

The upper parathyroids arise from the fourth branchial pouch. Eighty per cent are found on the posterolateral aspect of the thyroid, just above the termination of the inferior thyroid artery. The rest are posterolateral to the upper pole of the thyroid either just above or within the thyroid. The lower parathyroids arise from the third branchial pouch and are variable in position. Forty per cent are at the level of the lower pole of the thyroid, and another 40% are within the thymic tongue. The rest can be found lateral to the thyroid, within the thymus or, rarely, near to the carotid sheath. The glands are supplied almost exclusively by branches of the inferior thyroid artery.

The parathyroids play a vital role in calcium homeostasis. They are extremely sensitive to the level of serum ionised calcium. A fall in ionised calcium causes the chief cells of the parathyroid to secrete parathyroid hormone.

Parathyroid hormone causes increased:

- tubular resorption of calcium
- excretion of phosphate and bicarbonate
- osteoclastic resorption of bone
- intestinal absorption of calcium
- synthesis of 1,25-dihydroxycholecalciferol, the biologically active metabolite of vitamin D.

All of the above lead to a rise in plasma calcium. Levels of calcitonin (produced by the thyroid C cells) decrease. Calcitonin works antagonistically to parathyroid hormone and causes inhibition of osteoclastic bone resorption and increased renal excretion of calcium and phosphate.

DISEASES OF THE PARATHYROIDS

One of the most common endocrine diseases is hyperparathyroidism, with an incidence of about 1 in 1000 people, approaching 1 in 500 in females over the age of 45 years. It is the most common cause of hypercalcaemia in non-hospitalised patients and second to cancer in hospitalised patients.

PRIMARY HYPERPARATHYROIDISM

Surgical pathology

This is the abnormal secretion of parathyroid hormone

when there is a normal or increased calcium level. Patients present with the clinical effects of hypercalcaemia, the sequelae of long-term hypercalcaemia or non-specific symptoms, or they may indeed be asymptomatic, having only an incidentally found raised calcium.

The aetiology of primary hyperparathyroidism is unknown. It has been suggested that it may represent part of the ageing process, with the menopause playing a role. In addition, head and neck irradiation in childhood does lead to an increased incidence of adenoma and hyperplasia in later life.

In about 80% of patients, a single adenoma is responsible and its removal usually cures the condition (4% are due to multiple adenomata). Hyperplasia of the parathyroid glands accounts for approximately 10% of cases and carcinoma 1%.

Clinical features

'Painful bones, stones, abdominal groans and psychic moans' actually occur in less than 50% of patients with hypercalcaemia. The following are typical clinical features:

- *non-specific symptoms* – increased fatigue, anorexia, polydipsia, polyuria, weight loss
- *bone* – bone pain, arthralgias, pathological fractures
- *abdominal* – constipation, peptic ulcer disease, pancreatitis
- *renal* – renal calculi, nephrocalcinosis
- *neurological* – depression, confusion, neurosis, psychosis
- *cardiac* – hypertension, heart block
- *ophthalmic* – corneal calcification (in long-standing hypercalcaemia).

Investigations of hyperparathyroidism

Primary hyperparathyroidism only accounts for about 20% of all symptomatic patients with hypercalcaemia. A careful history and physical examination are required to exclude other causes, such as metastatic bone disease and multiple myeloma. The more important differential diagnoses are shown in Table 21.1.

To differentiate from the other causes of hypercalcaemia requires serum concentrations of:

- *calcium* – at least three repeatedly elevated calcium levels (preferably uncuffed specimens)
- *albumin* – quantified concurrently as albumin is the principal binding protein for calcium in the plasma

Table 21.1 Causes of hypercalcaemia

Cause	Frequency
Cancer — breast cancer — metastatic cancer especially squamous cell carcinoma — PTH-related peptide-secreting tumours (lung, renal carcinomas) — multiple myeloma	45%
Endocrine disorders — hyperparathyroidism — Addison's disease — phaeochromocytoma	45%
Other causes — milk–alkali syndrome — vitamin A and D overdosage — thiazides — TB — sarcoidosis — Paget's disease	10%

- *parathyroid hormone* – measured by radioimmunoassay of the intact molecule (which is more accurate than determination of either the initial or end fragment).

Further tests that are required are:

- *phosphate* – level decreased in hyperparathyroidism
- *creatinine* – raised level usually suggests renal impairment
- *alkaline phosphatase* – a normal level excludes bone disease
- *urinary calcium* – this is raised in hyperparathyroidism. However, if very high, pathology other than hyperparathyroidism is likely.

Radiological findings

Bones. Osteopenia is the main finding with subperiosteal resorption of the bone. This is best seen in hand X-rays, where loss of the terminal phalangeal tufts may occur. The most severe form of bone disease, Von Recklinghausen's disease or osteitis fibrosa cystica, with bone cysts and brown tumours (osteoclastomas) is rare.

Renal. Renal stones and nephrocalcinosis are radiological findings. An intravenous urogram may be indicated if a calculus is not seen on plain films.

Treatment

Severe hypercalcaemia (Ca >3.5 mmol/L) requires prompt medical management, which includes vigorous fluid hydration with i.v. normal saline (4–6 L/day) and correction of associated hypokalaemia and hypomagnesaemia. Bisphosphonates (particularly pamidronate) may be required to inhibit bone resorption and osteoclast activity. Corticosteroids are only of use if the underlying condition responds to corticosteroids (e.g. myeloma, sarcoidosis).

In *symptomatic* primary hyperparathyroidism, surgical treatment is indicated. This results in a decreased incidence of renal stones, subperiostal resorption resolves and bone and joint pain are relieved. However, well-established hypertension and renal impairment often progress despite successful treatment of the hypercalcaemia.

In *asymptomatic* patients, the following are indications for surgery:

- calcium persistently >2.9 mmol/L
- osteopenia or alkaline phosphatase >350 mmol/L
- renal calculi or nephrocalcinosis
- creatinine clearance reduced by 30%
- patients under the age of 50 years.

Preoperative localisation of the glands. Experienced surgeons can usually localise, by dissection, about 95% of pathological parathyroid glands. The following localisation techniques are therefore usually reserved for patients who have had an unsuccessful neck exploration.

Ultrasound. This is quick and inexpensive but unable to localise retrosternal glands and overall has poor resolution.

Computerised tomography (CT) or magnetic resonance imaging (MRI) have higher resolution but still detect fewer than 75% of diseased glands.

Thallium/technetium subtraction scanning. A scintigram of the thyroid is performed using technetium; thallium is then used to image both thyroid and parathyroid tissue. The images are digitally subtracted to demonstrate abnormal parathyroid tissue. This will identify around 75% of abnormal glands, but it has a high false-positive rate.

Selective venous sampling. This is the most reliable technique, with assay of parathyroid hormone in multiple cervical and mediastinal neck veins. A map can be drawn, and the vein draining the highest concentration of hormone can be found. This is a good *lateralising* rather than localising technique and is generally reserved for patients requiring re-operation.

Preoperative preparation of the patient. Patients with renal insufficiency must be adequately hydrated. Those with primary hyperparathyroidism and a raised alkaline phosphatase and most with renal bone disease should receive 1-α-hydroxycholecalciferol 2–3 days before the operation to prevent profound hypocalcaemia postoperatively from 'hungry bones'. Intravenous methylene blue may be used to aid intraoperative localisation as it is selectively taken up by the parathyroid glands.

Operation. The approach is similar to that for a thyroidectomy. The aim is to identify all four glands and any supernumerary glands. This can be done by following the course of the inferior thyroid artery, which usually supplies them, and gently palpating the area. The presence of other normal glands at operation indicates that the tumour is most likely to be adenomatous, and the histological presence of a compressed rim of normal parathyroid tissue within the abnormal gland is suggestive of an adenoma. If the other glands are enlarged they should also be removed.

With hyperplasia of all four glands, subtotal resection is performed in which three and a half glands are removed (leaving half of the most normal sized gland, identified by a surgical clip).

Recurrent hyperparathyroidism is seen in about 1% of patients who have had a single adenoma removed and in 5% of those with multigland disease. It is, however, higher for those with MEN I or familial hyperparathyroidism. An alternative strategy for these patients is to perform a total parathyroidectomy, with autotransplantation of one of the glands into the brachioradialis muscle of the nondominant forearm. This method allows easy access either to remove tissue if hyperparathyroidism persists or to add further tissue which has been cryopreserved at the time of the operation.

If neck exploration fails, patients should be given 6–8 weeks to recover. Extensive radiological investigation should then be performed and either a further neck exploration or a mediastinal exploration can be undertaken. In this setting, intraoperative ultrasound aids the surgeon in locating the diseased glands.

Postoperative care

Once the adenoma(s) or hyperplastic glands have been removed, serum calcium levels fall from 4 to 12 hours postoperatively, reaching a minimum level at 48–72 hours. Serum calcium must be measured 12 hours postoperatively and then daily for at least 3 days. Patients most likely to develop hypocalcaemia are patients with long-standing hyperparathyroidism, very high preoperative serum calcium levels or severe skeletal depletion, where skeletal demineralisation produces the 'hungry bones' syndrome.

Signs of hypocalcaemia include:

- Chvostek's sign – tapping on the facial nerve to produce facial spasm
- Trousseau's sign – inflating a blood pressure cuff to greater than the systolic blood pressure produces carpal spasm after 3 minutes.

In more severe cases, tetany, ventricular irritability and seizures may supervene.

Treatment of hypocalcaemia. With mild symptoms of hypocalcaemia, oral calcium supplements are sufficient. However, with severe hypocalcaemia, the use of intravenous calcium gluconate is indicated. It is also necessary to ensure concurrent hypomagnesaemia is corrected (normal levels of magnesium are required to ensure normal parathyroid hormone release).

HYPERPARATHYROIDISM IN PATIENTS WITH MULTIPLE ENDOCRINE NEOPLASIA (MEN)

Parathyroid hyperplasia occurs also in patients with MEN I, MEN IIa and MEN IIb (Table 21.2). In MEN I, parathyroid disease is difficult to manage and frequently recurs unless all parathyroid tissue is removed. In patients with MEN IIa, parathyroid disease commonly follows the development of medullary thyroid cancer and can usually be managed by subtotal parathyroidectomy. In MEN IIb, the medullary cancer is very aggressive and most patients die before developing either a phaeochromocytoma or hyperparathyroidism.

SECONDARY HYPERPARATHYROIDISM

This is the response of the parathyroid glands to low serum calcium levels; it is usually due to renal failure and, less often, chronic intestinal malabsorption. The kidney fails to excrete phosphate, which in turn causes a low calcium, and the parathyroid glands respond by hyperplastic change, typically in all four glands. The skeletal changes which occur are the same as those in primary hyperparathyroidism but more severe. Medical management is usually successful in controlling secondary hyperparathyroidism (by increasing calcium and reducing phosphate in the dialysate). Surgery is required when this fails and the patient is suffering with bone pain, pruritus or soft tissue calcification leading to ischaemic skin necrosis.

Table 21.2	Features of multiple endocrine neoplasia
Type	Clinical features
MEN I	Pituitary adenoma, pancreatic tumours, parathyroid hyperplasia
MEN IIa	Medullary cancer of the thyroid, parathyroid hyperplasia, phaeochromocytoma
MEN IIb	Medullary cancer of the thyroid (aggressive), parathyroid hyperplasia, phaeochromocytoma Characteristic facies and mucosal neuromas

TERTIARY HYPERPARATHYROIDISM

Long-standing secondary hyperparathyroidism can cause the hyperstimulated parathyroid glands to become autonomous. This is known as tertiary hyperparathyroidism and is most frequently seen in patients on long-term dialysis for chronic renal failure and after renal transplantation.

Tertiary hyperparathyroidism is less responsive to medical intervention, and total parathyroidectomy with autotransplantation (see p. 196) is becoming the treatment of choice.

PARATHYROID CARCINOMA

This is a rare tumour but should be suspected when patients present with a very high serum calcium and a palpable neck mass. At operation, the gland is hard with a whitish or irregular capsule. Ipsilateral thyroidectomy and lymph node dissection are required.

ADRENAL GLANDS

Adrenal pathology is relatively uncommon and usually becomes apparent through either excess or under functioning. The patient will therefore usually present either to a general practitioner or to an endocrinologist before being referred to a surgeon.

ANATOMY AND PHYSIOLOGY

The adrenals are paired structures found superomedially to the kidneys. They are extremely vascular, supplied by multiple, inconsistent adrenal arteries, but importantly they are drained by only one vein. The shorter right adrenal vein drains directly into the inferior vena cava, whilst the left adrenal vein receives the inferior phrenic vein and drains into the left renal vein.

Normal adult adrenal glands weigh 4–5 g each, and although the cortex and medulla are intimately related, they are anatomically and functionally quite separate.

The adrenal cortex, derived from mesoderm of the urogenital ridge, is a deep yellow colour due to its high fat content – the precursor for steroid synthesis. There are three defined zones (from the outside in): the zona glomerulosa, fasciculata and reticularis. The outermost zona glomerulosa is responsible for aldosterone production. The control of this mineralocorticoid is through the renin–angiotensin system. The zona fasciculata (approximately 80% of the total cortex) and reticularis produce the glucocorticoids (most importantly cortisol) and sex hormones (mainly androgens), and are under the control of adrenocorticotrophic hormone (ACTH) secretion by the anterior pituitary gland.

The adrenal medulla is derived from the neural crest and is very closely associated with the sympathetic nervous system. It secretes catecholamines, predominantly adrenaline, and also noradrenaline.

ADRENAL CORTEX

Surgery is indicated in those patients with hyperfunctioning tumours giving rise to Conn's or Cushing's syndromes or more rarely non-functioning malignant tumours.

PRIMARY HYPERALDOSTERONISM

The aetiology of this condition is unknown. It results from the excess secretion of aldosterone by an adenoma of the adrenal cortex (85%) or less commonly due to bilateral hyperplasia of the zona glomerulosa (15%). Bilateral adenomas and aldosterone-secreting cancers are very rare.

Aldosterone causes the retention of sodium in exchange for potassium and hydrogen in the distal nephron; hence raised aldosterone levels cause hypokalaemic alkalosis and hypertension due to intravascular fluid expansion secondary to sodium retention. Patients present with muscle weakness and cramps, polydipsia, polyuria and may have signs of chronic hypertension. Hypertensive patients who merit investigations for primary hyperaldosteronism are those with serum potassium less than 3.5 mmol/L (or less than 3.0 mmol/L and on diuretics) or those unable to remain normokalaemic despite potassium supplements.

It is critical that these patients are differentiated from those patients with renin-induced secondary hyperaldosteronism. This is seen in patients with hypertension secondary to renovascular disease and also severe essential hypertension.

Investigations

The diagnosis is usually made on the basis of:

- hypokalaemia in response to salt loading (1 g sodium chloride with each meal for 3 days)
- increased urinary potassium loss – inappropriately high urinary loss of potassium in the presence of hypokalaemia
- increased plasma aldosterone which is not suppressed by saline infusion
- decreased plasma renin which fails to rise with either salt or water depletion or after standing up from a night's recumbency.

It is important to differentiate between an adenoma and hyperplasia as the cause of hyperaldosteronism, as the management differs.

Imaging of these lesions may be performed using either CT or MRI. If equivocal, then *selective adrenal venous sampling* for aldosterone is required to differentiate between bilateral and unilateral disease. Alternatively, *labelled cholesterol (NP59) scintigraphy* (see p. 200) may be used to differentiate unilateral from bilateral disease.

Treatment

If left untreated, hyperaldosteronism leads to uncontrolled hypertension and hypokalaemia, causing profound weakness. The best available medical treatment is spironolactone, a specific antagonist to aldosterone, although its side-effects include nausea, rashes, gynaecomastia and impotence. Alternatively, the potassium-sparing diuretic amiloride can be used. These drugs may be used until the time of operation, in order to normalise the hypertension and hypokalaemia.

If primary hyperaldosteronism is due to an adenoma, a unilateral adrenalectomy is required. This will cure hypertension in 70% of patients (the remaining 30% of patients usually require less intensive antihypertensive therapy). Those with hyperplasia do not do well with surgery and therefore long-term medical treatment is the management of choice.

Postoperative management

Should the remaining adrenal gland, which has been suppressed preoperatively, not function initially after surgery, then replacement mineralocorticoid treatment with fludrocortisone should be used until it resumes normal function.

HYPERADRENOCORTICISM

This condition, also known as *Cushing's syndrome*, is a result of increased circulating levels of glucocorticoid. The most common cause now is iatrogenic (therapeutic synthetic steroid administration). Excluding this, Cushing's syndrome is most often due (70% of cases) to an ACTH-secreting microadenoma of the anterior pituitary gland, also known as *Cushing's disease*. Ectopic ACTH secretion, either from a benign source (e.g. bronchial carcinoid) or more commonly of malignant origin (in particular, small cell lung carcinoma or pancreatic cancer), comprises around 15% of cases. Primary adrenal causes (adenoma, adrenal cancer and adrenal hyperplasia) are rare and account for the rest.

Clinical features

These include:

- progressive truncal obesity
- acne, facial hirsutism, plethora
- thin skin with capillary fragility
- characteristic abdominal striae
- muscular weakness

- osteoporosis
- polydipsia and polyuria
- hypertension
- susceptibility to infections
- depression and/or psychosis.

The nature of Cushing's syndrome means that patients will present with non-specific symptoms in the early stages of the disease. It is important to recognise and diagnose the syndrome, since without diagnosis and treatment, 50% of patients die within 5 years.

Investigations

The aims of the investigations are firstly to confirm the diagnosis of Cushing's syndrome and then to identify its cause. A simple algorithm is shown in Figure 21.1.

24 hour urinary free cortisol measurement. This is a useful test for the confirmation of the diagnosis of Cushing's syndrome (95% accurate when elevated). False positive tests may occur in pregnancy, obesity and

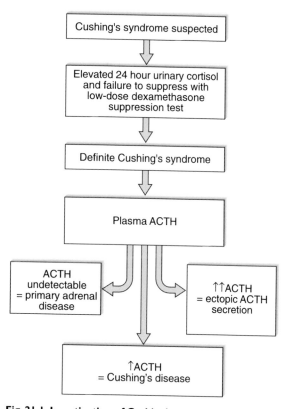

Fig. 21.1 Investigation of Cushing's syndrome.

oral contraceptive use. If the result is markedly elevated above normal, this should raise the possibility of either ectopic ACTH or adrenocortical cancer.

Low-dose dexamethasone suppression test. This is the gold standard for making the diagnosis in which administration of 0.5 mg of dexamethasone, four times a day for 2 days, fails to bring about suppression of urinary free cortisol.

Plasma ACTH (determined by radioimmunoassay) is useful in differentiating the cause of Cushing's syndrome. In primary adrenal disease, ACTH levels will be undetectable. In Cushing's disease, ACTH levels will be elevated. With ectopic ACTH production, ACTH levels are characteristically highly elevated.

Imaging

Pituitary CT/MRI. CT will visualise many pituitary tumours but MRI may be more sensitive.

Thoracic CT or MRI scanning. This may be required to detect bronchial carcinoma or carcinoid. However, these lesions may be small and all scanning modalities may be negative despite the presence of disease on biochemical grounds. *CT of the chest and/or abdomen* is required where ectopic ACTH secretion is suspected.

Abdominal CT is able to identify lesions >1 cm in diameter. It cannot, however, differentiate between adenoma and carcinoma (although most carcinomas are greater than 5 cm at presentation). CT may be able to demonstrate local invasion, periaortic lymph node enlargement or distant metastases, although MRI is now regarded as a superior means of demonstrating the interface between the tumour and associated soft tissues and its vascularity.

Labelled cholesterol (NP59) scintigraphy. NP59 is an isotope whose uptake reflects the level of corticosteroid production. There are characteristic imaging patterns with uptake of NP59 giving both anatomical and functional information. Bilateral increased uptake is seen in ACTH-driven Cushing's syndrome, either pituitary or ectopic in origin. In contrast, unilateral uptake is seen with adrenal adenomas where the opposite adrenal is suppressed. In addition, non-visualisation may be seen when an adrenocortical carcinoma fails to concentrate enough isotope to be imaged but the contralateral adrenal remains suppressed.

Treatment

Treatment varies with the cause of the hypercortisolism and severity of the disease. It is important to control the excess cortisol secretion preoperatively as the unprepared patient fares badly. Metyrapone, which inhibits the final step in the production of cortisol, is administered to render plasma cortisol to normal levels. Aminoglutethamide may be used as an alternative.

Cushing's disease. Trans-sphenoidal microsurgical adenoma excision is the treatment of choice. Implantation of radioactive yttrium needles may also be used. Radiotherapy produces good results in children (80% cure) but not in adults (20–50%) and is usually reserved for adults unfit for surgery. Should the above fail, then bilateral adrenalectomy offers a chance of cure. However, following bilateral adrenalectomy for pituitary disease, around 20% of patients will develop *Nelson's syndrome* – an enlarging pituitary tumour in response to adrenal resection with associated hyperpigmentation (from melanocyte-stimulating hormone (MSH) hypersecretion in association with ACTH). Visual field loss may ensue from optic nerve or chiasm compression.

Adrenal disease. Unilateral adrenalectomy is indicated when an adrenal adenoma is established as the cause and this usually produces cure. The previously suppressed contralateral adrenal recovers in 1–2 years and steroid replacement therapy must be given during this time. Bilateral adrenalectomy has limited use in primary adrenal disease and is reserved for those with primary adrenocortical hyperplasia.

Adrenocortical carcinoma. Fortunately, this is rare. It is a highly aggressive cancer with a poor prognosis; 50% of these cancers will present with a hypersecretory state and some are large (greater than 7 cm) at initial presentation due to inefficient steroid production. They produce hypercortisolism, excess androgens or oestrogens, or often a mixed picture. The other 50%, classified as non-functioning, will present with abdominal pain and abdominal mass with weight loss. Sadly, 75% of patients will have metastases at the time of diagnosis.

Treatment is by radical resection with removal of tumour and adjacent involved organs if possible. Even where cure is impossible, debulking surgery may be useful as a palliative procedure. This is particularly important when the cancer is functioning. Median survival is 15 months.

Adjuvant chemotherapy with mitotane (a DDT derivative), given in the immediate postoperative period or when surgery is not possible, produces selective necrosis of the zona fasciculata and zona reticularis. This induces tumour regression (and control of hormone secretion) in 20% of cases, but improved survival rates have not been shown and the drug is highly toxic.

Ectopic ACTH secretion. Ideally the ectopic ACTH source should be removed. Only occasionally is bilateral adrenalectomy indicated for slow-growing but unresectable primary tumours. Usually the poor prognosis from the patient's primary malignancy precludes adrenal surgery.

Postoperative care

With both adrenals removed, lifelong steroid replacement therapy is required. In the first few days after surgery, parenteral hydrocortisone is given in high doses. This is subsequently tapered to a maintenance dose of oral hydrocortisone 20–30 mg a day. Initially no mineralocorticoid is needed due to the mineralocorticoid effects of hydrocortisone. Fludrocortisone is commenced once the daily dose of hydrocortisone drops below 50 mg to prevent excess urinary electrolyte losses.

Patients must carry an 'I am a patient on steroid treatment' card or wrist badge stating their normal daily dose. Stress from infection or general anaesthesia can induce an Addisonian crisis and patients must be fully aware of the need to increase their normal dose at such times. Should adrenal insufficiency supervene, intravenous steroids and volume replacement with normal saline are required.

ADRENAL MEDULLA

PHAEOCHROMOCYTOMA

This tumour composed of chromaffin cells of the sympathetic nervous system is rare and is responsible for around 1 in 1000 cases of hypertension. These lesions can arise anywhere along the distribution of the neural crest derived sympathetic/adrenal system – from neck to pelvis. The most common extra-adrenal site is in the retroperitoneum or in the organ of Zuckerkandl in the region of the aortic bifurcation. Roughly 10% of phaeochromocytomas are bilateral, malignant, extra-adrenal, multiple, familial, occur in children or will recur or develop a further tumour after surgical resection. Familial phaeochromocytomas occur with MEN IIa and IIb (Table 21.2), when they tend to be bilateral, and may also occur with neurofibromatosis (von Recklinghausen's syndrome) and von Hippel–Lindau's syndrome (cerebellar, medullary and spinal haemangioblastoma, phaeochromocytoma and retinal angioma).

Clinical features

The symptoms and signs are due to the excess outpouring of catecholamines (noradrenaline and/or adrenaline) and may vary from mild, subclinical to a 'phaeochromocytoma crisis' presenting with stroke, seizures and even death.

The classical triad is headache, sweating and tachycardia in association with episodic hypertension. General symptoms include weight loss, anxiety, headache, tremor and excessive sweating.

Cardiovascular symptoms are common. Hypertension, sustained, episodic or paroxysmal, occurs and systolic blood pressure can exceed 300 mmHg. Postural hypotension and polycythaemia – due to a markedly decreased intravascular volume in a chronically vasoconstricted arterial and venous system – are characteristic. Arrhythmias, most commonly tachycardias, are common, as are angina and congestive heart failure. Cardiomyopathy, even acute myocardial infarction, can also develop.

Polydipsia and polyuria with hyperglycaemia and other features of diabetes due to the anti-insulin effects of catecholamines are also frequently seen.

Often these symptoms may be absent unless the patient is seen during an attack. These attacks may be precipitated by a number of events, e.g. trauma, exercise, emotional upset and even clinical palpation of the abdomen for a suspected phaeochromocytoma!

Phaeochromocytoma presenting in pregnancy deserves special mention. Unrecognised, the mortality for fetus and mother approaches 50%. The hypertension is usually ascribed to pre-eclampsia. The only accurate way to diagnose it is by measuring urinary catecholamines and imaging with ultrasound or MRI. Once recognised, the tumour may be removed either in the second trimester or 6 weeks after a caesarean section delivery.

Investigations

Twenty-four hour urinary excretion of meta-nephrines (MTA) and vanillyl-mandellic acid (VMA). – the major breakdown products of catecholamines – is the most useful screening test for phaeochromocytomas.

Clonidine suppression test. Clonidine suppresses neurogenically mediated catecholamine release (e.g. in anxious individuals) but will have no effect in the phaeochromocytoma patient.

Glucagon stimulation test. Catecholamine levels will rise within minutes of administration of glucagon.

Imaging

CT of abdomen and pelvis. As phaeochromocytomas are usually >2 cm diameter at presentation, the majority of tumours will be clearly seen on CT scanning.

MRI is the investigation of choice in pregnancy, as the fetus is not exposed to harmful radiation. MRI is also better able to demonstrate the interface between tumour and adjacent soft tissue.

Isotope scanning. ^{131}I-m-Iodobenzylguanidine (^{131}I-MIBG), a radioactive isotope and analogue of guanethidine, is taken up and concentrated in phaeochromocytomas. CT and ^{131}I-MIBG scanning together will identify over 95% of all phaeochromocytomas, both adrenal and ectopic.

Catecholamine venous sampling along the inferior vena cava may be used if imaging techniques fail to localise or lateralise the tumour.

Preoperative preparation

Excision of a phaeochromocytoma poses a challenge to both the anaesthetist and the surgeon. Unprepared patients are at extreme risk from catecholamine outpouring from tumour manipulation (levels may increase 600-fold), leading to arrhythmias and/or severe hypertension, and subsequently cardiovascular collapse when the tumour has its venous drainage clamped. The removal of circulating catecholamines causes the sudden expansion of the vascular bed which the contracted intravascular volume is unable to compensate for.

Careful preoperative preparation is required. Alpha-adrenergic blockade, to control blood pressure and restore plasma volume, is achieved with phenoxybenzamine, a long-acting α_1 antagonist. The adequacy of blockade can be assessed by serial haematocrits and normalisation of blood pressure with a small postural drop. This takes at least 1 week. Beta-adrenergic blockade is required for those patients who have arrhythmias or who develop a tachycardia with phenoxybenzamine. It is crucial that beta blockers are commenced only after alpha blockade, as a catecholamine outpouring in the absence of beta-adrenergic-induced vasodilatation would lead to a severe hypertensive crisis.

In those patients whose hypertension persists with alpha blockers, ACE inhibitors or calcium channel blockers may be used. Metyrosine, which inhibits tyrosine hydroxylase and reduces catecholamine synthesis, may also be required in refractory cases. Control of hypertension at least 1 week preoperatively with restoration of normal blood volume has been shown to be of major benefit to the patient and to reduce operative risk.

Treatment

The treatment of phaeochromocytoma is excision of the tumour. This produces a total cure in 75–90% of cases. Despite accurate preoperative localisation, the possibility of undetected extra-adrenal tumours – necessitating careful exploration along the paraspinal axis – and the need to avoid tumour manipulation have usually meant a transabdominal approach. Although extra-adrenal tumours always require an open abdominal approach, a number of surgeons advocate an extraperitoneal approach for adrenal lesions and several reports indicate that laparoscopic resection is appropriate for small adrenal tumours.

Operative strategy. The adrenal vein should be ligated early during the operation, if possible, to prevent a surge of catecholamines at the time of tumour removal. Anaesthetists must be prepared to deal with any arrhythmia and nitroprusside, a direct vasodilator, must be available to counter severe hypertension. Hypotension, once the phaeochromocytoma is removed, should be corrected with fluid replacement. If this is not effective, angiotensin II may be appropriate.

When the phaeochromocytoma is malignant (usually greater than 6 cm in size) radical resection with removal of adjacent involved organs is indicated. When curative resection is not possible, debulking may be performed for symptom control (the amount of catecholamine secreted is proportional to the size of the tumour). Radiotherapy and chemotherapy have little effect on this malignant tumour. ^{131}I-MIBG has had some success in treating residual malignant tumour or metastases, but remission is short-lived. The overall 5-year survival from malignant phaeochromocytoma is around 45% at best.

Postoperative care

Once the anti-insulin effects of catecholamines are removed, hypoglycaemia may develop and must be excluded as a cause of postoperative hypotension. Another cause of hypotension is catecholamine cardiomyopathy which can cause congestive cardiac failure. Hypertension may persist as a result of concurrent primary hypertension, but if blood pressure remains high 2 weeks postoperatively, then urinary excretion of catecholamine metabolites should be measured to exclude residual disease.

Patients require follow-up for life, with yearly blood pressure checks and urinary collections, as they are at risk of recurrence or developing a further tumour.

ADRENAL SURGERY

There are a number of approaches to the adrenal gland, and each has its advantages and disadvantages. The selection of approach is based upon the adrenal pathology, the patient's size and health, and the experience of the surgeon.

Anterior approach. This approach is via a midline, extended subcostal or bilateral subcostal incision and provides excellent exposure of both adrenals, the abdominal viscera and retroperitoneum. It is used for bilateral adrenal disease, removal of large or potentially malignant tumours and is frequently used for excision of a phaeochromocytoma (when tumours are particularly large a thoracoabdominal approach may be used). Disadvantages include ileus, atelectasis and poor wound healing in patients with Cushing's syndrome, who are at risk of wound dehiscence.

Posterior approach. This is via an oblique incision which passes through the bed of the 11th and 12th rib. This is the preferred approach when the exact location of the tumour is known and, due to the limited exposure this incision affords, the tumour is less than 5 cm in size.

Lateral approach. This approach through the bed of the 11th rib is occasionally used for Cushing's syndrome in obese patients with unilateral disease.

Laparoscopic technique. This is becoming increasingly popular as the approach of choice for benign tumours.

INCIDENTALOMAS

Ultrasound, CT and MRI are now commonly used in the investigation of abdominal disease. Occasionally an incidental mass will be seen in the adrenal. These incidentalomas are found in 1% of abdominal CT scans and this correlates with autopsy findings. The majority of these tumours will be non-functioning adenomas; however, it is important to determine whether incidentalomas are functioning or malignant – both are indications for their surgical removal.

Twenty-four hour urinary collections for cortisol, MTA and VMA should initially be performed. Investigations for hyperaldosteronism should only be undertaken if hypertension and hypokalaemia coexist.

When results are equivocal, isotope scanning with NP59 and ^{131}I-MIBG will differentiate between subclinically functioning and non-functioning tumours.

Having excluded a functioning tumour, it is necessary to decide whether the incidentaloma is malignant. Those less than 3 cm are highly unlikely to be malignant and can be followed with serial CT scans at 6-monthly intervals. Those greater than 5 cm have a 30% chance of being malignant and should therefore be resected.

CT-guided fine needle aspiration biopsy of the tumour – once phaeochromocytoma has been excluded (to biopsy this could cause a dangerous hypertensive crisis) – may be required for diagnosis. 'Chemical shift' MRI may be employed. In comparing signal intensity of the incidentaloma with that of the spleen, the likelihood of the tumour being an adrenocortical adenoma can be determined through its 'fat' (steroid precursor) content – adenomas are full of 'fat'.

FURTHER READING

Friesen S R, Thompson N W (eds) 1990 Surgical endocrinology: clinical syndromes, 2nd edn. J B Lippincott, Philadelphia

Mann C V, Russell R C G (eds) 1992 Bailey & Love's short practice of surgery, 21st edn. Chapman and Hall, London p 769–787.

22 Breast disease

Mark Kissin

OVERVIEW

As a secondary sexual organ, the female breast undergoes striking changes at the menarche and the menopause. In addition, it is subjected to a regular pattern of growth and involution with every menstrual cycle. These physiological disturbances contribute to a variety of benign breast disorders, which are a frequent source of anxiety and discomfort. Hormonal fluctuations may also play a part in the aetiology of breast cancer, which is the commonest malignancy in women. The growing collaboration between surgeons and oncologists and the advent of breast screening programmes are at last promising to improve the outcome in this lethal disease.

In the last 5 years, breast surgery has become recognised as a subspecialty within the framework of general surgery. The breast surgeon has become the leader of a multidisciplinary team consisting of surgeon, radiologist, cytologist, histologist, nurse counsellor and radiotherapy oncologist. As far as breast cancer is concerned, three major advances have recently occurred. Firstly, national statistics have shown that the mortality rate from breast cancer is starting to decrease. This decrease is probably due to wider employment of effective systemic adjuvant strategies delivered by well-organised breast teams. Secondly, improvements revolve around the national screening project, which has a target to reduce deaths by 25% in the target population by the year 2000. Finally, there have been enormous strides forward in understanding the genetics of breast cancer, which may be important in up to 10% of patients.

SURGICAL ANATOMY OF THE BREAST

THE BREAST

The breast takes origin from the skin and subcutaneous tissue from the second to the sixth ribs. It is not uncommon for the two breasts to be of different sizes, and the overall shape is remarkably variable. Accessory breast tissue may also develop in the axilla, with extra nipples being found anywhere along the milk line. Sometimes the breast fails to develop (amazia) and this in turn is sometimes associated with absence of the pectoralis major muscle (Poland's syndrome). The breast has 10–15 major ducts opening onto the nipple, each duct draining a segmental system of small ducts and lobules. At the smallest level the breast is organised into terminal duct lobular units.

LYMPH DRAINAGE

Most of the lymphatic drainage of the breast permeates through the breast itself to reach axillary lymph nodes. About 20% flows to the internal mammary (thoracic) chain, and this drainage may be important for medially based tumours. A small amount of lymph follows intercostal vessels or penetrates directly through the diaphragm to reach the liver.

Axillary lymph nodes may become enlarged in both benign and malignant conditions of the breast. They also may be palpable due to pathological conditions in the skin of the arm or back, or as a part of generalised disorder of the reticuloendothelial system. The nodes are aggregated into several groups: pectoral, scapular, central, lateral, apical and interpectoral. It is also convenient to divide the axillary nodes into three groups according to their relationship to the pectoralis minor muscle, with level 1 nodes lying lateral, level 2 nodes lying behind and level 3 nodes lying medial to this muscle.

INVESTIGATION OF BREAST DISEASE

Patients are referred to the breast clinic for a variety of reasons, ranging from the sudden discovery of a discrete lump to the need to have a discussion regarding the risk of developing breast cancer in an asymptomatic woman (see Table 22.1). All women attending such a clinic are in a state of anxiety, and considerable care is required to ensure that their visit is organised so that a working diagnosis can be established by the end of the day. This so-called one-stop diagnostic clinic should involve three main steps: an accurate history and clinical examination, breast imaging and needle biopsy. In addition, the patient should have access to a breast counsellor to help her understand the underlying diagnosis more fully.

MAMMOGRAPHY

Mammography should be carried out at any age when the clinical findings give rise to suspicion of breast cancer.

Table 22.1	Frequency of breast-related symptoms	
Symptom complex	Frequency	Underlying causes
Discrete lump	42%	Cancer, cyst, fibroadenoma
Generalised lumpiness	20%	Aberrations of normal development and involution
None	16%	Anxiety, starting HRT, (fear of cancer)
Pain	11%	Hormone imbalance, Tietze's syndrome, (cancer)
Inflammation	4%	Periductal mastitis, abscess, (cancer)
Nipple discharge	2%	Duct ectasia, duct papilloma, (cancer)
Developmental	2%	Accessory tissue or asymmetry
Miscellaneous	2%	Trauma, Mondor's disease, lipoma
Lumpiness in males	1%	Gynaecomastia

HRT, hormone replacement therapy (after menopause).

Under these circumstances, it is useful for examining both the palpable lump and also other areas of the same and the other breast, as there are sometimes impalpable synchronous lesions. Two views of each breast are taken, including a 45° oblique and a craniocaudal position. Sometimes extra views, using compression or paddle magnification, are used to show particular areas of the breast with greater clarity. Mammography is a safe investigation that exposes the breasts to less than 0.2cGy of radiation (at this level it may cause less than five cancers per million examinations per year). In general, the accuracy of mammography increases with the age of the patient, as dense glandular tissue is gradually replaced by radiolucent fat. Characteristic features of malignancy include a spiculate density, fine microcalcifications, especially those with branching and (less commonly) large, well-defined rounded opacities. Some cancers produce microcalcification alone, and these are usually non-invasive. Cancers that produce only architectural distortion are the most difficult to diagnose by mammography. The overall accuracy of mammography is more than 90%.

ULTRASOUND SCAN

Real-time ultrasound imaging of the breast is performed using a 7.5 MHz linear array transducer. It is especially useful for evaluating palpable masses and can easily distinguish a solid from a cystic lesion. A cyst is classically seen as a well-defined, round echo-free lesion with posterior enhancement, whereas a solid lesion has echoes within it and has no such enhancement. A fibroadenoma is usually seen as a well-defined, round abnormality with uniform echoes within it and no posterior effect, whereas a breast cancer usually has an ill-defined edge and is an echo-poor mass with posterior attenuation.

Ultrasound scan is not a good tool for breast screening as it cannot detect microcalcifications.

MAGNETIC RESONANCE IMAGING (MRI)

The role of MRI in breast diagnosis has yet to be established. It is a useful investigation but is still rather expensive. Nonetheless, it has a role to play in the previously irradiated breast and may eventually prove useful in screening familial cases of breast cancer where any form of X-rays could be potentially harmful (e.g. positive ataxia-telangiectasia gene or p53 gene).

FINE NEEDLE ASPIRATION BIOPSY (FNAB)

FNAB is carried out using a 10 or 20 ml syringe and a 21 (green) or 23 (blue) needle inserted directly into the breast abnormality. Local anaesthetic can be used to decrease the discomfort of the procedure without hindering the quality of the result. Cystic lesions are aspirated until dry and the fluid can be discarded unless it is bloodstained or if there is a residual mass. For solid lesions, seven to 10 passes are made through the lump to obtain a field sample for analysis. The material is smeared on to a microscope slide and is wet-fixed in alcohol and air-dried. Needle washings are spun down to give preparations that can be used for biological markers.

Cytodiagnosis is scored according to a five point systems as follows:

- C5 – definite cancer
- C4 – suspicious/probable cancer
- C3 – suspicious/probable benign
- C2 – benign
- C1 – inadequate smear.

C1 is insufficient for accurate diagnosis and should be repeated. This failure should occur in less than 10% of aspirations. The availability of a cytologist within the breast clinic reduces the C1 proportion, as the FNAB can be repeated there and then.

Stereotactic FNAB is used in the diagnosis of impalpable mammographically detected lesions. Scrape cytology is useful in the diagnosis of crusted nipple lesions, and fluid from the nipple discharge also provides material for cytodiagnosis. Cytology has an accuracy of more than 90%. It is a very cheap investigation but one that requires an experienced cytologist. Its main drawback lies in the difficulty of distinguishing between invasive and non-invasive cancer.

NEEDLE CORE BIOPSY

Core biopsy requires a bigger needle, produces enough material to permit histological assessment and can be obtained using a variety of pneumatic devices. The extra material it provides compared with FNAB may allow wider scope for histological subtyping and analysis of tumour grade and receptor status. However, it is more expensive and more uncomfortable, and it takes longer to process the result.

TRIPLE ASSESSMENT

Management of most breast lesions can be based on the results of clinical examination, mammography (and/or ultrasound) and FNAB. This triple assessment achieves a 95–99% sensitivity in the diagnosis of breast lumps. In addition, the texture transmitted through the needle during a biopsy process is a very useful indication as to the true nature of the underlying condition. Care should always be taken when there is a mismatch in the results of these investigations. Although false positive results are extremely uncommon, it would be unwise to proceed to definitive surgery if only one of the tests were positive. Where there is doubt and a preoperative diagnosis cannot be made, excision biopsy is required for palpable lesions or needle localisation biopsy for impalpable lesions. Frozen section analysis is now discouraged, except when it is used to assess preoperative margins of safety.

BENIGN BREAST DISEASE

In the past the subject of benign breast disease has been bedevilled by problems in nomenclature and in relating symptoms to precise pathological entities. This process has now been rationalised so that symptoms and age are correlated with pathology. Most benign disorders arise on the basis of dynamic change occurring in the breast throughout life. Seven ages of the breast are recognised according to the underlying physiological climate:

- neonatal
- prepuberty
- youth
- early adult life
- reproductive phase
- late premenopause
- menopause.

Most benign breast conditions can be regarded as part of a spectrum that extends from a normal state to overt disease. In between these extremes exist conditions so common in frequency and modest in severity that the term 'aberration' may seem more appropriate. This situation has led to the concept of *aberrations of normal development and involution* (ANDI), which is summarised in Table 22.2.

The development of dedicated breast teams together with triple assessment means that benign lumps in the breast should not be routinely removed. Providing that all investigations are satisfactory, the only overriding

Table 22.2 Aberrations of normal development and involution

Stage	Normal process	Aberration	Presentation	Disease state
Early reproductive period (15–25 yr)	Lobule formation	Fibroadenoma	Discrete lump	Giant fibroadenoma Multiple fibroadenomas
	Stroma formation	Hypertrophy	Large breasts	
Mature reproductive period (25–40 yr)	Cyclical change	Exaggerated cyclical change	Cyclical mastalgia and nodularity	
Involution (35–55 yr)	Lobular involution	Cysts Sclerosing lesions	Discrete lump X-ray abnormality	
	Ductal involution	Periductal inflammation	Nipple discharge Abscess	Periductal mastitis Abscess
		Duct dilatation Periductal fibrosis	Nipple discharge Nipple retraction	Duct ectasia
	Increased epithelial turnover	Mild epithelial hyperplasia	Found on histology report	Hyperplasia with atypia

indication for surgical intervention in benign disease is patient-driven. This plan contrasts with the previous dogma of removing every lump in every breast. This previous zeal is exemplified by the finding that 12% of women attending for breast screening have had a previous benign biopsy.

PRE-PUBERTAL DISORDERS

Physiological enlargement of the neonatal breast may occur in response to transplacental passage of maternal sex hormones before birth and secretion of hormones into milk after birth. It will usually settle without intervention. Rarely, a breast abscess may develop in this age group and require antibiotics. Before puberty, some girls develop a smooth, mobile, painless lump deep to the undeveloped nipple–areola complex. This process may be unilateral and represents the development of the breast bud. Strong reassurance is all that is required. Sometimes cystic change may develop, even at as young an age as 4 years. These cysts can usually be seen as a blue swelling close to the skin.

BENIGN NEOPLASMS (YOUTH)

Fibroadenomas are hard, mobile, smooth, solid lumps that usually present between the ages of 15 and 30 years. They are quite innocent and can be safely left in situ, providing that triple assessment confirms the diagnosis. No woman with a breast lump should be dismissed after only one outpatient appointment but should always have two clinical examinations and two separate FNABs of good diagnostic quality. Indications for removing fibroadeno-

mas (which can be done safely as a day case procedure with or without general anaesthetic) include patient preference, overall size more than 3 cm, continued growth or a lump presenting for the first time over the age of 40 years. The natural history of fibroadenomas is intriguing, as many will spontaneously disappear or calcify. Sometimes they can be multiple and can occasionally grow to enormous size, particularly around puberty.

Cystosarcoma phyllodes is an entity that is closely related to fibroadenoma. It usually occurs in the slightly older woman and is more cellular and exhibits mitotic activity. Its morphological appearances are leaf-like. All of these tumours have a capacity for local recurrence, and those with a high mitotic rate also have the ability to metastasise. The benign variety should be adequately excised, whereas the malignant ones (20%) may need quadrantectomy or even simple mastectomy for local control.

PAINFUL LUMPINESS (EARLY ADULT LIFE)

Cyclical mastalgia

Most women experience a cyclical change in their breasts according to the phase of the menstrual cycle. In the week before a period there tends to be an increase in the size and weight of the breasts, with painful nodularity most pronounced in the upper outer quadrants. Sometimes this response becomes exaggerated and causes a burning, aching discomfort that interferes with lifestyle (difficulty wearing a seatbelt, problems in cuddling children, alteration in sex life and going around clutching breasts when there is no one looking). The discomfort commonly radiates to the axilla and even down the arm.

Cyclical mastalgia requires investigation and treatment. Many patients' symptoms appear to resolve once they have been reassured that they do not have cancer. For those with persistent symptoms, a variety of therapeutic measures can be instituted according to the level of discomfort which, in turn, can be assessed with the use of a pain chart. For mild to moderate pain, the drug of choice is evening primrose oil, which contains gammalinoleic acid (an unsaturated fatty acid), which stabilises breast epithelium via the prostaglandin E_2 pathway. For breast discomfort resistant to evening primrose, stronger measures are required. Severe pain usually responds to danazol, which acts as an antigonadatropin and decreases LH and FSH secretions. This drug is also useful in treating recurrent breast cysts and duct ectasia. Side-effects include weight gain, menstrual irregularity, migraine, leg cramps and mood disturbance. Other important agents include bromocriptine (antiprolactin), low-dose tamoxifen (10 mg/day), thyroxine (50 ug/day) and Zoladex (an LHRH agonist).

Other conditions

Some breast pain (10%) appears to have no relationship to the menstrual cycle and may be related to sclerosing lesions or even breast cancer. One variety of non-cyclical pain is termed Tietze's disease, which is characterised by exquisite tenderness over the costochondral margin. This condition may be related to repetitive muscular strain during house-cleaning or sport and can be treated by anti-inflammatory agents. Some breast discomfort is referred pain, particularly from cervical spondylosis. Mondor's disease is a rare cause of sudden severe breast pain and is due to thrombophlebitis of a vein crossing the inframammary fold.

DISORDERS OF PREGNANCY AND LACTATION (REPRODUCTIVE PHASE)

Breast pain may be one of the earliest signs of pregnancy. As pregnancy develops, the breast enlarges and becomes engorged, and the nipple–areola complex darkens. Pregnancy usually stimulates the growth of underlying fibroadenomas. Breast masses appearing during pregnancy should be evaluated in the normal way and, if necessary, mammography can be carried out using lead shielding to protect the fetus.

Lactation can be suppressed by bromocriptine and fluid restriction. Bloodstained milk can occur at the onset of breast feeding and requires no investigation. Mastitis during lactation is caused by true bacterial infection and requires antibiotic therapy (flucloxacillin ± metronidazole). The baby can continue to feed quite safely. If a *breast abscess* develops, this should be managed initially by aggressive percutaneous needle aspiration; only if this measure fails to control the situation should formal incision and drainage become necessary.

After cessation of lactation, a milk-retention cyst may develop and require aspiration. Likewise, milk may continue to discharge spontaneously from the nipples for 2–5 years after lengthy lactation (*galactorrhoea*). Galactorrhoea outside this setting may be the first manifestation of a prolactin-secreting pituitary adenoma. It is investigated by measuring serum prolactin levels and imaging the pituitary fossa with MRI. Treatment with bromocriptine usually suffices, and operation is rarely required unless there is compression of the optic chiasma.

CYSTIC DISEASE (LATE PREMENOPAUSE)

From the age of 35–50 years, breast cysts may suddenly enlarge and present as discrete, uncomfortable lumps. They are often multiple and can range in volume from 2 to 40 ml. Some 7% of women in the Western world develop breast cysts. Some reports have linked cyst formation with later cancer formation, but this relationship is tenuous and controversial. Cysts can be divided into types according to the ratio of sodium and potassium within the cyst fluid. Fluid from flattened cysts has a high ratio compared with those from apocrine cysts, which are more likely to be associated with multiple cyst formation and a potential for subsequent cancer. Cysts also contain growth factors and proteins that may be important. Symptomatic cysts should be aspirated. The colour in the fluid ranges from yellow to dark green. Fluid does not need to be sent for cytology unless it is bloodstained or there is a residual lump. Abnormal cyst cytology may indicate an intracystic papilloma or, rarely, a carcinoma.

PERIDUCTAL MASTITIS COMPLEX (EARLY REPRODUCTIVE LIFE, LATE PREMENOPAUSE)

This complex of benign breast conditions can produce a variety of symptoms and clinical entities that are difficult to define. These include duct ectasia, periductal mastitis, mammillary fistula and non-lactational abscess. The predominant feature is dilatation of the main duct system. It is not known whether this results in or is caused by leakage of duct material into breast fat. This leakage can in turn cause chemical irritation, which may then be followed by secondary anaerobic bacterial infection. These conditions must be distinguished from an underlying inflammatory cancer.

Duct ectasia can be treated by metronidazole, danazol or operation (macrodochectomy or excision of major ducts). Like most of these inflammatory conditions, it can pursue a relentless chronic course and is worse in smokers. It is not infrequently bilateral. Symptoms include pain, nipple retraction or discharge. Periductal mastitis is characterised by inflammation at the edge of the areola and pain. It sometimes responds to anti-inflammatory agents as well as antibiotics. It may progress to fistula formation, which is particularly difficult to treat. The whole of the affected duct must be excised to prevent recurrence. Granulomatous mastitis is a rare condition that can be treated by steroids. A small percentage of patients with benign inflammatory conditions of the breast eventually come to mastectomy, as no other treatment seems to control their symptoms.

OTHER LESIONS

Sclerosing adenosis and a radial scar. These two pathological entities can mimic the mammographic features of cancer as they may have microcalcifications and a series of long spiculations. Rarely they are also associated with tubular cancers, which carry a very good prognosis for a malignant condition.

Fat necrosis. This is another condition that may mimic the clinical features of a cancer. Usually there is a history of severe trauma such as a seatbelt injury after a road traffic accident. Provided cytology is satisfactory, these lumps can be left alone.

Intraduct papillomas are characterised by blood-stained nipple discharge limited to a single duct. They are treated by excision of the relevant duct (microdochectomy).

BENIGN BREAST DISEASE IN MALES

Primary gynaecomastia is the commonest disease of the male breast. About 35% of the normal adult population and up to 70% of normal pubertal boys have some degree of breast enlargement. Pubertal gynaecomastia may be due to relatively high serum oestradiol/testosterone ratios, and senile gynaecomastia may be due to reduced testosterone production. Most of these patients do not require active treatment. If pubertal enlargement does not resolve within 2 years and is causing marked social embarrassment, an operation will be required. For minor degrees of enlargement, especially those associated with discomfort, it may be worth trying a 3 month course of either danazol or tamoxifen.

Secondary gynaecomastia may be due to a variety of causes, e.g. reduced production of testosterone such as in Klinefelter's syndrome or secondary hypogonadism; feminisation by testicular or adrenal tumours; and as a side-effect of drug therapy. Patients with prostatic cancer may develop gynaecomastia from oestrogen or anti-androgen treatment. Drugs such as alcohol, cimetidine, digoxin and cannabis cause breast enlargement by affecting the sex steroid receptor, whereas phenothiazines, tricyclic antidepressants, diuretics and antihypertensive agents disturb gonadotropin control. Bodybuilders develop breast discomfort from steroid abuse.

Other causes include refeeding after starvation and trauma from braces or jogging.

BREAST CANCER

INCIDENCE

Breast cancer is the commonest cause of malignancy among women. Each year there are approximately 30 000 new cases and 16 000 deaths from the disease in the UK, and it is estimated that 1 in every 11 women will eventually develop breast cancer during their lifetime. This figure compares with an annual total of all cancer deaths of 75 000 and deaths from diseases in women of 340 000. The UK mortality and incidence rates are amongst the highest in the world but are fortunately now starting to fall. Breast cancer is in general more prevalent in developed countries, although it is uncommon in Japan. It is uncommon under the age of 35 years and rare under the age of 20. Its incidence continues to rise with age.

RISK FACTORS

Apart from age and country of residence (Japanese

women moving to the West acquire the incidence of the country to which they move), the most important factors influencing a woman's likelihood of developing breast cancer are:

- a history of previous breast cancer
- first pregnancy after the age of 30 years
- late menopause and/or early menarche
- previous biopsy showing epithelial hyperplasia or atypia.

Other more modest risks include higher social class, postmenopausal obesity, body shape, smoking and caucasian race. Specific risk factors vary according to the menopausal status of the patient and are amplified in patients with a strong family history of breast cancer. Female breast cancer is 100 times more common than male breast cancer. Trials examining the possibility of preventing breast cancer with tamoxifen are currently in progress.

The place of the oral contraceptive pill (OCP) and hormone replacement therapy (HRT) as risk factors remains controversial. The use of OCP for more than 5 years confers an increased risk for the following 10 years. HRT taken for more than 10 years increases the risk by 1.4 times, but, paradoxically, those cancers developing on HRT seem to have better prognostic features. Breast cancer developing during pregnancy and lactation should be managed in the same way as in any other woman. Where possible the pregnancy should be allowed to continue. There is no reason why young breast cancer sufferers should not go on to have children after successful treatment of their disease.

Approximately 10% of breast cancers have a formal genetic basis. So far two autosomal dominant breast cancer genes have been isolated and cloned. BRCA1 is a complex piece of genetic material on the long arm of chromosome 17. In these families, breast cancer risk is also associated with increased ovarian cancer risk. BRCA2 abnormalities are associated with increased risk of male breast cancer and prostatic cancer and are more frequent in Ashkenazy Jews. The genetic abnormality here is on the long arm of chromosome 23. Other genetic breast cancer syndromes include Lynch type 2 syndrome (associated with colorectal cancer) and Li–Fraumeni syndrome (associated with sarcomas, melanomas and lymphomas).

PATHOLOGY

Histological types

The vast majority of breast cancers take origin from duc-

tal elements. Infiltrating duct cancer is the commonest type (more than 80%); it probably develops in a stepwise fashion from ductal hyperplasia to ductal atypia and on to ductal carcinoma in situ (DCIS). Tumours are graded according to the extent to which they resemble normal breast tissue and this assessment depends on the amount of tubule formation, the number of mitoses and the degree of pleomorphism. Most tumours are located in the upper outer quadrant of the breast. Other pathological varieties are less common and may be associated with either a better than average prognosis (medullary, cribriform, tubular, mucoid, lobular) or a worse than average prognosis (squamous and signet ring).

Since the introduction of breast screening (see below), the incidence of non-invasive cancer has increased sharply from a previous level of 4% to a current level of almost 20%. The aggressiveness of non-invasive cancer is assessed according to cell type and whether there is necrosis. Non-epithelial breast cancer (sarcoma) is rare and may be related to extreme varieties of the phylloides tumour or long-term side-effects of breast radiotherapy. Sometimes other tumours can spread to the breast, as a metastasis. Melanoma is particularly common in this respect.

Patterns of spread

In the 19th century it was assumed that breast cancer spread in an orderly fashion. This 'Halstedian' theory led to the concept of centripetal spread to the axillary lymph nodes and thence to the bloodstream; surgical management was designed to eradicate the disease by taking more and more tissue. In the 1960s, the early results of adjuvant chemotherapy dictated a fundamental change in the theories behind breast cancer spread. It then became widely assumed that breast cancer was a systemic disease from very early on in its genesis and that micrometastases within the bloodstream were responsible for later death in patients who had what seemed to be a total local cure. Recent evidence from the breast screening programmes now suggests that both theories may be true. It may now be possible to cure patients with very early disease by local means alone, whereas those patients with larger tumours may be best served by having a period of medical treatment before operation (neo-adjuvant therapy).

BREAST SCREENING

The notion that breast cancer found early in its genesis is

a more curable disease than if left until later has led to the concept of breast cancer screening. This concept was first investigated in New York more than 20 years ago. Results of this and other randomised studies suggested that the mortality rate of the cancer may be reduced by at least 25% as a result of early detection. The national project in the UK was set up in 1988 and is the most ambitious of any countrywide programme. In 1996, 6600 cancers were detected by the national programme.

Women aged between 50 and 64 years are invited to attend for two-view mammography every 3 years. When abnormalities are noted, women are recalled to regional assessment centres where further investigations are carried out, including compression and magnification views, ultrasound and needle aspirations and core biopsies. Those found to have cancer or features suggestive of cancer are referred to a surgical team. For each discipline involved with breast treatment, strict quality assurance targets have been set and are subject to review and inspection by quality assurance teams. Approximately six cancers are detected for every 1000 attending for screening, so that the vast majority of women can be reassured that there is nothing wrong. Screen-detected disease tends to be smaller and is more likely to be grade 1 and node-negative than disease in patients presenting with symptoms. This fact should lead to increased cure rates. Breast screening programmes pay close attention to the number of cancers developing between screens (interval cancers). Currently, the interval cancer rate is higher than anticipated, and this may mean that the screening frequency should be reduced to every 2 years rather than every 3 years.

Within the breast screening community, there is tremendous enthusiasm that a reduction in mortality rate of at least 25% will be achieved by the year 2000. Some evidence suggests that screening women over the age of 64 years is of value, particularly as the natural frequency at this age is double that of the younger age group. There is also interest in screening women between the ages of 40 and 50 years, although each cancer costs more to detect, as the breasts are denser and therefore mammographically less easy to define. The introduction of breast screening has led to a vast improvement in services for breast cancer sufferers throughout the country and to the development of breast specialist teams, which are the mainstay of the breast service.

CLINICAL FEATURES

Most symptomatic cancers present with a lump. Most malignant lumps are firm to hard in consistency, with an irregular and indistinct edge. These are likely to be the slow-growing grade 1 lesions (see below). Some cancers are more mobile, softer and well circumscribed, and these may be features of rapid growth or grade 3 lesions. Less frequent clinical features include a bloodstained nipple discharge, nipple retraction, breast distortion and breast pain. In some instances, the cancer simulates an acute breast infection. When a patient presents with a hot, oedematous and red breast that does not settle on antibiotics, the diagnosis of inflammatory cancer should always be entertained. This has a particularly poor prognosis, as it is associated with widespread permeation of the subdermal lymphatics. In some patients the only outward manifestation of a cancer is the presence of an eczematous-like scabbing of the nipple (Paget's disease of the nipple). This condition is usually associated with an underlying invasive or non-invasive true breast cancer. Some breast cancers are relatively asymptomatic and the patient presents with distant metastases, especially in bones. In other patients there are signs of metastases without an obvious breast primary, which can then only be detected by mammography.

STAGING

Several staging systems have been used in the past to help classify patients into broad types which can then be compared from different parts of the world. Accurate staging is also important in the design and running of clinical trials. Traditional staging methods for breast cancer include the Manchester or Columbia systems and the TNM system, but these systems are now to some extent redundant (see below).

Once a cancer has been diagnosed, simple cost-effective investigations are necessary to determine whether distant metastases are already in evidence. These include a full blood count, liver function tests and chest X-ray. The use of liver and bone scans should be restricted to patients who have high risk disease, i.e. those with positive lymph nodes. They should also be used to follow up patients with symptoms referrable to a particular area. Several serum markers have shown promise as being useful in monitoring breast cancer progress; the best of these is CA 15.3.

PROGNOSTIC FEATURES

Precise knowledge of a variety of prognostic or biological variables is extremely helpful in planning an individual's treatment and has now largely superseded more traditional staging. The most important predictor of long-term survival is the pathological state of the axillary lymph nodes. This is a time-dependent factor, as involvement of the axilla indicates probable shedding of a substantial tumour burden into the bloodstream. Other prognostic factors of similar importance include tumour grade and size. Grade assesses the tumour-dependent biological features of a given cancer. Tumour grade (G, scored as 1, 2 or 3) and lymph node status (N, scored as 1, 2 or 3) have been combined with tumour size (S, size in centimetres, $\times 0.2$) to give a mathematical assessment of prognosis designated as the Nottingham Prognostic Index (PI). $PI = G + N + 0.2S$. A low score (< 2.6) identifies a group of women with breast cancer whose long-term survival closely resembles age-matched patients without cancer. By contrast, a high score of more than 5.6 denotes a group who will do very badly indeed (Fig. 22.1).

More than 60% of new breast cancer patients do not have lymph node deposits, yet a third of these will still do badly. There is therefore a further need to identify prognostic features within the node-negative group. A wide variety of markers has been examined. These include steroid hormone assays (oestrogen and progesterone receptors), markers of proliferation (Ki67) and markers of cell death (apoptosis). Other factors showing promise as prognostic markers include DNA flow cytometry, pS2 expression, epidermal growth factor, alpha- and beta-transforming growth factors (TGF) and insulin-like growth factors. Hardly a month goes by without another new prognostic factor being advocated. Some of these tests, such as oestrogen receptors, were particularly difficult to perform by radioimmunoassay but are now much simpler to carry out using immunohistostaining. Nonetheless, steroid hormone receptor status is not as powerful in prognostic models as lymph node status or histological grade.

OPERATIVE TREATMENT OF BREAST CANCER

Operative treatment is still the preferred modality for all early breast cancers. Cancers unsuitable for operation include those with involvement of skin or pectoral muscle or those with distant metastases and inflammatory cancers. Once the diagnosis of cancer has been established, the patient should be interviewed with her spouse or partner in the presence of the surgeon and a breast care

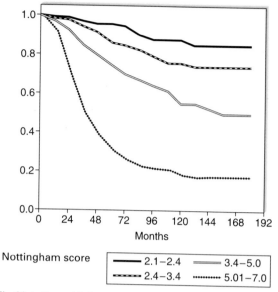
Cumulative proportion of patients surviving

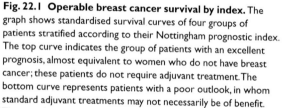
Nottingham score: 2.1–2.4, 2.4–3.4, 3.4–5.0, 5.01–7.0

Fig. 22.1 Operable breast cancer survival by index. The graph shows standardised survival curves of four groups of patients stratified according to their Nottingham prognostic index. The top curve indicates the group of patients with an excellent prognosis, almost equivalent to women who do not have breast cancer; these patients do not require adjuvant treatment. The bottom curve represents patients with a poor outlook, in whom standard adjuvant treatments may not necessarily be of benefit. Those with most to gain from adjuvant therapy are the intermediate groups. The prognostic index score is calculated by knowledge of node status, grade and size (see text).

nurse. Where possible, the patient should be given choices regarding her treatment and should be encouraged to participate in randomised controlled trials.

MASTECTOMY

Mastectomy is the definitive procedure for local surgical control. It has stood the test of time over the 20th century and is still carried out in 20–40% of patients in the UK. It involves removal of the whole breast, usually including the nipple, and is combined with axillary lymph node dissection. A radical mastectomy (Halsted) involves excision of the breast and the pectoralis major muscle. This mutilating operation is performed for males with breast cancer or when the tumour has penetrated into the pectoral fascia in a patient already treated by other means. A modified radical mastectomy (Patey) involves removal of the breast and pectoralis minor muscle only.

In a simple mastectomy, muscle is not removed but is reflected to gain access to the axillary lymph nodes. A subcutaneous mastectomy involves a small inframammary incision, but the lack of exposure risks failure to remove all the glandular elements of the breast; the operation is not to be recommended. There is an increasing trend to combine mastectomy with immediate breast reconstruction (see below).

BREAST CONSERVATION

Breast conservation involves removal of the tumour together with 1 cm rim of normal breast tissue. There is no difference in the survival prospects between breast conservation therapy and mastectomy, simply a difference in local control. Since breast conservation is associated with an increased risk of local relapse, it is usually important to give postoperative radiotherapy, although there may be some types of breast cancer that do not require radiotherapy (small grade 1 or certain node-negative cancers). The development of local recurrence seems to be directly related to the margin of surgical safety and to the presence of excessive amounts of DCIS within the surrounding tissue. Absolute contraindications to breast conservation include the patient's wish to avoid radiotherapy, multifocal invasive breast cancer (this is present in about 20% of cases), the presence of a large tumour in a small breast, the presence of widespread DCIS and patient choice. If the margins of safety are too slim after an attempted breast conservation procedure, either a further excision or conversion to mastectomy should be performed.

Breast surgery is well tolerated at any age, so that age by itself is no bar to surgical intervention. Although some studies have suggested that operations in the elderly (> than 75 years) should be avoided and the patient be given medical treatment alone, the evidence indicates that it is better to combine definitive surgery with medical treatment. There are controversies regarding the timing of operations in pre-menopausal patients. The long-term outcome may be worse if operations are carried out during the first half of the menstrual cycle when there are unopposed circulating oestrogens.

BREAST SURGERY FOR IMPALPABLE CANCERS

With the advent of breast screening, many impalpable cancers are being detected. Treatment for these tumours should be carried out in specialist centres. In order to remove the correct target zone, a needle should be placed into the area of abnormality to facilitate precise surgical removal. Alternatives are ultrasound-guided surgery or injection of carbon particles into the area of abnormality during screening. A variety of needles with differing hooks and wires can be used for the localisation procedure. Once the surgeon has removed the target, it is X-rayed to make sure that the relevant portion of breast tissue has been excised (Fig. 22.2). If a preoperative diagnosis of cancer has been established by stereotactic FNAB or core biopsy, then a definitive cancer operation can be carried out at one sitting. Otherwise, a second therapeutic procedure will be necessary once the diagnosis of an impalpable lesion has been established.

AXILLARY SURGERY

All surgeons agree that lymph nodes need pathological assessment, but there remains controversy as to the best means to achieve this aim. Pathological knowledge of axillary nodes is helpful in determining individual prognosis and planning adjuvant therapy. The average node yield after full axillary clearance is 15–20, and the node harvest can be increased by using fat clearance techniques in the laboratory. Axillary clearance can be achieved with or without removal of the pectoralis minor muscle. Full clearance is associated with an appreciable complication rate (notably swelling of the arm), but this procedure provides quantitative as well as qualitative information. For a lymph node sampling procedure, a minimum of five nodes is required to give a qualitative assessment of the axilla and 10 nodes for a more quantitative viewpoint.

BREAST RECONSTRUCTION

About 25% of women develop psychosocial complications after breast surgery. In those having breast conservation, the problem centres around the fear of local recurrence, whereas after mastectomy the problem is one of body image. Breast reconstruction may be carried out as either an immediate or a delayed procedure, but many experts believe that immediate reconstruction is preferable for the patient and more economical in health care terms. Reconstructive surgery can be carried out by the dedicated breast surgeon or an associated plastic surgeon. The method of reconstruction depends on the shape of the contralateral breast and chest wall, as well as previous use of radiotherapy.

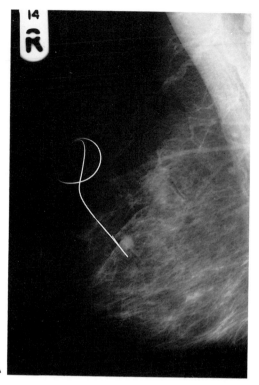
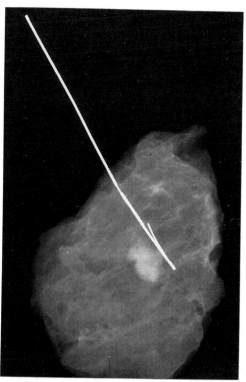

A

B

Fig. 22.2 Needle localisation biopsy. A. Needle inserted into breast close to impalpable density. **B.** Specimen X-ray showing the correct lesion removed with the needle. Histology showed a well differentiated tubular cancer.

Various types of reconstruction are now performed, as described below.

Silicone implant

This is the simplest reconstruction technique and involves the insertion of a silicone implant into a submuscular pocket. This technique is suitable for a small breast or a breast without ptosis, but it is contraindicated by previous radiotherapy. Despite previous concerns, it now appears that the use of silicone is safe. Nonetheless, other more biologically based implants are being developed.

Two-chamber implant

For a larger amount of breast tissue, expansion is required. Once again, a submuscular implant is used, but in this case it has two chambers. One of these can be expanded by the insertion of saline into a subcutaneous port. Inflation of the implant stretches the overlying tissues, so that when the excess fluid is eventually drained off, slight ptosis is produced (Fig. 22.3).

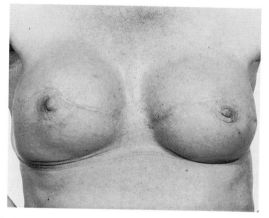

Fig. 22.3 A 55-year-old woman had bilateral breast cancer in 1990 and 1994. Each tumour measured 15 mm, was grade 3, and was associated with negative lymph nodes. Initial surgery on both occasions consisted of axillary dissection and wide local excision followed by chemotherapy and tamoxifen. After this was completed, she elected to have bilateral mastectomy with nipple preservation, with a breast reconstruction utilising immediate insertion of expanding implants in a submuscular pouch.

Myocutaneous flaps

The most complex form of reconstruction utilises myocutaneous flaps. The most reliable flap is obtained by swinging the latissimus dorsi muscle from the back to the chest wall and placing an implant or tissue expander beneath it. This operation produces excellent volume, shape and hang. The most life-like reconstruction is a TRAM (transverse rectus abdominis myocutaneous) flap; the fat from the lower part of the abdomen is rotated on a muscle pedicle to take the place of the previously removed breast. This technique gives the best cosmetic result, but the procedure is very time-consuming and ischaemia may cause the whole flap to be lost.

Other procedures

Other reconstructive procedures include a free tissue transfer of a buttock flap and reconstruction of new nipples from a variety of places. In order to produce a satisfactory cosmetic result, adjustments for symmetry to the contralateral breast are commonly required. Reconstructive techniques are now also being advocated for breast conservation when there is a need to remove a large amount of breast tissue. Latissimus dorsi flaps are becoming popular for filling these holes, although a simple alternative is to reduce the size of the contralateral breast in a mirror-image procedure.

POSTOPERATIVE COMPLICATIONS

Breast cancer surgery is safe, with a mortality rate below 0.5%. Death can occur from thromboembolism and appropriate measures should be taken to prevent this. Much of the postoperative morbidity relates to the axillary dissection rather than the breast surgery itself. The main short-term complications include:

- seroma formation (up to 50%)
- wound infection
- breast cellulitis
- flap ischaemia
- nipple ischaemia
- sensory disturbance in the distribution of T2 and T3 dermatomes
- oedema of the breast or the arm.

Long-term complications include:

- problems with scars
- cosmetic deformity
- breast or arm oedema

- atrophy of the pectoralis major muscle
- shoulder stiffness.

TREATMENT OF NON-INVASIVE BREAST CANCER

For widespread multifocal DCIS, the treatment of choice is mastectomy, which should be completely curative. For localised DCIS, local excision of the abnormality together with 10 mm of safety is all that is required, but patients will have approximately a 0.7% annual risk of further cancer in that breast. The role of radiotherapy and/or tamoxifen in treating non-invasive cancer is uncertain and is being addressed in randomised clinical trials.

Patients identified with a high risk of developing breast cancer because of a family history are now coming forward to have prophylactic mastectomy. Since it is possible to develop breast cancer even when the breast has apparently been removed, it is important that every last vestige of breast tissue is meticulously excised during such procedures.

RADIOTHERAPY

There is no evidence that the use of radiotherapy to the breast itself has any impact on overall survival, but radiotherapy is very effective at improving local control. As the local recurrence rate after mastectomy is <5%, radiotherapy should only be used for patients with aggressive cancers (histological grade 3) or those with tumours close to the underlying muscle. After breast conservation, radiotherapy should always be used unless the tumour is small, grade 1 and node-negative. With breast conservation, the whole breast is irradiated and then a boost is given to the tumour bed, using either external electron beams or implanted iridium wires.

Radiotherapy is given by two tangential fields, avoiding any exposure to the axilla as this will lead to an unacceptably high rate of lymphoedema. For medial tumours, an extra field should be added to cover the internal mammary chain of nodes. When the axilla is strongly positive, it may be important to irradiate the supraclavicular lymph nodes. Radiotherapy is given over a period of 5–6 weeks to a total dose of 15 cGy in 15–25 fractions. Short-term complications from radiotherapy include breast erythaema and ulceration; long-term problems include breast fibrosis, shoulder stiffness, arm or breast oedema, pulmonary fibrosis and, most important, brachial plexus neuropathy and radiation-induced angiosarcoma.

Radiotherapy is the treatment of choice to palliate symptoms of painful bone metastases and is invaluable in the management of spinal cord compression and cerebral metastases.

SYSTEMIC THERAPY

One 100 years ago, it was discovered that oophorectomy had a beneficial effect on breast cancer. This discovery led to the concept of hormonal therapy. Over the last 30 years, chemotherapy has also been shown to be highly effective in prolonging survival.

ADJUVANT THERAPY

With the realisation that many breast cancer sufferers have micrometastases at the time of presentation, systemic adjuvant therapy has been developed to treat any cancer cells that have escaped from the primary zone after surgical removal of the breast cancer and lymph nodes. The efficacy of adjuvant therapy has been tested in randomised control trials with more than 80 000 patients participating worldwide. The overall conclusions show that both chemotherapy and hormone therapy reduce the annual risk of death by 25%. This figure translates into an overall survival advantage of 8–10%. Use of adjuvant therapy should be stratified according to the prognostic index, as follows:

- Patients with an excellent prognosis should be left without treatment, as their natural survival prospects cannot be enhanced further.
- Although patients with a very poor prognosis have most to gain by adjuvant therapy, there are moral and ethical questions regarding the use of toxic treatment during what may be the last 2 years of life.

ENDOCRINE THERAPY OPTIONS

Tamoxifen binds selectively to oestrogen receptors on breast cancer cells but may exert its overall action by inhibiting growth messages between breast cancer cells. Although it is a well-tolerated drug in general, 5–10% of women experience troublesome side-effects, including nausea, hot flushes, weight gain, vaginal dryness and eye problems. There is a threefold increased incidence of endometrial cancer with the drug.

Response to tamoxifen may be predicted by knowledge of the oestrogen receptor status and expression of other markers such as PS2. Tamoxifen appears to decrease the incidence of contralateral breast cancer, and some of its beneficial side-effects include reduction in myocardial infarction and osteoporosis. The optimum duration of tamoxifen therapy is not yet established but is probably around 5 years; thereafter, the benefits may be overtaken by the potential complications. Tamoxifen is the drug of choice for the postmenopausal patient but probably has just as good effect in the younger patient as well (especially if the tumour is oestrogen receptor-positive).

Ovarian ablation is a more established treatment for the pre-menopausal patient. It can be carried out by irradiation, oophorectomy (preferably performed laparoscopically) or by using an LHRH agonist such as Zoladex. The advantage of a medical oophorectomy is that it is reversible and may therefore be of value in patients wishing to have children at a later date. Other useful hormonal agents, once tamoxifen or oophorectomy has failed, include aromotase inhibitors (Arimidex), progestogens (Megace), androgens, or even oestrogens themselves.

CHEMOTHERAPY OPTIONS

A variety of different chemotherapy regimes have been devised to improve breast cancer survival prospects. Since they are all associated with some troublesome side-effects, it is important to balance potential gain against impairment of quality of life. Drugs given in combination appear to produce better and longer-lasting responses than those given in isolation. The standard regime involves 6 months' therapy with CMF (cyclophosphamide, methotrexate and 5-fluorouracil), but combinations involving an anthrocycline drug have recently been advocated. Such regimes include FEC (5-fluorouracil, epirubicin and cyclophosphamide) and MMM (mitoxantrone, mitomycin-C and methotrexate). The optimum method of administration of chemotherapy has yet to be determined. There is current interest in the use of continuous intravenous chemotherapy infusions, particularly with the regime ECF (epirubicin, cisplatin and 5-fluorouracil) given via an implanted Hickman line.

For patients with very adverse prognostic features (>10 positive nodes), high-dose chemotherapy has been advocated. This treatment is extremely expensive and should only be used in the context of a clinical trial. The technique involves either marrow transplantation or autologous marrow rescue.

Table 22.3 Breast cancer management: local options

	Mastectomy	Conservative breast excision
Indications	Multifocal disease Larger tumours Extensive DCIS Smaller breasts Patient choice For salvage	Localised disease Larger breasts Impalpable disease Smaller tumours Patient choice
Radiotherapy	Grade 3 Breach of pectoral fascia	Grade 2 or 3 Lymph node positive

Table 22.4 Breast cancer management: systemic options

	Lymph node negative	Lymph node positive
Non-invasive disease	DCIS UK trial*	—
Grade 1[†]	?None required	Tamoxifen if >50 yr Chemotherapy if <50 yr
Grade 2[†]	Tamoxifen	Tamoxifen and/or chemotherapy if >50 yr Chemotherapy and/or oophorectomy if <50 yr
Grade 3[†]	Chemotherapy	Chemotherapy + tamoxifen if >50 yr Oophorectomy + chemotherapy if <50 yr (? + tamoxifen as well)

* For localised ductal carcinoma-in-situ (DCIS): no further treatment vs. tamoxifen vs. radiotherapy (DXR) vs. tamoxifen + DXR.

† Grading is according to a modification on the Bloom and Richardson grading scale where three parameters are scored on the basis of 1–3, and then the total score is added to give grade 1 (well differentiated), grade 2 (moderately differentiated) and grade 3 (poorly differentiated). The three parameters that are assessed are tubule formation, cellular pleomorphism and number of mitoses.

Chemotherapy is the treatment of choice for patients with visceral metastases, especially to the liver. It is also widely used in the management of inflammatory cancers, oestrogen receptor-negative and epidermal growth factor-positive cancers.

NEO-ADJUVANT THERAPY

The use of chemotherapy or hormone therapy before operation is now under investigation. As yet, there are no long-term data to show whether this treatment improves survival. Each technique can reduce the size of the cancer within the breast and thus diminish the mastectomy rate. At present, the frequency of local recurrence is uncertain, and likewise the effect of neo-adjuvant therapy on the natural history of the disease.

SUMMARY

The treatment of breast cancer remains controversial. Students may be confused by the differing opinions expressed by clinicians dealing with the disease. The summary of current thinking is shown in Tables 22.3 and 22.4. Despite the prevailing uncertainties, there is tremendous optimism within the breast cancer community that the multidisciplinary team approach will improve survival considerably.

FURTHER READING

Early Breast Cancer Trial, Collaborative Group 1995 The effect of radiotherapy and surgery in early breast cancer: an overview of the randomised trials. New England Journal of Medicine 333: 1444–1455

Fisher B et al 1995 Re-analysis of results up to twelve years of follow-up in a randomised clinical trial following total mastectomy with lumpectomy with or without irradiation in the treatment of breast cancer. New England Journal of Medicine 333: 1456–1461

Kertilowski K et al 1995 Efficacy of screening mammography, a metanalysis. Journal of the American Medical Association 273: 149–154

National Coordination Group for Surgeons Working in Breast Cancer Screening 1996 Quality assurance guidelines for surgeons in breast cancer screening. NHSBSP publication number 20, Sheffield

1995 Guidelines for surgeons in the management of symptomatic breast cancer in the United Kingdom. European Journal of Surgical Oncology 21 (suppl A): 1–13

Cardiothoracic surgery

Cardiothoracic conditions

Peter Smith

23

OVERVIEW

Cardiothoracic surgeons deal with conditions of the chest wall, pleural cavity and mediastinum, but especially with diseases of the heart and lung. This chapter concentrates upon the major aspects of their clinical practice: carcinoma of the bronchus, valvular disease of the heart (both congenital and acquired) and ischaemic heart disease. Modern surgical techniques are briefly discussed, including video-assisted thoracoscopy, coronary artery bypass graft and cardiopulmonary transplantation.

In the past 25 years the incidence of many intrathoracic lesions has changed. Infective lesions – pulmonary tuberculosis, lung abscess and bronchiectasis – which were previously common surgical conditions are now rarely seen in the West. Instead, thoracic surgery is increasingly concerned with the heart and great vessels and carcinoma of the lung.

The commoner surgical intrathoracic conditions will be dealt with in this chapter under the following sections:

- chest wall
- pleural cavity
- lung
- mediastinum
- heart.

Chest injuries, pulmonary embolism, oesophageal surgery and diaphragm are dealt with in separate chapters.

CHEST WALL

CLASSIFICATION

Intrathoracic conditions of the chest wall can be classified as follows:

- congenital pectus excavatum and carinatum
- chest injuries (Ch. 14)
- soft tissue tumours
  - lipomas, neurofibromas
  - fibrosarcomas, liposarcomas
- skeletal tumours
  - chondromas, fibrous dysplasia (bone cyst)
  - osteosarcoma, myeloma
- metastatic chest wall tumours
- infections of the chest wall
- thoracic outlet syndrome.

Soft tissue tumours and skeletal tumours will not be considered further in this chapter.

SURGICAL PATHOLOGY

Pectus excavatum ('funnel chest')

There is a varying degree of depression of the sternum and lower costal cartilages and ribs. It is often asymmetrical. If severe, there is deformity of the heart and often recurrent pneumonia in childhood. Surgical correction of the deformity is possible.

Pectus carinatum ('pigeon breast')

This is a rare deformity with a keel-like protrusion of the

sternum. In some cases it may be associated with Marfan's syndrome, a widespread disorder of elastic tissue which can lead to aortic rupture and lens dislocation.

Metastatic chest wall tumours

The involvement of ribs and sternum by a wide variety of metastatic growths is far more common than primary neoplasms of the bony thoracic cage. Direct extension occurs with breast and lung carcinomas. Lesions are often multiple and other primary sites include kidney, thyroid, prostate, stomach, uterus or colon. However, remember that a single 'hot spot' seen on a scintiscan is far more likely to be benign than malignant.

Infections of the chest wall

Infection of the chest wall is relatively rare, and nowadays infection is mostly associated with recent sternotomy or thoracotomy. Abscesses can occur in the subpectoral and subscapular spaces, and very rarely an empyema thoracis can 'point' through the chest wall ('empyema necessitans'). There are various conditions of costochondritis when the costal cartilages are painful and tender. These may be truly infective or may be associated with a non-suppurative swelling, e.g. Tietze's syndrome.

THORACIC OUTLET SYNDROME

This refers to a group of disorders associated with abnormal compression of the neurovascular structures at the base of the neck. The brachial plexus alone, the subclavian vessels alone, or both, may be affected.

The abnormal compressing structure may include:

- cervical rib
- scalenus anterior (scalenus anticus syndrome)
- anomalous ligament (costoclavicular syndrome)
- positional changes which alter the normal relation of the first rib to the structures that pass over it (hyperabduction syndrome).

The syndrome can also be associated with chest trauma including that involving the cervical spine.

The pathogenesis of arterial symptoms is due to post-stenotic dilatation, thrombus formation, microembolism and eventually arterial occlusion.

Clinical features

History

The primary cause of symptoms in most patients is intermittent compression of the lower trunk (C_8–T_1) of the brachial plexus, resulting in pain, paraesthesias and a feeling of numbness over the ulnar nerve distribution. When arterial involvement occurs, there may be symptoms of episodic digital ischaemia (secondary Raynaud's phenomenon) or upper limb claudication with exercise. In chronic cases, moderate to severe permanent ischaemia may lead to loss of digits from gangrene.

Examination

Peripheral sensory or motor deficits are rare and usually indicate severe compression of long duration. A bruit may be audible over the subclavian artery above the centre of the clavicle with the arm abducted.

Differential diagnosis

The differential diagnosis includes:

- cervical disc prolapse and/or arthritis of the cervical spine
- entrapment neuropathy
- Raynaud's disease
- Buerger's disease (rare in developed countries)
- superior sulcus tumours.

Special tests

Chest X-ray. This may demonstrate a cervical rib or an anomalous first rib. The incidence of cervical rib is 0.5% of the normal population, and in at least 70% of patients cervical ribs are symptomless.

Nerve conduction test. This is carried out to differentiate the condition from entrapment neuropathy.

Arteriography should be performed when vascular complications supervene and arterial surgery is contemplated.

Management

Mild neurological symptoms will usually respond to non-operative management by postural correction and physiotherapy directed at strengthening the shoulder girdle musculature.

If there are vascular complications or severe neurological symptoms and signs, the treatment of cervical rib and the scalenus anterior syndrome is surgical. Arterial reconstruction of the subclavian artery may very occasionally be necessary.

PLEURAL EFFUSION

The pleural cavity is a potential space in which normally no appreciable amount of fluid is found, due to an equilibrium between absorption and transudation.

CLASSIFICATION

Pleural effusion

Pleural effusion falls into two categories:

- Transudative
  — malignancy
  — congestive heart failure
  — cirrhosis
  — nephrotic syndrome
  — hypoalbuminaemia
- Exudative
  — infectious
  — malignancy
  — immunological
  — iatrogenic
  — chylothorax.

Pleural tumours

These are either primary, e.g. mesothelioma, or secondary.

Pneumothorax (see Ch. 14)

There are three types of pneumothorax:

- iatrogenic
- traumatic
- spontaneous.

SURGICAL PATHOLOGY

Malignant pleural effusion

About 50% of all patients with disseminated carcinoma of the breast or carcinoma of the lung develop pleural effusion during the course of their disease. Other primary sites include ovarian carcinoma and gastrointestinal tract tumours. Although in many instances there are associated pulmonary metastases, in some cases the intrathoracic metastatic lesions may be limited to the pleural cavity. Malignant pleural effusions are often bloodstained (serosanguineous), and cytology is positive in at least 70% and pleural biopsy in 80% of malignant effusions.

Chylothorax

Congenital chylothorax due to abnormal development of the lymphatic system is relatively rare. Leakage of lymph from the thoracic duct may result from penetrating or blunt injuries, or may follow complications of various forms of thoracic surgery.

Empyema thoracis

Empyema thoracis is pus in the pleural cavity. A wide variety of organisms can be responsible, including tuberculous (acid-fast) bacilli. Treatment can be medical, by repeated aspiration and instillation of antibiotics, but often surgical tube drainage and/or decortication with thoracotomy are necessary.

Mesothelioma

The localised form is usually benign, composed mainly of spindle cells, and well encapsulated. Diffuse malignant mesothelioma proliferates rapidly and is often associated with bloodstained effusion. There is a recognised association with exposure to asbestos.

CLINICAL FEATURES

Symptoms of pleural disease

Pleuritic pain associated with respiratory excursion is usually felt in the shoulder over the distribution of C3–5 segments but may also be felt peripherally anywhere in the chest wall. It may diminish when an effusion forms.

The extent of shortness of breath (dyspnoea) is dependent upon the size of the effusion, whether it is bilateral and the degree of pulmonary reserve. There may be a productive cough, particularly with complicated empyema.

Haemoptysis may be present with malignant infiltration.

Signs of pleural disease

On inspection, respiratory movements may lag on the affected side.

On palpation, there will be tenderness, local swelling, redness and heat with advanced empyema. Tactile fremitus is diminished with effusion, and with long-standing pleural disease, there may be immobility of the hemithorax. There is dullness to percussion with effusion.

On auscultation, breath sounds may be exaggerated and bronchial or absent with effusion.

Fever is likely, particularly with empyema and also malignancy.

Special tests

Chest X-ray. This will demonstrate the extent of an effusion, and there may be evidence of underlying lung disease.

Bronchoscopy. This may be useful in determining the primary disorder.

Thoracocentesis. This is used to identify the specific type of effusion – it depends on examination of the fluid, which should be sent for bacteriology and cytology.

Pleural biopsy. This should be performed especially if thoracocentesis is unsuccessful. Biopsy may be obtained either by needle or by an open method.

MANAGEMENT

Malignant pleural effusion

Although the prime objective is to obtain lung expansion and obliteration of the pleural space, this is limited by the very poor overall prognosis. The average duration of life in patients with malignant effusions is approximately 6 months. Closed intercostal tube drainage, maintained for several days, may permit re-expansion of the lung and result in obliteration of the pleural space. Instillation of various sclerosing agents causing pleurodesis may help. Repeated needle aspirations are unpleasant and recurrence of effusions is inevitable.

Chylothorax

In most instances, repeated thoracocenteses result in obliteration of the pleural space, as spontaneous closure of the leak occurs. Rarely, surgical division and ligation of the thoracic duct is required.

Mesothelioma

The localised form may be resected and the prognosis is good. Malignant mesothelioma is inevitably fatal, the results of radical surgery (e.g. pleuropneumonectomy) being poor.

In some countries (including the UK), mesothelioma is an industrial-related disease entitling the family of the affected patient to financial compensation. The determination of the exact histology of the malignant pleural infiltrate by the clinician is therefore most important.

Video-assisted thoracoscopy (VATS)

Increasingly, intrathoracic operations are being performed using thoracoscopic telescopes, cameras and television monitors. Usually three ports are used in the hemithorax, one for the telescope with the camera and light source and two for the instruments. The ports are made through 2 cm incisions in the chest wall.

The greatest use of these techniques is for pleurectomy and bullectomy to treat recurrent pneumothorax and also in open lung biopsies. In a limited number of cases, more radical surgery can be carried out in this minimally invasive fashion, e.g. lobectomy, intrathoracic sympathectomy, oesophageal resection or myotomy, spinal surgery or ligation of a patent ductus arteriosus.

Recently, in a few highly selected cases, coronary artery bypass grafting has been carried out using these techniques and without cardiopulmonary bypass.

LUNG DISORDERS

CLASSIFICATION

Disorders of the lung can be classified into:

- congenital bronchogenic cysts
- lung infections
  — lung abscess
  — tuberculosis
  — bronchiectasis
  — mycotic (fungal)
  — parasitic (hydatid)
- pulmonary embolism (Ch. 37)
- lung trauma (Ch. 14)
- hamartoma

- pulmonary metastases
- carcinoma of the lung (bronchus).

Lung cysts and infections will not be considered further.

CARCINOMA OF THE LUNG

This is the most common malignancy to cause death in men. The incidence in females is rising, so that it is the second commonest cancer next to that of the breast.

Aetiological factors

Cigarette smokers are statistically more likely to develop a bronchial carcinoma. Several environmental factors are known to be causally related: asbestos, arsenic, nickel, chromium, uranium, cobalt.

The epidemiology of the disease indicates that genetic factors may be important (the highest incidence of bronchial carcinoma in the world is in Scotland).

Surgical pathology

Squamous cell carcinoma. Approximately 60% of all lung tumours are derived from squamous cells, which have arisen by metaplasia of the normal bronchial mucosa. They may be centrally located near the hilum, or peripheral. The degree of differentiation depends upon the presence of keratinisation, formation of epithelial pearls, cell size and number of mitoses.

Adenocarcinoma. This group represents about 15% of lung carcinomas. Histologically, glandular elements are seen and may be acinar or papillary in type. Loss of differentiation produces pleomorphic or multinucleated cells. They often spread along vascular channels. Adenocarcinoma is more often seen in women and is more often peripheral in location.

Undifferentiated large cell carcinoma. This comprises another 15% of malignant lung tumours, though the incidence varies in reported series. Histologically, there is abundant cell cytoplasm and the cell pattern is highly variable, with anaplastic or squamous cell features. This group of tumours also tends to be peripheral.

Small cell carcinoma (including oat cell carcinoma). These are more often than not central in location and the frequency is about 10%. They are the most malignant of lung tumours, and on histology show small round or oval cells. They are the best-known group of tumours to produce ectopic endocrine secretion of ACTH or ADH. Small cell carcinoma most frequently invades the lymphatics and has the highest incidence of pleural effusion.

Clinical features

History. It is generally found in both men and women over 50 years of age; the incidence of bronchial carcinoma is still rising. Heavy cigarette smoking is likely to be a feature, or occupational exposure to known hazards, such as asbestos and cobalt.

Symptoms. About 10–20% are asymptomatic and are discovered as a chance finding on routine chest X-rays. Otherwise, symptoms are either thoracic or extrathoracic.

Thoracic. Thoracic symptoms include the following:

- cough, haemoptysis, dyspnoea
- pain – chest pain, pleuritic pain with pleural extension, and retrosternal pain with mediastinal involvement
- hoarseness of voice from recurrent laryngeal nerve involvement
- pain and loss of strength in the arm – Pancoast's syndrome, when an apical lung carcinoma involves the brachial plexus with or without involvement of the sympathetic ganglia at the base of the neck (Horner's syndrome: ptosis, miosis, anhidrosis, enophthalmos).

Extrathoracic. These include:

- metastatic symptoms, i.e. bone pains, symptoms of brain metastases, liver and adrenal metastases
- non-metastatic symptoms, i.e. progressive weight loss, anaemia with lethargy, hyperadrenocorticism (ectopic ACTH) and inappropriate antidiuresis (ectopic ADH).

Signs. Signs of carcinoma of the lung are:

- pleural effusion
- supraclavicular and cervical lymphadenopathy
- Pancoast's syndrome, Horner's syndrome
- swelling of the upper body and distended superficial veins from superior vena caval obstruction
- hypertrophic pulmonary osteoarthropathy.

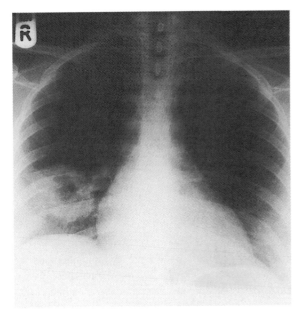

Fig. 23.1 Chest X-ray showing a typical cavitating squamous cell carcinoma in the right lung.

Special tests

Chest X-ray. This remains the most important method of diagnosis for lung carcinoma (Fig. 23.1). Posteroanterior and lateral views are essential to delineate which lobe the tumour occupies. Almost a third of thoracotomies performed are based on radiological findings, and errors are infrequent.

Computerised axial tomography (CT scan). This investigation is a cornerstone in the diagnosis and preoperative assessment of pulmonary malignancy.

Bronchoscopy and biopsy. Biopsy in the first instance is usually by flexible bronchoscope. Surgeons always like to assess a tumour before resection with a rigid bronchoscope.

Mediastinoscopy or anterior mediastinotomy. This allows direct biopsy of paratracheal and carinal lymph nodes. This technique is often used together with bronchoscopy to assess operability.

Lung biopsy using a needle. This is sometimes indicated where there is doubt as to the nature of a peripheral opacity seen on chest X-ray, e.g. carcinoma or non-malignant lesion.

Cytology. Sputum cytology is a useful investigative tool to confirm the presence of carcinoma and sometimes to determine its type.

Differential diagnosis

Carcinoma of the bronchus presenting as a solitary pulmonary nodule ('coin' lesion) needs to be differentiated from other circumscribed peripheral lesions including:

- non-specific granuloma
- hamartoma (mixed tumour of cartilage, muscle and epithelium)
- primary carcinoma
- metastatic carcinoma
- tuberculous granuloma.

It is generally advised that after all diagnostic procedures are done, it is still unwise to adopt a watch-and-wait policy in a peripheral coin lesion. This policy is based on the calculation that the risk of thoracotomy in the average patient is less than 1%, while the risk of malignancy is 5%. The probability of cure will outweigh the risk of thoracotomy.

Principles of treatment

Although the overall results are depressing in lung cancer the only treatment presently available that offers hope of survival is surgical resection.

Radiotherapy is of great value in the treatment of distressing symptoms such as pain from bony secondaries, superior vena caval obstruction, haemoptysis.

Approximately two-thirds of patients are incurable when first seen because of spread manifesting as:

- malignant pleural effusion
- enlarged supraclavicular nodes
- superior vena caval obstruction
- recurrent laryngeal nerve paralysis
- distant metastases.

In otherwise resectable tumours, the commonest contraindication to operation is poor respiratory reserve.

If there is no evidence of incurability, the surgical treatment of lung carcinoma consists of thoracotomy and resection of the involved lung or lobe of lung with regional nodes or contiguous structures. Where possible, lobectomy is the procedure of choice. Pneumonectomy is used when the tumour is sited at a fissure or in such a way as to require wide excision. About 30% of patients who have undergone resection are likely to live 5 years, and 15% are likely to live 10 years.

The best results are achieved with squamous cell carcinoma; next comes undifferentiated large cell carcinoma, then adenocarcinoma, and there are very few survivors after 2 years with small cell carcinoma. The presence of metastases in hilar glands considerably worsens the prognosis.

Multi-agent chemotherapy is useful particularly in small cell carcinoma. Immunotherapy may also be used in the treatment of pulmonary malignancy.

PULMONARY METASTASES

Secondary deposits in the lung are found in about 30% of all patients with malignancy. Both carcinomas and sarcomas metastasise to the lung.

Surgical pathology

Pulmonary metastasis may be solitary (see 'coin lesions') or multiple (particularly from genitourinary tract primaries giving rise to 'cannonball' lesions).

Common primary sites include colon, kidneys, uterus and ovaries, testes, malignant melanoma, pharynx and bone.

Diffuse infiltration of lung lymphatics is also seen in breast and gastric carcinoma.

Management

As long as the primary is controlled and there is no evidence of further metastases, it is reasonable to recommend surgical resection for solitary pulmonary metastasis. About 80% of solitary pulmonary metastases are found to be resectable, producing 5-year survival figures of up to 35%.

MEDIASTINUM

This is the midline space between the pleural cavities. It may be divided anatomically into four sections: superior, anterior, middle and posterior.

Surgery of the mediastinum is concerned mainly with the heart and great vessels, mediastinal mass lesions and (occasionally) trauma. The heart and great vessels are dealt with separately in the next section.

CLASSIFICATION OF MEDIASTINAL MASS LESIONS

These lesions are classified as follows:

* neurogenic tumours
* teratodermoids
* lymphoma
* thymoma
* intrathoracic goitre
* mediastinal cysts
* ganglioneuroma.

SURGICAL PATHOLOGY

Neurogenic tumours

These are the most common tumours of the mediastinum and are found almost exclusively in the posterior mediastinum. About 10% of neurogenic tumours are malignant, malignancy being more frequent in children. The most common variety is the nerve sheath tumour, neurilemmoma (schwannoma) and neurofibroma, usually attached to intercostal nerves or the sympathetic nerves. Neuroblastoma and ganglioneuroblastoma are malignant varieties. Neurogenic tumours may be multiple and may erode into the vertebral foramina with intraspinal extension.

Teratodermoids

These are the most common mass lesions of the anterior mediastinum and tend to be more frequent in the young. They range from solid tumours with a single epithelial lining (dermoids) to both solid and cystic tumours with elements of all three germ layers present (teratomas). Calcifications are often present and may contain hair or teeth. Occasionally these tumours rupture into the lung, pleura or pericardium.

Lymphoma

Mediastinal lymphoma is usually associated with concurrent disease outside the mediastinum. Both Hodgkin's disease and non-Hodgkin's lymphoma (lymphosarcoma, reticulum cell sarcoma) can arise as a primary mediastinal growth.

Thymoma

This is much more common in adults than in children.

About 30% of patients with thymoma have myasthenia gravis, and about 15% of patients with myasthenia develop a thymoma. The relationship is incompletely understood. Thymomas may be difficult to differentiate from lymphoma on histology; furthermore, it is extremely difficult to distinguish benign from malignant thymomas. Gross tumour invasion of adjacent structures defines malignancy in thymoma. About one-third of thymomas are malignant. Metastatic deposits may settle on the pleura.

DIAGNOSIS AND MANAGEMENT

Respiratory symptoms may be the presenting feature, particularly in children, but in adults mediastinal tumours are frequently discovered on incidental chest X-rays. Symptomatic tumours in adults are more likely to be malignant with symptoms related to compression of surrounding structures. Although CT scanning may be useful in evaluating mediastinal lesions, an extensive diagnostic work-up for mediastinal lesions is usually not productive and operation is required to establish the diagnosis. Most mediastinal tumours can and should be removed surgically. Adjuvant radiotherapy or chemotherapy may be indicated for malignant lesions. Thymectomy is occasionally performed for myasthemia gravis, even in the absence of a thymoma.

HEART

Since the introduction of cardiopulmonary bypass in 1953, 'open heart surgery' now offers a prospect of safe and effective treatment for many forms of congenital and acquired heart disease. In the last 20 years, coronary artery surgery for myocardial ischaemia has become well established; more recently, the surgical techniques of cardiac transplantation have been largely standardised.

CLASSIFICATION

Classification is as follows:

- congenital heart disease
  — coarctation of the aorta
  — patent ductus arteriosus
  — Fallot's tetralogy
  — septal defects
- acquired heart disease
  — valvular heart disease
  — ischaemic heart disease

- aneurysm
  — thoracic aortic aneurysm
  — dissecting aneurysm
- pericarditis
  — effusion
  — cardiac tamponade
- atrial myxoma.

SURGICAL PATHOLOGY

Congenital heart disease

Coarctation of the aorta. In most patients the coarctation is located adjacent to the ligamentum arteriosum or ductus arteriosus. It occurs twice as frequently in males as in females. The obstruction to flow is bypassed by collaterals opening up between the subclavian and intercostal arteries.

Patent ductus arteriosus. Failure of normal obliteration, which normally occurs at birth, results in a patent ductus arteriosus. With a patent ductus after birth, blood is shunted from the aorta to the pulmonary artery, with consequent increase in pulmonary resistance and pulmonary hypertension.

Fallot's tetralogy. This is the commonest lesion in the group of disorders in which there is a right-to-left shunt with a combination of an obstructive lesion of the right heart and a septal defect. The four characteristic features are:

- right ventricular outflow obstruction
- ventricular septal defect
- right ventricular hypertrophy
- an aorta which overlies both ventricles.

Septal defects. These consist of atrial septal defects or ventricular septal defects which may be membranous or muscular. Surgery is not necessarily indicated for small septal defects.

Acquired heart disease

Valvular heart disease. Valvular heart disease used to be commonly post-rheumatic in origin, with a certain number of congenitally abnormal valves also being seen. Today, however, more and more cases of degenerative valve disease are being operated on, particularly in the older population. The aortic and mitral valves are most commonly affected, with either stenosis or insufficiency. In many instances, the anatomical abnormality consists of a fixed orifice that may both restrict forward flow and fail to prevent backward flow.

Ischaemic heart disease. Atherosclerosis of the coronary vessels impairs myocardial perfusion with consequent myocardial ischaemia. The effects of myocardial ischaemia include:

- depressed ventricular contractility
- exertional chest pain – angina pectoris
- rest pain
- unstable angina – prolonged chest pain at rest without electrocardiographic or serum enzyme changes of infarction
- myocardial infarction
- deaths from arrhythmias or low cardiac output
- myocardial infarction may lead to post-infarction ventricular septal defect, mitral incompetence or indeed left ventricular aneurysm (Fig. 23.2) or rupture.

Dissecting aneurysm

A split in the wall of the aorta usually arises from an intimal tear either just distal to the aortic valve or adjacent to the origin of the left subclavian artery. Blood dissects along a plane of cleavage in the media.

Rupture may be:

- internal – into the true aortic lumen, thus decompressing itself
- external – into the pericardium with cardiac tamponade, or into the mediastinum, or into the abdominal cavity.

The pathogenesis is cystic medial necrosis. Predisposing factors are Marfan's syndrome (a complex connective tissue disease), atherosclerosis and hypertension.

The dissecting aneurysm can cause myocardial infarction, by occluding the coronary ostia, or heart failure owing to massive aortic valve regurgitation, the aortic valve being 'dissected' from its support.

In addition, branches of the intrathoracic or abdominal aorta may become occluded by the dissection, causing stroke, paraplegia, renal failure or an ischaemic limb, according to the artery involved.

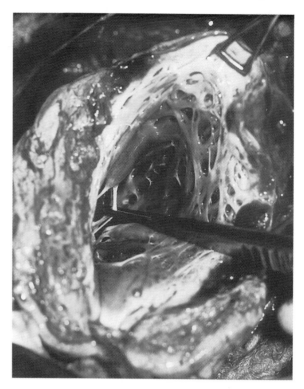

Fig. 23.2 A left ventricular aneurysm opened up at operation. The white fibrous tissue of the aneurysm wall is seen with the darker viable ventricular muscle below in the interior of the heart.

Atrial myxoma

This accounts for almost 80% of primary benign cardiac tumours. Macroscopically it may be either a smooth, firm, encapsulated mass, or a cystic gelatinous mass. Most atrial myxomas are found attached to the left atrial septum. Embolisation, particularly to the brain, may be the presenting feature.

DIAGNOSIS AND MANAGEMENT

Coarctation of the aorta

Infants with coarctation may have life-threatening heart failure. There may be other associated cardiac lesions. Hypertension in a child or young adult should raise the suspicion of coarctation. There may be diminished or delayed femoral pulsations in relation to upper limb pulses. A systolic murmur may be audible in the chest. Chest X-ray shows left ventricular enlargement, and rib notching may be seen, owing to enlarged intercostal collaterals.

Operative repair consists of excision and anastomosis or prosthetic replacement of the diseased aortic segment. The results of coarctation repair are good.

Patent ductus arteriosus

A machinery-like murmur is best heard over the second left interspace. Pre-term infants may present with heart failure. If left untreated, some 5% of full-term infants die from heart failure and pulmonary complications in the first year of life. The remainder are usually asymptomatic. Apart from chest X-ray, which may reveal left ventricular enlargement and increased pulmonary arterial markings, cardiac catheter studies are usually not required unless other congenital lesions are suspected. Surgical obliteration of the ductus by ligation or division is sometimes necessary.

Fallot's tetralogy

A cyanotic or hypoxic appearance is diagnostic of a right-to-left shunt in congenital cardiac disorders. Chest X-ray shows a small heart size with diminished pulmonary markings. Cardiac catheter studies are essential to assess the feasibility of a one-stage total correction under cardiopulmonary bypass or a two-stage procedure with initial palliative shunting, e.g. Blalock–Taussig shunt where the subclavian artery is anastomosed to the pulmonary artery. The overall long-term success rate for surgical correction is reported to be about 90%.

Valvular heart disease

Echocardiography, both transoesophageal and transthoracic, is the cornerstone of the diagnosis and assessment of cardiac valve disease. Cardiac catheter studies with angiography may be supplementally needed. Since the disease is one of mechanical failure of the valve, definitive therapy usually needs to be surgical. However, recently, 'balloon' valvuloplasty has been used to open up stenotic valves, particularly pliable mitral valves. The balloon catheter is inserted transcutaneously.

Conservative valve surgery, i.e. not using a prosthetic valve, is the method of choice for dealing with mitral valve disease, if possible.

Valve replacements may be of two types:

- mechanical prosthetic valves (Fig. 23.3)
- tissue valves (Fig. 23.4).

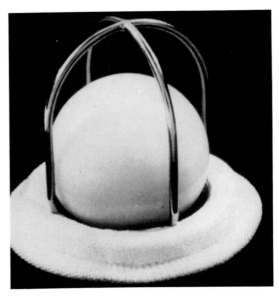

Fig. 23.3 A mechanical artificial heart valve. Starr–Edwards™ Silastic (Dow Corning) ball valve, Mitral model 6120.

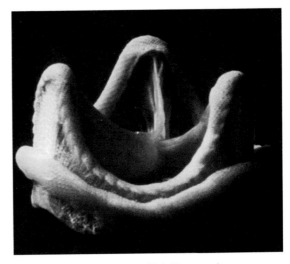

Fig. 23.4 A porcine tissue artificial heart valve. Carpentier-Edwards® Bioprosthesis, aortic model 2625.

The advantage of the first type is that they have excellent durability, although they do require lifetime anticoagulation. Tissue valves, on the other hand, are less thrombogenic, but suffer from the disadvantage that they may require replacement 10–15 years later.

Ischaemic heart disease – angina pectoris

History. The patient will have substantial chest pains

radiating to the arm, neck or jaw, occurring with exertion or exposure to cold; symptoms promptly disappear with rest and relief with nitroglycerin.

When severe, angina pectoris may progress to 'rest pain', indicating the need for urgent assessment and treatment.

Examination. The patient may be a known hypertensive and may have evidence of vascular disease elsewhere (e.g. carotid bruit).

Special tests. A graded exercise electrocardiogram (exercise stress test) may show ischaemic changes (ST segment depression) during or immediately following exercise. ST segment depression on resting ECG during episodes of chest pain indicates more severe coronary insufficiency.

Coronary angiography is carried out in most patients to define the anatomy of the coronary stenoses.

Management. This can be medical, surgical or by transluminal balloon angioplasty.

Medical management is as follows:

- nitroglycerine, beta-adrenergic blockers, calcium antagonists and/or angiotensin-converting enzyme (ACE) inhibitors may all be used
- control of hypertension or hyperlipidaemia if present

- stop smoking
- attain ideal weight.

Surgical. Indications for surgical management are:

- disabling angina pectoris refractory to medical management
- occlusion of the main stem of the left coronary artery
- triple coronary artery disease with depressed left ventricular function.

Ideal conditions for operation are: greater than 70% proximal stenosis of one or more major coronary arteries (greater than 1 mm in diameter), satisfactory distal vessels and acceptable left ventricular function.

Operation is by median sternotomy with cardiopulmonary bypass, using moderate hypothermia. Autogenous saphenous vein grafts are anastomosed between the ascending aorta and the coronary arteries. In addition, the internal mammary (thoracic) artery is used wherever possible to graft the coronary vessels, particularly the left anterior descending vessel (Fig. 23.5). A graft of this type has a greatly increased late patency compared with a saphenous vein graft. Coronary endarterectomy may also be necessary.

The saphenous graft patency rate is about 80% at 1 year. Prospective randomised studies show improved survival after operation in patients with lesions of the left main stem coronary artery and poor left ventricular function.

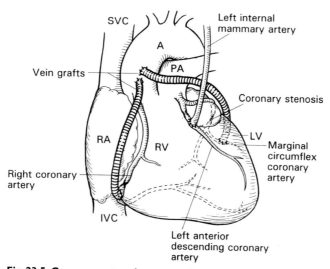

Fig. 23.5 Coronary artery bypasses × 3. There are vein grafts to the right and circumflex coronary arteries and the left internal mammary artery to the left anterior descending coronary artery.

Transluminal balloon angioplasty. This involves non-operative percutaneous passage of a fine balloon catheter into the coronary artery with dilatation of the stenosis. Balloon angioplasty is often combined with the insertion of a prosthetic stent into the coronary artery across the dilated stenosis. Results are encouraging in selected cases of coronary stenosis.

Dissecting aneurysm

History. The patient will have chest pain, often radiating to the back.

Signs. The patient may present with shock due to hypovolaemia associated with blood loss into the hemithorax or with cardiac tamponade due to blood loss into the pericardial cavity. Congestive cardiac failure can result from myocardial ischaemia or torrential aortic regurgitation. A cold, pulseless limb, hemiplegia or paraplegia can also occur.

Special tests. Chest X-ray may show mediastinal widening or haemothorax. CT or MRI, transoesophageal echocardiography or aortography can be used to confirm the diagnosis.

Differential diagnosis. Other causes of chest pain particularly myocardial infarction.

Management. This is by control of hypertension, usually using intravenous hypotensive agents. A central venous line, arterial line and urinary catheter should have been inserted on diagnosis.

Ascending aortic involvement with the dissection is an indication for emergency operation to prevent the high risk of rupture into the pericardium leading to tamponade. Severe aortic regurgitation and coronary occlusion may also be prevented. The ascending aorta is replaced with a tube graft, with repair or replacement of the aortic valve as necessary.

Atrial myxoma

The tumour may act as a ball valve and mimic mitral stenosis or regurgitation. Transoesophageal echocardiography is the investigation of choice. Atrial myxomas should be surgically removed.

Cardiopulmonary transplantation

Transplantation of the heart, lung or heart and lungs is an accepted form of treatment for end-stage cardiac or respiratory failure.

Common indications for heart transplantation are heart failure due to end-stage ischaemic heart disease and cardiomyopathy. It is possible to 'bridge' the patient who has untreatable heart failure to transplantation, using a mechanical left ventricular assistance device (LVAD) or a mechanical heart.

Patients who have received a heart or lung from other persons require long-term immunosuppression with attendant side-effects of the drugs concerned. Long-term follow-up is intense, and often psychological help is needed in the recipients.

The number of patients on the waiting list for heart transplantation is far greater than the availability of donor hearts. The financial cost of a heart transplant programme is considerable.

A heart transplant recipient can expect a 1-year chance of survival of approximately 70%.

FURTHER READING

Carpentier A et al 1980 Reconstructive surgery of mitral valve incompetence. Ten year appraisal. Journal of Thoracic and Cardiovascular Surgery 79: 338–348

Favoloro R G 1962 Saphenous vein graft in the surgical treatment of coronary artery disease: operative technique. Journal of Thoracic and Cardiovascular Surgery 58: 178–185

Kirklin J W, Barratt-Boyes B G 1992 Cardiac surgery, 2nd edn. Churchill Livingstone, Edinburgh

Sabiston D C, Spencer F C 1983 Gibbon's surgery of the chest, 4th edn. WB Saunders, Philadelphia

Shields T W 1994 General thoracic surgery, 4th edn. Lea and Febiger, London

Shields T W 1991 Mediastinal surgery. Lea and Febiger, London

Starr A, Edwards M L, McCord C W, Griswold H E 1963 Aortic replacement: clinical experience with a semi-rigid ball-valve prosthesis. Circulation 27: 779

Surgical gastroenterology

Oesophagus

David Gotley

24

OVERVIEW

The oesophagus is the conduit from mouth to stomach, disorders of which cause narrowing or diminished propulsion presenting as difficulty in swallowing (dysphagia). This chapter covers the benign and malignant causes of dysphagia with emphasis on carcinoma and peptic oesophagitis/stricture, caused by reflux, achalasia and perforation. Disorders of the diaphragm are covered, with a detailed discussion of hiatus hernia.

OESOPHAGUS

The purpose of the oesophagus is to control the passage of solids, liquids and gas between the pharynx and stomach. Disorders which interfere with this function most commonly present with *dysphagia*. Although there are many conditions which present with this symptom, the most sinister is oesophageal carcinoma, a disease which still carries a grave prognosis.

SURGICAL ANATOMY

The oesophagus is a muscular conduit from the pharynx to the stomach. The length of the adult oesophagus is about 25 cm and the distance from the incisor teeth to the gastro-oesophageal junction is around 40 cm. The tubercle of the cricoid cartilage (sixth cervical vertebra) marks the level of the origin of the oesophagus. It extends through the superior and posterior mediastinum and lies in close proximity to the thyroid gland, recurrent laryngeal nerves, carotid sheath and trachea in its cervical por-

tion. In the thorax, the oesophagus passes behind the aortic arch and the left main stem bronchus, enters the abdomen through the right crus of the diaphragm and joins the stomach at an angle. About 2.5 cm of oesophagus lies within the abdomen. The gastro-oesophageal junction lies at the level of the twelfth thoracic vertebra and is covered anteriorly and on its left side with peritoneum. It is related anteriorly to the anterior (left) vagus nerve and the left lobe of the liver, and posteriorly to the posterior (right) vagus nerve and diaphragmatic crura.

Structure

The musculature of the pharynx and upper third of the oesophagus is composed of striated muscle, while the distal two-thirds of the oesophagus is smooth muscle. Whereas the upper oesophageal sphincter (cricopharyngeus) is a distinct anatomical entity, the musculature of the lower oesophageal sphincter is macroscopically indistinct but highly specialised in ultrastructure and in function. It is detected as a high-pressure zone 2–3 cm in length.

The mucosal lining of the oesophagus consists of non-keratinising stratified squamous epithelium with scattered submucosal glands. It gives way to simple columnar epithelium marked by an irregular junction about 1 cm above the anatomical gastro-oesophageal junction. While the oesophagus is remarkably distensible, its thin wall and lack of serosa make it friable during surgical manipulation. Surgery of the oesophagus therefore demands meticulous technique.

Three anatomical areas of narrowing occur in the oesophagus:

- at the level of the cricoid cartilage
- in the midthorax, from compression by the aortic arch and left main stem bronchus
- at the level of the oesophageal hiatus of the diaphragm.

Most foreign bodies and caustic burns occur in proximity to these constrictions.

Anatomical weak points lie above and below the cricopharyngeus muscle posteriorly (where pulsion diverticula may form), and the left lateral wall of the lower oesophagus (where spontaneous rupture may occur).

Blood supply

The *cervical segment* is supplied by branches from the inferior thyroid arteries; the *thoracic segment* is supplied from the bronchial arteries, and has oesophageal branches directly from the aorta; and the *abdominal segment* is supplied from the inferior phrenic arteries and oesophageal branches of the left gastric artery.

Venous drainage

The upper two-thirds drains to the azygos and hemiazygos veins, while the lower one-third drains to the left gastric vein and subsequently to the portal venous system.

There is a large submucosal venous plexus as well as an external oesophageal venous plexus. When there is a rise in portal venous pressure, portal venous blood can flow into the systemic circulation via the azygos system. It is the external oesophageal venous plexus which gives rise to the shunts seen in portal hypertension, whilst the submucosal plexus, through perforating veins, forms oesophageal varices.

Lymphatic drainage

Plexuses in each of the layers of the oesophageal wall run predominantly longitudinally. Lymph from the oesophagus can drain in external collecting trunks as far cephalad as the cervical nodes and to the coeliac nodes below. A large number of nodes are distributed along the length of the oesophagus, and they connect with groups of nodes which drain adjacent intrathoracic organs. This pattern of lymphatic drainage explains the tendency for oesophageal cancer to disseminate widely in the thorax.

PHYSIOLOGY

Normal oesophageal function depends on the orderly integration of the motor activity of the upper and lower oesophageal sphincters and the oesophageal body. The most important role of the upper oesophageal sphincter is the prevention of oesophagopharyngeal regurgitation of gastric contents. Peristaltic contractions serve to propel food from the pharynx to the stomach and to return refluxed gastric contents to the stomach. As a bolus of food enters the oesophagus, a peristaltic wave sweeps distally at a speed of 4–6 cm/s and the lower oesophageal sphincter relaxes.

Primary peristalsis is a wave of contraction initiated by swallowing and which travels the entire length of the oesophagus. *Secondary peristalsis* is a peristaltic wave not initiated by the act of swallowing and which is triggered by food residues, distension (e.g. belching) and gastro-oesophageal reflux.

Simultaneous waves account for up to 5% of oesophageal contractions in normals. Up to one-fifth of peristaltic waves are not conducted over the full length of the oesophagus.

The lower oesophageal sphincter exhibits a resting tone of between 10 and 25 mmHg, which varies in individuals from minute to minute and relaxes in response to swallowing, oesophageal distension, belching and vomiting. The tone is controlled by the vagus nerve and is the most important component of the anti-reflux mechanism.

SYMPTOMS OF OESOPHAGEAL DISEASE

Oesophageal dysphagia

Dysphagia means 'difficulty in swallowing' and can be caused by local disease in the mouth and pharynx as well as in the oesophagus. Only oesophageal dysphagia will be discussed here. Intermittent, transient discomfort or hold-up of food during swallowing without the presence of a stricture is common in patients with gastro-oesophageal reflux disease. True persistent dysphagia, especially if progressive (i.e. to solids and then to liquids), virtually always indicates pathology.

Sudden and persistent complete dysphagia may be the first symptom of a stricture (benign or malignant) as a result of bolus obstruction.

Aetiology. The cause can be luminal, i.e. by foreign bodies lodging in the oesophagus, including food.

Lesions both in and outside the oesophageal wall can

also be responsible. Those in the oesophageal wall include the following:

- stricture
  — reflux oesophagitis
  — corrosives
  — irradiation
  — trauma
- carcinoma
- motility disorders
  — achalasia
  — diffuse oesophageal spasm
  — cricopharyngeal spasm
- benign tumours
- scleroderma
- Paterson–Kelly syndrome (sideropenic dysphagia)
- Schatski ring
- dermatomyositis
- bulbar paralysis
- myasthenia gravis
- globus hystericus
- congenital atresia (tracheo-oesophageal fistula)
- Crohn's disease
- tetanus.

Lesions outside the oesophageal wall include:

- pharyngeal pouch
- para-oesophageal hiatus hernia
- retrosternal thyroid
- mediastinal tumours and lymph nodes
- aortic aneurysm
- congenital vascular anomalies
- tight fundoplication
- postoperative oedema after fundoplication.

Of the causes mentioned above, the commoner ones are:

- *carcinoma of the oesophagus (and cardia)*
- *reflux oesophagitis with stricture*
- *achalasia.*

Oesophageal pain

Chest pain of oesophageal origin is usually retrosternal but may be felt anywhere from the epigastrium to the cervical region and may radiate to the back between the shoulder blades. It can be central and crushing and can mimic cardiac ischaemic pain. Spontaneous oesophageal pain may be due to gastro-oesophageal reflux, spasm, 'irritable' oesophagus or unknown causes.

Heartburn is a sensation of rawness or burning referred to the lower retrosternal or epigastric areas and can be stimulated by acid, alkali, gastric contents, cold water, high osmolality fluids and balloon distension. Individuals vary greatly in their oesophageal sensitivity, making heartburn an unreliable clinical indicator of the severity of oesophageal disease.

Regurgitation

Regurgitation is the transfer of gastric contents to the pharynx or mouth in the absence of vomiting. This symptom can be disabling in some patients with gastro-oesophageal reflux disease, and can result in repeated aspiration with cough, hoarseness, bronchoconstriction, pneumonitis or even pneumonia.

CARCINOMA OF THE OESOPHAGUS

SURGICAL PATHOLOGY

Oesophageal carcinoma occurs particularly in males over 65 years, but there is a higher incidence than in the general population among females with long-standing sideropenic dysphagia and in people suffering from long-standing chronic irritation of the oesophagus such as occurs in reflux oesophagitis, leukoplakia and achalasia.

Barrett's oesophagus, or columnar-lined oesophagus, is an acquired premalignant condition which is seen in as many as 10% of patients with long-standing gastro-oesophageal reflux. There is a prevalence of adenocarcinoma of about 15% in newly diagnosed cases of Barrett's oesophagus. The risk of malignant change in patients with known Barrett's oesophagus is very low, but still much higher than in the general population. Carcinomatous change is associated with an 'intestinal-type' morphology of the mucosa, in which dysplastic epithelium is found.

Squamous carcinoma of the oesophagus is interesting in having strong geographic links, particularly with southern Africa, the Caspian and parts of mainland China. Dietary factors such as nitrosamine (or nitrite) and mould (*Geotrichum candidum* and *Fusarium*) ingestion, chewing of betel nut, deficiency of trace elements (e.g. molybdenum) and iron brewing pots have been implicated in the causation of oesophageal carcinoma. Alcohol ingestion and tobacco smoking are associated with carcinoma of the oesophagus.

Macroscopically, the malignancy presents as an ulcer,

a protuberant lesion or a stricutre; the lower third, the middle third and the upper third of the oesophagus are involved in about 50%, 35% and 15% of cases, respectively.

Microscopically, most are squamous cell carcinomas but with little keratinisation. In situ carcinoma is found distant from the primary cancer in about one-seventh of cases, indicating the 'field change' nature of the disease and the necessity for wide surgical clearance. Adenocarcinoma of the oesophagus arises either from proximal gastric epithelium or from Barrett's oesophagus.

Spread of the carcinoma longitudinally in the submucous plane usually occurs, and direct spread through the wall of the organ can lead to involvement of vital structures such as bronchi, lung and aorta. In most cases the tumour has invaded full thickness of the wall of the oesophagus by the time of presentation. Lymphatic spread to regional lymph nodes is present in about 70% of operative cases. Metastases from upper oesophageal lesions may skip to the supraclavicular lymph nodes, and lower oesophageal lesions may involve subdiaphragmatic and coeliac nodes. Complications arising as a result of oesophageal carcinoma include obstruction and ulceration with bleeding, while spread to vital structures may lead to recurrent laryngeal and phrenic nerve paralyses, tracheo-oesophageal fistula, empyema, lung abscess, pneumonia, pericarditis and superior vena caval obstruction.

CLINICAL FEATURES

More than 90% of patients with carcinoma of the oesophagus present with dysphagia which is usually progressive and will have been present for 3–6 months. Weight loss is also a common complaint and symptoms of anaemia may occur (most often in association with adenocarcinoma at the gastro-oesophageal junction). Chest pain is experienced by some patients. Physical examination may reveal little else but evidence of weight loss. Palpable cervical lymph nodes, hepatomegaly or ascites may be found.

DIAGNOSIS

A *barium swallow* will reveal an irregular luminal filling defect (Fig 24.1A), obstruction to flow or a communication with the bronchial tree in cases of tracheo-oesophageal fistula. *Barium meal* is useful in lower third tumours to assess the extent of spread into the stomach.

Oesophagoscopy (usually with a flexible endoscope) and biopsy are required to confirm the diagnosis. The carcinoma will appear as a friable proliferative lesion with contact bleeding, as an ulcer or rarely as a rigid plaque. Cytology of cells obtained by brushing the lesion is a helpful adjunct, especially in cases of suspected early oesophageal cancer.

PROPHYLAXIS

Alteration of lifestyles and dietary habits of populations at risk is rarely feasible. Awareness of symptoms and screening have a growing impact in China and Japan. Patients with Barrett's oesophagus should undergo periodic screening, since the development of high-grade dysplasia portends carcinoma, and oesophagectomy in these patients is recommended.

TREATMENT

The long-term survival rate with carcinoma of the oesophagus is 5%. Hence, the main aim of treatment is to restore the ability to swallow. This is best achieved by surgical resection and replacement with the stomach or a segment of colon. The oesophagus may be surgically resected by sequential laparotomy and thoracotomy, or by transhiatal (abdominocervical) oesophagectomy in which the oesophagus is dissected via the abdomen and an incision in the neck, avoiding a thoracotomy. Surgical resection of the oesophagus gives the best hope for cure in cases where the tumour appears confined to the oesophagus. For lower third tumours the oesophagus and proximal third of the stomach together with draining lymph nodes are resected. The mortality for oesophagectomy is of the order of 5–10% and the median survival after surgery is about 16 months. Disease-free survival is improved by the addition of adjuvant preoperative chemotherapy (5-fluorouracil/cisplatin) and radiotherapy (36 Gy).

Postcricoid carcinoma in relation to Paterson–Kelly syndrome is more susceptible to cure, but this usually means pharyngolaryngo-oesophagectomy and anastomosis of the mobilised stomach to the mid- or upper pharynx. Permanent tracheostomy is necessary.

When the tumour is not resectable, when the patient is infirm or there are distant metastases (liver or lung), restoration of swallowing may be achieved either by dilatation of the tumour and placement of a plastic tube or expandable metal mesh stent using an endoscope or by

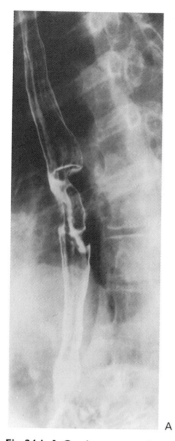
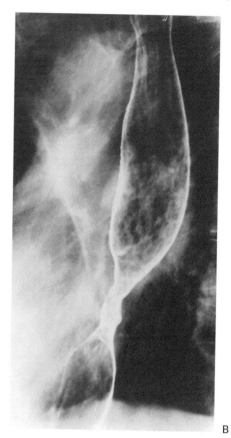

A

B

Fig. 24.1 A. Carcinoma oesophagus. Barium swallow showing irregularity and filling defects in mid-oesophagus.
B. Peptic stricture oesophagus. Barium swallow showing narrowing in lower oesophagus above a hiatal hernia.

laser recanalisation. Good palliation can also be obtained with combined chemotherapy and radiotherapy, which is sometimes used for the primary treatment of upper third tumours.

GASTRO-OESOPHAGEAL REFLUX

PATHOGENESIS

At rest, an intragastric pressure of 5–8 mmHg and intrathoracic pressure of –2 mmHg provide a gradient which favours reflux of gastric contents into the oesophagus. This is prevented primarily by a resting tone in the lower oesophageal sphincter and is aided by a length of intra-abdominal oesophagus (enclosed by the insertion of the phreno-oesophageal ligament and subject to the positive pressure environment of the abdomen), crural muscle of the diaphragm and angle of insertion of the oesophagus into the stomach (Fig. 24.2). Gastro-

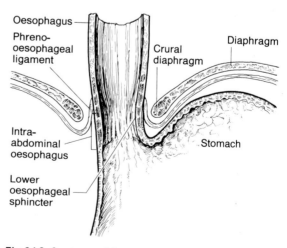

Fig. 24.2 Anatomy of the gastro-oesophageal region showing factors that prevent gastro-oesophageal reflux.

oesophageal reflux can only occur through a relaxed or hypotensive lower oesophageal sphincter. All normal individuals exhibit gastro-oesophageal reflux, which is usually postprandial in association with belching, asymptomatic and rapidly cleared by oesophageal peristalsis. Excessive gastro-oesophageal reflux occurs as a result of transient lower oesophageal sphincter relaxations or on the basis of defective lower oesophageal sphincter resting tone. Hiatus hernia may exacerbate lower oesophageal sphincter dysfunction, but many patients with severe reflux do not have hiatus hernia. Prolonged exposure of the delicate oesophageal mucosa to refluxed acid and pepsin produces ulceration – initially as vertical linear erosions which may become confluent ('reflux oesophagitis'). In severe cases, a fibrous stricture (Fig. 24.1B) or a metaplastic columnar-lined (Barrett's) oesophagus may develop.

CLINICAL FEATURES

Heartburn and regurgitation are the classic symptoms of gastro-oesophageal reflux. Some patients present with atypical chest pain or respiratory symptoms due to aspiration. The severity of the symptoms is not a reliable predictor of the degree of mucosal damage. Mild intermittent discomfort on swallowing or transient dysphagia in the absence of stricture is common in gastro-oesophageal reflux patients. Heartburn and regurgitation giving way to dysphagia may herald stricture development, but may also be a result of adenocarcinoma arising in a Barrett's oesophagus.

DIAGNOSIS

Endoscopy

Endoscopy is the mainstay of the diagnosis of reflux oesophagitis. It allows direct mucosal assessment and biopsy to exclude carcinoma.

Radiology

Whilst a barium swallow may demonstrate ulceration in the oesophagus, endoscopy with biopsy is usually required to exclude carcinoma. Since 60% of patients with severe symptomatic gastro-oesophageal reflux do not have oesophagitis, further investigation in endoscopically normal patients may be required. Gastro-oesophageal reflux seen on X-ray screening after gastric loading with barium may corroborate the diagnosis but is often insensitive.

pH monitoring

Twenty-four hour pH monitoring of the lower oesophagus is the current investigation of choice in these circumstances, especially if the symptoms are atypical. For this investigation, a pH electrode is placed in the oesophagus 5 cm above the lower oesophageal sphincter, and pH is sampled every few seconds over 24 hours and recorded by a portable datalogger carried at the waist. This test gives the number and duration of acid gastro-oesophageal reflux events, but most importantly allows for correlation between symptoms (which are recorded in a diary) and lower oesophageal pH.

Manometry

This may demonstrate a defective lower oesophageal sphincter but does not diagnose gastro-oesophageal reflux. It is used when an oesophageal motility disorder is suspected (e.g. achalasia) and prior to anti-reflux surgery to rule out abnormal oesophageal peristaltic function.

TREATMENT

Medical therapy

Most cases of mild gastro-oesophageal reflux are controlled by simple measures such as:

- weight reduction, avoidance of constricting belts and corsets
- sleeping with shoulders elevated (two or three pillows)
- cessation of smoking
- avoidance of foods that precipitate heartburn (spiced foods, alcohol)
- administration of antacids or antacid/alginate preparations.

Second-line therapy consists of H_2 receptor antagonists, sucralfate and prokinetic drugs (e.g. cisapride) and can heal oesophagitis and control symptoms in around 60% of cases. If these measures fail, H^+/K^+ ATPase inhibitors heal oesophagitis in 96% of cases within 8 weeks. Recurrence is the rule on cessation of therapy, however, and long-term maintenance therapy is required. Recurrence of oesophagitis occurs in 60% of those

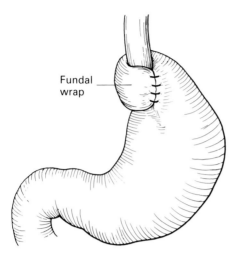

Fundal wrap

Fig. 24.3 Nissen fundoplication.

maintained on H_2 receptor antagonists and in 22% of those on H^+/K^+ ATPase inhibitors during the first year.

Surgical therapy

Anti-reflux surgery is indicated for cases of failed medical therapy (most often for persistent, severe regurgitation) or the development of complications (stricture, Barrett's oesophagus). Most anti-reflux operations incorporate a fundoplication, and the *Nissen fundoplication* is the most commonly used procedure (Fig. 24.3). In this operation, the gastric fundus is mobilised and loosely wrapped around the lower oesophagus and sutured, preserving the vagus nerves. A large-bore intra-oesophageal tube or bougie prevents the wrap from being sutured too tightly and thus protects against postoperative dysphagia and gas-bloat syndrome (inability to belch). The wrap functions as a 'flutter valve', reduces transient lower oesophageal sphincter relaxations, returns a portion of lower oesophagus to the abdomen and increases the angle of oesophageal insertion. If there is a large concomitant hiatus hernia, the diaphragmatic crura are approximated behind the oesophagus with sutures. The Nissen fundoplication eliminates acid reflux, heals oesophagitis and gives a satisfactory result in >90% of patients after 10 years of follow-up.

The *Angelchik prosthesis* is a gel-filled silicone collar which is placed around the lower oesophagus and secured with ties in front. Acid reflux is eliminated, but it is expensive and there is a 10% rate of re-operation for dysphagia, erosion, migration and recurrent reflux oesophagitis in the long term.

Peptic oesophageal stricture can be treated successfully in 95% of cases by dilatation and fundoplication. Resistant strictures require either resection and replacement with colon or complex plastic procedures such as Hugh's antral patch oesophagoplasty. The recent development of fundoplication without laparotomy using percutaneous laparoscopic techniques shortens hospital stay and speeds recovery. This has become an attractive alternative to the open operations, especially for patients who would otherwise require life-long maintenance drug therapy.

There is no strong evidence that either medical or surgical treatment of Barrett's oesophagus causes regression of the metaplastic epithelium or reduces its malignant potential in the long term.

ACHALASIA

SURGICAL PATHOLOGY

Achalasia (meaning 'inability to relax') is also known as cardiospasm or mega-oesophagus. Characteristically, the lower oesophageal sphincter fails to relax on swallowing and there is deficient oesophageal peristalsis. It is considered to result from a neuromuscular disorder which may be associated with degeneration of the oesophageal myenteric plexus. Infection with *Trypanosoma cruzi* (Chagas' disease), prevalent in South America, causes degeneration of the myenteric plexus and leads to motor changes indistinguishable from those of achalasia. In time, the oesophagus becomes dilated, thick-walled and sometimes tortuous. Patients with achalasia have an increased risk of developing carcinoma.

CLINICAL FEATURES

Whilst achalasia may become manifest at any time of life, it usually presents in the third to fifth decades and has an equal sex distribution. Symptoms develop very slowly, and classically they are dysphagia and regurgitation. The dysphagia varies from day to day. Regurgitation is postural and effortless, and undigested food is present; aspiration with respiratory symptoms may occur. About 50% of patients with achalasia develop chest pain of varying nature, and weight loss is a feature of advanced disease. Differential diagnosis includes carcinoma, peptic stricture and gastro-oesophageal reflux.

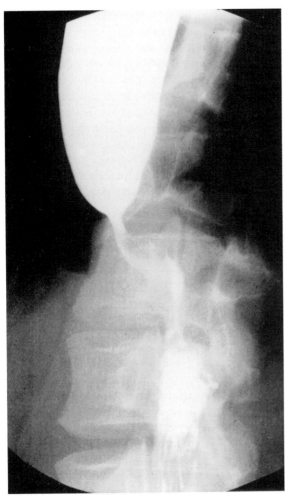

Fig. 24.4 Achalasia. Barium swallow showing proximal oesophageal dilatation with 'bird's beak' narrowing below.

DIAGNOSIS

Radiology

Plain chest X-ray may reveal an air–fluid level in the thorax and an absence of a gastric air bubble. Barium swallow may show a dilated oesophagus with abnormal peristaltic activity and a functional obstruction at the lower oesophagus which tapers and looks rather like a bird's beak (Fig. 24.4).

Endoscopy

This is required to rule out mechanical causes of obstruction such as carcinoma. A dilated oesophagus with food residue may be found. Often, in early cases, there will be no abnormal findings.

Manometry

The diagnostic feature of achalasia is failure of relaxation of the lower oesophageal sphincter in response to swallowing. Feeble or absent oesophageal peristalsis is characteristic and 50% of patients have an abnormally high resting lower oesophageal sphincter pressure.

TREATMENT

Treatment is by:

- medication
- endoscopic pneumatic balloon dilatation
- oesophagomyotomy (Heller's operation).

Medications including anticholinergics, nitrates and calcium channel blockers only give marginal short-term symptomatic relief, have problematic side-effects and do not improve oesophageal emptying. They are used for short periods prior to definitive treatment.

Endoscopic pneumatic balloon dilatation of the lower oesophageal sphincter gives good results in two-thirds of patients, but with an incidence of perforation of 1–5%.

Oesophagomyotomy involves a vertical division of the lower oesophageal sphincter muscle whilst preserving the integrity of the underlying oesophageal mucosa. It gives good results in over 80% of cases and is sometimes combined with fundoplication to prevent postoperative gastro-oesophageal reflux. A newer alternative is percutaneous laparoscopic oesophagomyotomy, which avoids a laparotomy.

OESOPHAGEAL TRAUMA AND PERFORATION

Untreated, oesophageal perforation is rapidly fatal. Mortality rates if treatment is undertaken within 24 hours are around 15%; this rises to 60% if there is more than 24 hours' delay.

Perforations of the oesophagus may be:

- from within
- from without
- postemetic.

From within. These types of perforation can occur as a

result of foreign bodies, including food (e.g. bones) and instruments. Instrumental perforation is associated with, for example, endoscopy (rigid and flexible), dilatation (bougie and pneumatic balloon), removal of foreign bodies, laser photocoagulation for tumours, sclerotherapy for varices and intracavity irradiation for oesophageal carcinoma. Perforations are most common at the natural sites of anatomical narrowing.

From without. This can result from penetrating and missile injuries, but these are rare.

Postemetic. 'Spontaneous' perforation (Boerhaave syndrome) occurs as a vertical tear in the lower left posterolateral aspect of the oesophagus. It follows violent vomiting or retching. A paroxysmal rise in intragastric pressure occurs so that a pressure cone is driven up into the lower oesophagus against a closed cricopharyngeus, resulting in full thickness rupture into the pleural cavity.

DIAGNOSIS

The cardinal symptoms and signs of oesophageal perforation are pain, fever and subcutaneous or mediastinal emphysema. The pain may be well localised, and cervical perforation may be associated with painful swallowing. Occasionally symptoms and signs develop insidiously, and hence a degree of suspicion needs to be maintained after difficult instrumentation procedures. Pain from postemetic rupture is sudden in onset and excruciating.

Radiology

Plain chest X-ray demonstrates mediastinal gas within hours of perforation in 90% of cases. A water-soluble contrast swallow demonstrates leakage from the oesophagus in 90%, but a negative examination does not rule out oesophageal rupture.

Endoscopy

This gives direct information about the site and size of the perforation and an indication of any associated pathology.

TREATMENT

Pleural and mediastinal drainage, nasogastric suction,

nutritional support and systemic administration of antibiotics are recommended for treatment of oesophageal perforations. Debridement and primary suture may be undertaken if the perforation is less than 24 hours old; oesophageal resection or exclusion manoeuvres are required for more delayed cases, with a consequently greatly increased mortality rate.

OTHER OESOPHAGEAL CONDITIONS

CAUSTIC OESOPHAGEAL INJURY

Ingestion of strong acid (HCl, H_2SO_4) or alkali (lye) may produce oesophagogastric lesions that vary from oedema to necrosis. Patients who have had a previous gastric resection (and removal of the pylorus) may have necrosis as far distal as the small bowel. After questioning about the type and amount of substance ingested, early endoscopy should be undertaken. Oedema and superficial erosions of the mucosa heal rapidly. Mucosal necrosis requires treatment with systemically administered antibiotics and parenteral nutrition together with repeated assessment. Around 50% of such patients develop a late stricture (3 months) which may be suitably treated by repeated dilatation, but which often requires resection and replacement with a segment of colon. Full thickness oesophageal necrosis (rare after acid ingestion) may be manifested by acidosis, leucocytosis, disseminated intravascular coagulation and shock; urgent oesophagectomy/gastrectomy is required in these patients. The oesophageal mucosa is subject to an increased risk of malignant change in the long term after severe corrosive injury. Strong acid ingestion tends to produce gastric rather than oesophageal necrosis; gastric perforation occurs in 3–10% of cases usually between 24 and 72 hours post-injury.

PHARYNGO-OESOPHAGEAL DIVERTICULUM (pharyngeal pouch)

Pulsion diverticula consisting of a mucosal sac may occur through an area of weakness between the inferior constrictor of the pharynx and cricopharyngeus posteriorly. The underlying abnormality seems to be pharyngocricopharyngeal dyscoordination during swallowing, or rarely cricopharyngeal spasm.

The condition usually occurs in those over 60 years of age and may present with dysphagia (which is localised to the cervical region), regurgitation of undigested food,

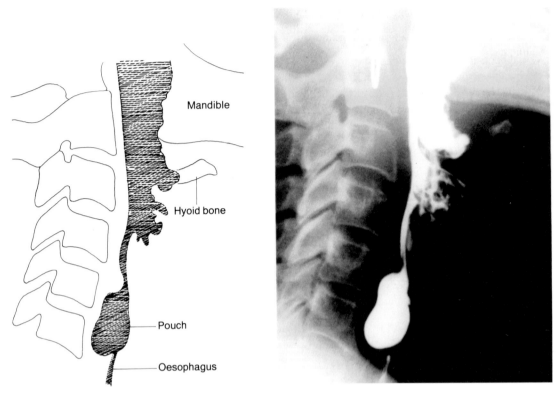

Fig. 24.5 Pharyngeal pouch. Barium swallow showing contrast filling the pouch in the upper oesophagus.

cough or respiratory symptoms associated with aspiration, a sensation of a lump in the throat, 'noisy' swallowing, halitosis and weight loss. Asymptomatic diverticula occur in 0.1–2% of populations. The diagnosis is made by barium swallow, where contrast is retained in the diverticulum (Fig. 24.5). Oesophagoscopy is generally contraindicated because of the ease with which the endoscope enters the diverticulum and the corresponding risk of perforation.

The treatment is surgical with excision via a cervical incision and suture closure of the neck of the diverticulum, together with cricopharyngeal myotomy. An alternative approach is internal pharyngo-oesophagotomy. Here, the septum – between the oesophagus and diverticulum – consisting of two layers of mucosa and the posterior part of the cricopharyngeus, is divided with diathermy through a pharyngoscope. This is suitable only for small pharyngo-oesophageal diverticula.

OESOPHAGEAL WEBS

These are congenital (found generally in the mid-oesophagus) or acquired (situated in the postcricoid region). They consist of a membrane of mucosa and account for around 5% of benign causes of dysphagia.

When associated with iron-deficiency anaemia, it is referred to as Paterson–Kelly (Plummer–Vinson) syndrome or sideropenic dysphagia. Diagnosis is made by barium swallow (a thin, horizontal shelf is seen) and endoscopy with biopsy to rule out malignancy. Treatment consists of correction of anaemia and oesophageal dilatation.

THE SCHATZKI RING

This consists of a fibromuscular shelf lined by mucosa and is found only at the squamocolumnar junction in the oesophagus. It is thought to be related to chronic gastro-oesophageal reflux but is an entity histologically distinct from a peptic stricture. Patients may present with symptomatic gastro-oesophageal reflux or with a history of intermittent bolus obstruction. The treatment is dilatation followed by fundoplication.

DIAPHRAGMATIC HERNIA

Diaphragmatic hernias are the main surgical condition of the diaphragm.

CLASSIFICATION

This condition can be classified into:

- congenital
  — hernia through foramen of Morgagni
  — hernia through the foramen of Bochdalek
  — eventration of the diaphragm
- traumatic
- hiatus hernia
  — sliding
  — para-oesophageal
  — combined sliding and para-oesophageal.

Congenital hernia will not be discussed here.

TRAUMATIC DIAPHRAGMATIC HERNIA
(see also p. 126)

Surgical pathology

Rupture of the diaphragm complicates severe blunt external trauma or crushing injuries to the abdomen (5%) or chest (1%). Concomitant injury to abdominal viscera (especially the spleen), thorax and lung occurs in two-thirds of these patients and one-third require assisted ventilation. Most diaphragmatic ruptures occur on the left side.

Clinical features

The clinical manifestations of diaphragmatic rupture are caused by acute blood loss and by herniation of abdominal viscera into the hemithorax. Acute cardiorespiratory compromise occurs in 10%; in the remainder, there may be a lapse of from weeks to years before substantial herniation ensues. Respiratory symptoms or obstruction to hollow viscera may occur with the necessity for urgent operation. At the time of injury, close scrutiny of the plain erect chest X-ray for diaphragmatic elevation or irregularity, pleural effusion, left lower rib fractures or shift of mediastinal structures may indicate diaphragmatic rupture. The diagnosis is obvious if abdominal viscera are seen in the hemithorax (Fig. 24.6). Computed tomography or contrast studies of the gastrointestinal tract may sometimes be needed to confirm the diagnosis.

Treatment

Reduction of the contents of the hernia and primary suture repair via the abdominal approach are usually all that is required. In cases of acute strangulation of gut, the mortality from operation may be as high as 20–30%.

HIATUS HERNIA

Sliding hiatus hernia is displacement of the gastro-oesophageal junction into the posterior mediastinum through the diaphragmatic hiatus (Fig. 24.7A). The phreno-oesophageal membrane is attenuated and forms the hernial sac in which the upper stomach and cardia usually move freely but are occasionally fixed. The incidence of sliding hiatus hernia increases with age, occurring in as much as 76% of the general population in their seventh decade. Obesity is also a predisposing factor.

Sliding hiatus hernia is not a disease; symptoms attributable to it are a result of gastro-oesophageal reflux. Less than 10% of subjects with hiatus hernia have symptoms of gastro-oesophageal reflux, although the presence of hiatus hernia increases the likelihood of having excessive gastro-oesophageal reflux, possibly by exacerbating lower

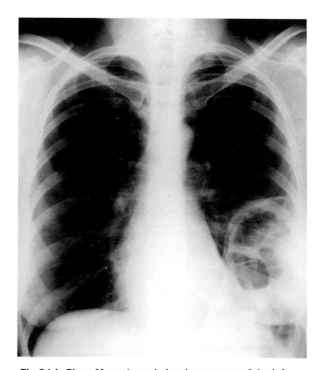

Fig. 24.6 Chest X-ray (erect) showing rupture of the left hemidiaphragm with loops of colon in the left chest.

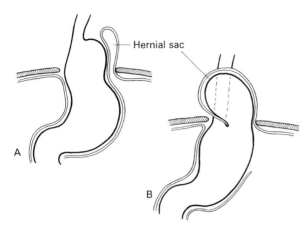

Hernial sac

A

B

Fig. 24.7 Types of hiatus hernia.

oesophageal sphincter dysfunction. Diagnosis and treatment are as for gastro-oesophageal reflux.

In a *para-oesophageal (rolling) hernia*, the gastro-oesophageal junction lies in the normal position, but the fundus of the stomach has herniated through the diaphragmatic hiatus into the posterior mediastinum and lies beside the oesophagus (Fig. 24.7B). Complications of para-oesophageal hernia are gastro-oesophageal obstruction, volvulus, strangulation/infarction, chronic or acute bleeding, peptic ulceration, perforation, cardiac or respiratory compromise and gastro-oesophageal reflux. Strangulation of the stomach may be precipitated by sudden rises in intra-abdominal pressure.

Patients with para-oesophageal hernia may present with epigastric discomfort and fullness, retrosternal pain and sometimes vomiting after meals. Dysphagia may be precipitated by gastric volvulus. The diagnosis of para-oesophageal hernia is made by plain chest X-ray (where a fluid level in the gastric fundus may be seen in the left hemithorax) and confirmed by a barium meal. The treatment is operative reduction of the stomach into the abdomen, approximation of the diaphragmatic defect around the oesophagus (which contains a bougie to prevent tight closure) and suture. A fundoplication is frequently added both to reduce the chance of recurrent herniation and to prevent gastro-oesophageal reflux.

In a *combined sliding and para-oesophageal hiatus hernia*, both the gastro-oesophageal junction and fundus have herniated into the posterior mediastinum. Complications and treatment are as for a para-oesophageal hernia.

FURTHER READING

Bennett G 1994 Oesophageal disorders. In: Pounder R (ed) Recent advances in gastroenterology 10. Churchill Livingstone, Edinburgh

Hennessy T P J, Cuschieri A 1992 Surgery of the oesophagus, 2nd edn. Butterworth-Heinemann, Oxford

Jamieson G G, Duranceau A 1988 Gastroesophageal reflux. W B Saunders, Philadelphia

Postlethwait R W 1986 Surgery of the oesophagus, 2nd edn. Appleton-Century-Croft, Norwolk

25 Stomach and duodenum

Paul O'Brien

OVERVIEW

Upper gastrointestinal surgery is an emerging subspecialty within general surgery and this chapter deals with two common problems faced by these surgeons, namely peptic ulcer and gastric cancer. Details of gastric secretion, mobility and mucosal defence are provided as background for the discussion of aetiology, pathogenesis, clinical presentation and management of peptic ulcer. The aetiology, pathology and staging for gastrointestinal cancer are followed by clinical assessment and management. Common operations and their sequelae are presented. Gastritis and the Zollinger–Ellison syndrome are also covered.

SURGICAL ANATOMY AND PHYSIOLOGY

The stomach is a J-shaped organ with a capacity of approximately 1500 ml. It is relatively fixed at the oesophagogastric junction and at the duodenum by the left and right gastric vascular pedicles. The mucosa of the body and fundus of the stomach is thick and vascular. The surface epithelium is invaginated by over 3 million pits. Three to six branched tubular glands arise from the depth of each pit, creating a total mucosal height of 1–1.5 mm. The oxyntic (acid-secreting) cells are located principally in the central portion of the gastric glands; the chief (pepsin-secreting) cells lie in the deeper portions. The gastric antrum is thinner and without the rugal folds of the fundus. The antral mucosa contains a simple epithelium folded into shallow glands with gastrin-secreting 'G' cells at the base. No oxyntic or chief cells are present.

GASTRIC SECRETION

The oxyntic cells secrete a primary acidity of H^+ concentration of approximately 150 mM/L (pH <1.0). The gastric juice in the lumen of the stomach in the fasting state is of reduced acidity, in the range of 10–100 mM/L (pH 1.0–2.0), due to admixture of the primary oxyntic cell secretion with secretions by the surface epithelium, back-diffusion of H^+ across the mucosa and dilution and neutralisation with saliva and refluxed duodenal secretions. The local endogenous stimuli of acid secretion are histamine, acetylcholine and gastrin. Their effects are synergistic, and blocking of one of these inhibits the influence of the others. Acetylcholine release occurs as the final transmitter of the parasympathetic nerves to the stomach. The right and left vagus nerves enter the abdomen through the oesophageal hiatus of the diaphragm, give fibres directly to the cardia and fundus of the stomach, and then branch to form the anterior and posterior nerves of Laterjet; these nerves pass along the lesser curve of the stomach, giving fibres to the remainder of the fundus and body before terminating as a 'crow's foot' at the junction of the antrum and body. Highly selective vagotomy is the surgical division of the numerous fine branches from the vagal trunks and from the nerves of Laterjet, thereby denervating the oxyntic cells of the stomach. Gastrin is secreted by the gastric antral 'G' cell as either a 17 amino acid form (little gastrin, 90%) or a 34 amino acid form (big gastrin, 10%) in response to amino acids in the gastric lumen, vagal stimulation or gastric distension.

GASTRIC MOTILITY

Functionally, the stomach can be divided into two regions:

- gastric fundus
- gastric antrum.

The fundus has a key role in regulating intragastric pressure and in emptying liquids from the stomach. It accepts the boluses of ingested food through properties of receptive relaxation and accommodation. These two properties permit a considerable increase in size with little change in intragastric pressure. The fundus demonstrates low sustained tonic contractions which exert steady pressure on the gastric content and thereby encourage gastric emptying. Loss of receptive relaxation and accommodation through resection or denervation leads to a rapid increase in intragastric pressure with eating, early satiety and an increased rate of emptying, particularly of liquids. Loss of tonic contractions of the fundus can result in delayed gastric emptying of liquids.

The gastric antrum reduces the solid food to small particles and mixes this food with gastric juice with a regular rhythm of peristaltic waves. Mainly 'to and fro' movements are generated to facilitate mixing and trituration of food. Intermittently, peristaltic contractions give complete occlusion of the lumen and propel the gastric content through the pylorus. Vagal activity enhances the contraction of the distal stomach.

The pylorus is best regarded as the end-point of the gastric antrum rather than as an independent structure. It does not act as a true sphincter as its lumen remains open at basal states and closes in association with antral peristalsis. It therefore works in concert with the antrum to control gastric emptying and to aid in tituration of the food. Generally only particles smaller than 0.1 mm are allowed to pass the pylorus. It further serves to prevent reflux of duodenal fluid into the stomach.

GASTRIC MUCOSAL DEFENCE

The normal gastric mucosa is resistant to damage by its own secretions. With gastric luminal fluid of pH 1.0, there is a concentration gradient for H^+ of 6 million to 1 across the gastric epithelium to the intracellular and interstitial environment of a pH of 7.4. This gradient is maintained or the back-diffusing acid is neutralised by a set of defences which can be divided into four main components:

- gastric mucosal barrier
- cellular mechanisms for neutralising acid
- role of the microcirculation
- restitution.

The gastric mucosal barrier

Diffusion of acid down the massive concentration gradient is discouraged by the mucus–bicarbonate barrier and by the impermeability of the gastric epithelial cell membrane. Gastric mucus consists of a hydrated array of glycoprotein polymers which provide an 'unstirred' layer between the epithelium and the lumen. The surface epithelial cells secrete HCO_3^- into this layer, creating a pH gradient from lumen to epithelium. The H^+ that does penetrate this layer must then diffuse across a relatively impermeable luminal border of surface epithelium to reach the intracellular environment.

Cellular mechanisms for neutralising acid

The gastric mucosal cells are specifically structured to cope with back-diffusing acid using the HCO_3^-/CO_2 buffer system with access to high levels of HCO_3^- generated from the process of acid secretion and high levels of carbonic anhydrase to catalyse the reaction.

Role of the microcirculation

With the transfer of each H^+ out of an oxyntic cell into the gastric lumen, there is an equimolar transfer of HCO_3^- into the interstitium. The capillaries of the fundic mucosa transfer that 'alkaline tide' to the surface epithelium before it passes into the venous drainage of the stomach so that, at times of maximal luminal acidity, the surface epithelium is provided with optimal acid–base conditions.

Restitution

Injury to the surface epithelium of the stomach is probably a frequent occurrence from ingested food or ingested irritants. If the injury results only in loss of surface epithelium with an intact basement membrane, rapid migration of healthy cells from the adjacent gastric pits leads to restitution of the intact mucosa within 15–60 minutes of injury. This process is rapid because it does not require new cell formation. During the interval prior to completion of restitution, a mucoid 'cap' of mucus and cellular debris limits acid back-diffusion across this vulnerable area.

PEPTIC ULCER DISEASE

FORMS AND FREQUENCY OF DISEASE

Peptic disease includes all conditions in which there is acid–peptic digestion of the mucosa of the upper gastrointestinal tract. *Erosion* involves loss of epithelium without penetration of the submucosa. *Ulceration* involves penetration through the submucosa. Common forms of chronic disease include gastric ulcers, duodenal ulcers and oesophagitis with erosions or ulceration. Acute diseases include erosive gastritis and stress ulcers. This group of conditions remains one of the most prevalent in gastroenterology. Although peptic disease of the stomach and duodenum are probably decreasing, there has been a matching increase in the clinical problems associated with reflux oesophagitis (Ch. 24).

AETIOLOGY AND PATHOGENESIS

Peptic ulceration results from an imbalance between the damaging effects of gastric acid and pepsin and the protective system of mucosal defences of the stomach and duodenum (Table 25.1). Specific agents and states contribute to this imbalance. Most important are infection of the mucosa with *Helicobacter pylori* and exposure to non-steroidal anti-inflammatory drugs (NSAIDs), which together probably account for more than 95% of peptic ulceration. Important special conditions are Zollinger–Ellison syndrome, with hypersecretion of acid and stress ulcers in the critically ill.

Helicobacter pylori

H. pylori is a Gram-negative spiral-shaped bacterium which colonises the mucus layer of the gastric antrum. Its presence is associated with a cumulative risk of 15–20% of developing a peptic ulcer and a 1–5% likelihood of developing gastric carcinoma. The prevalence of *H. pylori* in various clinical settings is shown in Table 25.2. The mechanism for the increased frequency and higher recurrence rates of duodenal ulcer when *H. pylori* is present in the antrum is unclear, but theories include increased acid secretion, gastric metaplasia in the duodenum and the production of irritants which cause duodenitis.

The presence of the organism can be established in those having gastroscopy by testing mucosal biopsies for the presence of urease and by histology and culture. For those not having gastroscopy, serological tests for IgG antibodies and breath tests measuring CO_2 release after urea ingestion can be used.

Eradication of *H. pylori* should be considered in patients when the organism has been demonstrated in association with peptic disease. Triple therapy with bismuth subcitrate, amoxycillin and metronidazole for 14 days will eradicate the organism in 80–90%. When used with antisecretory drug treatment for gastric and duodenal ulcers, the 1-year relapse rate for duodenal ulcer is less than 10%, compared with a rate of 75–95% without triple therapy.

Non-steroidal anti-inflammatory drugs (NSAIDs)

A single exposure to aspirin or another NSAID causes measurable damage to the gastric mucosa. Chronic use is associated with gastric ulcers in 20% of patients, an increased frequency of gastric and duodenal ulcer bleeding and perforation and an increased rate of ulcer deaths. Although the incidence of NSAID-induced gastric disease is low, the frequency of use of this group of drugs in the community is so high that its prevalence is considerable.

NSAIDs produce gastric mucosal injury by direct irri-

Table 25.1 Factors involved in mucosal attack and defence in the stomach and duodenum

Mucosal attack	Mucosal defence
Acid	Mucus
Pepsin	Bicarbonate
H. pylori	Cell membrane
Gastrotoxic drugs, especially	Cellular buffering
NSAIDS	Gastric microcirculation
Alcohol	Restitution
Duodenogastric reflux	Endogenous prostaglandin
Smoking	

Table 25.2 Prevalence of *H. pylori* in various clinical settings

Setting	Prevalence
Normal population	0–40%
Duodenal ulcer	90%
Gastric ulcer	65%
Chronic gastritis	80%
Non-ulcer dyspepsia	50%
Gastric cancer	65%

tation and by systemic effects through inhibition of cyclooxygenase, the enzyme centrally involved in the generation of prostaglandins. Most NSAIDs are weak organic acids which are non-ionised at normal levels of gastric acidity (pH 1.0–4.0) and so can easily diffuse into the mucosal epithelial cells. Within the neutral pH environment of the cell, ionisation occurs with release of intracellular acid. Intracellular pH decreases, osmotic pressure increases and the anion frequently acts as a metabolic toxin with uncoupling of oxidative phosphorylation. The endothelium of the gastric microvasculature is also injured, leading to initial ischaemic injury and subsequent reperfusion injury with free radical release.

Inhibition of prostaglandin production blocks a number of gastric mucosal defence mechanisms which are mediated by prostaglandin E_2, including mucus production, bicarbonate ion secretion, microvascular perfusion and epithelial proliferation.

Controversy exists regarding the relative importance of local and systemic effects. As the prostaglandin-linked effects are systemic, the toxic effect of NSAIDs may occur without direct gastric mucosal exposure and so alternative absorption sites such as the small gut with enteric-coated tablets and the rectum with suppositories do not provide complete protection against injury.

CHRONIC PEPTIC ULCERATION

The pain of both gastric and duodenal ulcers is described as dull, gnawing or burning, sharp, hunger-like, in the epigastrium and without radiation. It is quite variable in intensity, periodicity and time of onset. For duodenal ulcer, the pain frequently occurs in the early hours of the morning and is relieved by food or antacids. Gastric ulcer pain is more likely to be brought on by particular foods, usually spicy or acidic. Nausea, vomiting, anorexia and weight loss are less common symptoms. Occult bleeding leads to weakness and tiredness through anaemia. One-third of peptic ulcer patients who develop complications have no prior history of symptoms.

The diagnosis of peptic ulcer is made by upper gastrointestinal endoscopy. This provides good visualisation of the oesophagus, stomach and duodenum, the ability to biopsy gastric ulcers and any other potentially malignant lesion, biopsy for *H. pylori*, and some therapeutic options, particularly in the presence of bleeding. There is very limited need for barium meal if endoscopy is available. Study of gastric acid production is not helpful. Serum

gastrin should be measured if Zollinger–Ellison syndrome or retained gastric antrum after gastrectomy are to be excluded.

Medical management

Gastric and duodenal ulcers should be treated with acid-suppressing drugs and by eradication of *H. pylori*. Treatment with H_2 receptor antagonists such as cimetidine, ranitidine or famotidine for 6–8 weeks will result in healing of the ulcer in more than 90% of patients. If no additional measures are taken, recurrence of the ulcer will occur in 75–95% within a 12-month period. Eradication of *H. pylori*, in conjunction with the initial period of acid suppression, using 'triple therapy' (bismuth subcitrate, amoxycillin and metronidazole) for 2 weeks will reduce the relapse rate to less than 10%. If *H. pylori* is not present or is not eradicated by triple therapy, maintenance therapy with H_2 blockers may be indicated. For resistant ulcers or ulcers associated with hypersecretory states, therapy with proton pump inhibitors such as omeprazole or lansoprazole is indicated.

Surgical treatment

With the major improvements in medical therapy, there is now little call for the elective application of surgical treatment for chronic peptic ulcer disease. More commonly, surgical procedures are indicated in the treatment of the complications of the disease. Persistence of symptoms in spite of medical therapy, or rapid or multiple recurrences may be indications for considering surgical treatment. The two primary surgical modalities are:

- vagotomy, which removes the cholinergic stimulus to the parietal cell to secrete acid
- resection, which removes the antral source of gastrin.

For gastric ulcer, a more extensive resection may be performed to remove the ulcer-bearing area of the stomach as well.

Highly selective vagotomy. (Fig. 25.1). This is the preferred form of vagotomy for the elective treatment of chronic duodenal ulcer. This procedure divides those fibres of the vagus that innervate the parietal cell-bearing area of the stomach with preservation of vagal innervation to the gastric antrum and to the remainder of abdominal viscera. It may be performed by open or laparoscopic approach and is associated with very few side-effects,

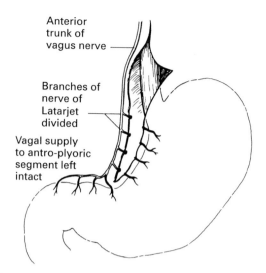

Fig. 25.1 Highly selective vagotomy. The diagram shows ligation and division of vagal filae supplying parietal cell mass.

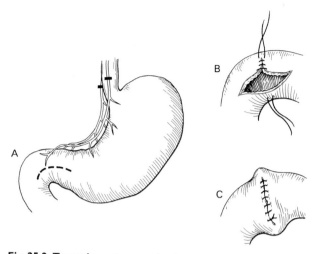

Fig. 25.2 Truncal vagotomy and pyloroplasty. A. Both trunks of vagus are divided, and the pylorus is opened longitudinally. **B.** Heineke–Mikulicz pyloroplasty: a full thickness longitudinal incision through the pylorus is closed transversely. **C.** Completed pyloroplasty.

but recurrence of the ulcer is found in 5–20% of patients in a 10-year follow-up.

Truncal vagotomy and pyloroplasty. This procedure is used more commonly for the emergency treatment of complication of duodenal ulcer, particularly perforation and bleeding. The anterior and posterior trunks of the vagus are divided as they pass along the intra-abdominal segment of the oesophagus (Fig. 25.2A), resulting in total vagal denervation of intra-abdominal structures. The delayed gastric emptying expected to result from denervation of the gastric antrum is overcome by the addition of pyloroplasty. This involves destroying the 'gate' effect of the pylorus. In the commonest type of pyloroplasty – Heineke/Mikulicz pyloroplasty – a longitudinal incision across and through the pyloric sphincter is closed in a transverse plane (Fig. 25.2B,C). This procedure is equally effective as the highly selective vagotomy, but because it destroys controlled gastric emptying, it is associated with a higher frequency of postgastric surgery sequelae (see Table 25.4).

Partial gastrectomy (Figs 25.3 and 25.4) is used most commonly for benign and malignant tumours of the stomach. It is a highly effective treatment of peptic ulcer with a recurrence rate of 1–2% achieved through removal of the antrum as a source of gastrin and removal of much of the parietal cell mass from the body and fundus. Restoration of gastrointestinal continuity can be

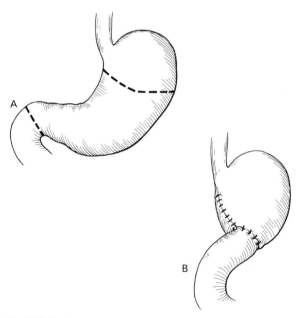

Fig. 25.3 A. Partial gastrectomy. B. Billroth I (gastroduodenal) reconstruction.

achieved through anastomosis with the proximal duodenum (Billroth I reconstruction) (Fig. 25.3) or with a loop of proximal jejunum (Billroth II or Polya reconstruction) (Fig. 25.4). The major changes to normal gastric function by this operation lead to postgastric surgery sequelae in

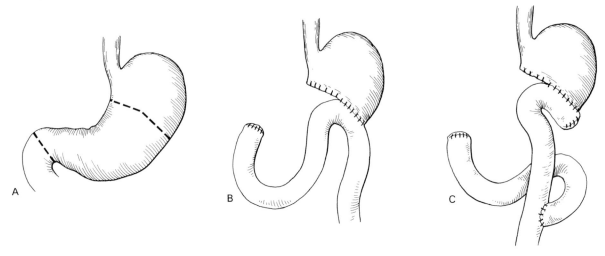

Fig. 25.4 A. Partial gastrectomy. B. Billroth II or Polya, with simple loop gastrojejunal reconstruction. C. With Roux-en-Y jejunal loop reconstruction.

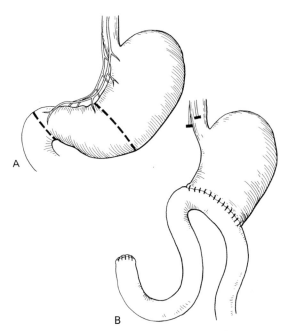

Fig. 25.5 Vagotomy and antrectomy. A. Truncal vagotomy and antrectomy (resection of antrum and pylorus). **B.** Billroth II gastrojejunal reconstruction.

20–30% of patients and these sequelae can be severe in about 5%.

Vagotomy and antrectomy (Fig. 25.5). This procedure combines the deletion of cholinergic stimulation of

acid secretion through vagotomy with the deletion of gastrin stimulation of acid secretion through antrectomy, and thereby achieves a very low rate of ulcer recurrence (<1%). It is an alternative to HSV in the treatment of chronic duodenal ulcer, or to partial gastrectomy in the treatment of low gastric ulcer. Restoration of continuity is by Billroth I or Billroth II type. Postgastric surgery sequelae are frequent.

BLEEDING PEPTIC ULCER DISEASE

This presentation is discussed in Chapter 33.

PERFORATED PEPTIC ULCER DISEASE

About 1 in 10 patients with chronic peptic ulcer will perforate that ulcer. The event is usually accompanied by the sudden onset of severe epigastric and then generalised abdominal pain. Peritonitis caused by the release of gastric fluid is intense, leading to abdominal wall rigidity and patient immobility. Shoulder tip pain is common due to diaphragmatic peritoneal irritation. The patient is distressed but is neither shocked nor toxic. There is generalised abdominal guarding to the point of board-like rigidity, and erect plain X-ray of the abdomen and lower chest should reveal free gas under the diaphragm in more than 80% of patients. If clinical or plain X-ray findings are equivocal, a gastrograffin meal is indicated.

Laparotomy or laparoscopy should be performed with

aspiration of fluid from the peritoneal cavity. It is common for the site of perforation to be oversewn and for reliance to be placed on medical therapy for healing of the ulcer disease. However, for the stable patient with chronic disease, it is preferable that definitive anti-ulcer surgery be performed for duodenal ulcer. This would consist of truncal vagotomy and a pyloroplasty, which includes closure of the perforation or a highly selective vagotomy with oversewing of the perforation. For perforating gastric ulcer, a gastrectomy is appropriate.

PYLORIC STENOSIS

Chronic ulceration in the region of the pyloric canal may cause narrowing to the point of gastric outlet obstruction. The narrowing is due in part to chronic inflammation with fibrosis and in part to acute inflammation with oedema.

The clinical picture is of episodic vomiting of large volumes of fluid containing partly digested food. The patient is dehydrated and malnourished. A succussion splash may be present. A grossly enlarged stomach may be visible on plain X-ray and contrast studies also demonstrate gastric outlet obstruction. A characteristic metabolic picture of hypochloraemic, hypokalaemic alkalosis with dehydration and malnutrition may be expected and should be actively corrected. Other causes of gastric outlet obstruction, especially malignancy, should be excluded.

Generally, relief of the obstruction in the short term can be achieved with anti-ulcer therapies which reduce the acute oedematous component of the process. Temporary benefit can also be achieved by endoscopic dilatation of the pylorus. Definitive surgical treatment involves treatment of the ulcer diathesis and clearing the obstruction. This can generally be achieved by truncal vagotomy and antrectomy (Fig. 25.5) or by highly selective vagotomy and duodenoplasty.

GASTRIC CANCER

EPIDEMIOLOGY AND AETIOLOGY

Gastric cancer is the second most common fatal cancer in the world with high frequency in Japan, Korea, Chile, Finland and Central America. The frequency of cancers in the body and antrum of the stomach have been decreasing in Western nations over the past 50 years, possibly associated with the introduction of refrigeration and better food hygiene. However, cancer of the fundic region and oesophagogastric junction is rapidly rising in frequency. The disease presents most commonly in the fifth and sixth decades of life. Survival rates after treatment vary greatly between countries with 5-year survival of greater than 50% in Japan, 20–30% in the USA and Australia, and around 12% in the UK. These differences appear to be due to the timeliness of diagnosis rather than a reflection on the efficacy of treatment.

Ingestion of carcinogens or their precursors is the main candidate for causation. Dietary nitrates are converted by gastric bacteria to nitrites, which react with amines, amides and urea to form carcinogenic N-nitroso compounds. Gastric colonisation with bacteria occurs in a setting of hypochlorhydria (e.g. atrophic gastritis) or the ingestion of contaminated food.

Other associations with gastric cancer include:

- *H. pylori* colonisation
- a diet high in dry, salted, or smoked foods
- blood group A
- the presence of adenomatous polyps.

PATHOBIOLOGY AND PATHOLOGY

Gastric cancer may arise in the antrum (50%), the gastric body (30%), or the fundus or oesophagogastric junction (20%). The macroscopic forms of gastric cancer are described by the Bormann classification which shows a correlation with survival (Table 25.3).

Microscopically the tumour is an adenocarcinoma with a range of differentiation. Lauren described two important subtypes on histological examination: intestinal and diffuse. The intestinal form is better differentiated, tending to form glands. It arises from a background of atrophic gastritis, dysplasia or intestinal metaplasia. It is more common in men and spreads haematogenously. The diffuse form is less differentiated, occurs more in females and younger people and tends more to locoregional spread.

Early gastric cancer is a special subtype which is defined as a cancer which is confined to the mucosa and

Table 25.3   Bormann classification (macroscopic forms) of gastric cancer
Polypoid
Ulcerating
Ulcerating/infiltrating
Diffuse infiltrating (Linnitus plastica)

submucosa, regardless of lymph node status. This stage is encountered in 50% or more of gastric cancers treated in Japan and fewer than 10% in Western countries.

Spread is by three primary routes:

- locoregional
- haematogenous
- lymphatic.

Locoregional spread is through the serosa into the greater or lesser sac, and into adjacent organs of liver, pancreas, spleen, and transverse colon. Transcoelomic spread can give specific metastases to the pouch of Douglas (Blumer's shelf), the ovaries (Krukenberg's tumour) or the umbilicus (Sister Joseph's nodule). Locoregional spread is responsible for 40% of recurrent disease.

Haematogenous spread is demonstrated by the presence of metastases in the liver, lung, bone and other organs and is the principal cause of 45% of recurrent disease.

Lymph node spread is an important marker of tumour stage but is probably not an important pathway of tumour spread. Lymphatic spread may sometimes be detected in the left anterior supraclavicular nodes (Troisier's sign).

PRESENTATION AND EVALUATION

The clinical features of gastric cancer may arise from local disease, its complications or its metastases.

Local disease. This may give no symptoms or only vague dyspepsia even when extensively involving the stomach. More typically, symptoms of epigastric pain, nausea and vomiting, anorexia, early satiety and weight loss are present.

Complications. The complications of the disease may provide the presenting features. Gastric outlet obstruction leads to copious vomiting and weight loss in association with a metabolic profile of hypochloraemia, hypokalaemia, alkalosis, dehydration and malnutrition. Oesophagogastric obstruction will lead to dysphagia. Bleeding from an ulcerating cancer can present as haematemesis and melaena or, more commonly, as occult iron deficiency anaemia. Perforation of a cancer will lead to presentation as an acute abdomen.

Metastases. These frequently provide the presenting features. An epigastric mass generally indicates exten-

sion of the tumour into surrounding structures. Peritoneal metastases may cause bowel obstruction and ascites and may be palpable on rectal or vaginal examination. Lymph node metastases may present with a lump in the neck (Troisier's sign) or jaundice due to compression at the porta hepatis. Liver metastases generate profound anorexia, weight loss and jaundice.

Investigations

The specific investigations required will be determined by the presenting features. Upper gastrointestinal endoscopy is the most important single test. It allows good visualisation of the nature and extent of the lesion, the taking of biopsies or brushings for cytology, the identification of obstruction or other complications, and the evaluation of other local disease. The extent of local disease and the presence of metastases are evaluated most effectively by CT scan of the chest and abdomen and by liver function tests. Endoscopic ultrasound is currently being assessed for its value in measuring the depth of invasion. If early gastric cancer can be demonstrated, more limited excision will be adequate. Prior to laparotomy, a laparoscopic evaluation of the upper abdomen can demonstrate unresectability, leading to change of the treatment plan.

TREATMENT OPTIONS

Surgical excision with curative intent is the mainstay of treatment of gastric cancer. The central goal of curative resection is to remove all disease, both macroscopic and microscopic, within the gastric wall, from the surrounding structures and from the draining lymph nodes.

Within the gastric wall. Because of the tendency for gastric cancer to infiltrate along the submucosal plane, it is recommended that there be a 6 cm margin of stomach from the palpable edge of the tumour to the line of resection. Infiltration into the duodenum is less extensive, making a 2 cm margin sufficient at the distal aspect of pyloric tumours.

Surrounding structures. Generally cure will not be achieved when the tumour is infiltrating the liver, pancreas, spleen or transverse mesocolon. However, as this is not invariable and as inflammatory adhesion can mimic malignant infiltration, excision is appropriate if feasible.

The extent of lymphadenectomy. This remains an area of controversy. Increasingly, both clinical and biological data indicate that tumour within a lymph node is a true metastasis and therefore is not intrinsic to the treatment of the primary tumour. If lymphadenectomy adds to the morbidity of the procedure, it should be justified by the demonstration that resection of metastasis is itself worthwhile. Prospective randomised trial of this for gastric cancer does not show a benefit. Limited lymphadenectomy (perigastric nodes alone) occurs as a part of routine resection of the stomach. More extensive lymphadenectomy probably does not improve survival.

Types of resection and reconstruction

Centrally placed or large tumours may require total gastrectomy to adequately clear the primary disease. Continuity of the gut is usually achieved by anastomosing the distal oesophagus to proximal jejunum (Fig. 25.6). Cancer in the upper body or fundus can be resected with the proximal two-thirds of the stomach and the antrum is then joined directly to the oesophagus (Fig. 25.7).

Cancer at the region of the oesophagogastric junction will also require partial oesophageal resection. This will usually require intrathoracic exposure of the oesophagus either by a left-sided thoraco-abdominal incision or by the combination of an upper abdominal incision and a posterior right-sided thoracotomy (Ivor Lewis procedure).

Cancer in the antrum of the stomach can usually be treated by a two-thirds distal gastrectomy with gastrojejunostomy (see Fig. 25.4).

Palliative procedures. The symptoms which most commonly require palliation are obstruction and bleeding. Obstruction at the upper stomach and oesophagogastric junction may be controlled by dilatation followed by placement of a stent or by destruction of the obstructing tumour using Nd/Yag laser, or alcohol injection. Stent placement is best achieved endoscopically. Obstruction at the gastric outlet is relieved by gastrojejunostomy (Fig. 25.8). Acute major haemorrhage is treated by resection if feasible. Chronic blood loss may be reduced by a bypass procedure which diverts the food from the ulcerated surface of the tumour.

Chemotherapy has generally been ineffective in controlling gastric cancer growth. Meta-analysis of randomised trials of its use as an adjuvant to surgery in potentially curative resection demonstrates no survival

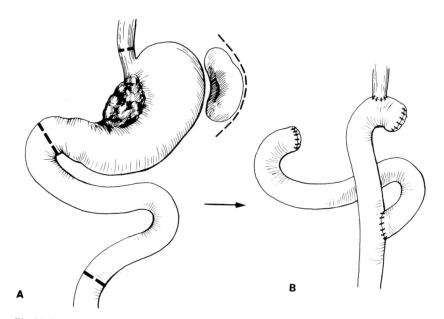

Fig. 25.6 Total gastrectomy for a large carcinoma of the body of the stomach. A. The resection generally includes the spleen, the entire greater and lesser omentum and several lymph node groups – pyloric, pancreaticosplenic, superior gastric, coeliac. **B.** Reconstruction is by oesophagojejunostomy Roux-en-Y.

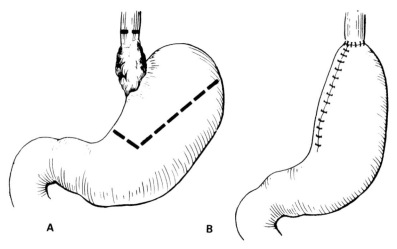

Fig. 25.7 Oesophagogastrectomy for carcinoma of the cardia. A. Extent of resection.
B. Reconstruction with oesophagogastric anastomosis.

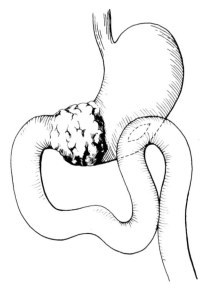

Fig. 25.8 Palliative antecolic gastroenterostomy for an irresectable cancer causing gastric outlet obstruction.

benefit. For locally advanced or metastatic disease, a trial of chemotherapy with 5-fluorouracil in combination with adriamycin, mitomycin-c or cisplatin may be considered, but a strong response is unlikely.

OTHER GASTRIC AND DUODENAL TUMOURS

A number of benign and malignant tumours other than

adenocarcinoma occur infrequently in the stomach and duodenum.

LYMPHOMA

Lymphoma of the stomach is considered primary if the patient presents with gastric symptoms and if the disease is entirely or almost entirely confined to the stomach. Otherwise it is considered to be part of a systemic disease. The symptoms are similar to those of gastric cancer with:

- vague dyspepsia or specific epigastric pain
- nausea and vomiting
- anorexia
- early satiety
- weight loss.

The diagnosis is made principally from endoscopic examination with biopsy and cytology. CT scanning is important in staging the disease. Well-localised disease should be treated by resection. More extensive disease should be treated with resection plus adjuvant chemoradiation or by chemoradiation alone.

LEIOMYOMA AND LEIOMYOSARCOMA

These tumours of smooth muscle may arise anywhere in the gastrointestinal tract but are most common in the stomach, representing 1% of gastric tumours. They may be sessile or pedunculated, the latter projecting into the gastric lumen or extragastrically or both (dumbbell tumour). They present due to blood loss anaemia, an epigastric mass or vague dyspepsia. Malignancy is suggested by the size (>5 cm in diameter) and confirmed by noting increased mitosis on histology.

GASTRIC AND DUODENAL POLYPS

These may be adenomatous, hyperplastic or hamartomatous. Adenomatous polyps are rare and usually single. Malignant risk correlates with size so that polyps greater than 2 cm should be excised. Patients with familial adenomatous polyposis, an autosomal dominant disorder characterised by colonic polyposis, also develop gastric and duodenal polyps and sessile adenomas which can undergo malignant transformation. Hyperplastic polyps are generally small (<1.0 cm in diameter) and multiple. They are found incidentally, do not cause symptoms and do not undergo malignant transformation.

Peutz–Jehger's syndrome is a rare, autosomal dominant disorder characterised by the development of hamartomatous polyps through the gastrointestinal tract in association with melanin pigmentation on the lips, buccal mucosa, hands and feet. The polyps may be of sufficient size to cause intestinal obstruction due to intussusception, or anaemia due to blood loss. The polyps have no malignant potential.

POSTGASTRIC SURGERY SEQUELAE

Operations on the stomach and its nerve supply alter the anatomy of the upper gastrointestinal tract and alter gastric motility and the control of gastric emptying. Postgastrectomy and postvagotomy syndromes (Table 25.4) are the product of these changes in anatomy and physiology. Common syndromes include:

- alkaline reflux gastritis
- early and late dumping syndrome
- diarrhoea
- delayed gastric emptying
- nutritional deficiencies.

Between 10% and 25% of patients having such surgery will be aware of some disability. The degree of disability tends to fade with time and, almost invariably, it is wise to allow at least 1 year after operation to pass before any decisions regarding re-operation are made. The various syndromes which may occur can at times be difficult to diagnose and even more difficult to treat successfully.

Table 25.4 Postgastrectomy and postvagotomy syndromes

Alkaline reflux gastritis
Dumping syndromes
— early dumping
— late dumping
Postvagotomy diarrhoea
Delayed gastric emptying
— gastric atony
— Roux stasis syndrome
Afferent loop syndrome
Nutritional deficiencies
— maldigestion/malabsorption
— anaemia
— bone disease

The keys to management are careful assessment based on history and investigations, and a treatment programme strongly biased towards non-operative measures.

ALKALINE REFLUX GASTRITIS

This problem arises after gastrectomy of the Billroth I or Billroth II type, or after drainage procedures such as pyloroplasty or loop gastrojejunostomy. Uncontrolled reflux or transit of duodenal and pancreatic fluids into the stomach exposes the gastric mucosa to a number of well known irritants such as bile acids and lysolecithin. Endoscopic examination of the gastric mucosa after a gastrectomy will generally reveal bile reflux-associated gastritis. However, significant symptoms occur in less than 10% of patients. The clinical syndrome is of burning epigastric pain, nausea, and bilious vomiting.

The diagnosis can be established from the clinical picture and the endoscopic findings. Medical therapy is usually ineffective. Binding of bile acids with cholestyramine or aluminium hydroxide may give partial relief and serves to support the diagnosis. Operative diversion of the bile and pancreatic fluids from the stomach or gastric remnant is required for patients with ongoing significant symptoms. A Roux-en-Y gastrojejunostomy (see Fig. 25.4C) of at least 45 cm in length is used and can be expected to give satisfactory control of the symptoms in 75% of patients. This condition represents an unusual situation in postgastric surgery syndromes in that the surgical therapy has a predictably good outcome.

DUMPING SYNDROME

This syndrome, which derives its name from the observation of rapid gastric emptying, is characterised by postprandial gastrointestinal and vasomotor symptoms. The gastrointestinal symptoms include epigastric fullness, cramping abdominal pains, nausea, vomiting, and explosive diarrhoea. The vasomotor symptoms include profuse sweating, weakness, dizziness, flushing, palpitations and a strong desire to lie down. Dumping is classified into early and late forms. In early dumping, the symptoms typically start within 30 minutes of ingestion of a meal and patients suffer a mixture of the gastrointestinal and vasomotor complaints. By contrast, late dumping occurs 2–3 hours after a meal and generally exhibits the vasomotor symptoms alone.

Early dumping arises from rapid emptying of hyperosmolar gastric content into the small bowel, leading to a large shift of fluid from the intravascular space into the lumen of the gut. The fluid shift, if sufficiently severe, leads to relative hypovolaemia and the vasomotor symptoms. The rapid distension of the bowel from this fluid generates the gastrointestinal symptoms.

Late dumping is thought to arise as a consequence of the delivery of high concentrations of carbohydrate into the proximal gut. Rapid glucose absorption leads to excessive insulin release which causes a reactive hypoglycaemia. The mechanism for excessive insulin release is unclear and other gut hormones may well contribute.

Disabling symptoms occur in less than 5% of patients. The syndrome is most unusual after highly selective vagotomy in which controlled rate of gastric emptying is preserved. It probably has a higher frequency in patients after resectional procedures than after vagotomy and drainage procedures.

POSTVAGOTOMY DIARRHOEA

Diarrhoea is a common sequel to many abdominal procedures. It typically fades away over the first few postoperative months and is generally not incapacitating, being neither urgent nor offensive. Patients should be investigated for:

- bacterial overgrowth
- antibiotic-associated colitis
- obstruction
- inflammatory bowel disease
- parasites
- malabsorption.

In some postvagotomy patients however, the diarrhoea can be persistent and it may be severely incapacitating in

1–2%. The condition is characterised by the frequent and sometimes explosive passage of watery stools with urgency. The bouts of diarrhoea tend to be episodic, several days of explosive diarrhoea being followed by weeks or months of normal bowel pattern. The condition may coexist with dumping syndrome.

DELAYED GASTRIC EMPTYING

A transient phase of delayed gastric emptying is relatively common after all gastric procedures but will generally resolve over a 3–4 week period. Gastric stasis beyond that postoperative period generally indicates the presence of gastric atony. In those patients in whom a Roux-en-Y gastrojejunostomy has been formed, a specific Roux stasis syndrome is possible.

Gastric atony is associated with rapid liquid but delayed solid emptying. The clinical syndrome is of nausea, vomiting of food, epigastric pain, abdominal distension, weight loss and altered bowel habits.

Investigations should include endoscopy to exclude a mechanical obstruction, and scintographic studies after ingestion of a radiolabelled solid meal. Prokinetic agents such as metoclopramide, cisapride, domperidone and erythromycin have been used with variable, but generally limited, success. For intractable gastric stasis, near-total or total gastrectomy may become necessary.

AFFERENT LOOP SYNDROME

This condition is generated by mechanical obstruction after a Polya type reconstruction. If it occurs in the early postoperative phase, catastrophic complications, including blow-out of the duodenal stump, may occur. It can, however, become evident as a chronic problem and generally arises because of a poorly constructed afferent loop with angulation at the anastomosis or with excessive length or by obstruction from extrinsic bands. The clinical syndrome is of postprandial abdominal pain and nausea followed later, at a variable time, by vomiting of food mixed with bile and immediate relief. This specific sequence is diagnostic and signals drainage of the distended afferent loop.

NUTRITIONAL DISORDERS

Any form of gastric surgery is liable to modify appetite and promote early satiety, and may modify digestion and absorption. For patients suffering postgastrectomy syndromes, the wish to avoid symptoms may lead to marked reduction of intake of food. Others may suffer specific disorders of digestion and absorption. Common problems after gastric procedures include:

- loss of weight
- early satiety
- iron deficiency
- vitamin B_{12} deficiency
- osteoporosis
- osteomalacia.

Maldigestion and malabsorption

Operations in which part or all of the stomach is resected or in which the controlled emptying of the stomach is destroyed are associated with increased steatorrhoea. Generally this is the consequence of maldigestion in the intestinal lumen because of rapid gastric emptying, loss of coordination between gastric emptying and pancreatic and other digestive enzyme release, and failure of the stomach to pass on only particles of food of less than 1 mm in diameter. Sequestration of pancreatic and biliary secretions may occur within an afferent loop. Stasis in the afferent loop permits bacterial overgrowth with consequent deconjugation of bile acids further impairing fat absorption.

Anaemia

At long-term follow-up after gastrectomy, up to two-thirds of patients will demonstrate at least moderate anaemia. Except for total gastrectomy, where vitamin B_{12} deficiency and consequent pernicious anaemia is inevitable without replacement therapy, the usual pattern is of an iron deficiency anaemia with secondary evidence of B_{12} deficiency in some patients.

Bone disease

Resectional procedures of the stomach accelerate the process of bone demineralisation that occurs with age in the normal population. Postvagotomy patients without resection do not appear to have this accelerated path. Both osteoporosis and osteomalacia are evident on bone biopsies. The mechanisms for this accelerated process are unclear. Reduced intake, relative lactase insufficiency as a result of duodenal bypass, rapid upper gastrointestinal transit and malabsorption of the fat-soluble vitamin D

have all been proposed. Frequency of pathological fractures has been noted in multiple studies to be at least three times higher than in control subjects. Screening for osteomalacia by measurement of serum alkaline phosphatase has been proposed. Calcium and vitamin D replacement in such patients would then be appropriate.

MISCELLANEOUS CONDITIONS

GASTRITIS

There are multiple form of gastritis, each of which has characteristic features.

Chronic gastritis

This is the commonest form, affecting 30–50% of the population. It is associated with *H. pylori* in the gastric antral mucosa. Generally there are no symptoms or only a non-specific dyspepsia. The condition is most efficiently diagnosed by endoscopy. However, neither diagnosis nor treatment of *H. pylori* is indicated unless significant symptoms are present.

Acute erosive gastritis

This type of gastritis results from acute exogenous injury to the gastric mucosa, most commonly by ethanol or NSAIDs. Multiple small erosions are present in the body and fundus of the stomach and may generate clinically apparent GI bleeding. Withdrawal of the injurious agent only is required for resolution.

Acute haemorrhagic gastritis – stress ulcers

This disease occurs in the critically ill, usually with hypotension or sepsis, and is characterised by major GI haemorrhage from diffuse fundic erosions. It arises from a failure of gastric mucosal defences to cope with normal amounts of acid in the gastric lumen and is almost totally prevented by maintaining the pH of gastric fluid above 4.0, preferably by administration of antacids.

Alkaline reflux gastritis

Gastric surgery reduces gastric acidity and allows free reflux of duodenal fluids, including bile, into the stomach. The gastritis produced is one of the postgastric surgery syndromes.

Chronic atrophic gastritis

This autoimmune disease is characterised by the generation of antibody against the acid-secreting cells of the stomach, failure of ileal absorption of vitamin B_{12} due to absence of intrinsic factor from the gastric fundus, subsequent pernicious anaemia and an increased risk of gastric cancer.

Hypertrophic gastritis – Menetrier's disease

This condition is characterised by the presence of giant gastric rugal folds and hypoalbuminaemia, and on histology there is marked elongation and tortuosity of the gastric pits with atrophy of the gastric glands.

ZOLLINGER–ELLISON SYNDROME

This syndrome consists of the triad of hypersecretion of gastric acid, severe peptic ulcer disease and the presence of non-beta islet cell tumours in the pancreas or duodenum. In one-quarter, it is part of the multiple endocrine neoplasia I syndrome (MEN). Ulceration is usually in the first part of the duodenum but may be present in the oesophagus, the stomach, the distal duodenum and even the jejunum. Diagnosis is based on the demonstration of a marked elevation of the serum gastrin levels. Treatment options include inhibition of acid secretion, excision of the tumour or total gastrectomy (see p. 197).

FURTHER READING

Ozmen M M, Patankar R, Johnson C D 1996 Helicobacter pylori: an update for surgeons. In: Johnson C D, Taylor I (eds) Recent advances in surgery 19. Churchill Livingstone, Edinburgh, p 61–77

Scott H W, Sawyers J L 1987 Surgery of the stomach, duodenum and small intestines. Blackwell Science, Boston

Wyeth J W, Pounder R 1994 Peptic ulcer. In: Pounder R (ed) Recent advances in gastroenterology 10. Churchill Livingstone, Edinburgh

26

Gallstones
Robin Williamson

OVERVIEW

Gallstones are one of the commonest abdominal conditions. They generally arise from a metabolic defect within the liver. Although many calculi are clinically 'silent', they can give rise to a wide range of problems including obstruction and infection of the gall bladder and biliary tree, acute pancreatitis and occasionally carcinoma of the gall bladder. Ultrasound scan is the mainstay of diagnosis. Symptomatic gallstones should be removed by means of cholecystectomy since the gall bladder is damaged by their presence. Nowadays most cholecystectomies are carried out by the laparoscopic approach, though an open operation may still be required in the presence of complications.

PATHOGENESIS

Non-malignant disease of the biliary tree is almost exclusively caused by the presence of gallstones. The formation of gallstones depends upon:

- secretion of lithogenic bile, i.e. bile which is supersaturated with cholesterol
- the occurrence of sepsis in the biliary tree
- anatomical abnormalities that predispose to stasis
- abnormalities of the gall bladder epithelium.

LITHOGENIC BILE

Cholesterol is 'solubilised' in bile as a micelle with lecithin (phospholipid) and bile salts. Only when the appropriate ratios of lecithin and bile salts are present will cholesterol remain in solution and be prevented from forming crystals (Fig. 26.1).

Metabolic abnormalities in the liver predispose to the secretion of lithogenic bile. Such abnormalities may be either inborn or conditioned by diet. Of the two, dietary factors seem more likely, and the 'Western' type of high-protein, high-fat diet has been incriminated. Other contributory factors are:

- the contraceptive pill
- pregnancy
- obesity
- low-residue diet with inadequate fibre
- loss of terminal ileum, which interrupts the enterohepatic circulation of bile salts.

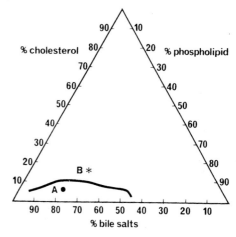

Fig. 26.1 The lipid composition of bile. The curve represents the maximum solubility of cholesterol. **A:** normal composition; **B:** 'lithogenic' bile supersaturated with cholesterol.

SEPSIS

The liver is thought to be constantly trapping small numbers of organisms from the portal or systemic blood. Some of these organisms may be excreted in the bile, and if they find an appropriate nidus (cholesterol crystals, mucus, epithelial debris) they will persist and proliferate. Local multiplication of organisms may then deconjugate and precipitate bile salts so that a 'mixed' stone results. Sepsis in a biliary tree that contains stones may cause bouts of:

- acute cholecystitis (gall bladder infection)
- acute ('ascending') cholangitis (bile duct infection).

A special form of sepsis is seen in the Far East, where primary common bile duct (CBD) stones (which are associated with precipitation of bile salts and pigment rather than with cholesterol deposition) give rise to severe ascending cholangitis, so-called oriental cholangiohepatitis. Extensive damage to the liver is common. The liver fluke *Clonorchis sinensis* is frequently present in the duct (as are roundworms occasionally), but its role in causation is uncertain.

ANATOMICAL ABNORMALITIES

The biliary tree is characterised by a remarkable frequency of anatomical variants and anomalies, which can make biliary operations difficult and occasionally hazardous. Any cul-de-sac or incompletely drained branch of the tree predisposes to sepsis and stone formation.

ABNORMALITIES OF THE GALL BLADDER EPITHELIUM

It is uncertain whether abnormalities of the gall bladder epithelium are primary or secondary. However, proliferation and detachment of cholesterol-laden epithelium may again form the starting point of a stone, as in the condition of cholesterosis of the gall bladder.

CLINICAL SYNDROMES

ASYMPTOMATIC STONES

The majority of gallstones are asymptomatic: 10–15% of all individuals over the age of 60 years in Western communities have gallstones, usually in a functioning gall bladder. Stones may be found during routine investiga-tions. If they occur in a functioning gall bladder there is no pressing indication to remove them. However, stones in a non-functioning gall bladder or in the common duct are very likely to cause trouble in the future and, other things being equal, are an indication for operation. Once symptoms develop, they tend to recur.

DYSPEPSIA

Gallstones predominantly produce episodic acute or sub-acute syndromes characterised by pain. Contrary to popular opinion, there is no evidence to support the idea that they are associated with fatty food intolerance or 'flatulent dyspepsia'. However, an acute attack of obstruction/infection can be precipitated by a fatty meal, presumably because the release of cholecystokinin causes forcible contraction against a potential or actual obstruction.

STONES WITHOUT INFECTION

Stones in the gall bladder present with attacks of 'biliary colic'. Stones in the main bile duct (common hepatic duct or common bile duct) can cause obstructive jaundice with or without pain. Stones or even small crystals passing down the bile duct and lodging at the papilla may precipitate acute pancreatitis (see Ch. 27).

Obstruction of the cystic duct without sepsis leads to distension of the gall bladder. Unlike acute appendicitis, the condition does not commonly progress to ischaemia and rupture of the wall, because one of the following occurs:

- the condition is self-limiting, the stone falling back into the fundus of the gall bladder as distension takes place
- a mucocele develops (i.e. gall bladder distended with mucus).

The clinical syndrome is called *biliary colic*. There is acute pain in the epigastrium and/or right hypochondrium, which may radiate to the back or right shoulder. Although called colic, the pain is more characteristically of distension type, rising rapidly to a peak and then persisting with little change for some hours or even a day or two. There is reflex nausea and often vomiting. Physical signs are limited because there is little transmural inflammation to generate peritoneal irritation. A mucocele may be palpable as a slightly tender globular mass protruding from under the right costal margin. Calculous obstruction of the common hepatic or common bile duct without sepsis is relatively uncommon, occurring mainly in primary common duct stones. Intermittent or unrelenting jaundice with mild pain of distension type is the rule (see p. 264).

STONES WITH INFECTION

Obstruction of the cystic duct with sepsis leads to acute cholecystitis (see below). The process does resemble acute obstructive appendicitis in many ways but again tends to be self-limiting. Macroscopically the gall bladder becomes inflamed on its serosal aspect; omentum and bowel may adhere, and the junction of cystic duct and common hepatic duct becomes involved in an inflammatory mass of varying density. On the internal aspect, varying degrees of mucosal ulceration take place. The sequelae may be:

- Resolution with or without episodic recurrence.
- Progression to gangrene and perforation, usually in the fundus but occasionally at the neck because of ulceration of a stone. Perforation may be:
  — local with abscess formation
  — into the peritoneal cavity
  — into a neighbouring viscus, most commonly the duodenum.
- 'Chronic cholecystitis', which is a pathological rather than a clinical entity.
- Empyema of the gall bladder – an intact wall but an intraluminal abscess, which can produce a varying amount of systemic disturbance and may occasionally progress to perforation.

Other clinicopathological associations of acute cholecystitis are:

- jaundice
- gallstone ileus.

Partial obstruction of the bile duct by a calculus lodged in Hartmann's pouch (the dilated neck of the gall bladder) with surrounding inflammation can cause a limited degree of *jaundice*. Jaundice can also result from a more generalised infective process involving the axial biliary tree.

Gallstone ileus follows perforation into the gastrointestinal tract with escape of a stone, which is then propelled down the small bowel to impact usually in the terminal ileum. Low small bowel obstruction ensues. The obstruction is incomplete, making this unusual condition difficult to diagnose. Plain abdominal X-ray shows dilated small bowel loops, air in the biliary tree and sometimes the obstructing calculus.

ACUTE CHOLECYSTITIS

HISTORY

Previous attacks of gallstone disease with upper abdominal pain have commonly been experienced.

SYMPTOMS

Pain. This is usually of sudden onset and severe in nature. At first it is situated centrally, but thereafter beneath the right costal margin and radiating to the back to the angle of the scapula. The pain may first be colicky, indicating the stage of obstruction of the cystic duct or neck of the gall bladder. Occasionally the attacks stop short at this stage, while progression to acute cholecystitis is associated with more constant and throbbing pain.

Vomiting and nausea. These are common but most often mild in nature.

SIGNS

General

Pyrexia and tachycardia are indicative of the infective nature of the process.

Local

Tenderness over the gall bladder is a constant sign. It is the presence of fever and tenderness that distinguishes acute cholecystitis from biliary colic.

Guarding and rigidity indicate involvement by the inflammatory process of the parietal peritoneum adjacent to the gall bladder. More generalised abdominal rigidity indicates that perforation has probably occurred and that the process has certainly spread beyond the limits of the gall bladder.

A palpable mass of globular proportions extending beneath the right costal margin and moving with respiration is due either to a pericholecystic collection of omentum and adjacent viscera or to an empyema of the gall bladder.

Murphy's sign is positive if the patient complains of pain on taking a deep breath while a hand is placed below the right costal margin and pressed onto the gall bladder fundus. This is merely a special way of testing for peritoneal irritation.

SPECIAL TESTS

Plain X-ray. An abdominal plain film may show radio-opaque calculi or a soft tissue mass in the region of the gall bladder. Occasionally there is evidence of small bowel or large bowel distension. The investigation is also advisable to exclude a renal or upper ureteric calculus causing pyonephrosis, the clinical features of which may closely resemble those of acute cholecystitis.

Urine and serum tests. The white cell count is raised. Serum bilirubin may be elevated, even without clinical jaundice, and bilirubin may be detected on urine testing. Serum amylase estimations are indicated if acute pancreatitis is considered an alternative diagnosis. Marked elevation of amylase occurs in acute pancreatitis, but moderate levels may be seen with cholecystitis and other abdominal conditions.

Ultrasound. This is the least expensive and least invasive test. Not only will it demonstrate abnormality of the gall bladder and common bile duct but, in expert hands, it can also give information about the liver and pancreas. For these reasons it has become the first-line investigation in biliary colic and acute cholecystitis. A stone may be seen, identified by the 'acoustic shadow' behind it; the gall bladder wall may be thickened, and there is often some fluid around the gall bladder.

Isotope excretion (HIDA) scan. This is a sensitive and also very specific test for demonstrating failure of the gall bladder to fill, but it requires adequate liver function plus the availability of a gamma camera.

Computed tomography (CT). Not a routine test for gallstones, CT scans may detect early calcification or show an inflammatory mass in severe acute cholecystitis.

DIFFERENTIAL DIAGNOSIS

Extra-abdominal

Myocardial infarction and acute right-sided lung conditions may offer some difficulty. Apart from obtaining a careful history and making a thorough examination, a chest X-ray and electrocardiograph should help. However, electrocardiographic abnormalities are not uncommon in elderly patients with biliary disease.

Abdominal

Acute appendicitis. A high retrocaecal appendix may cause concern, especially in a short thick-set person. If there is no suggestion of past gall bladder disease and there is a lack of characteristic radiation of pain, then the diagnosis may only be made at operation.

Perforated duodenal ulcer. This is now less often confused with cholecystitis because of the availability of the tests outlined above. A partly sealed perforation may cause diagnostic difficulty.

Acute pancreatitis. A constant boring pain with backache and a raised serum amylase help to differentiate this condition from cholecystitis, though the two may coexist.

Hepatic disease. Hepatic enlargement from viral hepatitis or cardiac failure causes a dragging pain in the right hypochondrium. Pyogenic infection (abscess) of the liver may be demonstrated by isotope liver scan or ultrasound.

TREATMENT

The treatment of acute cholecystitis is generally cholecystectomy. The timing of operation should be urgent, early or delayed, depending on the symptoms, as follows.

The operation is *urgent* if there are severe constitutional symptoms or local peritonitis suggesting empyema, gangrene or perforation of the gall bladder. Laparotomy should follow a short period of resuscitation.

The operation should be carried out *early* in the majority of cases. The acute inflammation is treated, the diagnosis is confirmed by ultrasonography and the operation is performed on the next available list. The policy of early cholecystectomy has largely superseded the tradition of delayed (interval) cholecystectomy, which risks a further attack of acute cholecystitis during the one-to-two period of waiting.

The operation should be *delayed* only if the attack settles and there is uncertainty about the diagnosis requiring a period of detailed investigation.

The initial *management* includes the following:

- intravenous fluids and nil (or fluids only) by mouth
- pain relief by parenteral opiate administration, provided this is carefully controlled to avoid masking of signs
- antibiotics are used in a short intensive course for 3–5 days, but they may damp down infection rather than abolish it.

Progress is judged generally by frequent observations of pulse, blood pressure, temperature and white cell count, and locally by frequent palpation of the right hypochondrium for tenderness and guarding.

Operation is indicated if:

- fever does not settle within 24–36 hours
- other systemic signs such as tachycardia and leucocytosis persist
- local tenderness or guarding remains unchanged or becomes worse
- cardiac, respiratory or combined cardiorespiratory problems are making management difficult. The additional demands thrown on the cardiorespiratory system by a large inflamed area are an indication for operation if there is limited reserve. Such patients are not too ill to undergo an operation but are too ill to do without one.

The nature of the operation is dictated by the clinical circumstances. If the biliary anatomy can be clearly identified and the patient is in good general condition, cholecystectomy is appropriate and such additional procedures as are judged necessary.

If the biliary anatomy is obscured by gross local inflammation and/or the patient is in poor general condition, cholecystostomy – drainage of the gall bladder – is followed at a later date by cholecystectomy. Nowadays, cholecystostomy can be performed by percutaneous intubation under ultrasound control, avoiding the need for general anaesthesia in a high-risk patient.

Subtotal cholecystectomy, leaving the neck of the gall bladder and sometimes its posterior wall, is an alternative to cholecystostomy in a difficult case; no further operation is needed thereafter.

ACALCULOUS ACUTE CHOLECYSTITIS

Approximately 10% of attacks of acute cholecystitis develop in the absence of gallstones. Acalculous cholecystitis can arise spontaneously, but it often occurs in a patient in the intensive therapy unit who has undergone recent major trauma or surgery and who may be septic. Biliary tract stasis may be contributory, resulting from opiates and parenteral nutrition. Fever and dehydration increase the viscosity of bile. It is unclear whether bacterial infection plays a primary or secondary role.

The clinical features of fever and local tenderness may be overshadowed by the concomitant illness or may be masked by sedation. A high index of clinical suspicion is required to make the diagnosis, which can be confirmed by ultrasound evidence of gall bladder dilatation and thickening of the wall. There is a major risk of gangrene and perforation of the gall bladder, which explains why the mortality rate of acute acalculous cholecystitis (approximately 15%) is 2–3 times higher than that of acute calculous cholecystitis. Rare variants of this disease are acute emphysematous cholecystitis (caused by gas-forming organisms) and torsion of the gall bladder (usually seen in elderly patients with visceroptosis).

CHOLECYSTECTOMY

INDICATIONS

Cholecystectomy is one of the commonest abdominal operations. It is indicated for the following conditions:

- symptomatic gall bladder stones
- acute cholecystitis, whether calculous or acalculous
- polyps or tumours of the gall bladder
- in selected patients with typical biliary pain in whom repeated tests fail to show gallstones.

It should be noted, however, that *carcinoma of the gall bladder* is seldom diagnosed at a resectable stage. In Western countries, almost all gall bladder cancers are associated with long-standing gallstones. There may be calcification of the wall of the gall bladder ('porcelain gall bladder', Fig. 26.2).

For patients with typical biliary pain in whom repeated tests fail to show gallstones, the gall bladder may show poor contraction with a fatty meal (or cholecystokinin injection) when visualised by ultrasonography or oral cholecystography. Some of the gall bladders removed in such cases will show cholesterosis ('strawberry gall bladder'), adenomyosis (diverticulosis) or chronic acalculous cholecystitis, in which case the operation may be curative.

ALTERNATIVE TREATMENTS

Dissolution therapy

This is occasionally indicated in unfit patients with radi-

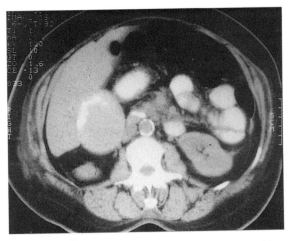

Fig. 26.2 CT scan showing calcification in the gall bladder wall of an elderly woman. The woman had developed carcinoma of the gall bladder after many years of symptomatic gallstones.

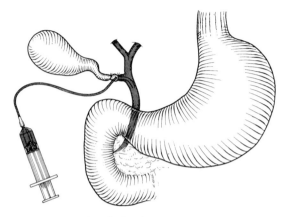

Fig. 26.3 Operative cholangiogram.

olucent calculi in a functioning gall bladder. Prolonged bile salt therapy is needed, e.g. with ursodeoxycholic acid, and there is a high recurrence rate.

Extracorporeal shock-wave lithotripsy

Expensive machines can be used to generate shock waves which are focused into the gall bladder and pulverise the stones. Generally no anaesthetic is required but, as with dissolution therapy, the cystic duct must be patent for clearance of the stones.

Percutaneous extraction or dissolution

Under ultrasound scan the gall bladder is punctured trans-hepatically and a catheter is inserted. The radiologist can then dilate up the track and insert instruments to extract the stones. Alternatively, methyl tert butyl ether can be instilled to dissolve them.

Each of these techniques has its own limitations, and all suffer from the drawback that the diseased gall bladder is retained with a strong potential to re-form calculi.

TECHNIQUES

Open cholecystectomy

The traditional and tested method involves opening the abdomen through an oblique subcostal or transverse or paramedian incision. The fundus of the gall bladder is

grasped to steady the organ. Careful dissection identifies the borders of Calot's triangle: cystic artery, cystic duct and common bile duct. Because of the association of ductal calculi (see below) in 10–20% of cases, routine *operative cholangiography* (Fig. 26.3) is performed by cannulating the cystic duct; these films also help to display the biliary anatomy and may reduce the risk of injury to the common duct. If filling defects are seen in the bile duct or if the main duct is dilated and fails to empty, the surgeon should proceed to explore the duct. Otherwise the cystic artery and cystic duct are ligated, and the gall bladder is peeled away from the liver.

Laparoscopic cholecystectomy

During the last decade, this technique has been introduced and has proved so popular that in most centres it is now preferred for the majority of patients needing cholecystectomy. Instead of one relatively long incision, there are four or five tiny incisions to allow introduction of the laparoscope and necessary operating instruments (see Ch. 9). The first stage is to create an adequate pneumoperitoneum using carbon dioxide gas rapidly instilled through a Verres' needle. The use of a miniature video camera allows a clear and magnified view of the operating field on a video screen. The great advantages of the laparoscopic procedure lie in the increased patient comfort, the minimal physiological disturbance and the reduction in hospital stay (usually not to exceed 24 hours). As with any new operative technique, there is an increased risk of technical errors during the surgeon's learning curve. One other slight drawback is that satisfactory operative cholangiograms are more difficult to obtain.

Minicholecystectomy

This variant of the open operation employs a very short (5–7 cm) transverse incision in the right upper quadrant. The gall bladder is dissected 'fundus first' using narrow retractors to provide adequate exposure. Although it is quite a difficult technique, it can produce results similar to those of laparoscopic cholecystectomy in terms of minimal postoperative pain and a speedy recovery.

COMPLICATIONS

Cholecystectomy has an excellent safety record with an operative mortality rate of less than 1% for elective cases. Complications include wound haematoma and sepsis and a collection of bile, blood or pus in the subhepatic space, which may need to be evacuated by percutaneous drainage. The most serious complications are bile leakage and injury causing stricture to the main bile duct.

Bile leaks may occur from the raw surface of the liver, in which case they are usually trivial and dry up after a few days. More profuse leakage stems from a slipped cystic duct ligature or an injury to the right or common hepatic duct. Occasionally bile may leak in substantial quantities following removal of a T-tube. The bile leak will usually be apparent in the form of an external biliary fistula, and if this persists radiological investigation is required – fistulography, PTC or ERCP as circumstances dictate. If no drain was inserted at operation or if it was removed prematurely, the patient may present with right upper quadrant pain and fever. Ultrasound scan may confirm a subhepatic collection that requires percutaneous drainage, thereby creating an external biliary fistula but relieving the patient's symptoms. Unless the fistula resolves with endoscopic sphincterotomy and/or stenting, re-operation is likely to be needed.

Bile duct stricture results from accidental ligature of one of the main ducts or from a laceration or complete transection of the duct that has been inexpertly repaired. The injury should be suspected if the patient develops postoperative jaundice with or without an external biliary fistula. This is a potentially catastrophic complication of cholecystectomy that can give rise to repeated and disabling attacks of acute cholangitis, sometimes ending in secondary biliary cirrhosis and portal hypertension. The best hope of avoiding this sequence lies in a careful repair carried out by an expert surgeon using a Roux loop of jejunum to anastomose to healthy proximal duct (see p. 266).

POST-CHOLECYSTECTOMY SYMPTOMS

Some patients fail to gain relief from their abdominal pain or dyspepsia following cholecystectomy. Possible explanations include the following.

Wrong diagnosis. Other abdominal conditions such as peptic ulcer disease, hiatus hernia and irritable bowel syndrome can produce symptoms that closely mimic those of cholelithiasis. The surgeon should resist the temptation to remove a gall bladder containing stones if the symptoms are atypical, at least not before conducting a full gastrointestinal investigation.

Retained bile duct stones. If no operative cholangiogram has been performed or post-exploratory films were omitted or are inadequate, this diagnosis should be suspected – especially if the patient develops jaundice. Occasionally stones will re-form in the bile duct, especially in the presence of chronic stasis. ERCP is the investigation of choice, and endoscopic sphincterotomy should deal with the problem of residual or recurrent ductal calculi. Following an open exploration of the bile duct, if the postoperative T-tube cholangiogram shows a retained stone, the tube should be left in place for 6 weeks to allow a mature track to form. Thereafter, the T-tube is removed and the stones are extracted under radiological control using a steerable catheter inserted along the T-tube track.

Pancreatic or papillary disease. Papillary fibrosis and minor degrees of chronic pancreatitis can produce pain that is indistinguishable from that of gallstones. ERCP may clinch the correct diagnosis. Endoscopic sphincterotomy or surgical sphincteroplasty can be successful in selected cases.

CHOLEDOCHOLITHIASIS AND CHOLANGITIS

SURGICAL PATHOLOGY

Most stones in the common bile duct have originated in the gall bladder; less commonly they arise in the intrahepatic ducts or common bile duct. These primary ductal stones are either black or brown in colour and are often crumbly.

Stones less than a few millimetres in diameter may be passed with or without the production of biliary colic. However, larger stones may cause a ball-valve obstruction in the distal common bile duct, while occasionally a stone may be impacted in the lower end of the duct and result in continuous obstruction. The association between ductal stones and acute pancreatitis is considered in Chapter 27.

After prolonged obstruction, the common bile duct dilates. Later infection may supervene with thickening of the duct wall and mucosal ulceration and, in cases of severe and prolonged obstruction, cholangitis can result in intrahepatic abscess formation.

When partial obstruction of the common bile duct occurs, ascending cholangitis can lead to secondary biliary cirrhosis, liver failure and portal hypertension (see 'bile duct stricture', p. 265).

CLINICAL FEATURES

Choledocholithiasis usually presents with jaundice. Fever occurs when the bile is infected. The triad of right upper quadrant pain, shaking chills and jaundice is characteristic of duct stones and was first described by Charcot. These three features of acute cholangitis do not always coexist.

Symptoms

Pain is usually colicky in nature and situated in the right hypochondrium; it often radiates through the back.

Jaundice is present if a stone is causing partial or complete obstruction of the bile duct. Jaundice is nearly always preceded by biliary colic and, when a ball-valve type of obstruction exists, the jaundice will tend to fluctuate from day to day; it will also be associated with pruritus, dark urine and pale stools (see Ch. 27 for a more general discussion of jaundice).

Fever is often associated with shaking attacks or rigors. The fever is intermittent in type, occurring every few days with exacerbation of pain and jaundice. The organism involved is usually *E. coli*, and sometimes the cholangitis is so severe that septicaemia results, with shock, vomiting and dehydration. Indeed, biliary sepsis is one of the commonest causes of Gram-negative septicaemia.

Signs

General. Patients present with fever plus weight loss, if jaundice has been present for a prolonged period. Jaundice is variable in degree.

Local. There is tenderness in the right hypochondrium.

SPECIAL TESTS

Serum bilirubin is elevated. Serum alkaline phosphatase is usually raised. Other liver function tests, including serum transaminase estimations, may indicate associated liver cell damage. Blood cultures and white cell counts are important when cholangitis is suspected.

Ultrasound scan may demonstrate dilatation of the bile duct and stones, but a stone at the lower end of the duct is quite often missed. Percutaneous transhepatic cholangiography (PTC) or endoscopic retrograde cholangiopancreatography (ERCP) will show the degree of dilatation and site of stones (see Ch. 27).

Oral cholecystography and intravenous cholangiography are of no value in the presence of jaundice.

DIFFERENTIAL DIAGNOSIS

Episodes of pain, fever and jaundice are typical of choledocholithiasis. However, in the absence of pain and fever, other causes of cholestatic jaundice must be considered and the appropriate investigations pursued (see Ch. 27).

MANAGEMENT

The initial management of acute symptomatic choledocholithiasis is supportive with:

- fluid and electrolyte replacement
- antibiotics if ascending cholangitis is present
- frequent reassessment of clinical state.

Urgent removal of the stone or stones in the CBD is called for if there is unabating cholangitis, with high fever, positive blood culture and systemic disturbance despite the above measures. There is less urgency in the patient with obstructive jaundice, but even here delay should not be allowed as damage to the liver parenchyma may follow prolonged obstruction, so making operations more dangerous.

Methods of removing the stones

Until recently, open operation was the only way of removing the stones. Now developments in endoscopy may permit removal after endoscopic incision of the papilla.

Endoscopic removal (ERCP with sphincterotomy). This should be considered in patients who present a very poor operative risk and cannot be improved in the short term. The technique is particularly popular in patients over the age of 70 years, in whom clearance of the duct may be followed by prolonged freedom from trouble, even though a diseased gall bladder remains in situ. The papilla is cut with a diathermy wire, and the stones either are expelled spontaneously or can be removed with the aid of a balloon catheter. Stones up to 2–2.5 cm in diameter can be extracted in this way, and the overall success rate is over 90%. There is a risk of acute cholangitis after endoscopic papillotomy unless the duct is cleared of stones or a nasobiliary catheter is left in situ.

Open operation. This is still appropriate in younger and fitter patients or where endoscopic expertise is not available. It must consist of:

1. Removal of the gall bladder and its contained stones.
2. Adequate duct exploration. It is sometimes necessary to open the duodenum and incise the papilla to achieve this (transduodenal sphincteroplasty).
3. Drainage of the biliary tree by a T-tube in the common bile duct – this is necessary to avoid leakage from a choledochotomy because of oedema at the lower end of the duct (Fig. 26.4).
4. In a patient with multiple ductal stones and/or stenosis at the papilla, consideration must be given to permanent drainage of the bile duct. Either the papilla is widened by means of transduodenal sphincteroplasty, or a side-to-side bypass is fashioned between the dilated bile duct and the duodenum (choledochoduodenostomy).

Postoperative management

This is the same as for any major abdominal procedure. There are special problems with jaundice (see Ch. 27) and management of the T-tube, which should not be removed until 8–10 days have elapsed. By this time, the patient's general condition should be satisfactory, bile drainage will be clear and non-infected and a postoperative T-tube cholangiogram will have been obtained to

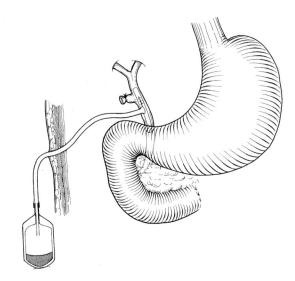

Fig. 26.4 T-tube drainage of the common bile duct.

ensure that there are no residual stones in the common bile duct or hepatic radicles.

BILE DUCT STRICTURE

TYPES OF STRICTURE

There are two forms:

- congenital
- acquired.

Congenital biliary atresia is a rare condition in which the ducts fail to develop either locally or in a widespread way thoughout the liver substance. It must be considered in the diagnosis of jaundice early in life. Sometimes the condition can be put right by simple operation, but usually it requires more complex surgery; extensive forms of the condition require liver transplantation.

Acquired stricture is often the result of a surgical accident during cholecystectomy. The causes are:

- failure to appreciate biliary tract anomalies
- anatomy that just cannot be unravelled at operation because of acute inflammation or chronic fibrosis
- surgical inexperience (especially in the presence of severe cholecystitis)
- haemorrhage with blind clamping.

There are other uncommon causes of bile duct stricture:

- *primary carcinoma of the bile duct*, i.e. cholangiocarcinoma
- *sclerosing cholangitis* – an ill-defined entity that may

be related to either 'true' inflammatory disease or malignancy. Both types are occasionally associated with ulcerative colitis. Secondary sclerosing cholangitis can complicate intrahepatic gallstones or iatrogenic strictures of the bile duct.

CLINICAL FEATURES

Iatrogenic stricture

Bile duct trauma may present as follows:

- At operation (see p. 263).
- Early postoperative:
  — a persistent discharge of large amounts of bile through a wound or a drainage tube indicates some loss of continuity or at best a lateral hole in the duct
  — rapidly developing obstructive jaundice implies a ligated bile duct (usually the common hepatic).
- Late postoperative – intermittent or progressive jaundice, often associated with cholangitis.

Carcinoma and sclerosing cholangitis

The mode of presentation is nearly always progressive obstructive jaundice. In sclerosing cholangitis there may be associated evidence of infection.

MANAGEMENT OF STRICTURE

Cause is all-important when managing stricture.

Traumatic stricture

The damaged area must be bypassed. There was formerly a vogue for reconstruction of the main bile duct. However, it is generally agreed that in most traumatic strictures a new communication should be made between healthy duct and healthy intestine. Therefore some form of choledochoenterostomy is appropriate. The usual one will be choledochojejunostomy Roux-en-Y (Fig. 26.5).

Malignant stricture

A malignant stricture can often be resected. For hilar cholangiocarcinoma, resection may entail either partial hepatectomy or local excision of the hilus, with reconstruction in each case by hepaticojejunostomy Roux-en-Y. Cure is unlikely but palliation is good. Otherwise, proximal decompression is used. Percutaneous insertion

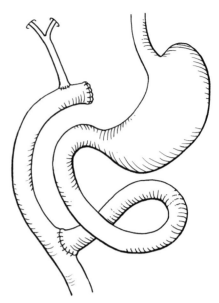

Fig. 26.5 Choledochojejunostomy – Roux-en-Y.

of an 'endoprosthesis' as an internal bypass, under X-ray control, is now available, giving palliation without operation. At the moment it is unclear whether operative or non-operative procedures are better. Distal cholangiocarcinoma resembles cancer of the pancreatic head and is treated along similar lines (see p. 276).

Sclerosing cholangitis

There is no satisfactory treatment for primary sclerosing cholangitis. Surgical excision is occasionally indicated for a 'dominant' stricture, while percutaneous dilatation under radiological control can be useful. Neither corticosteroids nor immunosuppression is helpful. Liver transplantation may eventually be required. The secondary type will sometimes be controlled by restoring adequate bile drainage.

CHOLEDOCHAL CYST

The condition is almost certainly a developmental anomaly, although presentation may be delayed. Choledochal cyst is associated with a long common channel between bile duct and pancreatic duct, i.e. a high (anomalous) pancreatobiliary ductal junction. The bile duct is thin-walled and dilated so that there is a lake of bile somewhere along its length. Occasionally the lake is in what appears to be a diverticulum, but more frequently the dilatation is fusiform.

The cyst may be:

- a cause of neonatal jaundice
- a cause of an upper right quadrant mass at any age
- associated with ascending cholangitis.

Choledochal cysts have a high incidence of malignant change, and this is the main reason for suggesting that the treatment of choice is excision of the cystic area with the appropriate reconstruction – usually a choledochoenterostomy.

FURTHER READING

Cheslyn-Curtis S, Russell R C G 1991 New trends in gallstone management. British Journal of Surgery 78: 143–149

Donovan J M, Carey M C 1993 Formation of cholesterol stones. In: Bouchier I A D, Allan R N, Hodgson H J F, Keighley M R B (eds) Clinical science and practice, 2nd edn. Saunders, London, vol 2, p 1702–1712

McGinn F P, Miles A J G, Uglow M, Uzmen M, Terzi C, Humby M 1995 Randomized trial of laparoscopic cholecystectomy and mini-cholecystectomy. British Journal of Surgery 82: 1374–1377

McMahon A J, Fullarton G, Baxter J N, O'Dwyer P J 1995 Bile duct injury and bile leakage in laparoscopic cholecystectomy. British Journal of Surgery 82: 307–313

Williamson R C N 1990 Acute cholecystitis, calculous and acalculous. In: Williamson R C N, Cooper M J (eds) Emergency abdominal surgery. Churchill Livingstone, Edinburgh, p 110–127

27

Pancreatic disorders and jaundice
Robin Williamson

OVERVIEW

Remote in its retroperitoneal fortress, the pancreas was a difficult organ to study until the advent of modern imaging techniques such as ERCP and CT scan. Pancreatic disease is all too common, in both medical practice (diabetes) and surgical practice (acute pancreatitis, carcinoma of the pancreas). This chapter also covers chronic pancreatitis and neuroendocrine tumours. Pancreatic cancer is one of the leading causes of obstructive ('surgical') jaundice. An understanding of the pathophysiology of jaundice allows a logical plan for diagnosis and treatment.

ACUTE PANCREATITIS

AETIOLOGY

Acute pancreatitis results from varying degrees of autodigestion of the pancreas by activated enzymes. The aetiology of the condition is still being worked out, but some causes – if not the exact mechanisms – are known.

Biliary tract disease

The passage of gallstones down the common bile duct with or without their impaction at the papilla is an undoubted cause of acute pancreatitis. The exact mechanism is uncertain, but reflux of bile or pancreatic juice could activate enzymes in the gland, especially if the pancreatic duct is partly obstructed.

Acute pancreatitis is associated with gallstones in at least 30–40% of cases in most reported series, and in some it has been placed as high as 90%.

Alcoholism

Excessive alcohol intake is associated with acute pancreatitis in at least 25% of patients in Australia and the USA; in the UK the relationship is a little less frequent. The nature of this association is unknown, although alcohol may cause a gastroduodenitis with oedema of the duodenal papilla and reflux.

Most patients with acute alcoholic pancreatitis are thought to have some permanent underlying damage to the gland, i.e. chronic pancreatitis.

Pancreatic duct obstruction

Obstruction to the duct of Wirsung by pancreatic calculi, tumours or congenital anomalies is a rare cause of pancreatitis and accounts for well under 5% of cases in most reported series.

Trauma

The pancreas may be damaged during endoscopic retrograde cholangiopancreatography (ERCP) or upper abdominal operations. Postoperative pancreatitis accounts for about 5% of cases. External abdominal violence, particularly crush injuries, can result in contusion, laceration or even division of the pancreas and the development of pancreatitis. Most traumatic pancreatitis is the consequence of damage to a major duct with extravasation and is more correctly a peripancreatitis.

Miscellaneous

Viral infection of the pancreas including mumps, allergic

phenomena, metabolic disturbances in association with liver disease, raised serum calcium (from hyperparathyroidism and other causes), hypothermia and hyperlipaemia with obesity are known associated factors. A number of drugs have been implicated, including steroids. The frequency of acute pancreatitis in the elderly suggests a possible role for arteriosclerosis.

Idiopathic

In about 20–30% of cases, there is no evidence of a definitive causative factor. Some patients in this group may be suffering from microcholelithiasis, because tiny gallstones or cholesterol crystals can be found by assiduous examination of the stools or duodenal juice.

SURGICAL PATHOLOGY

The changes seen in acute pancreatitis vary according to the severity of the attack. Oedema, exudation, haemorrhage, suppuration and necrosis may occur alone or in combination. In the mildest cases, there is oedema of the pancreas with minimal symptoms and signs. Pancreatic haemorrhage and necrosis may be associated with profound shock from loss of extracellular fluid and blood, because of exudation of fluid retroperitoneally and into other tissues as a consequence of increased capillary and cellular permeability.

Severe haemorrhagic pancreatitis is likely to be followed by necrosis, which also affects adjacent tissues. The result is a large retroperitoneal phlegmon which, if infected, leads to abscess formation, septicaemia and sometimes secondary haemorrhage from an eroded artery or false aneurysm. *Infected pancreatic necrosis* is a potentially lethal complication.

Fat necrosis, a common accompaniment of acute pancreatitis, is due to the combination with calcium of fatty acids liberated from hydrolysed fat and is seen as white flakes in the omentum, mesocolon and mesentery. Occasionally it may be metastatic and appear in subcutaneous tissues and periarticular fat as the result of circulating lipase.

A *pseudocyst* (so called because it does not have an epithelial lining) forms over a period of 2–3 weeks when fluid is walled off by fibrous tissue. There may be either a sympathetic effusion of fluid into the lesser sac from the surface of the inflamed gland or rupture of a major branch of the pancreatic duct.

MORTALITY AND PROGNOSIS

Approximately one in four attacks of acute pancreatitis is severe and gives rise to complications. The mortality rate varies between 6% and 20%, some patients dying rapidly before a diagnosis can be made. Death rates are not affected by the aetiological cause, except that postoperative pancreatitis is particularly dangerous. Death results from:

- hypovolaemic shock in the early stages of an attack, especially in the elderly
- multiple organ failure (lungs, heart, kidneys) as a consequence of infected pancreatic necrosis at a later stage.

Early prognosis

Early assessment of the severity of an attack is not only an indication of prognosis but will also identify those patients more likely to develop the complications listed above and therefore those that may benefit from aggressive conservative treatment or early operation.

A system of prognostic signs was shown by Ranson to predict outcome and may be used on admission to hospital and again after 48 hours of treatment. The bad prognostic signs are as follows:

- On admission
  - age greater than 55 years
  - blood glucose greater than 11 mmol/L
  - blood leucocyte count greater than 16×10^9/L
  - serum LDH greater than 70 i.u./L
  - serum AST greater than 60 i.u./L.
- At 48 hours
  - serum calcium below 2 mmol/L
  - blood urea, an increase of 10 mmol/L
  - haematocrit, a fall of over 10%
  - base excess greater than –4
  - arterial Po_2 below 8 kPa (60 mmHg)
  - estimated fluid sequestrated is over 6 L.

The presence of three or more of these signs at either time of assessment is associated with a greater incidence of haemorrhagic pancreatitis and death. Other scoring systems (Imrie, APACHE II) can give a similar discrimination between mild and severe attacks.

A severe attack is also indicated by:

- a high level of C-reactive protein (CRP) in the blood
- the finding of bloodstained free fluid on abdominal paracentesis

- the finding of a peripancreatic mass on an urgent CT scan (see below).

Late prognosis

In cases where biliary tract disease can be surgically eradicated, the ultimate prognosis is excellent. When alcoholism is a factor and can be successfully controlled, the outlook is also good.

In the idiopathic group, provided pancreatic duct carcinoma can be excluded, many will settle with the passage of time.

CLINICAL FEATURES

The clinical features of acute pancreatitis vary considerably, because this is a disease with an unpredictable sequence of pathological changes.

Symptoms

Pain. This is invariably present, but its severity is related to the degree of peritoneal irritation caused by haemorrhage and liberated pancreatic enzymes.

Pain is usually of sudden onset, intense, continuous and situated in the upper abdomen. Radiation to the back and the flanks is associated with spread of blood, enzymes or an effusion into the retroperitoneal space. The severity and location of the pain are rarely diagnostic but often suggest the diagnosis.

Patients with pancreatic pain often assume bizarre positions, while those with a perforated viscus are afraid to move.

Vomiting. Continuous retching is common. It may be prolonged and faeculent in nature as the disease progresses and becomes associated with paralytic ileus.

Signs

Signs associated with acute pancreatitis fall into two categories: general and local.

General

Shock. When pancreatitis is severe and associated with loss of blood and tissue fluid from the circulation, shock will be apparent. The patient is pale and sweating, with an elevated pulse rate and lowered blood pressure. Confusion and dyspnoea may be accompaniments.

Fever. This is occasionally present, but the temperature is commonly subnormal at first.

Jaundice. This may be present in the early stages if there is associated bile duct disease, or after a day or two if the inflammatory process causes oedema and obstruction.

Cyanosis. This indicates hypoxia and suggests that the attack may be severe.

Local

Peritonitis. Local or general abdominal wall rigidity and rebound tenderness are usually present but to a lesser degree than when due to a perforated peptic ulcer. Rigidity may in fact be absent.

Paralytic ileus. Abdominal distension, vomiting and absent bowel sounds indicate ileus.

Abdominal mass. This may become apparent a few days later and is due to pseudocyst, palpable omentum or pancreatic abscess formation.

Abdominal discoloration. Extravasation of blood from haemorrhagic pancreatitis to the periumbilical region is a rare occurrence, but when it does occur umbilical discoloration may be seen (Cullen's sign). Similarly, discoloration in the flanks has been described (Grey Turner's sign).

SPECIAL TESTS

Plain X-ray of chest and abdomen. This should always be performed, not as a diagnostic test but to exclude the presence of free gas which has originated from a perforated peptic ulcer. Occasionally, radio-opaque gallstones, a gas-filled right colon or a distended loop of small bowel (sentinal loop) may be seen. A left basal pleural effusion is not uncommon. Lung field mottling is a bad sign (and indicates ARDS).

Imaging. Ultrasound, CT and indium scanning have all been used, both for diagnosis and to assess progress. CT scan is used to assess the extent of swelling of the pancreas and surrounding retroperitoneal tissues. The failure of the pancreas to 'enhance' on the scans when intravenous contrast is given suggests pancreatic ischaemia and potential necrosis. Percutaneous aspiration of the phlegmon under CT guidance confirms bacterial infection in a patient with pancreatic abscess (infected pancreatic necrosis).

Serum amylase. Many laboratories now use the Phadebas tablet method for estimating serum amylase levels, the normal range being 70–300 i.u./L. A value of 1000 i.u./L or greater is virtually diagnostic of acute pancreatitis.

The serum amylase peak is reached within 48 hours, but the magnitude of the rise is not a guide to the severity of the attack. Similarly, the rate of fall gives little indication of the rate of resolution of the disease. A persistently raised amylase does usually indicate persistence of the process and/or the development of a pseudocyst.

Serum amylase levels may also be raised in cases of perforated peptic ulceration, acute cholecystitis and bowel obstruction, but the levels reached are seldom as high as those found with acute pancreatitis.

In doubtful cases a peritoneal lavage may produce bloody or turbid fluid with a raised amylase content.

Other blood tests. To make an early assessment of the severity of the attack, the following tests are recommended:

- full blood count and haematocrit
- blood glucose
- blood urea
- serum calcium
- liver function tests
- arterial blood gases.

DIFFERENTIAL DIAGNOSIS

It is seldom necessary to resort to laparotomy to make the diagnosis. Diagnostic laparoscopy should be considered in a suspected case if perforated viscus or ischaemic bowel cannot with confidence be excluded.

In *severe cases*, coronary occlusion may cause confusion, particularly when epigastric pain is severe. However, abdominal rigidity is unusual with cardiac disease and an electrocardiograph may show ischaemic heart changes.

In *less severe* cases, a perforated peptic ulcer may be difficult or impossible to exclude. The presence of free

gas beneath the right hemidiaphragm on X-ray examination is a most helpful sign of perforation.

In *milder cases* of pancreatitis, acute cholecystitis will require consideration. The situation and radiation of pain of cholecystitis and marginally raised serum amylase levels may give a clue.

TREATMENT

Treatment is usually non-operative in the first instance. Operative treatment should be reserved for specific indications (see below).

Conservative treatment

Conservative treatment may be described as the 'R' regimen and includes the following.

Relieve the pain. Intravenous opiate is given as required.

Rest the pancreas. Nothing is given by mouth. Parenteral fluid and electrolytes are administered.

Anticholinergic drugs used to suppress pancreatic secretion and spasm of the sphincter of Oddi have not proved to be of sufficient value to warrant their routine use.

Rest the bowel. Gastric suction is indicated in the presence of abdominal distension or persistent vomiting due to paralytic ileus.

Resuscitation. This is an essential requirement in the presence of hypovolaemia, when replacement therapy with blood, plasma expanders, saline and dextrose solution will be indicated. Large volumes of fluid, both colloid and crystalloid, may be required to correct the initial hypovolaemia. In such cases, fluid replacement should be monitored using a central venous pressure line.

Resist enzymatic activity. Many attempts have been made pharmacologically to block digestion. None has worked. Therapeutic peritoneal lavage has not been shown to be of value.

Resist infection. Septic complications and intra-abdominal abscess formation may occur. Broad-spectrum antibiotics are often given, although there is limited evidence that they reduce the mortality or morbidity rates.

Repeated examinations. Frequent assessment of the progress of general and local features is mandatory, and particular attention is paid to fluid balance and the progress of abdominal signs. The development of a mass will indicate a developing pseudocyst or abscess that may require operative intervention.

Repeated blood tests. Daily estimation of the serum calcium is of value in a severe attack. A fall of serum calcium below 2.0 mmol/L (corrected for albumin level) indicates severe disease, and levels below 1.5 mmol/L indicate a grave prognosis. Intravenous 10% calcium gluconate is given as often as is required in the presence of hypocalcaemia.

Frequent white cell counts are valuable, particularly when there is persistent elevation or resurgence of the temperature, indicating continuing activity or a developing complication. Likewise, serial CRP levels can be monitored.

Respiratory support. Falling Po_2 on arterial gas analysis may indicate pleural effusions, atelectasis (from abdominal distension) or even ARDS. Oxygen should be given by mask, and in a severe case endotracheal intubation may be needed to allow mechanical ventilation.

Renal output. Careful monitoring of urinary output to be greater than 30 ml/hour is needed, with an indwelling catheter if the attack is severe. A careful fluid balance chart should be kept. Incipient renal failure may respond to diuretic therapy, but in severe cases peritoneal or even haemodialysis may be needed.

Operative treatment

This should be reserved for the following specific indications.

Endoscopic papillotomy. There is growing evidence to suggest that this procedure can be beneficial in patients with severe gallstone pancreatitis. Gallstone disease may be indicated by raised liver enzymes in the blood and/or ultrasonography. If ERCP confirms calculi in the common bile duct, papillotomy (in expert hands) can safely relieve the obstruction.

Pancreatic debridement. Severe sepsis and incipient organ failure indicate the development of infected pancreatic necrosis (pancreatic abscess), which carries a high mortality rate of 20–25%. There is leucocytosis and there may be CT evidence of gas in the pancreatic phlegmon. Early laparotomy is required to allow radical debridement of the necrotic peripancreatic tissue (and sometimes part of the pancreas itself). At the end of the operation, the abdominal cavity is either closed with several drains to the lesser sac (for postoperative irrigation) or left open (so-called 'laparostomy'); the viscera are covered with moist packs and the abdominal cavity is inspected daily in the intensive therapy unit.

Internal drainage of pancreatic pseudocyst. Modern imaging techniques show that small peripancreatic effusions are common after an attack of acute pancreatitis but that most are resorbed spontaneously. A larger pseudocyst is suggested by renewed pain and hyperamylasaemia, epigastric mass and a fluid-filled swelling on ultrasound or CT scan. It is usually possible to wait for 4–6 weeks for the cyst to 'mature' and then to drain it internally into a Roux loop of jejunum. Percutaneous catheter drainage or endoscopic drainage into the stomach may have a role in symptomatic pseudocysts.

Subsequent treatment

If gallstones are confirmed in a patient recovering from acute pancreatitis, cholecystectomy should be performed during the same hospital admission to prevent a recurrent attack.

A recurrent attack of acute pancreatitis is an indication for ERCP to look for occult gallstones, underlying chronic pancreatitis, pancreas divisum or carcinoma of the ampulla or pancreas.

CHRONIC PANCREATITIS

AETIOLOGY

Whereas most patients who survive an attack of acute pancreatitis get restoration of a normal pancreas, chronic pancreatitis implies permanent injury to the gland. The diagnosis is suggested by pain, loss of endocrine and exocrine function and morphological abnormalities on pancreatic imaging (ERCP, CT scan). The causes are:

- alcoholism – in affluent countries this makes up at least two-thirds of cases
- recurrent acute pancreatitis – occasionally one or more severe attacks of acute pancreatitis (gallstone, idio-

pathic, etc.) will lead on to permanent pancreatic injury

- dietary – 'tropical pancreatitis' in southern India is thought to be caused by protein deficiency, at least in part
- idiopathic – as in acute pancreatitis, there may be no obvious predisposing factor.

SURGICAL PATHOLOGY

After repeated attacks of pancreatitis, the pancreas becomes atrophic and fibrotic. The pancreatic duct shows varying degrees of stenosis frequently at multiple sites along its length, proximal to which duct dilatation occurs with the formation of 'lakes' or cyst-like cavities. However, pancreatic ductal ectasia (dilatation) often occurs in the absence of main duct obstruction in this disease. Eventually calcification and intraluminal calculus formation occur, with loss of parenchyma and replacement with scar tissue. Endocrine and exocrine function deteriorate. Pseudocysts commonly develop, while progressive pancreatic fibrosis may lead to obstruction of the common bile duct, portal vein or duodenum.

CLINICAL FEATURES

As the natural history and pathological changes are variable, so are the clinical features.

Pain. Upper abdominal pain, which may be precipitated by alcohol or food, is the commonest symptom. The pain may become progressively severe and demand the daily use of opiates.

Backache. Severe and intractable backache, which proves resistant to various forms of therapy, is a common symptom.

Pancreatic failure. Gradual weight loss, anorexia, anaemia, steatorrhoea and diabetes occur, in the most severe cases leading to malnutrition and death.

Jaundice. Obstructive jaundice is quite a common complication of chronic pancreatitis and may be difficult to distinguish from jaundice due to carcinoma of the head of the pancreas.

SPECIAL TESTS

Except in those patients in whom pancreatic failure is obvious, chronic pancreatitis presents a diagnostic challenge. Biliary tract disease should be excluded by appropriate tests (Ch. 26).

The following tests are useful.

Plain X-ray of the abdomen. This may demonstrate pancreatic calcification.

Ultrasound and CT scan (Fig. 27.1). These may show swelling and calcification of the gland, pseudocysts, dilatation of the pancreatic duct and associated biliary tract disease.

Pancreatic function tests. The degree of permanent damage to the pancreas may be assessed by the following:

- reduced glucose tolerance
- increased faecal fat
- reduced electrolyte and enzyme content of duodenal juice after stimulation with secretin and cholecystokinin. Modern 'tubeless' tests of exocrine function (e.g. pancreolauryl test) are less unpleasant for the patient.

Endoscopic retrograde cholangiopancreatography. An endoscope is passed into the second part of the duodenum, and then both the common bile duct and the pancreatic duct are cannulated (under intravenous sedation).

ERCP is the most satisfactory method of confirming or refuting the diagnosis. The ducts may be dilated, strictured or truncated. Demonstration of the type of duct abnormality allows planning of operative treatment. Dilatation of the pancreatic duct may be amenable to a ductal drainage procedure (see below), whereas extensive narrowing may be better treated by pancreatic resection.

The congenital anomaly of *pancreas divisum* occurs when the ventral and dorsal buds of the pancreas fail to coalesce. ERCP demonstrates an abnormal ventral duct. Pancreas divisum may predispose to recurrent attacks of acute pancreatitis and thereby perhaps to chronic pancreatitis.

Angiography. Coeliac angiography is of limited diagnostic value but is an important preoperative test to

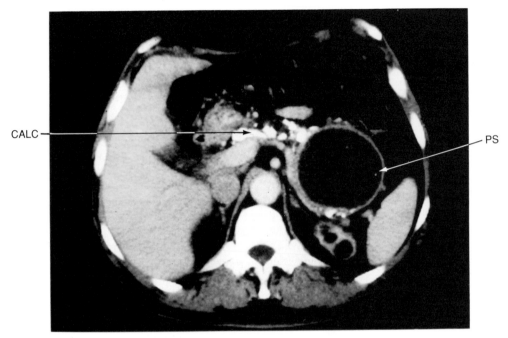

Fig. 27.1 Computed tomography (CT) scan showing pancreatic calcification (CALC) and a large pseudocyst (PS) in a patient with chronic pancreatitis.

show arterial anomalies or portal/splenic vein compression.

Pancreatic biopsy. Ultrasound or CT scan-guided needle biopsy can help to exclude carcinoma.

Chronic pancreatitis can usually be distinguished from pancreatic cancer because of the long history of pain and alcoholism and the presence of calcification. Sometimes operation and even resection are needed to exclude cancer, however.

TREATMENT

Correct predisposing factors

It is most important to eliminate any possible predisposing factor that could perpetuate pancreatitis. If gallstone disease is apparent, it must be corrected. Psychiatric and social support should be enlisted to combat alcoholism.

Non-operative

Alcohol should be forbidden. A low-fat, high-protein and high-carbohydrate diet is advocated and pancreatic enzymes may also be added.

Hypoglycaemic agents may be indicated if diabetes mellitus is present. Coexistent anaemia is treated by oral iron.

Relief of abdominal pain is provided by regular analgesics. Percutaneous coeliac plexus block, using a neurolytic agent such as 50% alcohol, should be considered in patients with severe pain who are poor candidates for operation.

Failure of conservative treatment is apparent if invalidism occurs as the result of severe and persistent pain or progressive pancreatic failure. In such circumstances drug dependency is likely, and in the alcoholic this produces a vicious cycle that is difficult to break.

Operative

The indications for operation are either intractable *pain* or a *complication* such as pseudocyst, stenosis of the bile duct or duodenum, pancreatic ascites or *suspicion of carcinoma*. Provided that the operation performed is individualised according to the nature of the pathological changes in the pancreas and its duct system, then good long-term results can be expected in 70% of patients. Failure is likely in alcoholics who continue to drink.

Operations such as splanchnicectomy that are

designed to relieve pain have no effect on the progress of pancreatitis, and they are often ineffective in relieving pain. However, thorocoscopic splanchnicectomy may have a temporising role. The surgeon must otherwise choose between a drainage procedure and a resection tailored to the extent of pancreatitis.

Drainage procedures. Approximately one-third of patients with chronic pancreatitis have either a grossly dilated pancreatic duct (at least 8 mm diameter) or a pseudocyst, or both, and may be suitable for internal drainage into a Roux loop of jejunum. Longitudinal pancreaticojejunostomy entails slitting open the pancreatic duct from head to tail, removing all calculi and carrying out a long side-to-side anastomosis to the Roux loop. It can effectively control pain without further impairment of endocrine or exocrine function. In appropriate cases a pseudocyst or obstructed bile duct can be drained into the same loop of jejunum.

Pancreatic resection. Depending upon the predominant site of disease, the following resections can be undertaken:

- distal pancreatectomy
- proximal pancreatectomy
- total pancreatectomy.

In distal pancreatectomy, which usually incorporates splenectomy, the pancreas is transected near the portal vein, and the stump is oversewn. In those with endocrine insufficiency, the operation may precipitate the need for insulin.

Proximal pancreatectomy usually incorporates duodenectomy but with preservation of the stomach and pylorus. Continuity is restored by anastomosing the pancreatic neck, transected bile duct and duodenal stump to the upper jejunum.

Total pancreatectomy combines distal and proximal pancreatectomies. This major procedure is reserved for those in whom lesser operations have failed or those with exocrine and endocrine failure. Afterwards there is a lifetime need for insulin and pancreatic enzymes.

CARCINOMA OF THE PANCREAS

PREDISPOSING FACTORS

In many developed countries the incidence of carcinoma of the pancreas has doubled over the last 30 years. It occurs with increased frequency in smokers and diabetics. The peak incidence is in the sixth and seventh decades, and men are more often affected than women.

SURGICAL PATHOLOGY

Ductal adenocarcinoma accounts for 90% of pancreatic tumours, two-thirds of which are located in the head of the gland. Islet cell (neuroendocrine) tumours (see below) and cystadenocarcinoma account for most of the remaining malignancies. Many ductal carcinomas are poorly differentiated, spread early into contiguous structures and metastasise to regional lymph nodes and the liver.

Spread may be:

- local, leading to
  — common bile duct obstruction and jaundice
  — invasion of the duodenum, stomach or small intestine
  — direct invasion of the portal vein, superior mesenteric vessels or coeliac plexus
- lymphatic to coeliac, para-aortic and even supraclavicular nodes
- through the blood, via the portal vein to the liver
- peritoneal and omental, causing ascites.

Peripapillary carcinoma is a term used for juxtapancreatic carcinomas that are biologically less aggressive and present early with jaundice and/or occult gastrointestinal bleeding. There are three forms:

- carcinoma of the ampulla
- carcinoma of the lower common bile duct
- duodenal carcinoma.

CLINICAL FEATURES

Because of the retroperitoneal site of the pancreas and because the symptoms are usually vague, delay in presentation and diagnosis is the rule. There is no reliable screening test, and the at-risk population is poorly defined. All too often patients present with features of advanced disease, especially those with carcinoma of the body or tail of the pancreas.

Modes of presentation

Weight loss is common, occurring in 70–90% of cases.

Pain. This is more often epigastric than lumbar and may be relieved by sitting forward. Back pain suggests an invasive and irresectable cancer.

Jaundice. This is the presenting feature in most patients with tumours in the head of the pancreas and may be associated with a non-tender palpable gall bladder. Courvoisier's law states that a palpable gall bladder in obstructive jaundice was previously normal and therefore unlikely to have been the seat of gallstones, but the more complete nature of the bile duct obstruction in pancreatic cancer may be more relevant. Pain may precede the jaundice, but the latter is usually unrelenting and associated with severe pruritus. The differential diagnosis of jaundice is discussed at the end of this chapter.

Steatorrhoea results from obstruction of the pancreatic duct and is a common feature of cancer of the body of the pancreas.

Diabetes mellitus of sudden onset in middle age with no family history may be associated with a pancreatic carcinoma.

Thrombophlebitis migrans (Trousseau's sign). This may also occur with other malignancies and is characterised by spontaneous thrombosis of peripheral veins that resolves only to recur elsewhere.

Acute pancreatitis. Acute pancreatitis due to pancreatic duct obstruction by tumour is an occasional presenting feature.

SPECIAL TESTS

Ultrasound scan. This is the non-invasive investigation of choice in the jaundiced patient; it may show intrahepatic duct dilatation and a mass in the pancreas.

CT scan. This gives better resolution of space-occupying lesions of the pancreas and is used as an adjunct to ultrasound. It may demonstrate portal vein involvement or hepatic metastases, i.e. evidence of irresectability.

MR (magnetic resonance) imaging. This is an alternative to CT scan. Modern scanners can show the ducts and blood vessels without the need for injection of contrast.

Fibreoptic endoscopy and ERCP. A peripapillary

lesion may be seen, duodenal aspirates can be taken for cytology and ERCP demonstration of the common bile duct and pancreatic duct may show obstruction or distortion.

Barium studies. These were much used in the past, but contrast radiography has little to offer now except in patients with incipient duodenal obstruction.

Histology and cytology. Differentiation of cancer from pancreatitis is not always easy, and ultimately the diagnosis rests on obtaining histological or cytological proof. This may be achieved *preoperatively* by:

- duodenal aspiration
- ERCP
- fine needle aspiration of tumour under ultrasound or CT control

and *intraoperatively* by:

- fine needle aspiration cytology
- transduodenal or direct pancreatic needle biopsy.

Angiography (coeliac, superior mesenteric). This procedure may be used to assess resectability before operation.

Laparoscopy. This has been advocated to improve staging of pancreatic cancer by showing unsuspected peritoneal seedlings.

TREATMENT

Most patients have overt or occult spread at the time of presentation and the overall 5-year survival is only 2%; therefore treatment is generally palliative. Invasive and non-invasive tests are often rigorously pursued in an attempt to make a diagnosis, to stage the disease and sometimes to avoid an operation.

Curative resection

This is often possible for peripapillary carcinoma as the 5-year survival after radical surgery in this subgroup can be as high as 40%. Partial pancreatectomy for localised ductal carcinoma is indicated in selected patients without evidence of distal disease, but recurrence often develops in 1–2 years. The standard operation of proximal pancreatoduodenectomy was carried out by the American surgeon Whipple in 1935 and bears his name. It includes a distal gastrectomy, but many surgeons now prefer to retain the pylorus and duodenal cap. Radical resections incorporating the portal vein (with reconstruction) and regional lymph nodes are of doubtful value.

Palliative management

Common duct obstruction may be relieved by a 'stent' inserted either transhepatically or with the endoscope, provided that the nature of the tumour and its irresectability have been clearly established. Expandable metal stents remain patent for longer than plastic stents but are more expensive.

The surgical alternative is to resect the dilated gall bladder and perform a high choledochojejunostomy. Gastrojejunostomy is often added because of the likelihood of duodenal obstruction as the tumour grows, but this precedes death from other causes in only about 15–20% of instances. Injection of the coeliac plexus with alcohol to relieve pain may be performed at the time of operation or percutaneously and can prove very effective.

Radiotherapy and chemotherapy

Neither form of treatment has, to date, prolonged survival. Combination chemotherapy may become more effective in the future.

NEUROENDOCRINE TUMOURS

Insulinomas and gastrinomas are usually diagnosed when they are small because of the biological effects of the peptides they secrete. By contrast, 'non-functioning' tumours of pancreatic islets present like pancreatic cancer with pain and jaundice, although they are relatively slow-growing and therefore carry a much better prognosis. Other peptides such as glucagon, vasoactive intestinal polypeptide (VIP) or somatostatin are very occasionally secreted in sufficient quantity to cause a typical syndrome.

INSULINOMA

The commonest islet cell tumour, insuloma is usually benign. Insulinomas arise from the beta cells of the pancreatic islets and consequently secrete insulin. Whipple's classic diagnostic triad is: hypoglycaemic symptoms produced by fasting, documented hypoglycaemia, and relief of symptoms by intravenous glucose. The diagnosis is confirmed by measuring circulating immunoreactive insulin and by the failure of insulin suppression by fast-

ing; most patients develop faintness due to hypoglycaemia within 24 hours of fasting.

This tumour may arise independently or as part of multiple endocrine neoplasia type I, which includes parathyroid, pituitary and gastrin-secreting tumours.

Preoperative localisation of the tumour is important because identification at operation can be difficult. A combination of CT scan and selective pancreatic angiography makes localisation more definite but does not always succeed. Surgical resection is the treatment of choice and this applies also to metastases, even when the disease is incurable. The alternative is suppression of insulin with diazoxide, which can give a fairly prolonged period of relief.

GASTRINOMA

Usually malignant, this tumour can arise in pancreatic islets, in the duodenal wall or sometimes further afield. It gives rise to the Zollinger–Ellison syndrome of intractable peptic ulceration and diarrhoea (see Ch. 25). The best treatment is to find and remove the gastrinoma.

NON-FUNCTIONING ENDOCRINE TUMOURS

These are rich in various peptides on immunohistochemical staining, but they fail to release biologically active hormones into the circulation. The diagnosis should be suspected when the patient presents with a large pancreatic mass without the systemic features that would be anticipated with a pancreatic ductal cancer of this size. Some of these tumours are hypervascular, and they may ulcerate into the gut and cause haemorrhage. Surgical resection may be appropriate, even in the presence of metastases.

JAUNDICE

Jaundice is a yellow staining of the body tissues produced by an excess of circulating bilirubin. Normal serum bilirubin concentration is 5–17 μmol/L, and jaundice is detected clinically when the level rises above 40 μmol/L. It is most evident in tissues that have a high elastic collagen tissue content (skin and sclera).

SURGICAL PATHOPHYSIOLOGY

Bilirubin is formed from haem, a compound of iron and protoporphyrin, and about 85% of that produced daily comes from the breakdown of haem from mature red cells in the reticuloendothelial system. The actual mechanism involved is still unknown. The remaining 15% is derived from marrow compounds incorporated into red cell precursors that have not been released into the circulation and from haem compounds in the liver that have not been incorporated into red cells. In states of increased haemolysis, excess haem is released from red cells that have a shortened life span, and an increased production of bilirubin causes acholuric jaundice (acholuria = no bile in the urine). Following its release, unconjugated bilirubin, which is insoluble in water, is transported by plasma proteins to the liver cell.

In the hepatocyte, lipid-soluble bilirubin is conjugated into water-soluble bilirubin glucuronide. Defective uptake or conjugation of bilirubin can occur in such conditions as Gilbert's disease and Crigler–Najjar's disease, with the result that unconjugated bilirubin appears in excess in the blood but not in the urine because it is water insoluble.

The transport of conjugated bilirubin from the liver cells into the bile ducts and bowel is probably an active mechanism, but the controlling influences are poorly understood. Disturbances of the flow of bile lead to stagnation and retention of conjugated bilirubin (cholestasis), which may occur in the intrahepatic biliary tree (intrahepatic cholestasis) or in the extrahepatic biliary tree (extrahepatic cholestasis).

Bacterial deconjugation of bilirubin occurs mainly in the colon to form stercobilinogen, which is partly reabsorbed into the circulation and re-excreted by the liver or kidneys (urobilinogen) and partly excreted in the faeces in an oxidised form (stercobilin).

CLASSIFICATION

The standard classification is into prehepatic jaundice, resulting from excessive red cell destruction; hepatic jaundice, due to liver damage; and posthepatic jaundice (obstructive or 'surgical'), due to obstruction of the biliary tree. Although useful, this classification is inadequate for two reasons:

- Obstruction (cholestasis) can occur without any evidence of a lesion requiring surgical correction (e.g. intrahepatic cholestasis due to drugs or early primary biliary cirrhosis).
- Little indication is given of the site of the disturbance of bilirubin metabolism.

In addition, classifications that ascribe diseases to particular types of jaundice are too rigid: a patient with viral hepatitis may have considerable cholestasis, while a patient with obstruction of a large duct may go on to develop a degree of hepatocyte insufficiency, which interferes with bilirubin conjugation or manifests itself in terms of increased levels of intracellular enzymes in the blood. Thus, separation of causes of jaundice in an individual patient may be difficult. What should always be borne in mind is that the diagnosis required is one that permits action of the appropriate kind – be this surgical or non-surgical (Fig. 27.2).

Increased bilirubin load

In this case jaundice results from an excess of unconjugated bilirubin. This is known as haemolytic jaundice and can occur as a result of:

- hereditary spherocytosis
- hereditary non-spherocytic anaemias
- sickle cell disease
- thalassaemia
- acquired haemolytic anaemia
- incompatible blood transfusion
- severe sepsis
- drugs.

Disturbed bilirubin uptake and conjugation of bilirubin

Jaundice resulting from disturbed bilirubin uptake is seen in:

- viral hepatitis
- hepatotoxins
- cirrhosis
- Gilbert's familial hyperbilirubinaemia
- familial neonatal hyperbilirubinaemia
- Crigler–Najjar's familial jaundice.

Disturbed bilirubin excretion

Jaundice due to an excess of conjugated serum bilirubin is known as *cholestasis*. This can be either intrahepatic or extrahepatic.

Intrahepatic cholestasis (without mechanical obstruction). This is found in:

- cirrhosis

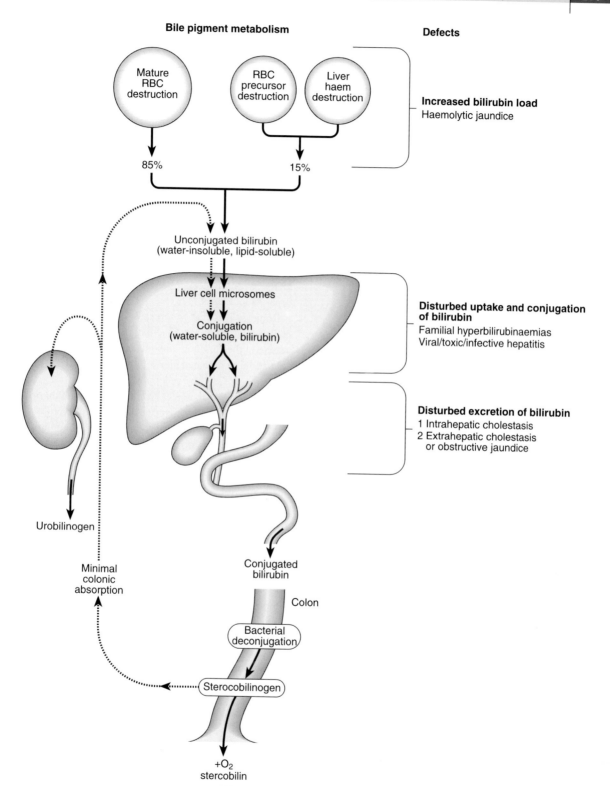

Fig. 27.2 Bile pigment metabolism and associated disorders.

- viral (chronic active) hepatitis
- use of certain drugs (e.g. chlorpromazine, methyl testosterone)
- Dubin–Johnson's familial conjugated hyperbilirubinaemia
- primary biliary cirrhosis (chronic, non-suppurative, destructive cholangitis)
- parenteral or enteral feeding with synthetic nutrients.

Extrahepatic cholestasis. This is obstructive or 'surgical' jaundice with mechanical obstruction of the common bile duct. The obstruction can be inside the duct, in the duct wall or outside the duct:

- inside duct
  — gallstones
  — foreign body, e.g. broken T-tube, parasites (hydatid, liver fluke, roundworms)
- in duct wall
  — congenital atresia
  — traumatic stricture
  — sclerosing cholangitis
  — tumour of bile duct
- outside duct
  — carcinoma of head of pancreas
  — carcinoma of the ampulla
  — pancreatitis
  — lymph node metastases.

The commoner causes of extrahepatic cholestasis are gallstones and carcinoma of the pancreas.

DIAGNOSIS OF CAUSE

The surgeon is mainly concerned with extrahepatic cholestasis, although occasionally he is called upon to perform a splenectomy for hereditary spherocytosis.

The diagnosis is established from a consideration of the usual triad of history, examination and special tests.

History

Occupation. Sheep farmers or allied workers are at risk of hydatid infestation in areas where the disease is endemic, which may result in extrahepatic cholestasis. Residence in developing countries may suggest an exotic cause.

Family history. A family history of anaemia, gallstones or splenectomy suggests hereditary spherocytosis.

A family history of anaemia and jaundice is present in the congenital hyperbilirubinaemias.

Personal history. Previous difficult biliary surgery suggests a traumatic stricture or a residual stone in the common bile duct, while heavy alcoholic intake points to cirrhosis or chronic pancreatitis. Drugs such as chlorpromazine or methyl testosterone may indicate a haemolytic or intrahepatic cholestatic cause for the jaundice. Intermittent pain of biliary type strongly suggests gallstones.

Symptoms

Jaundice. A relatively *sudden onset* of jaundice suggests gallstones or viral hepatitis. A gradual onset is more likely with cirrhosis, pancreatic carcinoma or porta hepatis metastases.

Remorseless and *progressive* jaundice is typical of malignant obstruction. Fluctuating jaundice is likely with a stone in the common bile duct, carcinoma of the duodenal papilla or repeated haemolytic episodes.

Pain. *Painless* jaundice may occur in viral hepatitis, although a dragging subcostal ache is common, the consequence of hepatic enlargement. In older people, painless but fluctuating jaundice suggests intermittent obstruction by gallstones or a necrosing ampullary carcinoma. Painless but progressive jaundice is usually due to malignant obstruction of the common bile duct.

Painful jaundice strongly suggests gallstones or pancreatic disease. Colicky right subcostal pain radiating beneath the costal margin to the shoulder blade suggests biliary colic.

Moderate boring pain passing through to the back can be associated with chronic pancreatitis or pancreatic tumour. There is sometimes relief with posture.

Fever and chills. Extrahepatic cholestasis with cholangitis causes fever and chills and is typical of bile duct stones.

Pruritus. Cholestatic jaundice is often associated with persistent pruritus, which results from the irritation of cutaneous nerves by retained bile salts.

Weight loss. Progressive weight loss suggests malignancy, but it also occurs in patients with chronic hepatocellular damage.

Signs

General. A particular search is made for the following.

Depth of jaundice. A lemon-yellow colour may suggest a haemolytic cause, an orange colour a hepatocellular cause and a deep mahogany hue is usual with prolonged obstructive jaundice.

Anaemia. This suggests a haemolytic, malignant or cirrhotic cause.

Liver failure. This may be apparent with palmar erythema, spider naevi, ascites, foetor hepaticus, gynaecomastia, testicular atrophy, finger clubbing, ankle oedema, bruising and a 'flapping' tremor.

Supraclavicular lymph node enlargement. This suggests metastatic carcinoma.

Skin. Scratches and xanthomas are seen in chronic cholestasis.

Pyrexia. This is caused by:

- cholangitis
- viraemia and hepatic involvement (e.g. infectious mononucleosis)
- septicaemia and haemolysis
- hepatic abscess.

Local (abdominal)

Scars. Scars may indicate previous operations on the biliary tree.

Caput medusae. Dilated periumbilical veins indicate portal hypertension and cirrhosis.

Sites of tenderness. Tenderness over the gallbladder indicates biliary inflammation.

Gall bladder. A palpable gall bladder in the presence of jaundice means that the jaundice is unlikely to be due to a stone (Courvoisier's law). In these circumstances, carcinoma of the head of the pancreas must be suspected.

Liver. A palpable hard nodular liver of large proportions suggests metastatic malignancy, while a small nodular liver indicates cirrhosis. A slightly enlarged smooth liver suggests chronic cholestasis. If the liver is tender, viral hepatitis must be considered.

Spleen. Splenomegaly may be evident in congenital haemolytic anaemia or portal hypertension.

Abdominal mass. A hard and irregular abdominal mass suggests malignancy.

Ascites. This may be due to either abdominal malignancy or liver failure.

Rectal examination. This is an essential requirement. It will indicate the colour of the stools and it may reveal the presence of a primary malignancy or of metastatic deposits in the pouch of Douglas.

Investigations

Preliminary tests. These include urine, faeces and blood tests.

Urine. Absent urobilinogen indicates obstruction to the common bile duct, while excess urobilinogen occurs in haemolytic jaundice and sometimes in liver damage.

Absent bilirubin indicates haemolytic jaundice and excess bilirubin is present in obstructive jaundice.

Faeces. Absence of bile pigment indicates biliary obstruction at any level; excess of bile pigment indicates haemolytic jaundice.

A positive occult blood test suggests an ulcerative lesion, carcinoma, bleeding oesophageal varices (cirrhosis) or an alimentary carcinoma.

Blood. A raised serum bilirubin level confirms the presence of jaundice and also gives some indication of its severity. However, it is unusual for the bilirubin to rise linearly, and in obstruction it often 'peaks out' to a plateau.

A high serum alkaline phosphatase is indicative of cholestasis if bone disease is absent. Serum albumin and globulin levels are reversed in chronic hepatocellular damage, and serum transaminase levels are particularly high in viral hepatitis.

Prothrombin time is normal in haemolytic jaundice; prolonged but correctable with vitamin K in cholestatic jaundice, provided there remains some functioning liver tissue; and prolonged and not correctable in advanced hepatocellular disease.

Spherocytosis, red cell fragility, reticulocytosis and a positive Coombs' test will establish a haemolytic cause.

In terms of immunology, autoantibodies may be elevated in primary biliary cirrhosis, especially antimitochondrial immunoglobulin, and in other connective tissue diseases that involve the liver.

Special tests. When biochemical studies clearly delineate a *parenchymal origin* of the jaundice, then liver biopsy will provide tissue for histological and immunofluorescent analysis.

The usual surgical situation is when *obstructive jaundice* is suspected. Ultrasound scan is the first step to establish the presence of dilated intrahepatic ducts implying extrahepatic obstruction. In expert hands, ultrasound will also give detailed information concerning the gall bladder, the common bile duct, the pancreas and, to a lesser extent, the parenchyma of the liver.

CT scan may give better resolution than ultrasound, particularly in:

● demonstrating pancreatic lesions
● obese patients
● patients with excess bowel gas shadows.

Dilated intrahepatic ducts. Percutaneous transhepatic cholangiography (PTC) is the next test of choice (Fig. 27.3).

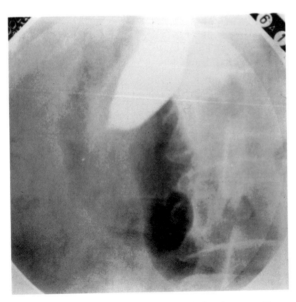

Fig. 27.3 Percutaneous transhepatic cholangiogram. Gross dilatation of the common bile duct above an ampullary carcinoma can be seen.

The coagulation profile is checked and the procedure is covered by parenteral antibiotics. A fine, pliable needle is inserted under local anaesthetic into the liver, a duct is entered and contrast medium is injected.

Should decompression of the biliary tree be desired pre-operatively, then a fine bore catheter may be left in the ducts to allow continuous drainage. If possible, the catheter is passed through the stricture to allow internal drainage of bile. The benefits of pre-operative drainage are yet to be proved and there are risks attached to the procedure (haemorrhage, cholangitis, etc.). Similarly, if an unresectable malignancy compressing the duct is suspected, then the percutaneous insertion of an endoprosthesis may avoid an operation, but there is a long-term risk of stent blockage resulting in acute cholangitis.

PTC is ideal for demonstrating the anatomy above an extrahepatic obstruction, which is most relevant to the surgeon.

Non-dilated ducts or equivocal ultrasound. Endoscopic retrograde cholangiopancreatography (ERCP) is the test of choice. Using a side-viewing fibre-optic endoscope, the duodenal papilla is cannulated and contrast medium is injected into either the common bile duct or the pancreatic duct, or both. Simultaneous endoscopic sphincterotomy and removal of common duct stones may be performed (see p. 265).

ERCP is ideal for demonstrating the anatomy distal to an extrahepatic obstruction. As with PTC, a temporary or permanent stent can be placed through a biliary structure at ERCP.

Both PTC and ERCP are effective techniques, and the choice, for either situation of duct dilatation, depends upon the expertise available.

SURGICAL TREATMENT

Clearly, this will relate to the cause, and various procedures have already been outlined in the previous sections of this chapter. Preoperative preparation is vital.

Preoperative preparation

The almost universal availability of ultrasound or CT scan has simplified the management of obstructive jaundice, and it is a rare occurrence when exploratory laparotomy is used as the definitive investigation for a patient with suspected extrahepatic obstruction.

Laparotomy on a patient who does not have extrahepatic obstruction usually worsens liver function and is thus harmful.

Laparotomy in patients with extrahepatic biliary obstruction carries three special risks, as described below.

Hypocoagulability. This occurs because of prothrombin deficiency, which is corrected by vitamin K administration in the days preceding operation.

Renal failure postoperatively. The exact cause is uncertain but it is probably a combination of:

- increased bile pigment load on the tubule
- increased postoperative distal tubular reabsorption of water because of the secretion of antidiuretic hormone
- perhaps most important, failure of the liver to trap endotoxins derived from bowel organisms
- dehydration in a deeply jaundiced patient.

The condition is prevented by pre-operative rehydration, and diuretic therapy can be used intra- and postoperatively either with mannitol (osmotic diuresis) or frusemide (loop diuretic). Mannitol is usually given at the time of induction in a dose of 100 ml of 10% mannitol; the infusion may be continued for 24 hours at a sufficient rate to give a urine output of 1 ml/min or more.

Sepsis. Stasis of bile, with or without calculi or other foreign bodies, will predispose to bacterial colonisation and overgrowth. A combination of biliary sepsis and renal failure is usually fatal. Antibiotic prophylaxis is therefore given, using an antibiotic to deal with coliforms.

FURTHER READING

Cheslyn-Curtis S, Sitaram V, Williamson R C N 1993 Management of non-functioning neuroendocrine tumours of the pancreas. British Journal of Surgery 80: 625–627

Cuschieri A 1995 Jaundice. In: Cuschieri A, Giles G R, Moossa A R (eds) Essential surgical practice, 3rd edn. Butterworth-Heinemann, Oxford, p 1182–1183

Grace P A, Williamson R C N 1993 Modern management of pancreatic pseudocysts. British Journal of Surgery 80: 573–581

Imrie C W, Buist L, Shearer M G 1988 Importance of cause in the outcome of pancreatic pseudocysts. American Journal of Surgery 156: 159–162

Poston G J, Williamson R C N 1990 Surgical management of acute pancreatitis. British Journal of Surgery 77: 5–12

Ranson J H C 1990 The role of surgery in the management of acute pancreatitis. Annals of Surgery 211: 382–393

Sarr M G, Cameron J L 1984 Surgical palliation of unresectable carcinoma of the pancreas. World Journal of Surgery 8: 906–918

Stapleton G N, Williamson R C N 1996 Proximal pancreatoduodenectomy for chronic pancreatitis. British Journal of Surgery 83: 1433–1440

Trede M 1987 Treatment of pancreatic carcinoma: the surgeon's dilemma. British Journal of Surgery 74: 79–80

Warshaw A L 1989 Pancreatic cysts and pseudocysts: new rules for a new game. British Journal of Surgery 76: 533–534

Watanapa P, Williamson R C N 1992 Surgical palliation for pancreatic cancer: developments during the past two decades. British Journal of Surgery 79: 8–20

Williamson R C N 1988 Pancreatic cancer: the greatest oncological challenge. British Medical Journal 296: 445–446

28 Intestinal obstruction

Bruce Waxman

OVERVIEW

The diagnosis and management of small and large bowel obstruction are based on an understanding of the pathophysiological changes that occur following either mechanical or non-mechanical obstruction of the bowel. It is vital to recognise the presence of strangulation and its associated clinical manifestations. This chapter deals mainly with the principles of surgical pathology and aims to give the student an understanding of how intestinal obstruction may present in a clinical setting, and then presents a logical approach to the non-operative and operative management of intestinal obstruction.

There are many ways of classifying intestinal obstruction:

- by the site of the obstruction in relation to the bowel wall – in the lumen, in the wall, outside the wall
- by the surgical pathology – simple, closed loop or strangulation
- by the level in the gastrointestinal tract – large or small bowel, high or low.

All have something to contribute, but the most useful is an understanding of surgical pathology.

SURGICAL PATHOLOGY

Obstruction may be either mechanical (dynamic), in which there is a bowel capable of contracting normally or excessively proximal to a local site of obstruction, or non-mechanical (adynamic, paralytic), in which obstruction follows cessation of peristalsis either locally or diffusely throughout the bowel.

MECHANICAL OBSTRUCTION

There are three main types: simple occlusion, closed loop obstruction and strangulation.

Simple occlusion. The bowel is usually occluded at one level and above the obstruction the bowel distends as the result of a raised intraluminal pressure from increased secretion of fluid and the accumulation of gas by air swallowing, and fermentation. At first the bowel above the obstruction shows increased peristalsis but this becomes uncoordinated and later may cease if the obstruction is not overcome.

Increased secretion of fluid into the obstructed bowel is associated with decreased reabsorption, and these losses, together with those from vomiting, deprive the patient of electrolytes and water (extracellular fluid). The higher the level of obstruction, the more severe are the fluid and electrolyte losses: the worst effects are seen with high small bowel obstruction while the least effects are seen with large bowel obstruction. The picture is that of acute, extracellular volume deficiency (p. 17).

Closed loop obstruction. This is a special type of simple occlusion where occlusion occurs at both ends of the loop of bowel, and the pathological processes are accelerated. A closed loop obstruction can occur with torsion of the small bowel, obstructed external hernia, colonic obstruction with a competent ileocaecal valve or volvulus of the sigmoid colon. In these cases there is rapid rise in intraluminal tension and gangrene or perfo-

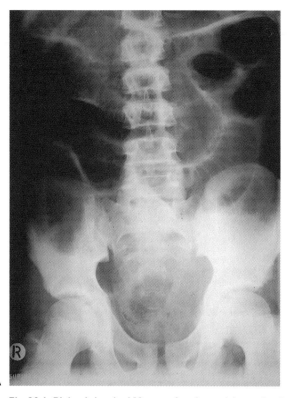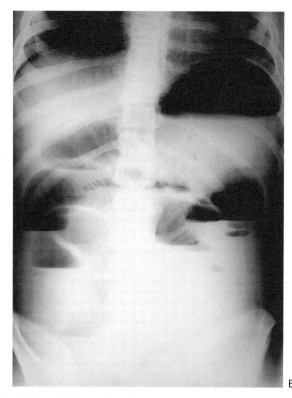

A   B

Fig. 28.1 Plain abdominal X-rays of patient with mechanical small bowel obstruction. A. Supine film showing multiple dilated loops of small bowel. **B.** Erect film showing multiple fluid levels in 'step-ladder' pattern typical of mechanical obstruction.

ration can occur more quickly. In such cases the contents of the bowel are always infected so the perforation produces severe peritonitis.

Strangulation. This is usually the end result of a closed loop obstruction when the major arterial supply to the affected bowel has been occluded, causing gangrene over a considerable area; a special variety is a superior mesenteric artery thrombosis or embolism, in which many metres of bowel may become gangrenous.

Common causes of mechanical small bowel obstruction

These include:

- adhesions and bands following previous abdominal surgery
- external hernia
- intussusception
- volvulus
- neoplasms (benign and malignant)

- obturation: bezoar, worms and gallstones
- stricture: inflammatory bowel disease (esp. Crohn's)
- internal hernia.

Common causes of mechanical large bowel obstruction

These include:

- large bowel cancer
- sigmoid diverticular disease
- sigmoid volvulus.

Adhesions and bands rarely cause a large bowel obstruction.

NON-MECHANICAL (ADYNAMIC, PARALYTIC) OBSTRUCTION

This form of obstruction occurs when bowel contraction ceases as a result of excessive sympathetic efferent discharge, peritonitis or drugs.

It is common after abdominal surgery for the return of bowel function to be delayed. Indeed, peristalsis returns to the small bowel approximately 16 hours after surgery, whereas peristalsis and emptying of the stomach is delayed up to 14–36 hours. Non-mechanical small bowel obstruction following abdominal surgery is often referred to as paralytic ileus.

Common causes of non-mechanical small bowel obstruction

These include:

- paralytic ileus after abdominal surgery
- localised intra-abdominal abscess or generalised peritonitis
- mesenteric embolism or thrombosis with small bowel infarction
- intestinal pseudo-obstruction.

Common causes of non-mechanical large bowel obstruction

These include:

- retroperitoneal haematoma following lumbar fracture or lumbar surgery
- metabolic causes, including drugs and potassium deficiency
- idiopathic causes.

MECHANICAL OBSTRUCTION

In detection, the following questions must be answered:

- Is it obstruction and, if so, at what level?
- Is strangulation present?
- Is dehydration (extracellular volume deficiency) present?
- What is the cause?
- What is the treatment for the individual case?

Is it obstruction, and if so, at what level?

The question is answered by considering the clinical features.

Symptoms. The cardinal features of bowel obstruction are pain, vomiting, constipation and distension.

Pain is usually colicky in nature but will become continuous if perforation or strangulation is present. Pain is absent in paralytic ileus.

Vomiting is early in high small bowel obstruction, late in low small bowel obstruction and delayed or absent in large bowel obstruction. Characteristically, in small bowel obstruction the vomitus is initially clear, and becomes discoloured and finally faeculent – dark and foul smelling.

Constipation is early with large bowel obstruction and is absolute in complete obstruction, but there may be an initial motion at the onset of obstruction. This may be bloodstained in a mesenteric occlusion, volvulus or intussusception.

Distension is usually epigastric or hypogastric in small bowel obstruction and generalised in large bowel obstruction. The patient often feels bloated and uncomfortable.

Signs. *General* signs may reveal evidence of dehydration and/or strangulation (see below)

The *local* signs in the abdomen are:

- On inspection
  - scars from previous operations
  - distension, which tends to be central in small bowel obstruction and peripheral in large bowel obstruction
  - visible peristalsis in a thin abdomen
  - irreducible swellings at external hernial orifices.
- On palpation
  - abdominal mass, which may suggest carcinoma or strangulated bowel
  - rigidity and rebound tenderness, which indicates peritoneal irritation
  - obstructed hernia.
- On percussion
  - resonance because of gas-filled bowel
  - tenderness on percussion indicates the presence of peritonitis and heralds early strangulation.
- On auscultation
  - metallic clicks as pressure is raised if much gas is present in the bowel
  - gurgling borborygmi if gas and fluid are present in the bowel
  - silence if generalised peritonitis or paralytic ileus is present.
- On rectal examination
  - impacted faeces
  - rectal tumour

— blood on finger, which may be present with mesenteric artery occlusions, intussusception or volvulus.

These clinical features are nearly always sufficient to permit a working diagnosis of mechanical intestinal obstruction to be made. Supplementary or confirmatory tests include the following.

Sigmoidoscopy. In large bowel obstruction sigmoidoscopy may reveal a carcinoma, sigmoid volvulus or inflammatory stricture. In sigmoid volvulus the procedure can be therapeutic.

Plain X-ray of the abdomen. This should be taken supine and erect, to show distended and fluid-filled coils of bowel. A closed loop obstruction may not contain gas and a low ileal obstruction may not show fluid levels (see Fig. 28.1).

Contrast X-rays. In doubtful cases, Gastrografin orally or thin barium rectally may outline the level of obstruction. However, more importantly, the latter may reveal a normal colon in a suspected large bowel obstruction (see 'pseudo-obstruction', p. 290).

Is strangulation present?

There are no cardinal signs of strangulation. However, the presence of marked shock, fever and tachycardia together with all or some of the following is strongly suggestive:

- abdominal wall rigidity
- abdominal wall rebound tenderness
- tense, hard and irreducible external hernia
- metabolic acidosis when clinical intestinal obstruction is diagnosed
- raised white cell count in similar circumstances.

Is dehydration present?

Examination must include a general assessment of the patient's condition and state of hydration (i.e. does the patient look well, relatively well, sick or very ill?). In small bowel obstruction particularly, persistent vomiting may result in dehydration, the features of which are:

- tachycardia
- hypotension
- dry skin

- dry mouth
- poor tissue turgor
- small volume of concentrated urine.

What is the cause?

Previous abdominal operation and features of small bowel obstruction suggest adhesions. The attacks may have been recurrent and managed non-operatively. Nevertheless the present attack may involve strangulation, so that great caution is needed in these cases.

Large bowel obstruction and a history of constipation, perhaps with intermittent mucus or bloody diarrhoea, suggest carcinoma of the colon. Diverticulitis of the colon is a much less common cause.

No previous abdominal operation and symptoms of small bowel obstruction suggest either an obstructed external hernia or an uncommon cause such as a congential band, gallstone ileus, internal hernia or mesenteric occlusion.

MANAGEMENT

In general, once bowel obstruction has been diagnosed, the treatment is operation, although there may be a delay while the severely dehydrated patient receives intravenous therapy. When strangulation is strongly suspected because of clinical signs and metabolic acidosis, the time taken for preoperative replacement therapy must be as short as possible.

Operation for bowel obstruction is contraindicated in the following circumstances:

- Paralytic ileus.
- Impacted faeces, when disimpaction by digital manipulation is all that is required.
- Volvulus of the sigmoid colon provided that the twisted loop of bowel can be negotiated with a rectal tube passed under vision through a sigmoidoscope. Colonoscopic decompression is also useful with good results. Endoscopic decompression allows elective sigmoid colectomy.
- When there have been many previous explorations for adhesions and there is confidence that strangulation is not present.

Preoperative preparation

If obstruction is detected early and there are no signs of

dehydration then special preoperative preparation is not necessary apart from starting nasogastric suction and intravenous therapy. A large nasogastric tube may be passed and the stomach emptied immediately before surgery. Alternatively, if it proves difficult or impossible to persuade the patient to swallow a tube, then anaesthesia can be induced while pressure is applied to the cricoid cartilage, which will prevent regurgitation from the oesophagus.

If obstruction is detected later, for example 24 hours after the onset of symptoms when signs of dehydration are present, then the following will be required.

Nasogastric suction. The stomach must be emptied so that the risk of inhalation of vomit is minimised. This also reduces the fluid which has collected in the small bowel.

Intravenous therapy. Correction of water and electrolyte losses must be effectively performed within a few hours. Adults who are clinically dehydrated require about 4 litres of fluid, while those who are hypotensive from reduction of extracellular volume may need up to 6–8 litres. Nearly all of this should be given as normal saline or Hartmann's solution.

Monitoring. A central venous line for measuring pressure may be useful in debilitated or elderly patients so as particularly to prevent too rapid or over-resuscitation.

Operation

This may entail removing the cause, e.g. division of adhesions, reduction of a hernia, resection of a gangrenous loop, excision of an obstructing carcinoma, proximal decompression by colostomy as in left-sided colon lesions, or bypass by anastomosis of proximal obstructed to distal unobstructed bowel. In addition, it is usual to empty the distended bowel either by direct aspiration or by milking its contents back to the stomach whence they can be removed by nasogastric suction. These manoeuvres allow the abdomen to be more easily closed.

Postoperative care

Nasogastric decompression is continued as is intravenous therapy until bowel function has recovered, as shown by normal bowel sounds, small aspirates and/or the movement of a colostomy.

Non-operative treatment

Simple occlusion caused by adhesions may be managed non-operatively provided that strangulation is certainly not present. The common circumstances in which non-operative treatment is considered are:

- immediately (2–10 days) after an operation when abdominal re-entry may be hazardous
- in patients with multiple prior attacks of adhesive obstruction
- when physical circumstances are unfavourable
- rarely in patients thought 'too ill' for an operation.

The principles are to institute nasogastric suction and intravenous therapy, the latter first for replacement and then for maintenance. If the obstruction persists, parenteral nutrition will have to be used. Indications of success are progressive resolution in abdominal distension; decline in nasogastric suction volume; return of bowel sounds to normal; and passage of flatus per rectum. Failure is indicated by persistent pain, increasing distension and the development of local signs. Particularly in the postoperative patient (see below) there should be no hesitation in switching from a non-operative to an operative policy.

LARGE BOWEL OBSTRUCTION

The onset is usually insidious because the most probable cause is a gradually encircling carcinoma. The final point may be impaction of faeces in the narrowed lumen and this may be dislodged by rising proximal pressure. In consequence, the condition is rarely an emergency which requires immediate operation unless there is unremitting complete distal obstruction and a competent ileocaecal valve, in which case the caecum distends and thins so that eventually its blood supply is imperilled and a patch of gangrene going on to perforation ensues. Clinical detection of this situation is by finding tenderness in the right iliac fossa and a grossly dilated (greater than 6 cm) caecal gas shadow on X-ray.

The site of obstruction in the large bowel is best detected using a limited barium enema with dilute barium, after sigmoidoscopy, to exclude any abnormality at or above the rectosigmoid junction. A colonoscopy is of limited value as bowel preparation is not practicable.

Treatment

Proximal large bowel obstruction (proximal to and including the splenic flexure). The treatment of choice in tumours of the caecum, ascending colon, transverse colon and splenic flexure causing large bowel obstruction is right hemicolectomy or extended right hemicolectomy (p. 325). Because of the better blood supply of the small bowel, a resection with primary ileocolic anastomosis is associated with a low leak rate.

Distal large bowel obstruction. Although extended right hemicolectomy or subtotal colectomy is an option, most surgeons prefer to conserve as much colon as possible with left-sided large bowel cancer. In most instances, the surgeon will perform a primary resection, with resection of the bowel containing the obstructive cancer at the time of surgery. Primary anastomosis in an unprepared, obstructed colon loaded with faeces is associated with a high leak rate. The surgeon then has the choice of performing one of the following:

- a double-barrel colostomy where both ends of the bowel are brought out on to the skin
- Hartmann's procedure (see p. 296) with end colostomy of the proximal bowel and closure of the distal bowel
- a primary anastomosis with a proximal stoma, either transverse colostomy or loop ileostomy
- on-table lavage of the colon via the terminal ileum or caecum with primary large bowel anastomosis.

POSTOPERATIVE MECHANICAL OBSTRUCTION

Although paralytic ileus is the common cause of intestinal obstruction in the first week after operation, the possibility of mechanical obstruction or sepsis must be considered after day 5. Thereafter, it can occur at any time up to at least 40 years.

SURGICAL PATHOLOGY

Postoperative mechanical obstruction can present as:

- strangulation through holes and cul-de-sacs left at operation
- volvulus of loop of gut attached to some fixed point, usually the abdominal wall or a vascular pedicle
- adhesions.

There are two types of adhesions: *fibrinous* and *fibrous*.

Fibrinous adhesions are delicate webs of exudate which glue the serosal surfaces of bowel together. They occur within the first few days of operation, particularly after an operation for peritonitis and usually resolve spontaneously.

Fibrous adhesions are dense, organised, strong vascular bands between coils of bowel or between the bowel and the abdominal wall. There appears to be little evidence that peritonitis itself causes these adhesions; more likely, they are outgrowths of blood vessels from adjacent tissues which act as vascular grafts into areas of poor blood supply.

CLINICAL FEATURES

Fibrinous adhesions. Features are postoperative 'windy' pains and occasionally vomiting.

Fibrous adhesions. These occur in small bowel obstruction, with abdominal pain, vomiting, distension, constipation and dilated coils of fluid-filled bowel on X-ray.

They also occur in cases of strangulating obstruction, when the features are as for small bowel obstruction but are seen in association with muscle guarding and rigidity.

MANAGEMENT

Prophylaxis

Prevention is by careful operative technique, avoiding the production of ischaemic and raw surfaces on the bowel and routine peritoneal lavage before closure.

Treatment

Fibrinous adhesions. These are treated non-operatively if possible as they will break down or be reabsorbed.

Fibrous adhesions. These require operation and relief of obstruction. In general, there is more of a danger in not operating in the early postoperative period than in operating.

PARALYTIC ILEUS

PREDISPOSING FACTORS

Paralysis of bowel movements is common in the first

24 hours after abdominal operations but may be prolonged if generalised peritonitis was present or if considerable rough handling of the bowel occurred. Under these conditions, the features of a small bowel obstruction become apparent. Other causes have already been mentioned.

CLINICAL FEATURES

Symptoms

Symptoms are of vomiting of large volumes of gastric contents, distended abdomen and lack of passage of flatus or faeces.

Signs

These include central abdominal distension, central abdominal tympany, absent bowel sounds, tachycardia and hypotension.

Special tests

Plain X-ray of the abdomen will demonstrate distended coils of bowel containing fluid levels, but these tend to be grouped at the same level rather than staggered as in mechanical obstruction.

MANAGEMENT

Prophylaxis

This is by peritoneal toilet (saline lavage) and gentle handling of bowel at the time of original operation. Restriction of oral feeding and gastric aspiration are routine postoperative care after many abdominal operations and this usually prevents paralytic ileus from developing.

Treatment

This is always non-operative and consists of intravenous replacement therapy and nasogastric suction, either continuously or intermittently, until the paralysis subsides, coordinated bowel sounds return and flatus has been passed. The use of parenteral nutrition has made prolonged conservative management much easier.

PSEUDO-OBSTRUCTION

This term has come to have different meanings depending upon whether it refers to the small bowel or large bowel and these conditions are best considered separately.

Pseudo-obstruction of the small bowel

Chronic or recurrent pseudo-obstruction affecting the small bowel occurs in patients with a wide variety of associated disease, including connective tissue disorders, drug abuse and radiation injury. A special form of pseudo-obstruction is associated with a familial visceral myopathy with degeneration of axons and neurons of the myenteric plexus.

The clinical features of chronic pseudo-obstruction include vomiting, cramping abdominal pains and distension and this disorder may also affect the oesophagus, stomach and large bowel and be associated with most abnormalities in the urinary bladder. Treatment is largely supportive, but some patients require long-term parenteral nutrition.

Pseudo-obstruction of the large bowel

This condition is usually an acute, non-mechanical obstruction of the colon associated with discoordinate contractions of the large bowel as a consequence of either inappropriate neural input or disordered metabolic environment. The common causes are hypoxia, anaemia, retroperitoneal haematoma, mesenteric malignant infiltration and potassium deficiency with hypokalaemia.

CLINICAL FEATURES

The patient is often elderly and may have been bedridden for several weeks or had recent spinal fracture, spinal surgery or other orthopaedic procedures. The history and physical signs are suggestive of large bowel obstruction, and X-rays show dilatation of both the large bowel and small bowel with no obvious 'cut-off', particularly of the distal colon as is often seen in large bowel cancer.

SPECIAL INVESTIGATIONS

The diagnosis is confirmed with a barium enema using dilute barium which usually shows contrast flowing around to the caecum and into the distal small bowel without obstruction.

The danger with this condition is distension of the caecum and caecal perforation.

TREATMENT

The treatment of choice is non-operative with supportive measures including nasogastric decompression and intravenous therapy.

Decompression of the colon can be achieved with colonoscopy following cleansing of the distal bowel using enemas and wash-outs. Laparotomy and colostomy are only indicated where there is evidence of bowel perforation.

FURTHER READING

Carty D, Ravichandram D 1996 The management of malignant large bowel obstruction. In: Johnson C D, Taylor I (eds) Recent advances in surgery 19. Churchill Livingstone, Edinburgh, p 1–18

Ellis H 1985 Intestinal obstruction. Appleton-Century-Croft, New York

Wangensteen O H 1984 Intestinal obstructions. C C Thomson, Springfield

29 Inflammatory bowel disease

Andrew Zbar   Witold Kmiot

OVERVIEW

Besides acute appendicitis, diverticulitis is the commonest type of inflammatory disease affecting the large intestine. Its acute and chronic forms are considered together with their various complications. Two idiopathic disorders – ulcerative colitis and Crohn's disease – share many clinical and pathological features and are occasionally indistinguishable ('indeterminate colitis'). Whereas the small bowel is most commonly affected in Crohn's disease (notably the terminal ileum), ulcerative colitis is confined to the large intestine. Colitis due to ischaemia, radiation and antibiotics is also discussed in this chapter.

The gastrointestinal tract can be affected by specific inflammatory disorders due to infections or infestations such as amoebiasis, tuberculosis or schistosomiasis. The incidence of these disorders is low in 'developed' Western communities but is still high where public health measures are rudimentary. More often bowel inflammation that affects surgical practice in the Western world is caused by conditions of uncertain aetiology. These conditions together with those following ischaemia have been collected under the heading of 'non-specific inflammatory colitides'.

The conditions considered in this chapter include:

- diverticular disease
- ulcerative colitis
- Crohn's disease
- indeterminate colitis
- ischaemic colitis
- pseudomembranous colitis
- radiation colitis
- diversion colitis.

DIVERTICULAR DISEASE

AETIOLOGY

Diverticular disease is regarded by most authorities as an acquired disorder of the colon induced by a relative lack of dietary fibre. This theory was advanced by Painter & Burkitt based on varying geographic differences in the incidence of complicated diverticular disease.

It is postulated that delayed colonic transit and disordered peristalsis lead to hypersegmentation of the colon, with high intraluminal pressures resulting in the development of mucosal 'blow-outs' or pulsion diverticula. However, studies of colonic transit and intracolonic pressures in patients with diverticular disease give conflicting results.

Diverticular disease is increasing in incidence and appears to be affecting a younger population, but the incidence of complicated diverticular disease may not be diminishing as a result of the introduction of dietary fibre as a treatment.

SURGICAL PATHOLOGY

Diverticular disease may affect any part of the colon; most disease is in the sigmoid colon. Isolated right-sided diverticular disease is uncommon, but it occurs in younger patients than those with left-sided disease. Diverticula develop between the mesentery and the two antimesenteric taenia coli where there is a potential weakened site of muscle at the entry point of the supply-

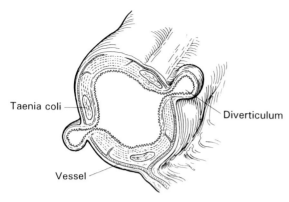

Fig. 29.1 Colonic diverticula.

ing vasculature (Fig. 29.1). In established disease, the muscularis propria and taenia are grossly thickened with histological evidence of hyperelastosis.

The natural history of uncomplicated diverticular disease is unknown, as previous studies document the number of hospital admissions for complicated disease. In patients admitted to hospital with symptoms, about one-third will have a prior history of diverticular disease. There is a 10% rate of mortality among hospital admissions, with the highest mortality rate in those patients who are elderly and those who present with perforation and faecal peritonitis. Over prolonged follow-up after hospital discharge with a diagnosis of acute diverticulitis, 50% of patients will be symptom-free, 15% will have further symptoms necessitating hospital admission, 20% will have severe complications requiring acute operation and 10% will die from their disease.

Diverticular disease presents acutely, chronically or with complications.

Acute diverticulitis

This inflammatory response occurs secondary to inspissation of stool within the neck of the diverticulum, with resultant bacterial proliferation and adjacent lymphangitis. This response may be localised to a solitary diverticulum or may spread to involve the adjacent mesentery, appendices epiploicae and peritoneum.

Chronic diverticulitis

Repeated attacks of acute inflammation are associated with fibrous tissue proliferation and the accumulation of fat in the submucosa and subserosa of the colon, the

appendices epiploicae and the mesentery. Contraction of the fibrous tissue in the colon and surrounding tissues leads to the development of a narrow rigid segment of bowel with a shortened mesocolon. Adhesions between the affected part of the colon and adjacent viscera may occur and give rise to a fixed rigid mass.

Complicated diverticulitis

Perforation. This may be a free perforation into the peritoneal cavity or a secondary perforation after the formation of a loculated abscess collection. Such secondary perforation may occur when the natural powers for localising intra-abdominal infection are inadequate (as in the debilitated, the aged and possibly those on steroid therapy). Peritonitis may be serous, seropurulent or faeculent.

Paracolic abscess/inflammatory mass (so-called 'phlegmon'). This condition follows a localised perforation.

Bowel obstruction. This is either large bowel obstruction as a result of a diverticular stricture or occasionally a small bowel obstruction, when a loop of adherent small bowel becomes kinked against a diverticular mass.

Lower intestinal haemorrhage. The usual source is an ulcerated vessel in the neck of a diverticulum.

Fistula formation. An external fistula (colocutaneous fistula) is rare. It may develop if a pericolic abscess points and discharges spontaneously or following operative or radiologically guided drainage of a pericolic abscess. Internal fistula formation occurs when a pericolic abscess points and discharges spontaneously into an adjacent and adherent viscus. The organ most commonly involved is the bladder, resulting in a colovesical fistula. Vaginal, uterine and tubal fistulas are less common.

CLINICAL FEATURES

Acute diverticulitis

Clinical features of acute diverticulitis include:

- pain, which is situated in the left iliac fossa, initially colicky and then constant
- an elevated temperature and pulse rate
- local left iliac fossa tenderness

- a palpable mass in the left iliac fossa
- leucocytosis and a raised erythrocyte sedimentation rate (ESR).

Plain radiology may show a localised ileus in the left iliac fossa or pelvis, or an air–fluid level within an abscess. Controversy exists over the timing of a barium enema to confirm the diagnosis and to exclude carcinoma. It is probably most safely performed several weeks after the inflammatory episode has settled down.

Chronic diverticulitis

Features include:

- recurrent pain in the left iliac fossa over many months or years
- irregular bowel habit, particularly constipation and bouts of diarrhoea
- the occasional passage of mucus per rectum.

Rigid sigmoidoscopy usually reveals no abnormality, but occasionally an oedematous mucosa and rigidity of the rectosigmoid junction are evident. Flexible sigmoidoscopy even in the unprepared state may reveal the orifices of diverticula.

Barium enema (Fig. 29.2) is useful to represent pictorially the extent of disease. Narrowing of the colon over several centimetres may be associated with a classical 'saw-toothed' appearance due to oedema and spasm. Open-mouthed diverticula are clearly seen, and in long-standing cases stricturing of the colon may be evident. Contrast will be retained in the cul-de-sac of the diverticulum after barium evacuation. The mucosal surface is intact, but carcinoma in a narrow segment can at times be difficult to differentiate accurately.

Colonoscopy is very helpful in excluding other pathology coincident with diverticular disease, most notably carcinoma. Colonoscopy may be difficult to perform because of distortion of the sigmoid colon and because lumina of large diverticula may be confused with the intestinal lumen. Great care must be taken because of the added risk of colonic perforation.

Complicated diverticulitis

Generalised peritonitis. Presentation is with sudden onset of lower abdominal pain, which becomes severe and continous. It is associated with vomiting, tachycardia and elevated temperature, board-like abdominal rigidity and absent bowel sounds. Plain radiology will demonstrate free intraperitoneal air in 30% of cases. Occasionally retroperitoneal air can be seen tracking along the psoas muscle shadow.

Pericolic abscess. This generally follows an attack of acute diverticulitis and causes marked local tenderness and guarding in the left iliac fossa. A mass of variable proportions is palpable in the left iliac fossa or within the pelvis on digital rectal examination. The patient is sys-

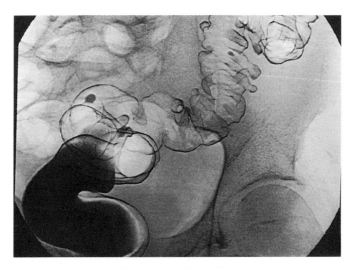

Fig. 29.2 Diverticular disease of the sigmoid colon shown on a double-contrast barium enema.

temically unwell with a swinging temperature and an elevated white cell count. CT scanning will differentiate between an inflammatory phlegmon and a pericolic abscess, as well as showing distant septic collections.

Percutaneous aspiration of pus collections under CT or ultrasound guidance has been advocated to diminish the need for acute operation and the chances of emergency stoma formation.

Large bowel obstruction. A past history of recurrent attacks of acute diverticulitis or irregular bowel habit may be associated with colicky abdominal pain, constipation and abdominal distension. Plain films suggest the presence of a low left-sided large bowel obstruction, which may be confirmed by an emergency water-soluble contrast enema.

Vesicocolic fistula. This should be suspected in a patient with a past history of chronic diverticulitis and a history of dysuria. Frequency, 'scalding' dysuria, haematuria, pneumaturia or faecaluria occur when the fistula is established. Microscopy of the urine shows pus, faecal debris and intestinal organisms; cystoscopy is usually non-specific but may reveal cystitis of the dome of the bladder. Actual visualisation of the fistula at cystoscopy is rare. Sigmoidoscopy is usually normal. Plain radiology may demonstrate an air bubble in the bladder, and barium enema reveals a diseased segment of chronic diverticular disease in close proximity to the bladder.

Massive bleeding. This is generally seen in the elderly patient, often without much history of chronic diverticulitis. When severe, it is usually right-sided in origin and is best demonstrated by emergency mesenteric angiography (see 'Gastrointestinal haemorrhage', Ch. 33).

DIFFERENTIAL DIAGNOSIS

Acute diverticulitis

The differential diagnosis includes acute salpingitis, acute appendicitis, gastroenteritis and irritable bowel syndrome.

Chronic diverticulitis

This can be difficult or impossible to distinguish from carcinoma of the colon, particularly if the segment cannot be negotiated at colonoscopy. The two conditions

occur in the same age group, produce similar symptoms and give rise to the same complications. They may also occur together.

Occasionally, other diagnoses such as ischaemic colitis, radiation-associated colitis and colonic endometriosis need to be considered.

Complicated diverticulitis

Generalised peritonitis. Other causes of generalised peritonitis include appendicitis and perforated ulcer.

Pericolic abscess. It may be impossible to exclude perforated carcinoma of the colon until the diseased segment has been excised.

Large bowel obstruction. Again, the distinction between carcinoma and diverticular disease can be difficult. It is wise after resection in the operating theatre to open the segment of bowel to examine the mucosa, but sometimes the diagnosis remains in doubt until microscopy.

Vesicocolic fistula. Other causes of vesicocolic fistula include carcinoma of the colon, carcinoma of the bladder, Crohn's disease and post-irradiation necrosis.

In summary, cancer and diverticular disease are *always* difficult to separate and may coexist. The maxim is: *do not miss cancer* by accepting diverticular disease as the diagnosis without full investigation.

TREATMENT

It has been suggested that since the widespread introduction of high fibre diets, the number of acute hospital admissions for complicated diverticular disease has fallen.

Acute diverticulitis

When the diagnosis is likely, treatment is conservative and includes bed rest and a fluid diet. Broad-spectrum intravenous antibiotics are employed with a mixed aerobic and anaerobic cover. When the diagnosis is uncertain and acute gynaecologic conditions or 'pelvic' appendicitis cannot be excluded, laparoscopy may be indicated to establish the diagnosis.

Once the acute phase has settled with or without operation, the full extent of disease and the exclusion of other pathology should be made by either colonoscopy or barium studies.

Chronic diverticulitis

Conservative management of chronic diverticulitis is the initial treatment of choice. Operation is indicated under the following conditions:

- doubtful diagnosis, when carcinoma of the colon cannot be excluded
- recurrent or chronic invalidism, repeated hospitalisation with attacks of acute diverticulitis.

There is no clear evidence that recurrent acute diverticulitis or a severe attack in a patient <50 years of age is a real indication for operation, but operative mortality and morbidity rates are higher in recurrent cases.

The operation performed is usually a segmental resection of the affected part of the colon and an end-to-end anastomosis. Resection must be extended down to the anatomical rectum to prevent recurrence of disease. The proximal extent of resection includes the diseased symptomatic area, since more proximal uninvolved diverticula may be left in situ. Mesenteric clearance of the colon should be as conservative as possible.

Complicated diverticulitis

The indications for operation include the following.

Generalised peritonitis/diverticular perforation.
Operation is carried out after a short period of resuscitation. The procedure involves peritoneal toilet and resection of the involved segment, usually without reconstruction. An end sigmoid colostomy is created (Hartmann's procedure; Fig. 29.3). Lesser procedures such as simple drainage and proximal colostomy, oversewing of a perforation or 'perforostomy' (where the perforation has been used as a stomal site) are not recommended. More recently, primary resection and bowel anastomosis with on-table colonic lavage (except in faecal peritonitis) have been advocated. It should only be considered in fit patients by surgeons experienced in these techniques.

Pericolic abscess.
Traditionally operation and evacuation of the collection of pus was advised with possible resection of the affected segment. There is no advantage in simple drainage with performance of a proximal transverse colostomy. CT drainage may be valuable but risks

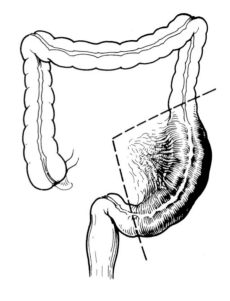

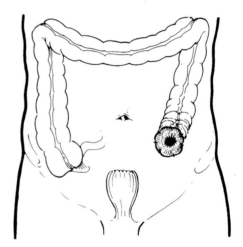

Fig. 29.3 Hartmann's procedure. Formation of end colostomy and closed rectal stump.

cutaneous fistula formation and the percutaneous drainage of an unsuspected carcinoma. It probably has not altered the resection rate for complicated disease.

Large bowel obstruction. Resection either with or without primary anastomosis is indicated.

Vesicocolic fistula. Resection of the affected portion of the colon with anastomosis and closure of the opening in the bladder is preferable as a one-stage operation. The alternative is to stage the procedure by means of a preliminary colostomy. The delayed morbidity of stomal closure and the need for multiple procedures make this approach less popular unless the patient is particularly unfit at the time of fistula presentation.

Massive haemorrage. Resection after delineation of the site of bleeding by angiography is indicated.

Persistent inflammatory mass. The presence of a mass is an occasional indication for elective operation.

Small bowel obstruction. Small bowel obstruction is usually temporary, with attachment of an enteric loop against an area of acute diverticulitis. Rarely, a chronic small bowel obstruction may result from a loop (or loops) of small bowel adherent to a diverticular mass and require operation.

ULCERATIVE COLITIS

Ulcerative proctocolitis is a non-specific continuous mucosal disorder of the large bowel which presents with either total or distal colonic involvement. It is a disease of unknown aetiology with remissions and relapses and a distinctive macroscopic and microscopic appearance that is separable from Crohn's colitis. It carries a well-defined risk of cancer development over a prolonged period of follow-up.

EPIDEMIOLOGY

The true incidence of ulcerative colitis is not known, as many cases of mild non-specific proctitis may not be included in disease estimates. Approximately 50 000 patients in the UK are thought to develop the disease, with an overall incidence of disease of between 2.5 and 15 cases per 100 000 population per annum.

The reported incidence of ulcerative colitis has increased slightly over the last decade. There is a relatively higher occurrence in Scandinavia, the UK and Australia when compared with Eastern Europe, Africa or Asia.

There is a slight female preponderance with a bimodal age distribution, the first peak occurring in the second to third decade, and the second peak in the sixth decade. Fifteen per cent of index cases will have a family history of disease (of either ulcerative colitis or Crohn's disease), suggesting some common factors in aetiology.

AETIOLOGY

Possible factors include the following.

Specific antigens

Animal models of either naturally occurring colitis or induced colitis do not have the same natural history as human ulcerative colitis. Experimental colitis has most often been produced by carageenan, a sulphated polysaccharide derived from seaweed, which in degraded form induces an active confluent colitis and in prolonged administration leads to dysplasia and frank carcinoma in rabbits.

Specific infection

The macroscopic and many of the microscopic features of ulcerative colitis are shared with those of specific infectious colitides (most notably *Campylobacter* colitis, amoebic colitis and salmonellosis). There is microbial evidence for transmission of colitis, although no specific bacterial or viral agent has been identified. Enteropathogenic *E. coli* have been found in higher than normal concentrations in colitic patients, and cross-reactivity has been identified between goblet cell antigens in colonic mucosa and bacterial wall proteins.

Autoimmunity

Disturbed immunology is a particular feature of ulcerative colitis, although this may be a secondary phenomenon. Both pro-inflammatory mediators (tumour necrosis factor, interleukin-2) and anti-inflammatory mediators (prostaglandins E_2 and I_2 and interleukin-4) are released from activated cells in the lamina propria and are thought to act as chemotactic factors for immunocompetent cells. The association of other autoimmune diseases such as systemic lupus erythematosus, autoimmune haemolytic anaemia and pernicious anaemia is well described, as is the presence of circulating anticolonic mucosal antibodies and immune complexes that bind to healthy colonic mucosa. These antibodies and circulating complexes do not correlate with disease activity. Perinuclear antineutrophil cytoplasmic antibodies are highly specific for ulcerative colitis, but again they do not correlate with disease activity or extent.

Allergy

Milk exposure has been linked to colitis relapse, but the incidence of anti-milk antibodies, the poor clinical response to milk-free diets and the lack of cutaneous hyperreactivity to intradermally administered milk proteins argue against a dietary allergen.

Altered mucosal barrier

Goblet cell depletion is a constant and early feature of ulcerative colitis. The mucosa of the large intestine provides a complex barrier to potentially injurious microbial proteins and dietary antigens present in the lumen. These defence mechanisms include surface immunoglobulins (surface IgA), proteolytic enzymes, the mucus gel layer and epithelial tight junctions. All these mechanisms may be disturbed in inflammatory colonic disease, allowing access of toxins to antigen-presenting cells in the lamina propria.

Psychogenic factors

Different behaviour patterns have been implicated in disease activity and aetiology. Many psychiatric factors may prolong or aggravate attacks and are probably consequent upon severe symptomatology and frequent hospitalisation in young patients.

SURGICAL PATHOLOGY

The disease is mucosal and tends to be most severe in the rectum. Inflammation may remain localised to the rectum for many years, although there is a trend in many patients towards proximal progression. The disease develops in continuity, with no free areas between disease sites. Relative rectal sparing rarely occurs, when the proximal colon appears worse than the rectum or when the rectum has minimal disease.

Macroscopic features

Disease may be classified as proctitis, proctosigmoiditis, left colitis, subtotal colitis and total colitis. In those patients with total colitis, there is frequently an active ileitis (so-called 'backwash ileitis') which is histologically indistinguishable from the colonic pathology. The mucosa is reddened and oedematous with a granular friable change associated with contact bleeding on passage of a sigmoidoscope. Despite its eponym, frank ulceration is not common, the mucosa being denuded between pinpoint shallow erosions with intervening islands of surviving oedematous mucosa. These islands give the appearance of polypoid protrusions (pseudopolyps) and are a feature of active disease.

Microscopic features

Disease is histologically confined to the mucosa with a characteristic polymorphonuclear infiltrate in the crypts, forming crypt abscesses. Goblet cell depletion is a common finding. Histological appearances can be divided into active, resolving and quiescent phases. When healed, the mucosa shows shortened bifid regenerating crypts of Leiberkuhn with disturbance of nuclear cell polarity. In fulminant disease, inflammation can become transmural as a preliminary event to colonic perforation and toxic dilatation of the colon. Chronic colitis is associated with a thickened muscularis mucosae as well as haustral loss which leaves the colon foreshortened, rigid and featureless (so-called 'lead-pipe' colon; Fig. 29.4).

COMPLICATIONS

These fall into two categories: local complications and extraintestinal manifestations.

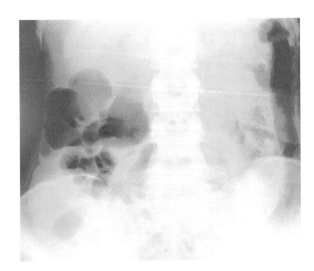

Fig. 29.4 Plain abdominal X-ray in a patient with active left-sided ulcerative colitis. The descending colon is straight and featureless with some mucosal oedema.

Local complications

Perforation. This is frequently a first presentation of disease. It occurs as a result of fulminant colitis or with toxic megacolon. Signs may be masked in patients receiving steroid therapy, making early diagnosis difficult.

Toxic dilatation (megacolon). This is seen particularly in the transverse colon. It is an acute transmural inflammation of the colon and may be induced in severe colitis by the use of narcotics or anticholinergic medication.

Perianal disease. A mixture of fissures, anorectal suppuration and fistulas may occur which mirrors disease activity in the rectum. Fissures occur at unusual sites and are often multiple. Anorectal suppuration may be extensive.

Stricture. This is uncommon and occurs as a consequence of hypertrophy of the muscularis mucosae. Strictures are smooth, frequently multiple and are rarely completely obstructing. They must be distinguished from carcinoma.

Dysplasia and carcinoma transformation. See below.

Haemorrhage. Massive life-threatening intestinal haemorrhage is rare.

Extraintestinal manifestations

These can mirror intestinal disease activity (joint and cutaneous manifestations) and may predate the diagnosis of colitis. They include:

- Musculoskeletal
  - focal arthritis
  - ankylosing spondylitis (HLA B27 negative)
  - clubbing*
  - hypertrophic osteoarthropathy
- Cutaneous and mucous membranes
  - erythema nodosum*
  - pyoderma gangrenosum*
  - non-specific vasculitis
  - oral aphthous ulceration*
  - exfoliative dermatoses
- Ocular episcleritis
  - iritis/uveitis
  - retrobulbar neuropathy (rare)

---

* More common in Crohn's disease.

  - corneal ulceration/keratitis (rare)
- Hepatobiliary
  - primary sclerosing cholangitis
  - pericholangitis
  - cirrhosis
  - cholangiocarcinoma
  - fatty hepatic infiltration
  - hepatic granuloma
  - focal hepatic fibrosis
- Other systems
  - hypercoagulability
  - growth retardation.

CLINICAL FEATURES

The clinical features of colitis are dominated by relapsing bloody diarrhoea and profuse mucous discharge. Three distinct disease patterns are recognised:

- acute fulminating colitis (5%)
- chronic continuous colitis (10%)
- chronic relapsing colitis (85%).

Single isolated attacks are uncommon. Total colitis is generally more severe and is more frequently complicated, requiring operation. Slow disease progression in patients with proctitis is common, with proximal advancement of disease in 10% at 5 years and 20% at 10 years.

Mild colitis

The patient's general health is not disturbed. Remission is usually complete and the disease is confined to the rectum and sigmoid. The cancer risk for this group is unchanged from the normal population, and extraintestinal manifestations are rare.

The patient will have several loose bowel actions per day (usually < 6), containing blood and mucus. Abdominal discomfort is unusual. Mild tenderness over the affected colon is common. Marked abdominal discomfort and distension are not seen.

Sigmoidoscopy reveals friable granular mucosa with intraluminal mucopus. The vascular architecture of the mucosa is lost, with haemorrhage on passage of the scope (contact bleeding). Biopsy is recommended to exclude unsuspected Crohn's disease or amoebic colitis, and a stool culture is taken to exclude an infective colitis.

Colonoscopy or barium enema is used to define the extent of colitis and to exclude associated pathology such as a carcinoma or polyps. Barium enema is generally less accurate than colonoscopy and shows loss of normal colonic distensibility, absent haustration and occasional fine serrated ulceration.

Acute and severe colitis

These patients are ill, with systemic features such as tachycardia, fever and leucocytosis.

A patient will experience up to 20–30 bowel actions per day, with considerable fluid and electrolyte losses, as well as blood loss accompanied by tenesmus and colicky abdominal pain. There will be signs of large bowel distension or peritonitis, or both.

The severity of illness is quantified according to the number of bowel actions per day, the presence of systemic signs of illness, the basal haemoglobin and the ESR (Table 29.1).

Flexible sigmoidoscopy may be performed without bowel preparation. This should be performed with the utmost care by an experienced endoscopist.

Barium enema is absolutely contraindicated in severe cases, particularly when toxic dilatation is suspected. Patients in this category are assessed by daily or twice daily plain abdominal X-rays to determine colon calibre and morphology. Dilatation of the transverse colon beyond 6 cm in diameter indicates the development of toxic megacolon. The plain film may reveal extensive ulceration, pseudopolyp formation and even intramural gas.

MEDICAL TREATMENT

There is no truly specific therapy for ulcerative colitis. Treatment is based on supportive therapy aimed at terminating the acute attack and preventing further attacks. Someone with mild disease can be treated as an outpatient, but severe attacks must be regarded as a medical emergency and admission to hospital is required. General measures in severe disease are:

- Rest the patient – this may include gentle sedation if necessary.
- Rest the colon – intravenous fluid therapy with nil by mouth. After recovery a low residue diet with enteral protein and vitamin supplementation is required.
- Replacement therapy – correction of anaemia and potassium losses.

Special agents are used alone or in combination. These include:

- corticosteroids
- sulphasalazine and aminosalicylates
- immunosuppressants.

Corticosteroids

Systemic steroids are used in fulminant or active total colonic disease. Intravenous hydrocortisone in a routine dose of 100 mg 6-hourly is advised without rectal steroid preparations. Once the disease comes under control, hydrocortisone is replaced by oral prednisolone (usually 40–60 mg orally daily). There is no evidence that steroids prevent relapse, so they should be tailed off as appropriate depending on the severity and extent of disease at presentation.

Topical steroid preparations (hydrocortisone acetate foam: Colifoam) is used once or twice daily. Disease confined to the rectum and sigmoid colon rarely requires systemic steroid therapy and is adequately controlled by topical steroid or salicylate enemas.

Sulphasalazine and aminosalicylates

Following remission, sulphasalazine is employed to prevent relapse. It consists of a sulphapyridine compound bound to 5-amino salicylic acid. Its use is confined to mild-to-moderate disease and for patients who have responded to parenteral steroid therapy after a severe attack. It should be introduced slowly in patients while observing for side-effects; these are mostly nausea and rash, but a small proportion of males may experience oligospermia. Genetic determinants govern the rate of salicylate acetylation in patients and the likelihood of side-effects. For sulphasalazine-sensitive patients (about 25%), oral $5\text{-}NH_2$ salicylate (mesalazine) or a diazo-linked $5\text{-}NH_2$ salicylate dimer (olsalazine) have been shown to be as effective as the parent compound.

Table 29.1 Severity of ulcerative colitis (after Truelove)		
	Mild–moderate	Severe
Bowel actions (no/day)	<4–6	>6
Temperature (°C)	<37.5	>37.5
Pulse rate (beats/min)	<90	>90
Haemoglobin (g/dL)	>10	<10
ESR (mm/h)	<30	>30

Immunosuppressants

Neither azathioprine nor 6-mercaptopurine (which have proven effectiveness in severe Crohn's disease) has been shown to be of benefit in ulcerative colitis. More recently, cyclosporin A, which has been used extensively as an immunosuppressant in organ transplantation, has been employed successfully in severe steroid-resistant colitis, particularly when a steroid-sparing effect is required because of either steroid complications or growth retardation.

SURGICAL TREATMENT

Indications for emergency and elective operation

Up to 25% of patients may require operative treatment for colitis; usually those with subtotal or total colitis.
   Relative indications include:

* failure of medical therapy – patients in whom severe colitis over years has resulted in chronic ill health and invalidism, repeated hospitalisation, persistent anaemia and weight loss; disease that is disruptive to normal education, career or social functioning or that is complicated by steroid-induced complications
* growth retardation in childhood colitis
* relapsing severe colitis with potential life-threatening complications, particularly in the elderly
* severe extraintestinal complications – resistant or severe monoarticular arthritis or severe ocular manifestations; pyoderma gangrenosum may also respond to colectomy
* long-standing extensive colitis – colitis of more than 10 years' duration with subtotal or total involvement, particularly when rectal and colonic biopsies have demonstrated persistent severe dysplasia in the absence of active disease.

   Absolute indications include:

* toxic dilatation of the colon
* perforation of the colon
* severe haemorrhage (rare)
* supervening carcinoma of the colon.

Operative approaches

The main procedures are:

* total colectomy and ileorectal anastomosis
* panproctocolectomy with permanent end ileostomy
* restorative proctocolectomy with ileoanal reservoir.

Additional procedures include:

* total colectomy, oversew of rectal stump (or rectal mucous fistula) and end ileostomy – this is the procedure of choice in fulminant colitis or toxic megacolon; a decision about the ultimate fate of the rectum should be made within 12 months based on disease activity, capacity or the presence of dysplasia
* loop ileostomy or split ileostomy – either of these procedures may be used to protect an anastomosis or reservoir
* Kock 'continent' ileostomy – this procedure for permanent ileostomy patients has fallen out of favour because of a high morbidity and revision rate.

The advantages and disadvantages of each procedure are outlined in Table 29.2.

Total colectomy and ileorectal anastomosis. This should be considered in the older patient, particularly if there is relative rectal sparing, adequate rectal capacity, good anal sphincter function and no rectal dysplasia. Patients need to be closely followed for dysplastic changes in the remaining rectum.

Panproctocolectomy and permanent ileostomy. This single-stage procedure was for many years the procedure of choice for ulcerative colitis. It will cure the disease and remove the risk of carcinoma development but necessitates a permanent stoma. There is a moderate incidence of prolonged perineal wound complications, particularly in patients with perirectal sepsis or those on steroids. It is still advocated in elderly patients with severe disease and poor sphincteric function, who would do less well with an ileoanal reservoir, and in patients who have accepted a permanent ileostomy.

Restorative proctocolectomy and ileoanal reservoir. Popularised by Parks and Nicholls in 1978, this is becoming the preferred elective operation for severe ulcerative colitis. It involves construction of an ileal reservoir proximal to either a hand-sutured or stapled ileoanal anastomosis.
   Much work has centred on pouch design and the need for and extent of anal mucosal resection. The two-limbed

Table 29.2 A comparison of three different elective operations for ulcerative proctocolitis

	Panproctocolectomy	Ileorectal anastomosis	Restorative proctocolectomy
Advantages	Curative one stage	One operation Sphincter preserved Minimal bladder/sexual dysfunction No stoma	Curative Sphincter preserved Small risk of bladder/sexual dysfunction
Disadvantages	Permanent ileostomy	Carcinoma risk Non-curative	Failure in 10% Covering stoma Moderate morbidity
Complications	Stoma revision Perineal wound dehiscence Small bowel obstruction	Small bowel obstruction Anastomotic dehiscence	Pouch fistula Pelvic sepsis Anastomotic dehiscence Stricture, small bowel obstruction Pouchitis
Contraindications	Desire to avoid ileostomy	Sphincter incompetence Rectal dysplasia/carcinoma	Crohn's disease Sphincter damage Rectal dysplasia Poor rectal capacity

J pouch is the most favoured design, being easily constructed with the luminal stapler and fitting well into the pelvis of most patients, although its capacity is less than other designs with a W (four-loop) or S (three-loop) configuration. (Fig. 29.5)

The anastomosis is usually performed without a deliberate transanal mucosal stripping, leaving at least 1 cm of transitional anal mucosa above the dentate line for added anorectal sensation.

Contraindications

There are several important groups of patients in whom the restorative proctocolectomy and ileoanal reservoir operation should *not* be performed because of poor short- and long-term results, namely those with:

- inadequate anal sphincter function
- unequivocal Crohn's colitis
- prior extensive small bowel resections
- rectal dysplasia/carcinoma
- poor nutrition
- attendant comorbidity (elderly patients)
- fulminant colitis or toxic dilatation of the colon – in this case, the operation should not be performed as a single-stage procedure.

Results

The procedure is safe and effective in expert hands trained in the techniques and salvage of complicated

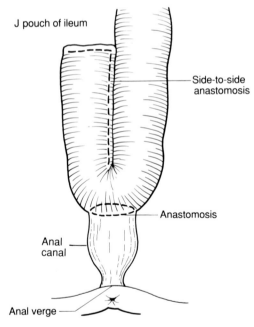

Fig. 29.5 Ileo-anal anastomosis. The J pouch provides a reservoir which decreases the frequency of defaecation. More complex pouches of 'S' or 'W' configuration have been widely used, but they increase the incidence of complications without improving clinical results.

pouch surgery and backed up by an experienced team in counselling and stoma care. It is wisest to cover the anastomosis with a loop ileostomy, which may be closed at a later date following pouch radiology.

Morbidity. About 20% of patients develop complications and about 10% of patients require ultimate pouch removal.

Early complications. These include:

- small bowel obstruction (15%, half require operation)
- pelvic sepsis (5%)
- wound sepsis (5%).

Late complications include:

- stricture (5%)
- pouch–vaginal fistula/pouch fistula (2%)
- pouchitis (7%).

Pouchitis is increasing in incidence and recognition. It is an inflammatory condition that is recognised both endoscopically and histologically in the pouches of patients with previous ulcerative colitis, although the appearance does not correlate well with symptoms. Patients present with crampy abdominal pain associated with diarrhoea, urgency, malaise and occasionally fever. Most patients develop symptoms within 12 months of operation. Although there is no uniform definition of pouchitis, endoscopic examination reveals mucosal oedema, friability and occasional frank ulceration. Histology shows patchy infiltration with both acute and chronic inflammatory cells, villous atrophy and colonic metaplasia.

The aetiology is obscure; there is no increase in bacterial content of the stool in patients with pouchitis and no evidence of delayed pouch emptying based on radionuclide studies. Increased deconjugated pouch bile acids, a decrease in pouch short chain fatty acids and immunological mechanisms have also been implicated.

The condition has been well recognised by the use of ^{111}In-labelled mixed granulocyte scanning. Metronidazole is successful in at least 80% of patients. There is some secondary response to topical steroid and salicylate preparations. Functional studies of patients after restorative proctocolectomy, including pouch physiological assessment, have shown an acceptable quality of life, with a mean daytime call to stool of 5–6 times per day and only occasional nocturnal bowel activity. The functional volume of the pouch tends to enlarge for the first 2 years, and nocturnal bowel urgency tends to diminish.

Reasons for pouch failure include serious perioperative complications (bleeding, pouch ischaemia), persistent pelvic sepsis, pouch–vaginal fistula, recurrent severe pouchitis unresponsive to therapy or intractable anastomotic stricture.

CANCER RISK IN ULCERATIVE COLITIS

There is a low cumulative incidence of cancer (<2%) within 10 years of diagnosis of colitis, with a steady increase after a decade of disease. The risk is increased with:

- total or near total colitis
- younger age of cancer development
- a more even distribution of carcinoma throughout the colon
- multiplicity of carcinoma
- a higher proportion of less well differentiated carcinomas
- infiltrative and flat carcinomas
- associated colonic and rectal dysplasia.

The risk may have been overestimated in the past, particularly with less extensive forms of colitis. Dysplasia has been advocated as a marker for cancer development, but this can be difficult to define and there is much interobserver error between pathologists. It is recommended that patients should undergo repeated colonoscopic surveillance after 10 years and that persistent severe dysplasia in the absence of active disease is an indication for operation. Those patients under surveillance tend to have earlier stage carcinomas and a better overall survival rate.

CROHN'S DISEASE (regional enteritis, granulomatous enterocolitis)

The incidence of Crohn's disease has increased over the last four decades, with an increasing recognition of Crohn's colitis. It is a disease of unknown cause characterised by discontinuous full thickness inflammation involving any part of the gastrointestinal tract.

AETIOLOGY

Possible aetiological factors include:

- infection
- allergy and antoimmunity
- ischaemia.

Infection

The faecal flora of patients with Crohn's disease contains

a higher concentration of obligatory anaerobes. Crohn's disease bears a histological resemblance to intestinal tuberculosis, and *Mycobacterium paratuberculosis* has occasionally been cultured from Crohn's tissue. There is an increase in non-specific humoral and cell-mediated responses to several mycobacterial species in vitro in Crohn's patients.

It has recently been suggested that persistent measles virus may cause a focal granulomatous vasculitis, and paramyxovirus particles have been demonstrated in the vascular endothelium of the tissues of some patients with acute Crohn's disease. Measles DNA has been shown in the granulomas of some Crohn's specimens.

Allergy and autoimmunity

Many of the microscopic features of Crohn's disease suggest an allergic type reaction: oedema and infiltration of the bowel wall with lymphocytes, plasma cells, eosinophils and giant cells. The changes could be secondary to an allergen, but detailed immunological studies have so far failed to reveal anything specific. Some patients show abnormal humoral responses to milk proteins and an increase in circulating antibodies to wheat and maize grain antigens.

Ischaemia

An abnormal gut microcirculation has been postulated with increases in procoagulant activity, notably an increase in thromboxane B_2 production and a decrease in factor XIII.

SURGICAL PATHOLOGY

Macroscopic features

The hallmark of Crohn's disease is its segmental or discontinuous nature. The disease is transmural; characteristic deep fissures penetrate adjacent structures and lead to abscesses and fistulae. Lymphadenopathy is prominent, and the involved segment has mesenteric encroachment of fat (so-called fat wrapping) as well as fine corkscrew vessels on the serosal surface.

The bowel is woody to feel because of extensive thickening. On its opened surface there is a classical cobblestone oedema and an ulcerated appearance to the mucosa. The differences in macroscopic features between Crohn's disease and ulcerative colitis are shown in Table 29.3.

Microscopic features

The inflammatory process is transmural. There is a chronic inflammatory infiltrate, lymphoid hyperplasia and extensive fibrosis. Although crypt abscesses may occur, acute inflammatory infiltration is not extensive. The muscularis mucosae and muscularis propria are both hypertrophied; lymphatic dilatation and fissures extend across the full depth of the involved segment.

Table 29.3 Differentiation between Crohn's colitis and ulcerative colitis

Macroscopic features	Ulcerative colitis	Crohn's disease of colon
Distribution in colon	Continuous	Discontinuous (segmental)
Ileal involvement	Rare if ever	30% and may be extensive
Rectal involvement	Always	50%
Serosa	Normal	Granular, fibrous or 'flared'
Ileocaecal valve	Normal or dilated	Often narrowed or thickened
Mucosa of bowel	Granular, ulcerated or continuous	Cobblestoned, fissured (cracked), patchy ulceration
Pseudopolyps	Usual	Not uncommon
Internal fistulas	None	80%
Anal lesions	25%	75%
Extent of inflammation	Mucosal and submucosal	Transmural (full thickness)
Granulomas	Absent	75%
Full thickness fissuring	Absent	Common
Fibrosis	Absent or minimal	Present
Lymphoedema and lymphoid hyperplasia	Absent	Present
Mesenteric nodes	Reactive hyperaemia	Granulomatous foci 25%
Carcinoma	Common in long-standing disease	Rare

Non-caseating (sarcoid-like) granulomata with Langhans type giant cell infiltrates and associated neuromatous hyperplasia are common in both the involved bowel and adjacent lymph nodes. The common sites for Crohn's disease are the ileocaecal region (40%), the isolated small bowel (29%), the colon (27%) and the perineal area (10%).

COMPLICATIONS

Calculi

Crohn's disease of the small bowel may be complicated by gall bladder calculi, which arise from impaired enterohepatic circulation of bile salts in disease of the terminal ileum or after ileal resection. There is an increased incidence of oxalate urinary calculi secondary to relative hyperoxaluria after small bowel resection.

Perianal disease

This is a particularly troublesome feature of Crohn's disease, impairing sphincter function and thus quality of life. Primary manifestations include eccentric and multiple anal fissures, oedematous cyanotic skin tags and painful cavitating ulcers. Secondary changes such as complex anal fistulas, strictures and deep anorectal abscesses are common.

Toxic dilatation

This is less common than in ulcerative colitis, but free perforation of the colon is more frequent, particularly in patients on corticosteroids.

Extraintestinal manifestations

These are similar to those observed in ulcerative colitis. Aphthous ulceration of the mouth, erythema nodosum and clubbing are more common in Crohn's disease, but sclerosing cholangitis is rare.

Urological disease

This is a particular feature of Crohn's disease and may present as hydronephrosis (particularly right-sided), enterovesical fistula, pyelonephritis, retroperitoneal abscess or renal amyloidosis.

CLINICAL FEATURES

Acute regional enteritis

The features are often indistinguishable from those of acute appendicitis, with right iliac fossa tenderness and an elevated temperature. The diagnosis is generally made at operation. Serology for *Yersinia enterocolitica* should be performed to avoid mislabelling certain patients with acute infective ileitis as Crohn's disease.

Chronic regional enteritis

Ulceration and fibrosis at the ileocaecal angle produce a clinical syndrome of chronic ill health, anaemia, abdominal pain and diarrhoea. Subacute or acute small bowel obstruction can supervene. A mass may be palpable representing loops of encased small bowel. The differential diagnosis in such cases is from caecal carcinoma or sometimes ileocaecal tuberculosis. Such disease may be complicated by the presence of intra-abdominal abscess(es).

Enteric fistula

This can be simple or complex. It may be enteroenteric, enterocolic, urinary-enteric or enterocutaneous.

Colonic Crohn's disease

Diarrhoea is the usual presentation. It is frequently intermittent and semi-formed, and bleeding is not profuse. Weight loss and general ill health are common. Perianal disease is frequent in this group of patients, with occasional destructive perianal pathology and complex fistulas.

INVESTIGATIONS

Radiology

The traditional small bowel meal and follow-through has been replaced by the small bowel enema (or enteroclysis), in which the proximal jejunum is intubated. The findings include oedema and separation of involved small bowel loops, extensive stricturing, usually of the terminal ileum (so-called 'string sign'; Fig. 29.6), and mucosal ulceration ('rose thorn' ulcers).

Fistulas may be evident between adjacent bowel loops or into the bladder. Skip lesions are a classical feature.

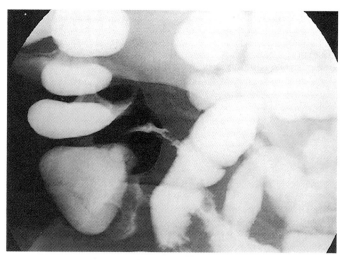

Fig. 29.6 Small bowel enema showing the classical 'string' sign caused by Crohn's disease of the terminal ileum.

On barium enema, patchy involvement of the colon and stricturing help to distinguish Crohn's disease from ulcerative colitis. Strictures are smooth and tapered, unlike those seen in carcinomatous or radiation-induced strictures.

Endoscopy

The rectum is often spared. There is cobblestone oedema of the mucosa. Segmental involvement may differentiate Crohn's disease from ulcerative colitis, but endoscopy may not be able to distinguish ischaemic colitis or radiation colitis in some cases.

MEDICAL MANAGEMENT

Sulphasalazine and derivatives

Sulphasalazine and aminosalicylates have not been shown to be of value in small bowel Crohn's disease, but they are the mainstay of treatment for Crohn's colitis. Their role in maintaining remission in colonic disease is uncertain.

Corticosteroids

Trials have shown a benefit with corticosteroid therapy in all forms of active Crohn's disease. Steroids should be used in acute colitis with associated systemic illness, extraintestinal disease and in proximal colonic disease unlikely to be reached effectively with topical agents.

There is no evidence that steroids maintain remission or prevent recurrence after operation. Budesonide, a corticosteroid structurally related to 16-α-hydroxyprednisolone with high affinity for corticosteroid receptors and little systemic activity, has recently been shown to be effective in active Crohn's disease of the distal ileum and proximal colon.

Immunosuppressants

Azathioprine (2–2.5 mg/kg) and 6-mercaptopurine (1.5 mg/kg) have no proven benefit in acute disease, but they can prevent relapse as well as exert a steroid-sparing effect in patients with steroid-related complications. Both drugs are particularly toxic to the bone marrow.

Cyclosporin A has been used with success in steroid-resistant acute disease. It needs close monitoring because of nephrotoxicity.

Antibiotics

Intermittent and prolonged low-dose metronidazole is beneficial in recurrent and destructive perianal disease.

Nutrition

Besides specific therapy, attention must be paid to fluid and electrolyte imbalance, the correction of anaemia and nutritional supplementation. Malnutrition is a prominent feature of many patients. It reflects poor oral intake, malabsorption, gastrointestinal bypass in internal fistulas or excess nitrogen losses from diarrhoea, short gut syndrome or external high output fistulas.

Enteral supplementation is best whenever possible, but the relative merits of elemental or low-residue polymeric diets are debated. Total parenteral nutrition (TPN) is occasionally needed in patients whose gut is unavailable for use, in short bowel syndrome after multiple small bowel resections or in certain high output fistulas.

INDICATIONS FOR OPERATION

Operative treatment is required in 80% of patients. It is not curative and recurrence is almost invariable given sufficient follow-up. It is usually indicated for complications of Crohn's disease, particularly obstruction, abscess and fistula.

Acute regional ileitis

Laparotomy is often performed for a suspected diagnosis of acute appendicitis. At operation, once the condition has been diagnosed, it is usually safe to perform an appendicectomy. The small bowel segment should not be resected unless it is complicated by fistula or abscess, but the entire small bowel should be carefully examined if possible to define the extent of disease.

Chronic regional enteritis

Resection of the involved segment is required for obstruction, fistula, perforation with abscess or ileocaecal disease that is poorly responsive to medical therapy and is causing chronic ill health, recurrent low-grade obstruction or a mass.

Resection is generally favoured as it provides histology for accurate diagnosis and prevents sepsis in the bypassed segment. Bypass of the inflamed segment has fallen out of favour as it may result in chronic bacterial overgrowth and unrecognised carcinomatous transformation in the excluded segment. Strictureplasty has been used since the early 1980s, particularly for very short segment disease in multiple sites where resection is ill-advised. A longitudinal incision is made through the strictured segment and then closed transversely. It is a safe procedure that gives marked symptomatic improvement but has a higher recurrence rate than resection.

Crohn's colitis

Operation may be performed for fulminating colitis, colonic perforation or toxic dilatation. Procedures include segmental colectomy, resection without anastomosis and proctocolectomy (for severe perirectal stricture, sepsis or fistulas).

Chronic perianal disease

Perianal sepsis should be drained. Formal operations are best avoided in extensive fistulous disease because of the risk of incontinence, but seton drainage may be used to prevent further abscess formation. Proctectomy should be considered in destructive disease of the sphincter with recurrent sepsis, although long-term complications with both the perineum and the stoma may be expected. It is important to define the state of the sphincters before operation by means of anorectal physiology and endoanal ultrasonography.

SURGICAL RECOMMENDATIONS

When surgery is indicated, the following recommendations are applicable:

- Deal only with the site(s) of complication provided by the operative indication – i.e. treat symptomatic and not radiological disease.
- Limit resections to macroscopic disease only. Recurrence rates are not increased if there is histological evidence of disease at the resection margins, so resections must be conservative.
- Attempt to use restorative resections in colonic Crohn's disease.
- Operate sparingly and conservatively for perianal disease.

INDETERMINATE COLITIS

About 10% of patients with inflammatory bowel disease have clinical and histological features that do not permit a clear distinction to be made between Crohn's disease and ulcerative colitis. With time, they may gravitate into one or other group as the disease progresses. If the diagnosis continues to be difficult on follow-up, most patients will behave as ulcerative colitis and their long-term outcome after restorative proctocolectomy is good.

ISCHAEMIC COLITIS

Ischaemic colitis is an inflammatory response in the colon that follows a local arterial or venous insult and has a spectrum of clinical presentations with a diverse aetiology. The outcome depends upon the severity and extent of ischaemia, the status of the collateral circulation and the bacterial flora present in the bowel.

PATHOPHYSIOLOGY

Ischaemia occurs at sites of vascular watershed such as between the terminal branches of the superior and inferior mesenteric arteries (at the splenic flexure), between the internal iliac and inferior mesenteric arteries (at the rectosigmoid junction) and in the right colon (where there may be absent middle or right colic arteries). In the right colon, the marginal artery is often poorly developed, with end vessels (vasa recta) that are more prone to non-occlusive mesenteric ischaemia. Ischaemic colon injury may be transient, chronic or acute.

The causes of ischaemic colitis may be broadly divided into occlusive or non-occlusive (Table 29.4). Occlusion of blood vessels supplying the colon can follow trauma, thrombosis, embolism or ligation of the inferior mesenteric artery during aortic operations. Diffuse disease of the small vessels of the colon may occur as part of a vasculitis or in hypercoagulable states where there is extensive mesenteric venous thrombosis.

Non-occlusive ischaemia may occur during shock, cardiac failure or extreme sepsis. Small vessel vasoconstriction and shunting within the mesenteric circulation contribute to colonic ischaemia, which often persists even when normal haemodynamics have been restored.

SURGICAL PATHOLOGY

The severity of changes depends upon the cause of vascular embarrassment, the adequacy of the collaterals and the speed of ischaemia. The anatomical extent of vascular anastomosis determines the degree of ischaemia. The most obvious changes affect the mucosa and submucosa.

Ischaemic colitis with gangrene

The condition has two phases:

- infarction of the colon causing varying degrees of mucosal gangrene, oedema and haemorrhage with intravascular platelet thrombi
- secondary invasion with organisms capable of accelerating the gangrenous process under anaerobic conditions and leading to full thickness bowel wall necrosis.

Transient ischaemic colitis

This is the mildest form of ischaemia. The mucosal ulceration and transmural inflammation resolve as collaterals open up.

Ischaemic stricture of the colon

Incomplete recovery from ischaemia can lead to full thickness inflammation of the colon with fibrosis and formation of a smooth stricture. Histologically the area shows fibroblastic proliferation with infiltration by haemosiderin laden macrophages. Strictures are short and never complete.

CLINICAL FEATURES

There are no pathognomonic signs of ischaemic colitis. Most patients are in their sixth or later decades, and

---

Table 29.4 Aetiology of colonic ischaemia

Occlusive factors
Large artery occlusion
— main stem SMA or branch embolus/thrombosis
— IMA ligation
— IMA trauma
— constricting tumour/adhesions/other mechanical factors

Small artery disease
— vasculitis
— radiation injury
— diabetes mellitus

Venous occlusion
— hypercoagulability
— portal hypertension
— severe intra-abdominal inflammatory process (pancreatitis)
— malignancy

Non-occlusive mesenteric ischaemia (NOMI)
Idiopathic
— profound shock (cardiogenic, neurogenic, septic)
— Iatrogenic: catecholamines, digitalis, mesenteric angiography

SMA = superior mesenteric artery; IMA = inferior mesenteric artery.

there is often a history of widespread atheromatous disease.

Ischaemic colitis with gangrene

The following are usually present:

- acute left-sided abdominal pain
- abdominal tenderness and rigidity
- abdominal distension
- shock and toxaemia
- gastrointestinal haemorrhage.

Sigmoidoscopy may reveal blood in the lumen, but the rectum and lower sigmoid colon will appear normal. Plain X-ray of the abdomen may show an ileus, toxic colonic dilatation, intramural bowel gas, free intraperitoneal air or rarely air in the portal venous system.

Transient ischaemic colitis

The following are usually present:

- transient abdominal pain of sudden onset
- rectal bleeding which subsides in several days
- diarrhoea which subsides in several days.

Sigmoidoscopy usually reveals no abnormality. The rectum is always spared. Early colonoscopy shows areas of mucosal pallor interspersed with hyperaemia, petechial haemorrhage or punctate ulceration. Colonic biopsy shows loss of the normal crypt architecture, loss of mucin, mixed inflammatory infiltrate in the lamina propria and intravascular thrombi in lamina propria vessels.

For diagnosis by barium enema, a high index of suspicion is required. Thumbprinting and areas of submucosal oedema and haemorrhage are classical features. The upper left colon is the typical site to be involved and there may be narrowing of the colon.

Ischaemic stricture of the colon

In this condition there are usually symptoms of sub-acute large bowel obstruction. Colonoscopy will reveal a smooth benign stricture with mucosal atrophy. Biopsy shows a relative blunting of crypts with extensive lamina propria fibrosis. Very occasionally an active vasculitis is seen surrounding intraluminal thrombus. Barium enema may show a tapered stricture, with saccular variants.

MANAGEMENT

Patients with abdominal pain but no evidence of peritonitis should be treated conservatively with intravenous fluids, broad-spectrum antibiotics and analgesia. Colonoscopy should be performed early to make the diagnosis and to assess the severity and extent of disease. Patients should be followed for the development of a colonic stricture.

Those patients who deteriorate should have a laparotomy, with resection of the ischaemic segment and exteriorisation of both colonic ends. This operation has a high perioperative mortality rate, particularly if it occurs secondary to major aortic reconstructive surgery. In such patients, clinical suspicion of colonic ischaemia is evident by severe abdominal pain, evidence of toxicity and metabolic acidosis. Aortography before aortic reconstruction may provide a clue to potential ischaemia by the absence of filling major visceral vessels or by the presence of a meandering mesenteric vessel supplying the colon. At operation, poor backflow through the inferior mesenteric artery may necessitate its reimplantation.

Provided a confident diagnosis of ischaemic stricture can be made and carcinoma eliminated, operation should be avoided since these strictures are incomplete.

PSEUDOMEMBRANOUS ENTEROCOLITIS

This condition is also known as antibiotic-associated colitis or *Clostridium difficile* colitis.

SURGICAL PATHOLOGY

Pseudomembranous enterocolitis (PMC) is an acute disorder of bacterial overgrowth secondary to short- or long-term antibiotic usage. Lincomycin and clindamycin were the first antibiotics to be incriminated in its causation. The organism responsible is *Clostridium difficile*, a Gram-positive spore-forming anaerobe which was identified as the causative agent in 1980. PMC is more common after oral rather than parenteral administration of antibiotics and may occur after only a single dose. Culture of normal adult faeces is usually negative for *C. difficile* although the organism is commonly found in neonates. Nowadays, PMC most commonly follows penicillin or cephalosporin usage. The hallmark of the disease is the appearance of grey-white pseudomembranes spread between inflamed parts of the mucosa.

These are usually located in the rectum, but there is relative rectal sparing in 10% of cases.

CLINICAL FEATURES

Diarrhoea after antibiotic administration is common, and causes other than *C. difficile* infection should be distinguished. Symptoms of PMC include watery diarrhoea, abdominal pain, fever and leucocytosis, but not usually bloody diarrhoea.

Diagnosis is made by sigmoidoscopy and the presence of positive *C. difficile* toxin in the faeces. Although *C. difficile* is readily cultured, toxin assay is available by latex agglutination in less than 1 hour. There is no correlation between disease severity and toxin concentration.

TREATMENT

Vancomycin has proven value when used orally in a dose of 125 mg four times daily. It is minimally absorbed and is excreted in high faecal concentration. Symptomatic control is high, but recurrence occurs in 5–55% of cases.

Metronidazole has been shown to be as effective as vancomycin in a recent randomised controlled trial. Other effective agents include oral bacitracin and anion exchange resins such as cholestyramine and colestipol which bind toxin and which may be used in recurrent disease. Competitive bacterial solutions (*Lactobacillus* sp. and *Saccharomyces boulardii*) have recently been shown to be effective and are inexpensive.

Operation is only required in fulminant PMC with associated toxic dilatation. The cause of recurrent PMC is unclear. It may be the result of vancomycin resistance, intermittent spore formation between antibiotic courses, subinhibitory vancomycin concentrations or reinfection.

RADIATION COLITIS

EPIDEMIOLOGY

There is an increasing incidence of radiation injury, particularly to the rectum, because of a general increase in the use of adjuvant pelvic irradiation for advanced rectal cancer and the combined use of intracavitary and external radiotherapy in gynaecological cancers. Radiobiological factors affecting the outcome include the total body dose, the use of fractionated therapy, the volume of tissue irradiated and the inherent tissue tolerance to radiation.

PATHOPHYSIOLOGY

Radiation has early direct effects on actively replicating cells and delayed indirect effects that follow late obliterative endarteritis in small and large vessels. Submucosal hyalinisation, fibrinoid vascular necrosis and infiltration of tissue with 'bizarre' fibroblasts are often associated with this 'endarteritis obliterans'. These delayed effects induce poor healing in irradiated tissue, with the development of stricture, radionecrotic ulceration and fistula, often many years after the radiation treatment. Consequently, surgical treatment in these patients has a high complication rate.

RISK FACTORS

These include:

- radiation-related parameters – total dose, overlapping radiation portals
- body morphology – radiation effects are worse in children and thin patients, whose pelvis contains a large amount of small bowel
- previous pelvic or abdominal surgery
- associated medical disorders – hypertension and diabetes mellitus aggravate the vascular damage
- chemotherapy – prior treatment with actinomycin D, doxorubicin or 5-fluorouracil.

INCIDENCE AND INJURY PATTERN

Approximately 5–10% of patients with radiation exposure develop the disease, and 20% will require operation. The rectum is involved in 75%, the small bowel in 35% and the ileum in 80% of cases. In general, patients who present with obstruction or bleeding have a better prognosis than those who present with fistula or free perforation.

CLINICAL FEATURES

Radiation disease can be acute or chronic.

Acute radiation enteritis

Between 50% and 75% of patients undergoing abdominal radiotherapy will experience some form of acute radiation enteritis, with abdominal pain, diarrhoea and occasional bleeding. This is self-limiting and will almost always recover within 6 months. It may require flexible sigmoidoscopy and stool culture to exclude other pathology. Treatment is supportive: reducing the dose of radiotherapy and using steroid or sucralfate enemas.

Chronic radiation enteritis

It may present in variable fashion with:

- chronic blood loss
- torrential rectal haemorrhage
- rectal ulceration
- stricture
- rectovaginal or other fistula
- chronic coloproctitis
- faecal incontinence.

Endoscopy reveals a pale oedematous mucosa with occasional contact bleeding and petechial haemorrhage. Total colonoscopy can be technically difficult in rigid bowel. There are no pathognomonic features on barium enema, but changes include lack of distensibility of the bowel, rectal and sigmoid foreshortening and fixed smooth stenoses. Occasional fistulas can be seen entering the bladder or vaginal vault.

MANAGEMENT

This includes the use of sucralfate enemas, oral sulphasalazine and occasional steroid enemas. Supportive therapy may include elemental diets and rarely (in severe cases) total parenteral nutrition. Laser photocoagulation with an Nd YAG laser or the use of 3% formalin enemas may stop recurrent severe haemorrhage from radiation proctosigmoiditis.

PRESENTATION

When radiotherapy of the abdomen or pelvis is planned, certain preventative manoeuvres can be used to diminish radiation exposure. Techniques described include:

- small bowel exclusion from the pelvis
- peritoneal closure after proctectomy
- pelvic omental transposition
- absorbable pelvic prosthetic meshes and inflatable reservoirs to fill the pelvis
- rotational radiation fields with Trendelenburg position to keep the bowel out of the pelvis
- pelvic conformational computerised fields
- smaller dose of high-fractionated therapy.

The *indications for operation* include:

- fistula
- perforation
- painful intractable rectal ulceration
- intractable proctocolitis/faecal incontinence
- stricture
- ischaemic enteritis (rare)
- life-threatening haemorrhage (rare)
- associated carcinoma – it appears that radiation confers an increased risk of carcinoma many years later. It is well described and tends to occur in younger patients, with a mucinous histology and a worse overall prognosis.

At operation, bowel that is damaged by radiation appears thickened with a dull grey-white appearance. The loops are often closely matted together with loss of planes of dissection and extensive interloop adhesion. In general, surgical resection of diseased bowel is advised. The alternatives of bypass or diversion are restricted to recurrent technically difficult cases.

SURGICAL RULES IN RADIATION ENTERITIS

When carrying out surgery for this condition, it is important to abide by certain rules:

- use bowel preparation
- avoid irradiated skin for incisions or stomas
- avoid excessive or unnecessary dissection of irradiated bowel
- cover anastomoses with stomas
- avoid irradiated bowel (often the terminal ileum) in stoma usage
- consider pre-operative ureteric stenting.

DIVERSION COLITIS (bypass colitis, disuse colitis, exclusion colitis)

This is an inflammatory colitis arising in a segment of the large intestine that is excluded from the faecal stream. Most cases are asymptomatic, but if symptoms develop they usually occur within 2 years. Very occasionally, patients will experience extraintestinal manifestations with low-grade fever and pelvic pain. Endoscopic changes are non-specific, including aphthous ulceration, pseudopolyps and rarely stricture formation.

Histologically there is a non-specific patchy infiltration of lymphocytes and plasma cells, but crypt architecture is maintained. The aetiology may be bacterial overgrowth or a deprivation of trophic short-chain fatty acids. Both surgical reanastomosis and topical fatty acid therapy (acetate, butyrate and propionate) have been shown to reverse the changes seen.

FURTHER READING

Au J, Smith A N, Eastwood M A 1988 Diverticular disease of the colon in Scotland over 15 years: any benefit from fibre advocacy so far? Journal of the Royal College of Surgery of Edinburgh 18: 271–276

Brynskov J, Freund L, Rasmussen S N et al 1989 A prospective double-blind randomized trial of cyclosporin therapy in active chronic Crohn's disease. New England Journal of Medicine 321: 845–850

Choi P M, Nugent F W, Schoetz D J et al 1993 Colonoscopic surveillance reduces mortality for colorectal cancer in ulcerative colitis. Gastroenterology 105: 418–424

Fazio V W, Tjandra J J 1993 Strictureplasty for Crohn's disease with multiple long strictures. Diseases of the Colon and Rectum 36: 71–72

Galland R B, Spencer J 1987 Natural history and surgical management of radiation enteritis. British Journal of Surgery 74: 742–747

Greenberg G R, Feagan B G, Martin F et al 1994 Oral budesonide for active Crohn's disease. New England Journal of Medicine 331(13): 836–841

Kamm M A, Senapah A 1992 Drug management of ulcerative colitis. British Medical Journal 305: 35–38

Kohler L W, Pemberton J H, Zinsmeister A R, Kelly K A 1991 Quality of life after proctocolectomy; a comparison of Brooke ileostomy, Kock pouch and ileal pouch-anal anastomosis. Gastroenterology 101: 679–684

Lichtiger S, Present D H, Kornbluth A et al 1994 Cyclosporin in severe ulcerative colitis refractory to steroid therapy. New England Journal of Medicine 330: 1841–1845

Longo W E, Ballantyne G H, Gusberg B J 1992 Ischaemic colitis: patterns and prognosis. Diseases of the Colon and Rectum 35: 726–730

O'Brien J J, Bayliss T M, Bayliss J A 1991 Use of azathioprine or 6-mercaptopurine in the treatment of Crohn's disease. Gastroenterology 101: 39–46

Painter N S, Burkitt D P 1971 Diverticular disease of the colon: a deficiency of western civilization. British Medical Journal ii: 450–454

Sartor R B 1995 Current concepts in the aetiology and pathogenesis of ulcerative colitis and Crohn's disease. Gastroenterologic Clinics of North America 24(3): 475–507

Tedesco F J 1986 Pseudomembranous colitis: pathogenesis and treatment. Medical Clinics of North America 66: 655–664

Truelove S C 1988 Medical management of ulcerative colitis and indications for colectomy. World Journal of Surgery 12: 142–147

30 Acute appendicitis and mimicking disorders

Robin Williamson

OVERVIEW

Appendicitis is such a common cause of the acute abdomen that all students and practising doctors should be aware of its presenting features. The diagnosis is still a matter of clinical judgment in most patients, some of whom present with an inflammatory mass. Ultrasound scan and laparoscopy can be useful to corroborate the diagnosis or provide an alternative explanation for the symptoms and signs, particularly in women of reproductive age who have many other potential causes of right iliac fossa pain. Mimicking conditions also include mesenteric adenitis and inflammation of a Meckel's diverticulum.

One person in six or seven develops appendicitis at some time, so that this condition is the commonest abdominal surgical emergency. Appendicitis is a 'disease of civilisation'; it is relatively uncommon in developing rural communities.

SURGICAL ANATOMY OF THE APPENDIX

The appendix is attached at the point of convergence of the three taeniae coli of the caecum on its posteromedial wall. The meso-appendix is a peritoneal fold containing a variable amount of fat and the appendicular artery, which generally arises from the posterior caecal branch of the ileocolic artery.

Like the hands of a clock, the appendix may be long or short and may occupy any position radially from its base (Fig. 30.1). It is commonly situated behind the caecum

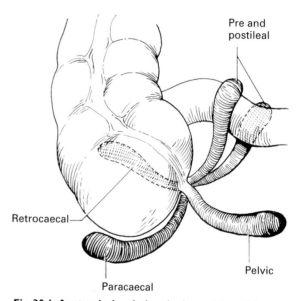

Fig. 30.1 Anatomical variations in the position of the appendix.

(retrocaecal) or lying on the psoas major muscle at or below the pelvic brim (pelvic) and rarely in other positions (pre-ileal, postileal, paracaecal).

SURGICAL PATHOLOGY

PREDISPOSING FACTORS

There are two major factors: obstructive agents and infective agents.

Obstructive agents. These include foreign bodies – animal (e.g. threadworms, roundworms), vegetable (e.g.

seeds, date stones) or mineral (e.g. faecoliths; this is the commonest cause) – and submucous lymphoid tissue. The latter is most abundant in childhood and adolescence. Lymphoid hyperplasia may cause obstruction of the appendix lumen.

Infective agents. Mixed intestinal organisms can usually be cultured from an inflamed appendix. Infection could be primary, leading to lymphoid hyperplasia, or secondary when bacteria gain access to the wall of the appendix through an area of epithelial erosion caused by pressure of an obstructing agent. Both aerobic and anaerobic organisms are involved, including coliforms, enterococci, bacteroides and other intestinal commensals.

TYPES OF ACUTE APPENDICITIS

There are three clinicopathological types of appendicitis, in each of which obstructive and infective factors play a part:

- acute appendicitis
- acute appendicitis with an inflammatory mass
- acute appendicitis with generalised peritonitis.

Acute appendicitis

Organisms enter the wall of the appendix and lodge in the submucosa, where they proliferate rapidly or slowly depending upon their virulence. Eventually the full thickness of the wall is involved, becoming reddened and turgid. The rate of acceleration of the inflammatory process is increased in the presence of obstruction to the lumen of the appendix.

Acute appendicitis with an inflammatory mass

In the presence of obstruction together with severe infection, the appendix becomes distended with pus, which causes an increase in intraluminal pressure. If the process is allowed to proceed, venous occlusion, further oedema and then arterial occlusion result in gangrene of part of the wall of the appendix. Commonly, gangrene develops close to the tip of the appendix, where the blood supply is precarious, or at the site of frank obstruction, where pressure necrosis plays a part. Perforation follows, but infected material is rapidly localised by the defence mechanisms, in particular the greater omentum and coils

of small bowel. An appendix mass is formed, which can undergo suppuration to produce an appendix abscess.

Acute appendicitis with generalised peritonitis

Free perforation occurs when severe degrees of obstruction and infection are followed by developing gangrene, especially in patients with poor powers of localisation (the young and the old). Perforation of the appendix allows infected material to disperse widely in the peritoneal cavity, causing an intense peritoneal reaction with outpouring of fluid, which is initially clear but which rapidly becomes purulent. The serosal surfaces of the bowel become injected and flaked with clotted lymph.

CLINICAL FEATURES

These vary depending on the clinicopathological type of appendicitis, as described above.

ACUTE APPENDICITIS

Symptoms

Abdominal pain may vary considerably in type and situation. It is classically periumbilical at first – the result of appendicular obstruction – followed by movement to the right iliac fossa (RIF) within a few hours, where it becomes persistent. However, it may start in the RIF. The onset is usually sudden, particularly if there is a high degree of obstruction to the lumen of the appendix, but there may be a preceding 12–24 hour period of nausea and of vague abdominal discomfort. The initial pain may be colicky in nature if a marked degree of obstruction is present, or continuous and nagging like a toothache. Retrocaecal appendicitis may cause pain in the loin.

Vomiting may be early and repeated if obstruction to the appendix is present. Otherwise it is not an outstanding feature. Loss of appetite is an early symptom of acute appendicitis.

Diarrhoea is more likely in the presence of an inflamed pelvic appendix irritating the rectal wall or a retro-ileal appendix irritating the terminal small bowel. Frequency or dysuria may also occur with an inflamed pelvic appendix.

Signs

General. The patient may look unwell and have a coated tongue and foul breath. Moderate pyrexia and tachycardia indicate an infective process, but their absence does not exclude appendicitis.

Local. Tenderness of a localised and persistent nature is the most important abdominal finding. It is situated over the appendix, at some place in the RIF and classically at McBurney's point (the junction of the middle and outer thirds of a line from umbilicus to anterior superior iliac spine).

Rigidity of the abdominal muscles overlying the right iliac fossa indicates involvement of the underlying peritoneum. Guarding may be absent in early, retrocaecal or pelvic appendicitis. Rebound tenderness also indicates peritoneal inflammation. The sign is best elicited by percussion.

Tenderness on the right side during rectal examination indicates involvement of the pelvic peritoneum by the inflammatory process. This may be the only sign with a pelvic appendicitis.

Special. Many tests have been described to determine the presence or absence of local peritonitis, but none is reliable. Some of these are described here.

Rovsing's sign. Deep pressure in the left iliac fossa causes pain in the RIF. However, there is no evidence to confirm the thought that pain is produced by distension of the caecum with gases forced into it from the left colon.

Blumberg's sign. Deep pressure in the left iliac fossa may be associated with pain in the RIF when the hand is suddenly released. This 'crossed' or 'rebound' tenderness is said to be strongly suggestive of local peritonitis.

Cope's sign. Flexion and internal rotation of the right hip may cause pain if the obturator internus muscle is in close relation to an inflamed pelvic appendix.

Psoas sign. Extension of the right hip may cause pain if the psoas muscle is in close relation to a retrocaecal or pelvic appendix.

Straight leg raising sign. With digital pressure over the tender spot in the abdomen, elevation of the right leg may cause increased pain. This is suggestive of a retrocaecal appendicitis.

Laboratory and other investigations

Abdominal X-rays are seldom helpful.

The white cell count is often raised, due to a neutrophilia.

The urine should always be examined by ward test and by microscopy in a doubtful case. Red or white blood cells may be found if the inflamed appendix abuts against the ureter or bladder.

Ultrasound scan may show a dilated lumen and thickened wall of the appendix, but its greatest value is to delineate an appendix mass or rule out gynaecological pathology.

Laparoscopy is discussed below.

Differential diagnosis

Usually there is little difficulty in diagnosing acute appendicitis. However, one must remember other possibilities, particularly in a young female. These conditions may be divided into extra-abdominal and abdominal.

Extra-abdominal. Right basal pneumonia and diaphragmatic pleurisy may be associated with abdominal symptoms, but the presence of respiratory symptoms and specific signs in the chest should cause little difficulty with the diagnosis.

Abdominal. Almost any abdominal condition can mimic acute appendicitis. Some of these are discussed here.

Mesenteric adenitis. Approximately 5% of all operations performed for suspected acute appendicitis discover mesenteric adenitis. The presence of enlarged pink and fleshy lymph nodes in the mesentery of the terminal ileum associated with a normal appendix are the characteristic features.

Probably viral in origin, mesenteric adenitis usually occurs in children and may be suspected when there is a history of recent sore throat together with a high fever, attacks of pain with complete relief between attacks, a tender spot medial to and above McBurney's point, shifting tenderness and little or no muscle guarding. Under these conditions it may be permissible to observe the patient, particularly if the abdominal signs are minimal in degree. However, if there is any doubt, operation is indicated. In all cases the appendix should be removed to avoid future confusion when confronted with an appendicectomy scar and RIF pain.

Pyelitis. Right-sided abdominal and loin pain associated with rigors and urinary symptoms is suggestive of a urinary tract infection. The absence of abdominal rigidity and the presence of pus in the urine indicate the diagnosis.

Ureteric colic. A calculus in the right ureter may cause confusion, but the radiation of the pain along the line of the ureter and the presence of blood in the urine should eliminate any doubt. A plain X-ray of the abdomen or an intravenous urogram will demonstrate the stone.

Gastroenteritis. Diarrhoea, vomiting, central abdominal pain and fever, without local tenderness or rigidity over the appendix region, suggest gastroenteritis.

Crohn's disease. Terminal ileitis may present with RIF pain (See Ch. 29).

Non-specific ileitis. This may cause a similar picture and *Yersinia* or *Campylobacter* sp. may be identified.

Meckel's diverticulitis. In this rare condition the clinical picture is very similar to appendicitis. Meckel's diverticulum and its disorders are discussed below.

Acute cholecystitis. Right upper abdominal pain associated with acute cholecystitis may be confused with high retrocaecal appendicitis (see also Ch. 26).

Diverticulitis. Acute diverticulitis of the sigmoid colon may be confused with pelvic appendicitis (see also Ch. 29). The sigmoid colon may lie centrally or even on the right of the midline. Rarely a solitary caecal diverticulum becomes inflamed.

Gynaecological conditions. Pelvic inflammatory disease, which includes salpingitis, pyosalpinx, tubovarian abscess and parametritis, is the commonest condition to exclude when considering appendicitis as the cause of abdominal pain in non-pregnant women of reproductive age. Gonococcal and chlamydial infection are the commonest underlying causes. This condition is particularly common in large city hospitals where promiscuity and prostitution are frequent predisposing factors. A further variant is FitzHugh–Curtis syndrome, in which infection spreads up the right paracolic gutter to involve the surface of the liver. The clinical features may mimic either acute appendicitis or acute cholecystitis. Pelvic examination of women who may have appendicitis is therefore mandatory. Torsion of a fallopian tube, torsion, haemorrhage or rupture of an ovarian tumour and endometriosis may have to be considered. Pain of sudden onset in the right iliac fossa, on the day a period begins, may be caused by the rupture of or minor haemorrhage from a corpus luteal cyst. Midcycle pain (mittelschmerz) may occur from rupture of a follicular cyst at ovulation.

During early pregnancy, abortion, retroverted and impacted uterus, degeneration of uterine fibroids and ectopic pregnancy require consideration. It should be remembered that acute appendicitis complicates 1 in 1000 pregnancies.

During late pregnancy, labour, abruptio placentae, ruptured uterus, fulminating pre-eclampsia and rectus sheath haematoma require consideration.

Women often develop recurrent acute or subacute RIF pain, particularly in their teens and twenties. Frequently no cause is found, but irritable bowel syndrome may be suspected. Appendicectomy should be avoided because it does no good.

Extra diagnostic techniques

All the above add up to a formidable list of possibilities, which is daunting for the student to remember and confusing for the surgeon when confronted with an individual patient. Sometimes no clear pathological lesion is identified, the symptoms subside and the diagnosis is one of *non-specific abdominal pain.* There are three ways around the problem in the differential diagnosis of the acute abdomen, when appendicitis or another common condition is suspected but the diagnosis after clinical evaluation remains uncertain. These are described below.

Computer assistance. The data obtained from the patient is matched against a data base of previous patients held in a computer. The computer calculates the probabilities of the existence of various conditions, given the findings, and feeds these back to the clinician. The accuracy of diagnosis of appendicitis can be increased by this means, and the incidence of both unnecessary operations and perforated appendicitis is reduced.

Fine catheter aspiration of the abdominal cavity. This is a relatively new technique in which a small plastic cannula is introduced and an aspirate of peritoneal fluid is obtained. Significant quantities of blood or leucocytes indicate that operation is required.

Laparoscopy. Although more invasive than the first two techniques, this is probably the most reliable in the doubtful patient. It has the additional advantage of often providing a positive diagnosis – such as FitzHugh–Curtis syndrome – which allows treatment to be instigated and the patient to be discharged from hospital. The tactic most commonly used is to divide the patients with acute abdomen into three groups: those who definitely need operation; those who definitely do not; and those in whom doubt remains. The last group is submitted to laparoscopy. Moreover, the appendix can now be removed laparoscopically.

ACUTE APPENDICITIS WITH AN INFLAMMATORY MASS

Symptoms

These are similar to those of acute appendicitis but pain is often more severe, entirely right-sided and present for 3 or more days. In addition the patient feels ill and nauseated.

Signs

In addition to those already described, there may be:

- a tender mass, sometimes not well defined, in the RIF; after 5 or 6 days there is usually little rigidity, and the mass is more easily felt
- a tender extension of the mass into the pelvis on rectal examination.

Differential diagnosis

An appendix mass may be confused with other masses in the RIF such as the following.

Carcinoma of the caecum. A history of large bowel symptoms, anaemia and weight loss may give a clue, but the diagnosis may not be apparent until operation. A perforated carcinoma of the caecum with pericaecal abscess formation will be indistinguishable from an appendiceal abscess until operation. If an elderly patient with a suspected appendix mass is treated conservatively, a barium enema or colonoscopy should be performed before interval appendicectomy.

Carcinoma of the left side of colon. With obstruction to the left colon, the caecum will be distended in the presence of a competent ileocaecal valve and present as a compressible and tympanitic mass in the right iliac fossa. Rarely, the caecal wall becomes attenuated or even gangrenous, and appendicitis is even more accurately mimicked (see Ch. 31).

Empyema of the gall bladder. Pain in the right hypochondrium radiating to the back, together with a tender globular mass projecting from beneath the costal margin and moving on respiration, indicates an empyema.

Renal mass. A right perinephric abscess should be suspected if loin pain and tenderness are associated with rigors and a possible distant staphylococcal focus (see Ch. 35).

Hydronephrosis may present as a uniform mass in the loin which moves on respiration. It may be associated with a classical band of colonic resonance anteriorly.

Miscellaneous. Ovarian cyst, fibroid uterus, psoas abscess, Crohn's disease and ileocaecal tuberculosis may need to be considered on occasions.

ACUTE APPENDICITIS WITH GENERALISED PERITONITIS

The clinical features often follow obstructive appendicitis with increasingly severe colicky abdominal pains and vomiting. When the appendix perforates, it is said that initially the symptoms abate somewhat. However, spreading abdominal pain rapidly develops and there are signs of peritonitis, with rebound tenderness, rigidity and ultimately abdominal distension from paralytic ileus. The patient becomes progressively more toxic.

There are three distinct stages.

Stage of shock. During this stage the following are seen:

- the patient is pale, sweating and anxious
- pulse rate is elevated
- blood pressure is lowered
- temperature may be subnormal
- respirations are rapid and shallow
- pronounced local tenderness is present in the RIF.

Stage of peritoneal reaction. At this stage, shock has improved and the following become apparent:

- severe local tenderness in the RIF
- rebound tenderness
- 'board-like' rigidity
- marked rectal tenderness.

Stage of frank peritonitis. Rigidity is less but paralytic ileus becomes apparent with the following features:

- abdominal distension
- absent bowel sounds
- faecal vomitus and later dehydration with 'Hippocratic facies' (hollow cheeks, sunken eyeballs and a 'pinched' expression).

Differential diagnosis

Any cause of generalised peritonitis commencing in the lower abdomen is part of the differential diagnosis. The list is extensive, but frank peritonitis means operation, so that a precise differential diagnosis is not all that vital (see Ch. 6).

TREATMENT

Once again, this depends on the type of appendicitis.

ACUTE APPENDICITIS

Once appendicitis has been firmly diagnosed the treatment is appendicectomy. We have already referred to methods of resolving doubt and avoiding unnecessary operations.

Appendicectomy is performed through an oblique or transverse incision centred over the site of maximal tenderness in the RIF unless there is serious doubt about the diagnosis, in which case a vertical incision may be preferred. The major steps of appendicectomy are illustrated in Figure 30.2. Recently, growing experience with laparoscopic appendicectomy suggests that this technique may also be appropriate.

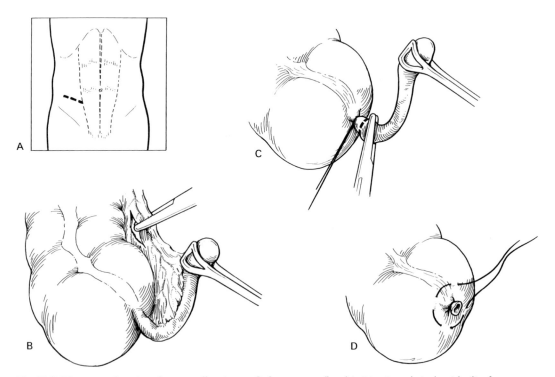

Fig. 30.2 The operative steps in appendicectomy. A. A transverse (Lanz) incision is made in the right iliac fossa.
B. Clamping the mesoappendix (containing the appendicular artery). **C.** The base of the appendix has been ligated and clamped, and the appendix will be cut off flush with the undersurface of the artery forceps. **D.** The stump of the appendix is invaginated into the caecal wall by means of a purse-string suture.

ACUTE APPENDICITIS WITH AN INFLAMMATORY MASS

The early stage is a mass comprising the inflamed appendix with surrounding coils of bowel and greater omentum; later a frank abscess may form or the mass may resolve without pus formation.

There are two schools of thought on the treatment of acute appendicitis with an inflammatory mass: non-operative and operative.

Non-operative treatment

This policy relies on the fact that natural processes have already limited the extent of inflammation and should not be disturbed.

The method entails the following:

- Ensure the patient is in a semi-upright position (in bed).
- Administer fluids only, by mouth or intravenously if necessary.
- The pulse rate should be observe 4-hourly, or more frequently, and the temperature should be recorded twice daily.
- Palpate the abdominal mass regularly and mark its limits on the skin surface daily. Ultrasound scan may increase the accuracy of measurement.
- Broad-spectrum antibiotic and metronidazole will probably aid resolution of an appendiceal mass. It will not alter a frank appendiceal abscess, athough it may suppress the systemic signs.
- Purgatives are forbidden.

With this regimen, the following may happen:

- *Resolution.* The patient recovers and the mass subsides in about 80% of cases.
- *Deterioration.* Elevation of the pulse rate, increased pain, tenderness, muscle guarding and size of the mass indicate failure, and operation becomes essential. This probably occurs in 10% of cases, and at operation generalised peritonitis may be found.
- *Abscess formation.* Rectal or vaginal examination may reveal a fluctuant mass, indicating that the abscess should be drained at these sites. Very rarely the abscess may point suprapubically and require drainage from this direction.
- *No change.* In a small percentage of cases, the inflammatory mass remains unchanged for days or even weeks and the decision as to what should be done may be difficult. The possibility of a wrong diagnosis and the presence of some other condition such as Crohn's disease or caecal carcinoma usually indicates that operation should be carried out.

Interval appendicectomy should be performed about 3 months later in those patients in whom resolution occurred or simple drainage of an appendical abscess was performed.

The *advantages* of the non-operative method of treatment are that a difficult and perhaps dangerous operation in an infected field is avoided and an elective appendicectomy can be performed months later when the patient's general condition has improved and when technical difficulties are no longer a hazard.

The *disadvantages* of the method are as follows. It should not be employed in young or elderly patients, who have inadequate ability to localise the inflammation. General peritonitis may result during the 'watching' period. Furthermore, there remains uncertainty of diagnosis on some occasions and there is a necessity for a second admission to hospital at a later date for appendicectomy.

Operative treatment

This method of treatment is preferred by many surgeons. At operation one of two procedures will be carried out:

- Appendicectomy and drainage of an abscess cavity is usually possible
- Drainage alone, when for technical reasons it is decided that appendicectomy may involve excessive hazards; an elective appendicectomy would then be performed 3 months later.

The *advantages* of the operative approach are that a certain diagnosis is made, a second admission to hospital can usually be avoided, and the stay in hospital is shorter.

The *disadvantages* are that manipulation through a mass or an abscess to remove the appendix may cause dissemination of infected material, haemorrhage or a faecal fistula; and postoperative complications such as wound infection and residual abscess are more frequent than after an elective appendicectomy.

ACUTE APPENDICITIS WITH GENERALISED PERITONITIS

The treatment is operative after a short period of resuscitation. Pre-operative nasogastric suction, intravenous replacement therapy, analgesics and antibiotics are administered.

At operation, peritoneal toilet is performed when generalised peritonitis is present. Whenever possible, the appendix is removed and a tube drain is placed to the site of the appendix bed. In all cases of generalised peritonitis it is common practice to carry out intraoperative peritoneal lavage with saline and an antibiotic.

Wound complications are reduced by perioperative antibiotics, i.e. by a short course of metronidazole (to treat anaerobes) and (in grossly contaminated cases) by leaving the wound open.

MECKEL'S DIVERTICULUM

The surgical problems of this remnant of the vitello-intestinal duct are considered here because it is frequently encountered in relation to acute appendicitis.

INCIDENCE

Between 2% and 3% of individuals have some form of Meckel's diverticulum, but clinical problems are very much less common. The diverticulum arises from the antimesenteric border of the terminal ileum within 1 m of the ileocaecal valve.

TYPES OF PROBLEM

Persistence of umbilical connection

Very rarely, an *open duct* is present at birth and causes an ileal fistula. This duct requires surgical closure.

An *umbilical sinus* without an opening into the ileum can also occur in rare instances. There is umbilical discharge of watery bloodstained material and this is also usually from birth. Treatment is by excision.

Closure of both ends of the umbilical cord may produce a midline subumbilical cyst (*vitellointestinal cyst*) at any age but it commonly occurs in infancy or childhood. It is usually asymptomatic and easily removed.

The *attachment of the diverticulum* or a cord from its apex to the umbilicus provides a fixed point around which torsion may occur, so producing volvulus and acute intestinal obstruction. Alternatively, *herniation* of small bowel through the gap between the attachment and the abdominal wall may take place with the same effects. Acute intestinal obstruction can occur at any age.

Acute inflammation

A narrow-mouthed diverticulum can become inflamed, usually because of retained content. The condition mimics acute appendicitis both clinically and pathologically. Resection is required, but care must be taken not to narrow the ileal lumen.

Consequences of heterotopic gastric musoca

For a reason that is far from clear, Meckel's diverticulum may contain acid–pepsin-secreting gastric mucosa. Consequently, the adjacent small bowel mucosa may develop a peptic ulcer either within the diverticulum or nearby in the ileum. Both bleeding and perforation can occur, although bleeding is much more common.

Bleeding has been described at any age but is commonest before the age of 20 years. There are usually episodes of bright red or slightly altered blood being passed per rectum. Haemorrhage can be brisk enough to cause shock. No cause is found on conventional investigation by barium enema or colonoscopy. The gastric mucosa in a diverticulum can be outlined with radiolabelled technetium, and the diverticulum itself is visualised with the same material when bleeding is occurring. Treatment is by prompt excision.

Perforation presents in the same manner as perforated appendix or Meckel's diverticulitis.

FURTHER READING

Berry J, Malt R A 1984 Appendicitis near its centenary. Annals of Surgery 200: 567–575

Cooper M J, Williamson R C N 1985 The continuing challenge of acute appendicitis. Survey of Digestive Diseases 114–128

Leaper D J, Kissin C, Virjee J, Johnson C D 1990 New diagnostic techniques in the acute abdomen. In: Williamson R C N, Cooper M J (eds) Emergency abdominal surgery. Churchill Livingstone, Edinburgh, p 1–20

Mackey W C, Dineen P 1983 A fifty year experience with Meckel's diverticulum. Surgery, Gynecology and Obstetrics 156: 56–64

Nitecki S, Assalia A, Schein M 1993 Contemporary management of the appendiceal mass. British Journal of Surgery 80: 18–20

Olsen J B, Myrén C J, Haahr P E 1993 Randomised study of the value of laparoscopy before appendicectomy. British Journal of Surgery 80: 922–923

Tate J J T, Chung S C S, Dawson J, Leong H T, Chan A, Lau W Y, Li A K C 1993 Conventional versus laparoscopic surgery for acute appendicitis. British Journal of Surgery 80: 761–764

Thomas W E G 1990 Complications of small bowel diverticula. In: Williamson R C N, Cooper M J (eds) Emergency abdominal surgery. Churchill Livingstone, Edinburgh, p 191–208

31

Large bowel cancer
Robin Phillips

OVERVIEW

Colorectal carcinoma is second only to lung cancer in man and breast cancer in women among leading causes of cancer death. Virtually all cancers of the large bowel are thought to arise from pre-existing benign adenomas. Screening for faecal occult blood can detect tumours at an earlier stage before they metastasise to the lymph nodes and liver. Surgical resection then provides an excellent chance of cure.

In many affluent countries, colorectal cancer is the second commonest cancer in men after lung cancer and now third commonest in women after breast and lung cancer. Large bowel cancer is common in the West and is uncommon in parts of the developing world, such as Africa. In the West there are areas of remarkably high prevalence, e.g. the west of Scotland in the UK. Epidemiologists and laboratory scientists have implicated lack of dietary fibre and an excess of dietary fat (especially beef fat) as important determinants of risk. There is probably a genetic susceptibility to bowel cancer in some people which, when combined with environmental factors, leads to expression of the phenotype. If this is so, some people will not develop bowel cancer almost regardless of what they eat (unless they consume a potent intestinal carcinogen such as methylazoxymethanol or its precursors), while others are at risk, though the actual development of cancer might be prevented by appropriate attention to environmental influences.

AETIOLOGY

In clinical practice there are identifiable precursors of colorectal cancer. These are:

- adenomatous polyps
- long-standing extensive ulcerative colitis.

POLYPS

Polyps are raised areas of pathological mucosa. They may be relatively flat (sessile) or on a stalk (pedunculated). Commoner intestinal polyps are metaplastic, hamartomas and adenomas. Other examples of polyps may be lymphomas or non-neoplastic polyps, e.g. postinflammatory.

Metaplastic polyps

These are usually very small, smooth, shiny polyps, and they have no malignant potential.

Hamartomas

These may be either juvenile polyps (which can be solitary or part of the extremely rare juvenile polyposis) or part of the Peutz–Jeghers syndrome (a dominant hereditary condition which comprises circumoral pigmentation, intestinal hamartomas that can occur from the stomach to the rectum, and a risk of various intestinal and extraintestinal cancers). In both juvenile polyposis and the Peutz–Jeghers syndrome there is a real risk of intestinal cancer developing, probably preceded by adenomatous or dysplastic change within the hamartoma.

Adenomas

It is likely that most bowel cancers develop out of adenomas, but that few adenomas go on to become carcinomas. Those that do are likely to be large and multiple and to have a villous architecture. Tubulovillous adenomas have a lesser risk, and tubular adenomas the least risk, of malignant change. A patient with a colorectal adenoma needs colonoscopic examination to exclude other adenomas and allow endoscopic removal. Such patients need regular colonoscopic follow-up. The frequency depends on the size and number of polyps: perhaps repeat examination at 1 year followed by examinations every 2–4 years.

Familial adenomatous polyposis. Familial adenomatous polyposis (FAP) is a dominant hereditary condition characterised by the development of more than 100 colorectal adenomas (usually many thousand) in the teenage years. Cancer is virtually inevitable. Adenomas also occur in the duodenum. New mutations occur so that sometimes there may be no family history. Treatment is aimed at preventing/reducing the risk of death from intestinal cancer. Operation is undertaken in the late teens. The options are:

- proctocolectomy and ileostomy
- colectomy and ileorectal anastomosis (followed by 6-monthly surveillance of the remaining polyps in the rectal stump)
- proctocolectomy and formation of an ileal pouch with pouch–anal anastomosis (see Ch. 28).

It is important to appreciate that roughly half the current and future members of the family will need treatment at some time or other. A prophylactic operation that results in a permanent ileostomy is likely to lead to the rest of the family defaulting from follow-up. A high complication rate such as may be seen after pouch surgery may have a similar effect, which explains the continued popularity of the lower morbidity colectomy with ileorectal anastomosis.

ULCERATIVE COLITIS (see also Ch. 28)

Patients with extensive ulcerative proctocolitis of more than 8 years' duration are at increased risk of colorectal cancer. Historically, extensive colitis has been diagnosed by barium enema, but nowadays there are patients with a normal barium enema examination of the proximal colon whose colonoscopy shows involvement of this segment.

There are even some whose colonoscopy appears macroscopically normal but in whom biopsy shows evidence of extensive colitis. It is not known whether extensive colitis detected in these other ways also carries an increased cancer risk, but some suspect it does.

Precancer in ulcerative colitis is called dysplasia. Unfortunately dysplasia cannot be seen reliably with the naked eye; it is patchy within the colon and may even be otherwise absent when a cancer is present. One can either perform prophylactic surgery or enter the patient into a programme of colonoscopic surveillance with its attendant problems.

SURGICAL PATHOLOGY

Large bowel cancers are adenocarcinomas.

THE SPREAD OF CARCINOMA

Carcinomas are spread by:

- direct extension
- lymphatic permeation
- blood-borne dissemination
- transcoelomic spread (across the peritoneal cavity).

ESTIMATION OF PROGNOSIS

The prognosis of a patient with cancer can to some extent be predicted according to how biologically aggressive the inherent cancer cells are (the umbrella term *grade* can be used to describe this) and how far in a geographical sense the cancer has already spread (which is called its *stage*).

One has to be careful to appreciate that the patient is interested in only one prognosis (his or her own); the dispassionate therapist is interested in the prognosis of groups treated in one way or by one institution with the prognosis of others treated in another way or by another institution.

The way in which prognosis is established is by examining the results of groups and arriving at an estimate of 'probable' outcome. Few patients are comfortable with probability, and this should be borne in mind. The endpoints that may be estimated are survival, local recurrence of disease, death in hospital and the ultimate quality of life.

Survival

This is largely determined by pathological factors. The

most critical factor in large bowel cancer is whether the liver is already involved. If it is extensively involved then modern treatment will not cure the patient, but a solitary liver metastasis may be resected with benefit (and sometimes three or four when the situation is otherwise favourable).

It is not always obvious whether or not the liver is involved. Each extra level of imaging of an otherwise apparently 'normal' liver will demonstrate cases with unsuspected occult hepatic metastases. Thus ultrasound and CT scanning will reveal more than careful intraoperative palpation, and postmortem slicing of the liver in the occasional circumstance of an unforeseen postoperative death may reveal even more still. Clearly, even the most sophisticated developments will still leave some patients with microscopic liver involvement undetected.

It is possible to obtain an idea of the chance that there already are occult hepatic metastases by examination of the resected specimen. Cuthbert Dukes was the histopathologist at St Mark's hospital and was responsible for devising a staging system in 1932 for rectal cancer which bears his name (Fig. 31.1):

- Dukes' A – tumour confined to the rectal wall
- Dukes' B – tumour penetrates the entire thickness of the rectal wall and is invading pararectal tissues/fat
- Dukes' C – lymph nodes are involved.

Dukes did not concern himself with incurable cases so did not have a 'D' category.

The approximate survival of Dukes' A cases is 90%, of Dukes' B cases 50% and of Dukes' C cases 35%.

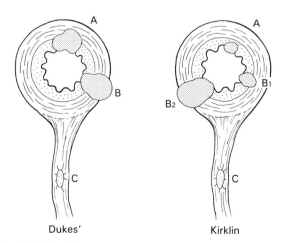

Fig. 31.1 **Two different staging systems, Dukes' and Kirklin, for carcinoma of the large bowel.**

Presumably the stage is reflecting the probability of undiagnosed (occult) metastases present at the time of resection.

There are many modifications to the original Dukes' staging system, so that there is no uniform standard worldwide. The Australian clinicopathological staging (ACPS) system includes ACPS A, B, C and D categories, D referring to metastases distant to the bowel and lymph nodes. In the USA, the Kirklin modification is used with A (confined to muscularis mucosa), B_1 (penetrating into but not through the bowel wall) and B_2 (the same as Dukes' B). Lymph node status can be subdivided according to the status of the apical lymph node at operation (C_1 = uninvolved, C_2 = involved) (Dukes), the number of lymph nodes involved (C_1 denotes ≤ 4, C_2 denotes > 4) (Gastrointestinal Tumour Study Group) or the depth of primary tumour penetration (C_1 = confined to the bowel wall, C_2 = through the bowel wall) (when used in conjunction with the Kirklin modification of A and B tumours, this is known as the Astler–Coller system).

Tumours that appear poorly differentiated are more likely also to be Dukes' C and have a worse prognosis than 'other' tumours (previously classified as well or moderately differentiated). Aggressive tumours tend to have an excess DNA content. This can be detected by flow cytometry, and such tumours are known as aneuploid (the opposite is diploid).

Local recurrence

Even if the patient cannot be cured of cancer, control of the local symptoms is important. Failure to control local symptoms is in part determined by pathological factors, such as Dukes' stage and tumour differentiation, but it is also determined by the expertise of the surgeon.

Death in hospital

This largely depends on clinical factors. Old and sick people do poorly, particularly if they are rushed to the operating theatre in the middle of the night without adequate preparation. It is essential to realise that the more unstable the patient (unless exsanguinating haemorrhage is the cause), the more is gained by a period of pre-operative optimisation.

Quality of life

It is important that the cure is not worse than the disease, but it is essential to learn how awful the consequences of failed therapy can be before one is in a position to judge. In colorectal cancer surgery, the key issue is the restoration of intestinal continuity by anastomosis or the construction of a permanent stoma on the anterior abdominal wall. It is not reasonable to expect the average patient to have thought about these issues in a clear-headed fashion before being struck by the disease, and afterwards the emotional maelstrom precludes rational deliberation. The surgeon, knowing both the disease and the cure, must often be a firm guide to the best choice.

SCREENING

If the gap between developing an early cancer and its metastasising is quite wide, then earlier diagnosis by screening holds out the hope of dealing just with a local problem, which would mean an improvement in survival rates. If, however, the cancer metastasises shortly after it has developed, then it is less likely that diagnosis a few months earlier will make much difference. One way of detecting colorectal cancer earlier is by looking for occult blood in the stools (for example, by the Haemoccult test). Whether the use of Haemoccult testing will improve the survival of a population at risk of colorectal cancer is the subject of considerable interest and a number of trials. It may just diagnose the disease earlier and thereby give an apparently longer survival because the disease has been known about for longer (lead time bias). It may pick up predominantly tumours that have a long natural life span and give false reassurance when screened patients are found to have a better prognosis. This is because if screening is repeated at intervals, many aggressive tumours will grow so rapidly that they present clinically between the screening intervals, which leaves the biologically more favourable tumours to be detected by screening (this is called length bias).

CLINICAL FEATURES

Large bowel cancer may present with the effect of the primary, the effect of secondaries, the general effects of malignant disease, and very rarely with a skin condition called acanthosis nigricans.

EFFECTS OF THE PRIMARY

Bleeding. This may be fresh, altered or occult depending on where the cancer is situated within the colon. It is a common cause of iron deficiency anaemia. An important indication that visible bleeding is not anal (i.e. from haemorrhoids) is blood that is darker or mixed with the stool. Even when anal bleeding is suspected, a thorough examination of the rectum and sigmoid colon is mandatory.

Mucus. Particularly seen with rectal villous adenomas (where malignant change is not uncommon), mucus may lead to potassium deficiency.

Tenesmus. This is a sense of inadequate evacuation, more commonly seen with rectal tumours.

Change in bowel habit.

Lower abdominal colic.

Large bowel obstruction. The features are pain, vomiting, distension and absolute constipation (see Table 31.1 for a contrast between small bowel and large bowel obstruction). See also Chapter 28.

Large bowel perforation.

Presence of a mass. Common causes of a right iliac fossa mass are appendix mass/abscess, caecal carcinoma, Crohn's disease; rarer causes include ileocaecal tuberculosis and actinomycosis.

EFFECTS OF SECONDARIES

These commonly go to the liver or transcoelomically to the peritoneum or ovaries (one cause of Krukenberg tumours, along with secondaries from the stomach and breast). Other rarer sites include lung, bone and brain.

Table 31.1 A comparison of the clinical features of small bowel obstruction and large bowel obstruction

Small bowel obstruction	Symptom	Large bowel obstruction
Midgut (central)	Pain	Hindgut (lower)
Early (within hours)	Vomiting	Late or absent
Mild, central	Distension	Marked
Bowels may open	Constipation	Marked

GENERAL EFFECTS OF MALIGNANT DISEASE

These are general malaise, weight loss and normochromic normocytic anaemia and tend to indicate advanced disease.

DIAGNOSIS

CLINICAL HISTORY

This should be related to the possible effects of the primary, secondaries or general effects of malignant disease. A family history of bowel cancer (particularly for right-sided cancer in patients aged < 40 years) or of cancer of the breast, uterus or ovary may suggest site-specific colorectal cancer or the cancer family syndrome, which have a dominant inheritance.

CLINICAL EXAMINATION

Examination is for the primary, secondaries and the general effects of malignant disease. In addition, the patient's general fitness for surgical intervention must be assessed. Clearly, rectal examination and sigmoidoscopy are necessary in all cases of suspected colorectal cancer.

INVESTIGATIONS

The large bowel must be visualised either by double-contrast barium enema examination or by colonoscopy. It is not always possible to obtain good views of the colon proximal to a carcinoma because of obstruction in some cases leading to poor bowel preparation. This is important as synchronous cancers are present in 3% of cases and, if small, may be overlooked. Anaemia should be sought. Examination of the liver by ultrasound may show unsuspected mestastases. The serum carcinoembryonic antigen (CEA) level may be raised.

TREATMENT

PREPARATION FOR OPERATION

Except for the most hopeless case, treatment is surgical. Operations on the colon usually result in an anastomosis. Anastomotic healing is safer if the bowel is empty of stool, so pre-operative bowel preparation with laxatives is performed. In the case of emergency operations, intra-operative lavage of the colon is possible. It may be necessary to have blood available for transfusion. Perioperative antibiotics that are effective against faecal organisms are used to reduce the rate of wound infection, and steps are taken to decrease the risk of deep vein thrombosis and pulmonary embolism (e.g. by using subcutaneous heparin and support stockings). The operation must be clearly explained to the patient and/or relatives and consent obtained. If either a temporary or permanent stoma is a possibility, this must be discussed with the patient, a stoma care nurse should see the patient, and an appropriate site for the stoma should be marked on the skin pre-operatively using an indelible marker.

SURGICAL TREATMENT

The surgical aim is to remove the area of bowel containing the tumour complete with its lymphatic drainage. As the lymphatic drainage follows the arterial blood supply, the axial artery is ligated at its origin. This procedure creates an ischaemic segment of bowel for excision that is somewhat larger than is strictly necessary for the removal of the primary tumour itself and gives rise to the various terms:

- right hemicolectomy – excision of caecum and ascending colon; division of ileocolic and right colic arteries
- transverse colectomy – excision of transverse colon; division of middle colic artery
- left hemicolectomy – excision of distal transverse colon and descending colon; division of left colic artery/inferior mesenteric artery
- sigmoid colectomy – excision of sigmoid colon; division of inferior mesenteric artery and/or sigmoid branches.

The ends of the bowel are joined together again by anastomosis using either sutures or surgical staples.

In the case of the rectum, the inferior mesenteric artery is ligated. If there is enough remaining rectum below the tumour to allow an anastomosis, the operation is performed abdominally and is called an *anterior resection*. Sometimes, especially in emergencies, the proximal colon is brought out as an end colostomy and the rectal stump is oversewn and returned to the abdomen. This is called *Hartmann's operation*; the colostomy can be reversed by further operation when the patient is well again. When the cancer is so low that the anal sphincter mechanism must be removed to obtain clearance, the operation is performed both from the abdomen and from the perineum. This is called an *abdominoperineal excision* and results in a permanent end sigmoid colostomy situated in the left iliac fossa.

POSTOPERATIVE MANAGEMENT

After major abdominal operations there is a period of 2–3 days when the gut cannot be relied upon for absorption and an intravenous infusion is required. During this time great attention must be paid to the prevention of chest infection occasioned by retention of sputum because of fear of the pain provoked by coughing. Thereafter, feeding is commenced, normal micturition is re-established and the patient is mobilised and sent home, usually between 6 and 8 days postoperatively. The patient can carry the shopping by about 4–6 weeks, but it is often many months before an elderly patient is finally able to put the effects of the operation behind them.

ADJUVANT THERAPY

There is now evidence that patients with Dukes' C colon cancer benefit from adjuvant chemotherapy with 5-fluorouracil (5-FU) and levamisole or folinic acid. Radiotherapy is used by some as an adjuvant for rectal cancer surgery, either pre- or postoperatively.

FOLLOW-UP

Patients are at risk of local recurrence (anastomotic) or an overlooked synchronous cancer in the bowel. They have a 3% risk of developing a metachronous carcinoma, so regular colonoscopy is indicated (within the first 12 months and then 3–5 yearly). Recurrence of the original tumour may be detected by finding an elevated serum CEA (although the test is not specific) or by scanning the liver and abdomen with ultrasound or CT. It is unclear at present whether intensive follow-up is cost effective.

TREATMENT OF RECURRENCE

Surgery is the only effective treatment of local recurrence, but the results are poor. Solitary liver metastases (or a cluster in one lobe of the liver) are amenable to liver resection with a 5-year survival of 30–40%, but few patients are candidates for resection. Chemotherapy with 5-FU and folinic acid or levamisole has better response rates in advanced disease than 5-FU alone, but no patients are cured. Of 100 patients presenting with colorectal cancer about 55% will have a curative resection; of these, 50% will live for 5 years.

ANAL CANCER

Squamous cell carcinomas may arise from the anus and can metastasise to the inguinal lymph nodes. Current treatment is primarily combination chemotherapy and radiotherapy (Nigro regimen) with about 60% of cases being controlled in this way. Residual cancers are treated either by local excision or rarely nowdays by abdominoperineal excision. Inguinal lymph node metastases are treated by block dissection as they tend to arise in salvage cases who have already undergone inguinal radiotherapy at the time of their original chemoirradiation.

FURTHER READING

Abulafi A M, Williams N S 1994 Local recurrence of colorectal cancer: the problem, mechanisms, management and adjuvant therapy. British Journal of Surgery 81: 7–19

Barlow A P, Thompson M H 1993 Colonoscopic follow-up after resection for colorectal cancer: a selective policy. British Journal of Surgery 80: 781–784

Caffarey S M, Broughton C I M, Marks C G 1993 Faecal occult blood screening for colorectal neoplasia in a targeted high-risk population. British Journal of Surgery 80: 1399–1400

Moertel C G, Fleming T R, MacDonald J S 1990 Levamisole and fluorouracil for surgical adjuvant therapy of colon carcinoma. New England Journal of Medicine 322: 352–358

Phillips R K S, Hittinger R, Blesovsky L, Fry J S, Fielding L P 1984 Large bowel cancer – surgical pathology and its relationship to survival. British Journal of Surgery 71: 604–610

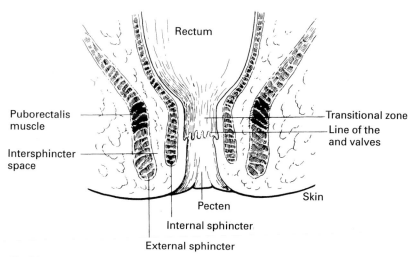

32

Perianal conditions
Robin Phillips

OVERVIEW

The anal canal and perianal skin are a frequent site for disease, which is painful and embarrassing to the patient yet relatively simple to cure if sensible measures are taken. This chapter considers some of the commonest anal and perianal lesions: haemorrhoids, perianal haematoma, anal fissure, anal fistula and anorectal abscess, pilonidal sinus, perianal skin conditions and faecal incontinence.

ANAL ANATOMY (Fig. 32.1)

The anal canal is about 4 cm long. It extends from the anal verge (hair-bearing skin with sebaceous glands) to the anorectal junction (columnar epithelium). The part of the external anal canal that is exposed by traction on the rim of the anus is hairless and is called the pecten or anoderm. The junction between the pecten and the large bowel mucosa is marked by the line of the anal valves and is otherwise known as the pectinate or dentate line. Above this there is a transitional zone of variable extent (usually 1 or 2 cm) which contains sensitive epithelium, above which is the insensitive large bowel mucosa.

The anus can be sketched simply as in Figure 32.2. The arrow denotes the 12 o'clock (anterior) position which corresponds to the vagina in women and the scrotum in men.

Rectum

Puborectalis muscle

Intersphincter space

Transitional zone

Line of the and valves

Skin

Pecten

Internal sphincter

External sphincter

Fig. 32.1 Cross-sectional anatomy of the anal canal and lower rectum.

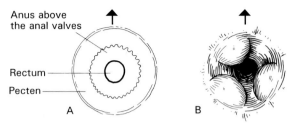

Fig. 32.2 A. Schematic representation of the anus as seen from below with the patient in the lithotomy position. B. The typical positions for haemorrhoids at 3, 7 and 11 o'clock.

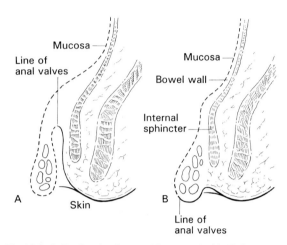

Fig. 32.3 A. Prolapsing internal haemorrhoids. B. Intero-external haemorrhoids.

HAEMORRHOIDS

These are vascular cushions that sit in the vicinity of the anorectal junction but may slip and descend to protrude through the anus. Classically they are situated at 3, 7 and 11 o'clock when the surgeon is looking at the anus with the patient in the lithotomy position (Fig. 32.2). These sites correspond to the left lateral, right anterior and right posterior positions. They were once thought to be determined by the terminal branches of the superior rectal (haemorrhoidal) artery, but this is no longer considered true.

CLASSIFICATION

Haemorrhoids may bleed, prolapse or strangulate. They are of varying degrees.

1° Haemorrhoids

These are small haemorrhoids which simply bleed. Bright blood may be seen on wiping the anus or it may be noticed to drip from the anus into the lavatory pan. Blood that is mixed with the stool or is darker red in colour should not be dismissed as bleeding from haemorrhoids, especially if there is any uncertainty.

2° Haemorrhoids

These prolapse from the anus but will return. In some classifications, those that return spontaneously are termed 2° and those requiring digital replacement are called 3°. As treatment for both varieties is the same, it is probably better simply to lump them both together as 2° haemorrhoids.

3° Haemorrhoids

These prolapse from the anus and despite attempts to replace them fall out again. Where 2° haemorrhoids have been subdivided into 2° haemorrhoids and 3° haemorrhoids, these are then called 4° haemorrhoids.

External skin tags

Any degree of haemorrhoids may be associated with an untidy anus caused by skin tags. Skin tags contain normal sensory nerve endings, so that an anaesthetic must be employed for their removal. Large 3° haemorrhoids having their outer margin covered by skin and their inner margin covered by mucosa are sometimes referred to as intero-external haemorrhoids (Fig. 32.3).

Strangulated haemorrhoids

Haemorrhoids that prolapse may be tightly gripped by the anus, which impedes venous return and leads to thrombosis and ultimately gangrene of the haemorrhoids. Such haemorrhoids present as an emergency and are described as strangulated or thrombosed.

Other terms used

External haemorrhoids are skin tags. The terms thrombosed external haemorrhoids and perianal haematoma are synonymous. The term 'piles' is generally reserved for internal haemorrhoids but is sometimes used loosely to describe any painful or bleeding lesion in the anal canal or perianal region.

SYMPTOMS

Besides symptoms defined by their classification (bleeding and prolapse), haemorrhoids may cause itching (see pruritus ani). Pain may also be described: in the absence of strangulation, be on the look out for another condition such as a fissure, perianal haematoma or abscess. Also, be aware that the patient may use the word pain to mean 'I don't like it' rather than 'it hurts'.

DIAGNOSIS

The diagnosis is made by history and clinical examination, which must include proctoscopy and sigmoidoscopy. Haemorrhoids are common but so is cancer, and the two may easily coexist in the same patient. It is clearly not feasible to investigate the large bowel in all patients with slight anal bleeding, nor is it wise: these investigations carry a morbidity and occasional mortality of their own which could exceed the benefit of their indiscriminate application. But if there is any doubt, particularly in patients over the age of 50 years where the blood is not clearly coming from the anal canal, or where there is a change in bowel habit or on sigmoidoscopy altered blood or mucus is seen, then barium enema examination or colonoscopy is indicated.

TREATMENT

Treatment varies according to the classification.

1° Haemorrhoids

Classically these have been treated in the outpatient department by injection of a sclerosing agent (such as 5% phenol in almond or arachis oil) into the area of the pedicle to cause fibrosis and destruction of the blood supply. Treatment is painless as the rectal mucosa is insensitive to injection. Alternatives are infrared photocoagulation and dietary advice plus the use of a bulk laxative. There is little evidence that any of these treatments is particularly effective. Indeed at 6 months, about half the patients treated either by injection sclerotherapy or by the use of a bulk laxative are still bleeding. Once the diagnosis has been confirmed and a more sinister cause has been deemed unlikely, simple reassurance may suffice.

2° Haemorrhoids

These may be treated by injection or rubber band ligation. Rubber band ligation is more effective and involves the application of a tight rubber band over the pedicle using an ingenious applicator. This serves to draw the prolapsing haemorrhoid back up into the anal canal and may also lead to its destruction. Banding should not immediately be painful, although there is often some discomfort.

Complications include haemorrhage when the band separates, sepsis (which is very rare but potentially life-threatening) and pain. This pain usually comes on some hours later and lasts for a number of days. It occurs in perhaps 5% of cases and is probably caused by thrombosis affecting a haemorrhoidal branch supplying blood to the sensitive pecten. The patient should be reassured and treated expectantly.

3° Haemorrhoids

These are best treated by haemorrhoidectomy. This treatment is also the best advice when the anus is untidy and the piles are 2°. The haemorrhoids are removed surgically and the wound is either left to heal by secondary intention or sutured. Pain should not be extreme, particularly if an anal canal dressing is avoided and any ligature does not incorporate any internal sphincter. When left open, the wounds take about 6 weeks to heal completely. Besides pain, complications of haemorrhoidectomy are rare. They include acute retention of urine (seen after many painful anal conditions/operations), secondary haemorrhage (which can be serious) and later anal stenosis if too much skin has been removed; anal stenosis usually responds to an anal dilator used regularly for 2 months.

Strangulated haemorrhoids

Treatment may be conservative (bulk laxatives, analgesics, local applications of soothing substances, e.g. ice packs) or operative. Conservative management usually results in loss of major discomfort within a week and resolution of the haemorrhoids, perhaps with some residual skin tags, by 6 weeks. Operations include manual dilatation of the anus and various forms of emergency haemorrhoidectomy. When the haemorrhoids are gross, the operation may have to be extensive, which is why some surgeons prefer a conservative approach.

PERIANAL HAEMATOMA

This condition, which is also known as thrombosed external haemorrhoid, presents as a painful perianal lump that usually appears acutely after an episode of straining. It is situated on the pecten and is very tender but without other signs of inflammation to suggest the diagnosis of a perianal abscess.

TREATMENT

If seen within 24 hours of the onset, the blood clot can be evacuated under a local anaesthetic. Thereafter, organisation of the blood clot makes removal incomplete. The natural history being rapid resolution over a few days, it is usually wise to leave alone those that present later.

FISSURE

This is a tear involving the pecten, which explains why it is painful.

Fissures are most commonly seen at 6 o'clock and 12 o'clock, i.e. in the midline anterior or posterior position. Rarely, they may be associated with other diseases, such as Crohn's disease or herpes simplex infection in HIV-positive individuals.

SYMPTOMS

There is pain and bleeding on and after defaecation. Constipation leads to a hard stool tearing the anus, thereby causing pain and making the patient avoid defaecation; thus further constipation develops, and a vicious cycle is established.

DIAGNOSIS

As the pecten is obscured unless the rim of the anal canal is opened up by traction, a fissure is not readily apparent. Fissures may be simple, or they may be associated with a sentinel skin tag or a fibroepithelial anal canal polyp. Seeing a skin tag should alert the doctor to the diagnosis, as should feeling an anal canal polyp, particularly if the examination has been painful and there is a streak of blood on the glove. However, the mainstay of diagnosis is adequate inspection. There is spasm in the anal sphincter, and appropriate traction on the anal verge will allow the pecten to be inspected and the fissure to be diagnosed.

TREATMENT

Simple fissures may be treated by a combination of a local anaesthetic cream and a bulk laxative, the intention being to break the pain/constipation cycle. There is a higher than normal resting pressure, caused by internal and sphincter spasm, and this prevents a good blood supply from reaching the pecten, thereby making any traumatic tear relatively ischaemic. The local application of a nitric oxide donor, such as GTN, relaxes the internal sphincter and may be of use. Experience has shown that when a skin tag or fibroepithelial anal canal polyp is present, recurrence is frequent unless operation is performed. Operations are designed to reduce the resting anal pressure and include manual dilatation of the anus or the more aesthetic lateral internal sphincterotomy with removal of any tags or polyps.

ABSCESS AND FISTULA

A patient may develop a boil that happens to be situated next to the anus. *Staphylococcus aureus* is the usual pathogen. This should be treated in the same way as a boil at any other site: diabetes or any other immune deficiency should be excluded, and if suppuration has occurred the boil should be drained. However, most infections in this area grow intestinal organisms and there is a communication with the anal canal. The acute version is an abscess, and the chronic version is a fistula-in-ano. Thus a chronic abscess is a fistula, while an acute fistula is an abscess.

AETIOLOGY

Some fistulas arise because of Crohn's disease, ulcerative colitis, cancer or tuberculosis. The vast majority arise from infected anal glands. There are between 15 and 20 of these glands. They open at the line of the anal valves and penetrate the internal anal sphincter to a varying depth, some lying in the intersphincteric space. When one of these deeper glands becomes infected, an intersphincteric abscess develops. The abscess may present perianally, or rupture through the external anal sphincter to lie in the fat of the ischiorectal fossa (Fig. 32.4). If chronic infection ensues, an intersphincteric fistula can develop from a perianal abscess, while a transsphincteric fistula can develop from an ischiorectal abscess. Rarely, the intersphincteric infection may pass proximally to become a supralevator abscess. This in turn may rupture

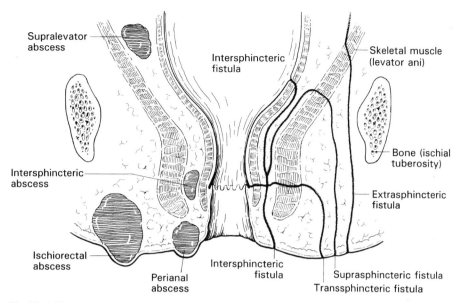

Fig. 32.4 The anatomical sites of anorectal abscesses and fistulas.

back into the bowel (a fistula of this sort, although it has a high internal opening, nevertheless remains an intersphincteric fistula which is easy to treat surgically), or it may break through the levator ani back into the ischiorectal fossa and then to the outside skin. If this latter becomes chronic, it results in a suprasphincteric fistula that encircles the whole anal sphincter mechanism and which is very difficult to treat. Finally, a pelvic abscess (from diverticular disease or Crohn's disease, for example) may drain perianally, and if a chronic track follows it is described as extrasphincteric.

INVESTIGATION

Digital rectal examination is usually all that is required. In complex cases, fistulography can be employed, but except when it demonstrates an extrasphincteric tract, it is confusing and often unhelpful. Ultrasound is less helpful than MRI (particularly when fat suppression sequences are used), which is very accurate but expensive.

TREATMENT

Abscesses should be drained, the pus sent for culture (gut organisms suggest an underlying fistula) and a sample of the abscess wall examined histologically (to exclude a rarer cause for the abscess). A sigmoidoscopy should always be done. Fistulas are treated by laying them open, i.e. by passing a probe through them and then cutting down on to the probe. Most fistulas can be treated in this manner, but when a substantial portion of the external anal sphincter needs to be cut, faecal incontinence is likely and more specialised techniques must be considered.

PILONIDAL SINUS

These commonly occur in the midline over the sacrum some distance from the anus. In barbers they can occur between the fingers. The chronic sinus contains hairs and is susceptible to infection. Their origin is uncertain: they may be congenital, or acquired when hairs drill their way into the soft tissues.

TREATMENT

An infected pilonidal sinus may contain a large quantity of pus which must be drained surgically. A chronic sinus can either be laid open, when healing can be slow, or excised with primary suture of the skin, which may include the use of a local skin flap transfer to flatten out the natal cleft and reduce recurrence.

WARTS

Condylomata acuminata are viral warts that affect the

genitalia and perianal region. Patients can be reinfected by their sexual partner.

TREATMENT

Local application of 25% podophyllin with an orange stick two or three times a week by a nurse may be effective. The caustic can cause damage if not carefully applied and washed off. Surgical removal can be used for persistent warts, but recurrent warts are not unusual and operation may need to be repeated.

PRURITUS ANI

Perianal itching is a particularly frequent and distressing symptom.

AETIOLOGY

Causes include:

- dermatological conditions (rare)
- sensitivity to local anaesthetic creams (common)
- dependence on steroid creams (common)
- threadworms (not very common)
- perianal leakage of stool (very common).

Perianal stool can be identified by wiping the anus with a damp piece of gauze and noting the discoloration. The causes of perianal stool are:

- high fibre diet (very common)
- poor hygiene (common)
- haemorrhoids, fissure, fistula (less common).

TREATMENT

Treat the cause. Avoid creams, although a short course of a steroid cream can be helpful. If there is perianal leakage, reduce the fibre in the diet, wash with water (not soap) and plug the anus with a small piece of cotton wool.

FAECAL INCONTINENCE

Faecal incontinence is common, but patients may be too embarrassed to mention it outright. Continence may be measured as:

- grade 1 – continent to solid, liquid and gas
- grade 2 – incontinent only to gas

- grade 3 – incontinent to gas and liquid
- grade 4 – totally incontinent of faeces.

Causes are rectal urgency, from rectal ulceration owing to inflammatory bowel disease or cancer or the irritable bowel syndrome and a weak anal sphincter (sphincter injury at childbirth or operation, pudendal neuropathy, rectal prolapse). Patients with rectal urgency are frequently more incontinent to solid stool than they are to flatus, whereas it is the other way round with a weak sphincter.

INVESTIGATION

Anal ultrasound is an accurate method of determining sphincter integrity. Anorectal physiology studies determine the following:

- resting pressure – internal sphincter function
- voluntary squeeze pressure – external sphincter function
- anal and rectal mucosal electrosensitivity – sensory neural pathway
- the pudendal nerve terminal motor latency – the motor neural pathway.

TREATMENT

If there is rectal urgency, the cause should be treated, although treatment of the irritable bowel syndrome is frequently unsuccessful. A weak sphincter caused by sphincter division should be treated by anal sphincter repair. Pudendal neuropathy is caused by a traction injury of the pudendal nerve through straining either at parturition or at stool. The sphincter being weak can hold solid stool most easily, so constipating agents are useful. Surgery is less successful for pudendal neuropathy than it is for a sphincter division but it has a place.

ANAL PAIN

Some patients complain of anal pain for which no cause can be found. When fleeting in young people the pain is known as proctalgia fugax. Most frequently affected are the elderly, when the pain may be described as burning, or like a ball, and the patient may have trouble sitting. Alternative terms are the levator syndrome and idiopathic anal pain.

TREATMENT

This is usually unsuccessful. Patients may become suicidal, so general support should always be maintained. The pain may be likened to phantom limb pain after amputation (where the pain persists despite the cause having been removed).

FURTHER READING

Allen-Mersh T G 1990 Pilonidal sinus: finding the right track for treatment. British Journal of Surgery 77: 123–132

Eu K-W, Seow-Choen F, Goh H S 1994 Comparison of emergency and elective haemorrhoidectomy. British Journal of Surgery 81: 308–310

Grace R H 1990 The management of acute anorectal sepsis. Annals of the Royal College of Surgery of England 72: 160–162

Loder P B, Kamm M A, Nicholls R J, Philips R K S 1994 Haemorrhoids: pathology, pathophysiology, and aetiology. British Journal of Surgery 81: 946–954

Parks A G, Gordon P H, Hardcastle J D 1976 A classification of fistula in ano. British Journal of Surgery 63: 1–12

33 Gastrointestinal haemorrhage

Bruce Waxman

OVERVIEW

Bleeding from the gastrointestinal tract often presents as a surgical emergency. Whether the bleeding is from the upper or lower gastrointestinal tract, the management is similar, involving: resuscitation, determining the source of bleeding and controlling the bleeding. The management is a combined effort of gastroenterologist and surgeon, with an emphasis on early intervention. This chapter deals with these management issues and provides both the principles and details of treatment.

Gastrointestinal haemorrhage is essentially a management problem needing both the right decision at the right time and close cooperation between gastroenterologist and surgeon. Only by defining accurately the source of bleeding, defining the high-risk group of patients and acting quickly will a successful outcome be achieved.

From a management point of view it is useful to divide gastrointestinal haemorrhage into two groups:

- upper gastrointestinal bleeding
- lower gastrointestinal bleeding.

UPPER GASTROINTESTINAL BLEEDING

The vomiting of blood, often associated with melaena, may be a serious and alarming event, necessitating rapid judgement and technical skill for successful management. However, haemorrhage may be less severe, so that diagnosis and definitive management can be performed more at leisure.

Haematemesis must be distinguished from haemoptysis. With the latter, the blood is bright red, frothy and alkaline in reaction and it may be associated with symptoms of respiratory disease. Occasionally, the vomiting of port or claret may be confused with upper gastrointestinal hemorrhage!

Melaena is the inevitable consequence of a substantial haemorrhage into the upper gastrointestinal tract. A varying degree of digestive alteration in the spilt blood makes the bowel content dark. Melaena may follow haematemesis or, particularly in bleeding beyond the pylorus (as, for example, a posterior duodenal ulcer), it may be the only symptom and sign. It is dangerous to assume that melaena is less serious than haematemesis or that the occurrence of one or the other identifies the source of the bleeding. Because melaena implies digestion, it is not usually associated with bleeding from a site beyond the ileocaecal valve. Bleeding from the caecum, however, may sometimes be difficult to distinguish from more proximal bleeding.

CLASSIFICATION OF CAUSES

The causes of upper gastrointestinal bleeding can be classified into:

- Oesophageal
  - varices
  - peptic oesophagitis
  - carcinoma (rarely)
  - foreign body
- Stomach
  - peptic ulcer
  - gastric erosions and gastritis

- — carcinoma
- — hiatus hernia
- — Mallory–Weiss syndrome (oesophagogastric tear)
- — foreign body (e.g. nasogastric tube).
- Duodenum
  - — peptic ulcer
  - — diverticulum
- Miscellaneous
  - — disorders of gastrointestinal blood vessels, e.g. pseudoxanthoma elasticum, Ehlers–Danlos syndrome
  - — aneurysm of the splenic artery
  - — generalised disorders such as uraemia
  - — arteriovenous malformations.

The *commoner causes* of upper gastrointestinal bleeding are:

- peptic ulcer (70–90% of instances)
- Mallory–Weiss syndrome
- acute gastric erosions or multiple ulcers
- portal hypertension (perhaps 5% of cases, but this varies with geographical location).

Less common causes are:

- carcinoma of the stomach
- hiatus hernia and peptic oesophagitis.

SURGICAL PATHOLOGY

Chronic peptic ulcer

Around 80% of all bleeding ulcers are duodenal. Haemorrhage may come from hyperaemic mucosa at the margin, from granulation tissue in the base, or from eroded blood vessels which may be either in the wall of the stomach or duodenum, or outside these organs. Haemorrhage in the latter situation is always caused by a large penetrating ulcer, and torrential haemorrhage is likely to occur from the left gastric, splenic or gastroduodenal arteries. The magnitude of the haemorrhage bears no relationship to the presence or absence of atherosclerosis but is dependent upon the degree to which the vessel is held open or encased by fibrous tissue.

Acute lesions

Acute gastric and duodenal lesions, variously labelled acute peptic ulcer, acute gastritis, acute gastric erosions and haemorrhagic duodenitis, are known to occur. Ulcers may follow burns (Curling's ulcer), head injuries and intracranial operations (Cushing's ulcer), administration of steroids and non-steroidal anti-inflammatory drugs (NSAIDs) such as aspirin, indomethacin and ibuprofen. Acute ulceration has also been noted after myocardial infarction, severe temperature changes, severe infections and physical or emotional stress. The causation of these lesions is discussed in more detail on page 337.

Portal hypertension

Obstruction of the portal venous system causes the development of a collateral circulation to transport portal blood into the systemic system. A most important and potentially dangerous collateral circulation is that in the submucosa of the oesophagus and stomach, which is formed by anastomoses of tributaries of the left gastric and short gastric veins with oesophageal veins. These anastomotic channels become varicose in the presence of an elevated portal venous pressure and may rupture, causing severe haemorrhage.

Carcinoma of the stomach

A slow ooze of blood from an ulcerated malignancy is not uncommon. However, more invasive tumours can be associated with erosion of larger gastric or extragastric vessels, leading to profuse haemorrhage.

Hiatus hernia

Peptic oesophagitis associated with a sliding hiatus hernia can lead to ulceration and haemorrhage from the lower oesophagus.

Mallory–Weiss syndrome

When vomiting occurs, there is usually a relatively orderly sequence of events in which paroxysmal contraction of the abdominal wall is associated with diaphragmatic relaxation and reverse peristalsis in the stomach. The oesophagus usually offers no bar to the ejection of stomach contents. Occasionally the oesophagus may not relax, either because coordination is lost (as in a very drunk individual) or when social pressures lead to inhibition. In such circumstances, the early changes of vomiting take place: there is a dramatic rise in intragastric tension so that a pressure cone is driven up into the lower oesophagus. The consequence is either full thickness rupture into the pleural cavity, known as the Booerhave syndrome, or a mucosal tear. The latter gives rise to bleeding, which constitutes the Mallory–Weiss syndrome.

CLINICAL FEATURES

Chronic peptic ulceration will be suspected when there is a long history of dyspepsia with pain related to meals. There may be a history of previous haemorrhages, requiring admission to hospital, and a past barium meal or endoscopy may have shown a duodenal or gastric ulcer. Though suggestive, this evidence should not automatically lead to the assumption that the bleeding is from an ulcer.

Alternatively, the patient may be a known cirrhotic and/or alcholic, when portal hypertension should be suspected. The presence of hepatomegaly, splenomegaly, palmar erythema, spider naevi, gynaecomastia, testicular atrophy, ascites, jaundice and a tremor indicate liver insufficiency. Again, bleeding may be coming from another source.

On other occasions, a history of non-steroidal anti-inflammatory drug ingestion, in the absence of other features, may suggest an acute erosion.

In Mallory–Weiss syndrome, characteristically there has been a drinking bout and either frank vomiting or retching. The latter may have been forgotten. If vomiting occurs it does not initially contain blood. After a varying period of minutes or hours, there is haematemesis which may be single or multiple. Clinical examination is, as in most circumstances of bleeding, often negative. Stigmata of alcoholic liver disease may divert attention away from an oesophageal tear and suggest varices.

SPECIAL INVESTIGATIONS

The introduction of fibre-optic endoscopes makes it possible to ascertain the source of upper gastrointestinal bleeding with some ease. Although as yet there is little evidence to suggest that overall mortality and morbidity rates are much altered by early and precise anatomical diagnosis, it is rational to find a cause as soon as possible. In the individual patient this may be of great importance. Thus, where facilities are available, endoscopy should be carried out:

- at once when bleeding continues; it may be necessary to wash the stomach out vigorously to see a lesion
- as early as is convenient if the bleeding has stopped.

Fibre-optic oesophagogastroduodenoscopy establishes the diagnosis in upwards of 90% of instances. If more than one lesion is present, it identifies which is bleeding and it may also be therapeutic as well as diagnostic. Barium meal is less reliable (60%) and has the slight disadvantage that it may demonstrate a lesion such as a duodenal ulcer, which is not the source of the bleeding.

MANAGEMENT

Early consultation between physician and surgeon is the basis upon which proper management of haematemesis is conducted. The surgeon's role may be to act immediately when life is threatened, but more commonly the haemorrhage is less catastrophic and operation is not urgently required. He may later be asked to operate to control repeated haemorrhages or to undertake a curative procedure.

There are three common groups of patients with haematemesis: those with a history indicative of chronic peptic ulceration, those with portal hypertension and those with no ulcer history. The latter usually have an acute erosion, Mallory–Weiss syndrome or a silent chronic peptic ulcer.

All patients with haematemesis should be admitted to hospital. When blood loss is minimal, time may be taken for a detailed history and examination, but in the presence of a seriously depleted circulating blood volume, no time should be lost before resuscitating the patient.

The management of haematemesis may be considered under the following headings:

- resuscitation
- establishment of a diagnosis
- specific management to secure haemostasis and treat the cause.

Resuscitation

An initial assessment must be made to determine whether or not blood transfusion is necessary. The patient's account of the amount of blood lost is often misleading, and the decision to transfuse may need to be made from other considerations. In all cases, cross-matching should be done so that transfusion is available if needed.

Thus, transfusion is certainly required if the patient is in shock with pallor, sweating, a lowered blood pressure and an elevated pulse rate, or if he is not, but has a haemoglobin below 10 g/dl and an elevated blood urea concentration or is showing signs of continuing haemorrhage. The indications may need to be modified for patients known to be previously hypertensive or anaemic.

If transfusion and treatment of shock are necessary, the following routine may be used:

1. Strict rest in bed.
2. Establish an intravenous line for volume replacement. It is desirable to have a central line to measure central venous pressure, which may provide a more sensitive way of assessing changes in blood volume.
3. Draw blood for grouping and cross-matching, for haemoglobin estimation and baseline values of electrolyte and urea concentrations.
4. Administer an opiate (morphine, pethidine) in small doses and preferably intravenously.
5. A nasogastric tube may be passed to empty the stomach and to provide early warning of further bleeding. Opinion varies about the advisability of this.
6. Arrange for repeated observations of pulse, blood pressure and respiration and for the recording of any blood lost.
7. Nil by mouth.
8. If ulcer bleeding is suspected or diagnosed start intravenous histamine H_2 blockade with cimetidine or ranitidine.

The further signs of continued or repeated bleeding are:

- falling central venous pressure
- rising pulse and respiration rate and falling arterial blood pressure
- increased restlessness, sweating and pallor
- failure of blood pressure during transfusion
- fall of blood pressure after an initial response to transfusion
- repeated or persistent aspiration of fresh blood from nasogastric tube
- repeated melaena, particularly if reddish rather than black, indicates fast continued bleeding.

Establishment of a diagnosis

Once shock and hypovolaemia have been corrected, time can be taken to elicit a detailed history and make a thorough physical examination. An endoscopy should be arranged.

Bleeding peptic ulcer

For this condition, operation is indicated in the following circumstances:

- when bleeding is massive and continuous
- when a patient who has bled has a further haemodynamically significant bleed (i.e. fall in CVP or arterial pressure, rise in pulse rate)
- when there is a coexistent systemic condition – incipient heart failure, poor respiratory function – which will make survival less likely if the patient bleeds again
- earlier in older patients; above the age of 60 years, prolonged bleeding is poorly tolerated and early operation may improve the chance of survival
- usually when there is pyloric stenosis
- when at endoscopy there is a visible vessel – bleeding or not – in the ulcer base and this cannot be treated satisfactorily at endoscopy.

Age is closely related to most of these factors. Endoscopic techniques used to try to stop the bleeding in the base of the ulcer are laser photocoagulation, bipolar diathermy and adrenaline injection. This latter is currently the preferred method.

Choice of operation. Unlike perforation, where a simple operation on the ulcer may be all that is necessary, control of bleeding requires reduction in acid secretion.

Duodenal ulcer. In this case, a Polya gastrectomy is effective, but is a large operation for a patient who is often not in a good condition. Alternatively, a vagotomy, under-running of the bleeding point and drainage, either by pyloroplasty (using the incision made to get at the ulcer) or gastroenterostomy may be performed, or a highly selective vagotomy and under-running of the bleeding point.

Gastric ulcer. This condition requires either a Billroth I gastrectomy or a vagotomy and pyloroplasty with local excision of the gastric ulcer.

Acute erosive bleeding, stress ulcer and Mallory–Weiss syndrome

In patients at risk of erosive bleeding/stress ulceration (chiefly burns, massive trauma and those in the ITU/ICU with severe sepsis), prophylactic H_2 blockade or high-dose alkali therapy should be used.

Erosive bleeding. Obviously operation should be avoided in this case. However, if H$_2$ blockade does not work, a subtotal gastrectomy with Billroth I reconstruction is the best procedure. Very occasionally, the patient bleeds from the gastric remnant and a total gastrectomy has to be done.

Stress ulcer. Again, operation should be avoided in these often seriously ill and septic patients. If required, vagotomy, under-run and a drainage operation is the treatment of choice, but the mortality is high.

Mallory–Weiss syndrome. Only rarely do these patients need operation. However, procrastination can be fatal. It is a relatively simple matter to under-run the tear after opening the stomach.

Bleeding oesophageal varices

The management of this condition can be considered in three phases:

- acute or emergency management
- prevention of further bleeding episode
- ongoing management.

Management of acute bleeding. There are four stages:

- resuscitation
- prevention of intraluminal protein breakdown
- securing haemostasis
- definitive management.

Resuscitation. Haemorrhage from oesophageal varices is often massive and repeated and the patient is often unstable and in a serious condition. Initial resuscitation includes establishing an airway, providing adequate ventilation and restoring circulation. The last involves securing intravenous access, resuscitation with intravenous fluid and subsequent blood transfusion. Because of underlying poor liver function and the large volume of blood lost, blood transfusion is supplemented with clotting factors, including fresh frozen plasma, platelets and vitamin K.

It is often best to manage these patients in the ICU/ITU setting as they require close monitoring and may require airway protection with endotracheal intubation.

The patient is managed jointly by a gastroenterologist, surgeon and intensivist.

Prevention of protein breakdown. In liver disease and when there are portosystemic communications, products of bacterial digestion (one of which is ammonia) can escape more readily across the liver 'barrier' into the general circulation. When there is a large amount of blood in the gut, the production of these substances increases and 'portosystemic encephalopathy' or 'hepatic coma' may develop. To prevent this, the number of organisms in the bowel and their multiplication should be reduced, as follows:

- the bowel is washed out from below, and lactulose is given both as a laxative and to change the faecal flora
- neomycin is given by mouth (1 g every 4 hours) because this agent is poorly absorbed and can significantly reduce the number of organisms in the gut
- the patient is placed on a low protein oral intake.

Secure haemostasis and reduce portal pressure. There are several methods that are used but the following are the most recent developments, in order of priority:

1. diagnostic endoscopy involving variceal sclerotherapy or banding
2. octreotide infusion
3. Sengtaken–Blakemore (Minnesota tube) and its modifications
4. invasive methods of reducing portal pressure and reducing re-bleeding.

In the case of the first method, the initial gastroscopy is usually performed with the patient's airway secured with endotracheal tube and the patient sedated. This not only provides airway protection but also gives the gastroenterologist freedom of access to the oesophagus and stomach to perform either injection sclerotherapy of the varices or, as is more frequently performed now, rubber band ligation (similar to treatment of haemorrhoids).

Octreotide (somatostatin) is a peptide which has been demonstrated to reduce the portal pressure. An infusion of octreotide, usually given by an infusion pump, is often combined with variceal sclerotherapy and banding. Infusion may be continued for up to 3 days.

The *Sengtaken–Blakemore (Minnesota) tube* comprises a double, triple or quadruple lumen balloon tube (Fig. 33.1). The tube is placed by mouth and the lower balloon in the stomach locates the upper balloon above the varices. The balloons should be deflated after 24 hours as

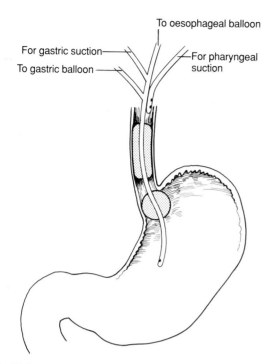

Fig. 33.1 **Four-lumen Sengstaken–Blakemore tube.** This is used for the control of bleeding varices.

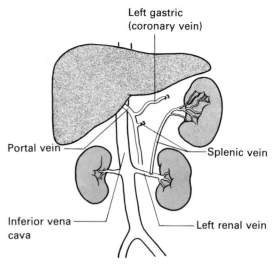

Fig. 33.2 **Distal splenorenal (Warren) shunt for portal hypertension.**

pressure necrosis may occur, both in the stomach and in the oesophagus. In the majority of centres, balloon tamponade is combined with the above-mentioned techniques.

Again, it is advantageous to have the patient's airway protected with an endotracheal tube during the use of this balloon.

There are three currently advocated *invasive methods* of reducing portal pressure and reducing re-bleeding:

- TIPS (transjugular intrahepatic portasystemic shunt)
- surgical transection of the oesophagus with devasculisation (Sugrura procedure)
- laparotomy and surgical portosystemic shunt.

TIPS has now replaced most surgical attempts at reducing portavenous pressure and can be performed percutaneously in the radiology department using specially designed catheters. The objective is to create a portosystemic connection through the liver parenchyma by inserting an expandable metal stent, thus creating a portosystemic shunt. A special balloon catheter is floated over a guide wire through the internal jugular vein superior vena cava into the hepatic vein and 'railroad-

ed' through into a portal radical within the liver. The new tract is dilated with the balloon and an expanding metal stent is placed across the artificial communication.

The Sugrura procedure is a direct attack on the varices at the gastro-oesophageal junction by circular stapler transection of the oesophagus with re-anastomosis. This is combined with devasculisation of the oesophageal varices by ligation of the left gastric vein and splenic vein. Good results have been achieved with this technique in Japan.

The procedure of laparotomy and surgical portosystemic shunt has now been superseded by TIPS and the Sugrura procedures. However, the operation is still performed in some centres.

The more established techniques of end-to-side direct portacaval shunting have been replaced by shunting operations that reduce incidents of portosystemic encephalopathy such as the distal splenorenal (Warren) shunt (Fig. 33.2).

Liver transplantation offers the ultimate treatment in those patients who are carefully selected and are predicted to have a more favourable outcome. This is particularly the case for patients with chronic hepatitis C or chronic hepatitis B.

Prevention of further bleeding. Most patients who have survived the initial acute bleeding episode are placed in a programme of ongoing sclerotherapy or banding over a period of several weeks.

Ongoing management. The long-term management of patients with portal hypertension and potential bleeding oesophageal varices includes the following:

- oral beta blocker therapy which may reduce portal venous pressure
- glyceryl trinitrate patch, also shown to reduce portal venous pressure
- reducing the primary insult to the liver by changing lifestyle, reducing alcoholic intake and improving nutrition.

The prognosis and outcome in patients with portal hypertension can be classified using the Child's grading (see Table 33.1). The majority of patients in grade A are suitable for the more definitive procedures of TIPS shunting and the Sugrura procedure. Some patients in grade B may also be suitable, but the prognosis for grade C patients is poor.

LOWER GASTROINTESTINAL BLEEDING

The causes and management of bleeding per rectum of bright blood and associated symptoms are dealt with in Chapters 29 (inflammatory bowel disease), 31 (large bowel cancer) and 32 (perianal conditions). This section will deal with the problem of massive lower gastrointestinal bleeding.

Blood that enters the gastrointestinal tract proximal to the duodenal jejunal junction, particularly proximal to the ileocaecal valve, mixes with liquid intestinal content and also undergoes some degree of digestive alteration. Therefore, unless the bleeding is massive, the passage of bright blood per rectum is unusual and the blood is usually a maroon colour but is often confused with and described as melaena. Bleeding from any lesion distal to the duodenal jejunal flexure can therefore usually be dif-

ferentiated from upper gastrointestinal bleeding by a close examination of the stool.

CLASSIFICATION OF CAUSES

The causes of lower gastrointestinal bleeding can be classified as follows:

- Small bowel
  - Meckel's diverticulum
  - intussusception
  - mesenteric infarction
  - aorto-enteric fistula
  - tumours
- Large bowel
  - diverticular disease
  - angiodysplasia (arteriovenous malformations)
  - ulcerative proctocolitis
  - Crohn's colitis
  - ischaemic colitis
  - carcinoma
  - neoplastic and hamartomatous polyps
  - endometriosis.

The *common causes* of massive lower gastrointestinal bleeding are:

- diverticular disease
- angiodysplasia (vascular ectasia)
- Meckel's diverticulum.

SURGICAL PATHOLOGY

Diverticular haemorrhage

The source of bleeding is usually a small ulcer overlying an intramural vessel; coexistent pericolic inflammation or abscess is unusual. The patient is characteristically elderly and hypertensive with no recent bowel symptoms and presents with an acute explosive passage of fresh rectal bleeding. The bleeding usually resolves spontaneously in all but 10% of cases.

Table 33.1	Child's grading of severity of liver disease in portal hypertension		
	Serum bilirubin	Serum albumin	Clinical stigmata (ascites, encephalopathy)
Grade A	Normal	35 g/L	None
Grade B	20–50 μmol/L	30–35 g/L	Mild, easily controlled
Grade C	>50 μmol/L	< 30g/L	Severe and uncontrolled

Angiodysplasia (vascular ectasia) arteriovenous malformations

These hamartomas occur both in the small and large bowel, but are more commonly localised in the caecum and right colon. They are increasingly recognised as the source of bleeding in massive colonic haemorrhage. The patient is characteristically elderly and may have associated aortic valve disease.

Meckel's diverticulum

Ectopic gastric mucosa in the neck or base of the Meckel's diverticulum may cause ulceration and bleeding. The condition is commonest in children and young adults. Abdominal pain usually precedes the passage of blood per rectum, whereas adults may present with either massive bleeding or anaemia.

Ischaemic bowel disease

Ischaemic bowel disease presents in two patterns.

Acute infarction. This is usually the result of an arterial embolism or thrombosis but may also occur with mesenteric venous obstruction. The superior or inferior mesenteric arteries may be occluded with either small bowel or large bowel infarction. Predisposing causes include atrial fibrillation, recent myocardial infarction with sluggish perfusion and atherosclerosis. Patients present with acute abdominal pain, shock, profuse diarrhoea and the passage of blood per rectum. The outcome is often poor.

Ischaemic colitis. This refers to small vessel occlusion of the colon, usually occurring in the region of the splenic flexure or upper descending colon, and results in infarction of the colon and possible later stricture formation. Bleeding may occur from the ischaemic mucosa, and on occasions this may be severe.

Aorto-enteric fistula

Erosion of an aortic prosthesis into the third part of the duodenum and subsequent fistula formation may follow aortic reconstructive surgery, particularly aneurysm repair. The diagnosis should always be kept in mind in patients presenting with bleeding per rectum or haematemesis who have had previous aortic surgery. Often a small initial haemorrhage heralds a more massive haemorrhage per rectum.

MANAGEMENT OF MASSIVE LOWER GASTROINTESTINAL BLEEDING

The principles of surgical management are similar to those for acute upper gastrointestinal bleeding, namely:

- resuscitation
- diagnosis of source
- definitive surgical treatment.

Resuscitation

This involves stabilising the circulation with intravenous fluids and blood transfusion and monitoring the response by assessing the vital signs of blood pressure and pulse, measuring urinary output and, in some instances, measuring central venous pressure.

Diagnosis of the source

This is the most difficult aspect, as the investigations for establishing a source of bleeding in the lower gastrointestinal tract have variable reliability.

It is important to exclude the upper gastrointestinal tract as a source with *gastroscopy* and to measure the clotting profile to exclude a bleeding diathesis. Moreover, the majority of patients with massive lower gastrointestinal bleeding will stop spontaneously and may be investigated electively with colonoscopy.

Special tests available to localise the source are described below.

Scintillation scan. This is a technetium-labelled red blood cell scan. It has been used as the initial investigation to assess the source of lower gastrointestinal bleeding. A sample of blood is taken from the patient, and the red cells are labelled with technetium then injected. Scans are taken with a gamma camera and extravasation of contrast into the bowel lumen may demonstrate the site of bleeding.

Selective angiography. Selective coeliac axis, superior mesenteric or inferior mesenteric angiography may be used to give more accuracy as to the source of bleeding. For best results, the patient needs to be bleeding at the time of angiography.

Colonoscopy. This form of endoscopy has become the most commonly used investigation in establishing the source of bleeding. The majority of patients stop bleeding, and this procedure can be performed in the elective setting after adequate bowel preparation. In some centres, colonoscopy is used in the acute phase but bleeding makes definition difficult.

On-table colonoscopy can be used in the operating theatre (see below).

Double contrast enema. This plays little role in the acute management of massive lower gastrointestinal bleeding.

Definitive surgical treatment

Although the majority of patients stop bleeding spontaneously, approximately 10% continue bleeding and require surgical intervention. The criteria for surgical treatment include:

- continued bleeding > 24 hours
- re-bleeding in hospital
- blood transfusion requirements > 6 units
- persistent shock.

Surgery in small bowel bleeding. If the small bowel is the source of bleeding, then the site is usually obvious at laparotomy. If the source is not obvious, the small bowel may be isolated into a number of segments with clamps and the segment containing the bleeder becomes distended and this is resected. Alternatively, an enterotomy may be performed and a flexible endoscope, either colonoscope or gastroscope, passed into the lumen of the bowel to isolate the source of bleeding. Segmental resection is then performed.

Surgery in large bowel bleeding. The objective is to perform, where possible, a segmental resection of the large bowel. However, best results are obtained with either right hemicolectomy or subtotal colectomy and ileorectal anastomosis. Poor results occur after left hemicolectomy.

When the source has not been identified pre-operatively, on-table colonoscopy may be performed. In this situation, antegrade on-table lavage of the colon is performed and the colonoscope is passed per anum. If no obvious source of bleeding is found, then subtotal colectomy and ileorectal anastomosis is the operation of choice.

FURTHER READING

Dykes P W, Keighley M R B 1981 Gastrointestinal haemorrhage. Wright, Bristol

Hunt P S 1986 Gastrointestinal haemorrhage. Clinical surgery international. Churchill Livingstone, Edinburgh

Sugawa C, Schuman B M, Lucas C E 1992 Gastrointestinal bleeding. Igaku-Shoin, New York

Genitourinary surgery

Testis and epididymis

Villis Marshall

34

OVERVIEW

Conditions affecting the male genitalia usually present with pain or a swelling. This chapter covers the common conditions of the testes and epididymis, with emphasis on clinical assessment and treatment. Undescended testes, epididymo-orchitis, hydrocele and testicular tumours are covered in detail.

Disorders of the testis and epididymis are common and, with the exception of imperfect testicular descent, they all give rise to solid or cystic scrotal swellings.

CLASSIFICATION OF DISORDERS

These can be classified as follows:

- Testis and epididymis
  - imperfect descent
  - inflammation
  - tumours
  - torsion
  - cysts
  - trauma
- Spermatic cord
  - varicocele
  - lipoma
- Tunica vaginalis
  - hydrocele
  - haematocele.

TESTIS AND EPIDIDYMIS

IMPERFECT DESCENT

The testis develops from coelomic epithelium and mesoderm of the urogenital ridge in the posterior wall of the coelomic cavity. It joins with the mesonephric duct system which forms the epididymis and the vas deferens and descends to reach the internal inguinal ring at 7 months' gestation; it then passes along the inguinal canal to reach the external ring at 8 months and enters the scrotum at birth.

During its descent the testis is preceded by a prolongation of peritoneum (processus vaginalis) which projects into the fetal scrotum. The testis slides down behind the processus vaginalis, which normally becomes obliterated at birth to form the innermost covering of the testis (tunica vaginalis).

A strand of fibromuscular mesoblastic tissue (the gubernaculum) attaches itself to the lower pole of the testis during fetal life, preceding it into the scrotum and, together with intra-abdominal pressure, probably brings about normal descent of the testis. It is also believed that Müllerian duct inhibitory substance is important in this process, as it may control gubernacular enlargement. In a recent review, it was stated 'that in most boys with cryptorchidism the cause is unknown but is probably mechanical, which honestly reflects the state of our knowledge at the present time'.

Testicular descent may be imperfect and result in:

- undescended testis
- ectopic testis
- retractile testis.

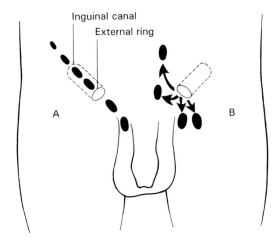

Fig. 34.1 Classification of undescended testes. A. Arrested in line of descent. Testes may be intra-abdominal, inguinal or high scrotal. The higher the arrest, the more hypoplastic are the testes. **B.** Ectopic. Testes have emerged from the external ring, and may be inguinal, penile, perineal or upper thigh in site; they are usually only mildly hypoplastic or normal.

Undescended testis (Fig. 34.1). Descent may be arrested along the normal pathway as the result of some local factor causing mechanical obstruction. Histological studies have shown that germ cell maturation and spermatogenesis are impaired in an undescended testis at age 2 years. There have been suggestions based on electron-microscopic findings that changes may occur within the first year of life. Hence it is believed that to minimise these changes, the testis should be placed in its normal position between the first and second year of life.

Unilateral undescended testes are about four times as common as bilateral testes; occasionally bilateral undescended testes are associated with some general endocrine abnormality, with hypogenitalism and obesity.

Complications of an undescended testis include all diseases peculiar to a normally placed testis, but in addition there is an increased risk of the following:

- defective spermatogenesis and sterility if bilaterally undescended
- torsion
- trauma
- inguinal hernia, which occurs in about 90% of cases
- malignancy, which is 4–10 times commoner than in a normally placed testis and which occurs most often in an abdominally situated testis.

Ectopic testis. Testicular descent takes place along the inguinal canal and beyond the external ring, but the testis is guided to an ectopic position (probably by gubernacular fibres) so that it comes to be superficial to the external oblique muscle at the root of the penis, in the perineum or in the upper and medial part of the thigh.

Retractile testis. Testicular descent occurs normally, and excessive cremasteric muscle activity draws the testis up into the inguinal canal. This does not represent a significant problem but may be difficult to exclude clinically from an undescended testis.

History

The mother should always be asked whether two testicles were present at birth. The newborn's scrotum is lax and both testicles are usually clearly visible. If the parent's answer is 'yes', a provisional diagnosis of retractile testes can be made.

Clinical examination

The proper clinical examination of a child who is said to have an undescended testis is critical. Relaxation of both child and mother must be achieved! The crucial manoeuvre is to get above the testis by putting the hand over the inguinal canal just lateral to the external ring. Firm pressure is exerted downwards and medially so as to trap a testis that lies outside the ring and push it towards the scrotum. In such circumstances the retractile testis will nearly always be displaced into the scrotum. An inguinal ectopic testis will slip under the fingers.

The following suggest an undescended testis rather than a retractile one:

- a testis cannot be felt in the conscious child
- the scrotum on the affected side is underdeveloped
- a hernia is present; sometimes the bulge of a hernia may be mistaken for a testis.
- if the testis can be felt, it is small and does not remain in the scrotum after manipulation.

It is important to remember to assess the child for endocrine or genetic abnormalities, particularly if there is bilateral imperfect descent.

Treatment

Treatment of undescended and maldescended testes is as follows.

Undescended testis. Operation is indicated in the first or second year after birth if both endocrine and reproductive functions are to be preserved. The principle of this operation is careful placement of the testes in the scrotum. Repair of the associated inguinal hernia may be necessary. Numerous methods have been devised for securing the testis in the scrotum, but these are much less important than that the testis should be freely mobile and able to be placed in the scrotum without tension on the cord structures. The major concern about very early surgery is that the cord structures are particularly delicate, making them vulnerable to surgical damage.

Ectopic testis. An ectopic testis, like the undescended testis, must be placed in the scrotum before it is damaged by defective maturation. The cord is usually of normal length and the operation easy.

Retractile testis. In this case, the parents should be reassured and the child left alone.

Hormone therapy. While there was once a vogue for gonadotrophin therapy in the management of this condition, this approach has now been virtually abandoned.

INFLAMMATION

Inflammation of the testis may present in the following forms:

- acute epididymo-orchitis
- chronic epididymo-orchitis.

Acute epididymo-orchitis

This inflammatory process of the epididymis and testes frequently occurs in young men without the isolation of any organism. If an organism is isolated, it is usually of the coliform species or a gonococcus. In the absence of an organism on culture, *Chlamydia trachomatis* is the likely causative agent. The mumps virus is well known for its ability to produce orchitis and in some instances it has been postulated that reflux of urine along the vas results in a chemical epididymitis.

Infecting organisms are believed to travel along the vas deferens in a retrograde manner to reach the epididymis before spreading to involve the testis. Alternative routes of infection are the bloodstream and lymphatics of the vas

deferens, but the exact means by which infection occurs has not been clearly established.

Clinical features. The clinical features of acute epididymo-orchitis are as follows.

Symptoms. These include:

- malaise and fever
- painful swelling of the testis of gradual onset and increasing in severity over several days
- dysuria and frequency – common
- urethral discharge – rare.

Signs. These include:

- pyrexia
- reddened and oedematous scrotum
- thickened cord
- painful swollen testis and epididymis which cannot be distinguished separately
- the common presence of a small secondary hydrocele.

Special tests. Microscopy and culture of urine are carried out to exclude a urinary tract infection and to establish a potentially causative agent.

Microscopy and culture of any urethral discharge should also be carried out, and a testicular ultrasound should be performed if the clinical diagnosis is in doubt.

Intravenous urography or renal and bladder ultrasound and cystourethroscopy should be carried out if bladder or bladder-neck disease is suspected.

Differential diagnosis. Torsion of the testicle may be difficult to distinguish from acute epididymo-orchitis but features of the former include the following:

- It occurs almost entirely in children and adolescents.
- There is occasionally a history of previous attacks of pain.
- There is a sudden onset of severe testicular pain, often accompanied by vomiting.
- There is an absence of urinary symptoms.
- The testis is usually situated high in the scrotum.
- There is absence of the cremasteric reflex.

Pyrexia may be present in both conditions, but it is usually greater in epididymo-orchitis. If there is any doubt, the testis should be explored.

Treatment. The patient should rest in bed, with the

scrotum elevated and analgesics administered. A broad-spectrum antibiotic should be administered after urine and any urethral discharge have been sampled for microscopy and culture. If the causative organism is isolated, the appropriate antibiotic is given.

Incision and drainage are required if abscess formation occurs, but this is a rare complication.

Chronic epididymo-orchitis

This may follow acute epididymo-orchitis, particularly in elderly patients with recurrent urinary tract infections. It may also be a sequel to urogenital tuberculosis, especially when the kidney is involved. Spread of infection is initially to the globus minor of the epididymis and later, by way of the vasa efferentia, to the testis.

Tuberculous epididymo-orchitis. The possible modes of infection of the epididymis by tubercle bacilli are the same as for acute epididymo-orchitis. In some cases, particularly young adults, blood spread from a primary infection in the lung appears most likely, especially when tuberculosis is also present at other sites.

Tuberculous epididymo-orchitis progresses slowly; it may be bilateral and associated with involvement of the prostate and seminal vesicles. The epididymis becomes hard and nodular but as caseation progresses, it softens and becomes adherent to the posterior scrotal skin where a sinus may form. The cord becomes thickened and nodular, and spread to the testis results in the formation of an irregular mass filling the scrotal compartment. There is sometimes a small hydrocele.

When tuberculosis exists elsewhere in the urogenital tract, there may be a 'sterile pyuria', in the sense that the urine is sterile to the usual culture methods, but usually tubercle bacilli can be cultured from the urine by an appropriate technique.

Treatment. A combination of isoniazid and rifampicin is the usual drug regimen. Second-line medications include streptomycin, ethambutol and cycloserine.

Surgery and epididymectomy or epididymo-orchiectomy will be indicated for a chronic scrotal sinus.

TUMOURS OF THE TESTIS

These usually occur in men under the age of 40 years. The majority are malignant, but they are rare and represent less than 1% of all male cancers.

The testis has two functions: the production of spermatozoa and the production of hormones. There are three cell types concerned in these processes:

- germ cells
- Sertoli cells
- Leydig cells.

Germ cells are spermatogenic cells which line the seminiferous tubules and produce spermatozoa in four stages (spermatogonia, primary spermatocytes, secondary spermatocytes and spermatids).

Sertoli cells are the cells in the seminiferous tubules which provide a supporting framework and perhaps nourishment for the developing spermatozoa. The Sertoli cells have been suggested as the source of a number of androgens and also oestrogens. Perhaps the most important product is androgen-binding protein, which is thought to be regulated by follicle-stimulating hormones and testosterone.

Leydig cells are interstitial cells in the lobules of the testis specialised to produce androgens which stimulate and maintain sex characteristics. They are probably stimulated by the luteinising hormone of the pituitary gland.

Surgical pathology

Imperfect descent is thought to be an important predisposing factor to malignant change.

Neoplasms of the testes may be either primary or secondary. The primary tumours are derived principally from the germinal epithelium. It is believed that the germinal tumours arise from a totipotent germ cell. This totipotent cell is thought to be capable of giving rise to either a seminoma or an embryonal carcinoma, which in turn can develop along either 'extra-embryonic' lines (yolk sac tumour, choriocarcinoma) or 'intra-embryonic' lines (teratoma).

Germinal tumours. Germinal tumours represent more than 96% of all tumours:

- seminoma
- non-seminomatous – including tumours that were described as embryonal, teratoma and choriocarcinoma.

Seminoma. This is the commonest tumour. It arises from the germinal epithelium of the seminiferous tubules in a patient usually between 20 and 30 years of age.

Macroscopically, it is a hard, smooth, fleshy tumour;

its cut surface is homogeneous and creamy, and fibrous septa give the appearance of lobulation.

Microscopically, there is considerable variation, with large clear polyhedral cells resembling spermatogonia and small lymphocyte-like cells with dark nuclei resembling spermatids. The cells are arranged in clumps or sheets.

Spread is usually by the lymphatics accompanying the cord to reach the para-aortic nodes. The inguinal lymph nodes are not involved unless local spread to the tunica vaginalis or scrotum has occurred. Bloodstream spread, particularly to the liver and lung, is generally a late manifestation.

Hormone effects may occur infrequently and cause feminisation.

Non-seminomatous tumours. The histological appearance of these tumours is varied. Some have cells that resemble embryonal fetal germinal epithelium, while others may have structures from all three germinal layers: ectoderm, mesoderm and endoderm. Rarely, some may contain chorionic tissues.

Macroscopically, the appearance is variable, but often there are areas of cystic spaces and haemorrhage. Occasionally, there may be hormone effects and often there are high levels of chorionic gonadotrophins.

Hormone effects are often pronounced and high levels of chorionic gonadotrophins may be excreted in the urine.

Non-germinal tumours. These represent less than 4% of all tumours:

- Sertoli cell tumour (sertolioma, tubular adenoma)
- Leydig cell tumour (interstitioma)
- orchioblastoma (gynandroblastoma)
- supporting tissue tumours: fibroma, lipoma, rhabdomyoma, neurofibroma, sarcoma, carcinoma of the rete testis, lymphoma.

Non-germinal tumours are exceedingly rare benign tumours, but they are of interest because of their hormonal effects.

Sertoli cell tumour. This is a common tumour in dogs; when it occurs in man, feminisation results.

Microscopically, Sertoli cells occur in compact alveolar masses. They are slender and pyramidal in shape with oval nuclei, and cytoplasm extends to the lumen of the seminiferous tubules as slender processes to which may be attached heads of spermatozoa.

Leydig cell tumour (interstitial cell tumour). This accounts for about 1% of all testicular tumours and is by far the most remarkable.

Microscopically, the tumour consists of large, round, slightly acid-staining cells with dark, round nuclei arranged in a pattern strongly suggestive of liver cords.

There is excess androgen production, and it is responsible for the production of precocious puberty when it appears in prepubertal years. However, for some unknown reason, feminisation occurs in about 50% of cases when it appears in postpubertal years.

Supporting tissue tumours and orchioblastomas. These are very rare and are not associated with hormone production.

Clinical features

Symptoms. Testicular tumours may present the following features:

- a painless testicular lump apparently only noted after minor trauma
- a slightly painful testicular lump growing rapidly over weeks or months
- a hydrocele, which is associated with 5% of testicular tumours
- weight loss, malaise, cough due to metastatic spread to lungs and lymph nodes
- feminising effects, particularly gynaecomastia.

Signs. These fall into two categories: local and general.

Local. These include:

- a painless, swollen and hard testis
- a small secondary hydrocele.

General. A search is made for metastases, particularly in the para-aortic chain of lymph nodes, and for evidence of feminisation.

Staging. Perhaps the single most important step in the management of a testicular tumour is its staging. To stage a tumour adequately, the following investigations are required:

- serum alpha fetoprotein (tumour marker)

Table 34.1	Stages of testicular tumours
Stage	Finding
Stage I	No clinical or radiological evidence of spread. Tumour markers return to normal after orchidectomy
Stage II	Demonstrable involvement of the para-aortic nodes
Stage IIa	Elevated markers and normal CT
Stage IIb	Mass <5 cm found on pre-operative scan
Stage IIc	Mass >5cm found on pre-operative scan
Stage III	Involvement of the mediastinal lymph nodes and parenchymal metastases

- serum human chorionic gonadotrophin (tumour marker)
- chest X-ray (all prior to orchidectomy)
- CT scan of the chest and abdomen.

The different stages are described in Table 34.1 in relation to findings of the above investigations.

Unfortunately, not all tumours are associated with elevated tumour markers. Consequently, there is considerable interest in finding other markers; some that have shown promise are lactate dehydrogenase and ferritin.

Treatment of malignant testicular tumours

Treatment depends on the type and stage of the tumour.

Seminoma

Stage I. Treatment is by inguinal orchidectomy and radiotherapy to the para-aortic nodes (25–30 Gy). Recently, the use of low-dose radiotherapy has been questioned; however, uncertainty exists about the possible long-term morbidity of this treatment. Leukaemia at this stage is potentially the only second tumour that may have a higher incidence after radiotherapy.

Stage II. In this case, treatment is by inguinal orchidectomy and radiotherapy to the para-aortic and mediastinal nodes.

Stage III. This stage will require elements of the above and chemotherapy. The agents in common use are cis-platinum, vinblastine, isosamide, etoposide and bleomycin.

Non-seminomatous tumours

Stage I. Treatment is by inguinal orchidectomy. In most centres, node dissection has been abandoned for a 'surveillance' policy. However, it is imperative, if this policy is to be adopted, that a proper follow-up protocol is used. This protocol requires frequent CT scans and measurement of tumour markers. It is also important to ensure that the patient is compliant.

Stage II. Chemotherapy which consists of three to four cycles of a regime containing cis-platinum, etoposide and vinblastine may be combined with surgery or radiotherapy. This is followed by further CT scans, and if there is a residual nodal tissue then para-aortic node dissection with removal of the mass is the usual form of treatment. Sometimes, a further cycle of therapy is given.

Stage III. The initial treatment is usually the same as for stage II. In patients failing to respond, high-dose chemotherapy with peripheral cell blood transplants has been tried. However, this approach is still being evaluated.

Prognosis

Seminoma. For stage I and II disease, the 5-year survival rates are 98% and 85%, respectively.

Non-seminomatous tumours. For stage I and II disease, 5-year survival rates of 90% and 80%, respectively, can be anticipated with the advent of triple-agent chemotherapy.

TORSION

This is a surgical emergency which is commonly referred to as torsion of the testis, although the twist is always in the lowest part of the spermatic cord or the mesorchium.

Predisposing factors

Abnormalities, which are often bilateral, said to predispose to torsion include:

- long mesorchium
- horizontal testis
- ectopic testis
- capacious tunica vaginalis
- well-developed spiral cremaster muscle.

Surgical pathology

The cord usually twists from without inwards; occasionally the cord may untwist spontaneously, but in the majority of cases necrosis of the testis will occur unless operation is performed. Operation must be performed as rapidly as possible if damage is to be minimised.

Clinical features

There is a sudden onset of lower abdominal and testicular pain. The localisation of the pain to the T_{12}, L_1 segment of the abdomen (the development origin of the testes) can cause diagnostic confusion unless the condition is thought of and the testis and scrotum are carefully examined.

The testis is swollen and drawn up and a small hydrocele is often present in an oedematous scrotum.

Differential diagnosis

Refer to the section on epididymo-orchitis.

Treatment

This is always operative when the diagnosis is certain or when epididymo-orchitis cannot be excluded. The operational procedure is as follows:

1. expose the testis and untwist the cord or mesorchium
2. establish viability – return of colour and free bleeding
3. fix the testis by opening the tunica vaginalis
4. perform orchidectomy if the testis is not viable
5. fix the opposite testis as the predisposition is a bilateral phenomenon.

CYSTS OF THE EPIDIDYMIS

These are common and may be unilateral or bilateral, single or multilocular cysts. They lie above and behind the testis and contain crystal clear fluid or opalescent fluid and spermatozoa.

They most probably arise from vestigial remnants in the epididymis or vasa efferentia; the pedunculated hydatid of Morgagni; the appendix of the epididymis; and the paradidymis or organ of Giraldes (all being remnants of the mesonephric or Wolffian duct system); or the sessile hydatid of Morgagni or appendix testis (remnants of the paramesonephric or Müllerian duct system). Alternatively, they may be acquired as retention cysts of the vasa efferentia.

Cysts which communicate with the seminiferous tubules and contain spermatozoa are sometimes referred to as spermatoceles, but the differentiation is of no practical value.

Treatment by excision is indicated if cysts are large enough to cause persistent pain or discomfort, but most do not require any treatment.

SPERMATIC CORD

VARICOCELE

It is commonly held that a varicocele is a dilatation and elongation of the pampiniform plexus of veins. The plexus is a mass of intercommunicating veins accompanying the testicular artery in the spermatic cord which joins to form two or three testicular veins in the inguinal canal and one testicular vein at the level of the internal inguinal ring. Almost invariably, the left side is involved. While the angle of entry of the left spermatic vein into the renal vein has been invoked to explain this left-sided preponderance, this seems to be an overly simplistic explanation.

Clinical features

A 'worm-like' collection in the scrotum is visible and palpable on standing. There is also pain of a dull dragging nature which may extend into the groin. Depression of spermatogenesis may occur and is presumably due to impaired heat loss in the scrotum. It is said that unless the testes are kept at a temperature of 2.5°C below rectal temperature, normal spermatogenesis will not occur.

Treatment

Conservative. Reassurance usually suffices and tight underpants may relieve ache and discomfort.

Operative. This is indicated rarely for infertility or continuing pain and discomfort. The standard operation entails ligature of testicular veins in the inguinal canal. An alternative method is to explore the scrotum and divide the cremasteric veins, but damage to the testicular artery is a hazard of this approach.

TUNICA VAGINALIS

HYDROCELE

This is a collection of fluid within the tunica vaginalis.

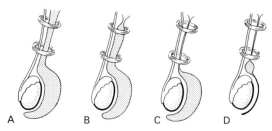

Fig. 34.2 Types of hydrocele. A. Congenital. **B.** Infantile. **C.** Vaginal (commonest). **D.** Encysted hydrocele of cord.

Primary hydrocele. There is no associated disease of the underlying testis or epididymis and the hydrocele may be:

- congenital
- infantile
- vaginal
- an encysted hydrocele of the cord (Fig. 34.2).

Secondary hydrocele. There is underlying inflammation or a neoplasm of the testis or epididymis.

Surgical pathology

In a primary hydrocele of the congenital type, there is incomplete obliteration of the processus vaginalis, and the tunica vaginalis is distended with peritoneal fluid. In the infantile and the encysted types, there is partial obliteration of the processus vaginalis. In the common vaginal type of hydrocele, the tunica vaginalis is distended with varying amounts of straw-coloured fluid, the origin of which is unknown. In long-standing cases, the tunica vaginalis becomes thickened and the underlying testis and epididymis become flattened.

In secondary hydroceles, the fluid collection in the tunica vaginalis may be rapid as in acute epididymo-orchitis or torsion of the testis, or slow as with chronic inflammation or testicular tumours. The fluid is usually an exudate, which in the presence of a tumour is often bloodstained.

Clinical features

A hydrocele presents as a tense or lax unilocular translucent scrotal swelling which may be emptied on lying down if it is congenital in type. The testis cannot be clearly separated from the hydrocele which lies anterior to it.

Diagnosis

A confident diagnosis can usually be made on clinical grounds. However, as the hydrocele may be secondary to testicular pathology, it is necessary to establish that the testis is normal. If the hydrocele is tense, ultrasonography is particularly useful in achieving this. If ultrasonography is not available, the only option is to aspirate the hydrocele so that the testis can be more easily palpated; however, this is definitely a second best option.

Treatment

Aspiration. The site for aspiration in the scrotum is usually anterior but it must be carefully determined by transillumination so that the testis can be avoided. Aspiration may be repeated for recurring tense hydroceles associated with discomfort, and techniques have been described for the installation of sclerosing agents into the hydrocele, which will prevent the reaccumulation of fluid.

Operation. This is the method of choice when repeated aspirations fail to control the hydrocele.

The tunica vaginalis can be partially excised and everted behind the epididymis if it is thin-walled (Jaboulay's operation); alternatively it can be completely excised if it is thick-walled and chronic. Meticulous haemostasis is particularly important, to prevent scrotal haematoma or haematocele.

HAEMATOCELE

This may follow trauma to the scrotum or it may follow an inguinal or scrotal operation or aspiration of a hydrocele.

A tense, painful swelling occurs which is treated by scrotal elevation, bed rest and analgesics.

Its major importance is often in the differential diagnosis of an enlarged testis.

TRAUMA

Trauma to the testes is not uncommon, particularly in contact sports such as football.

History

The history is usually of a severe blow to the testes with the onset of severe pain and swelling.

Examination

Depending on the extent of the injury, the whole scrotum may be swollen and tense, and no testes palpable. In minor degrees of injury, the testis may be only slightly enlarged and tender.

Management

The management will to a large extent depend on the degree of damage to the testis. In this regard, *ultrasonography* has been particularly helpful in demonstrating whether the testis has been significantly disrupted. In general, if the testis has been ruptured and there is a haematoma, exploration, removal of the blood and devitalised tissue, and closure of the tunica if possible without tension will result in the best long-term outcome.

FURTHER READING

Bullock W, Sibley G, Whitaker R 1994 Essential urology, 2nd edn. Churchill Livingstone, Edinburgh

Hutson J M, Beasley S W 1992 Descent of the testes. Edward Arnold, London

MacFarlance M T 1994 Urology, 2nd edn (House Officer Series). Williams & Wilkins, Baltimore

35

Urinary tract disorders
Mark Laniado   Paul Abel

OVERVIEW

Urological surgery is considered in detail in this chapter. It starts with common urological symptoms and their management: haematuria, acute micturition difficulty (retention of urine) and both voiding and filling symptoms of the lower urinary tract. Much of modern urology concerns prostatic disease, both benign hyperplasia and carcinoma. Other conditions that cause bladder outflow obstruction include urethral stricture and bladder neck stenosis. Urothelial tumours (notably carcinoma of the bladder) are considered separately from renal tumours (carcinoma, nephroblastoma). Calculous disease and urinary infection are aetiologically linked. Common conditions of the penis are described. The chapter ends with functional disorders of the bladder, especially incontinence.

MANAGEMENT OF COMMON SYMPTOMS

HAEMATURIA

The aetiology of haematuria can be usefully divided into medical and surgical causes, and the origin of blood into prerenal, renal and postrenal sites. Clinically, haematuria is divided into painful and painless haematuria. Blood at the beginning or the end of the stream suggests bleeding from the bladder neck, prostate or urethra. A congenital abnormality of the urinary system may be present if bleeding follows minor trauma to the loin, pelvis or perineum.

Painful haematuria. The common causes of painful haematuria are as follows:

- Unilateral loin pain suggests a tumour, hydronephrosis or cystic disease. Pain radiating to the groin suggests colic due to a calculus or clot.
- Pyrexia suggests pyelonephritis, which may be unilateral or bilateral.
- Frequency, urgency and pain passing urine suggest lower urinary tract infection in women and children, and bladder outflow obstruction in men.

Painless haematuria. Common causes are:

- cancer within the kidney, the tissues lined by urothelium, or the prostate; exposure to carcinogens and a history of smoking may be present
- drugs – anticoagulants, cyclophosphamide and D-penicillamine
- glomerulonephritis, the possibility of which is raised by a recent sore throat or URTI in association with oedema or joint pains.

Rarely, painless haematuria can occur as a result of:

- a bleeding tendency due to inherited disorders (haemophilia, sickle cell disease)
- a purpuric rash with bleeding secondary to idiopathic thrombocytopenic purpura or Henoch–Schönlein disease
- blackwater fever (malaria)
- exercise, e.g. running, which leads to 'jogger's haematuria'
- travel abroad to a country where schistosomiasis is endemic.

Other causes include reactive or secondary haemorrhage

following prostatectomy, urethral dilatation, prostatic biopsy or even injection of haemorrhoids or insertion of foreign bodies.

Examination

General signs to observe are:

- pyrexia, which suggests infection, but also inflammation, e.g. glomerulonephritis
- bruising or purpura
- hypertension and oedema, which suggest renal impairment in glomerulonephritis
- cardiac rhythm – atrial fibrillation resulting in the formation of emboli that lodge in the kidney (rare).

Abdominal examination may show an enlarged bladder due to chronic retention of urine (common), or very occasionally a bladder tumour. A kidney with a tumour, polycystic disease or hydronephrosis may occasionally be palpable if very large. Splenomegaly may also be seen because of a haematological disorder with impaired clotting, although this is rare.

Vaginal examination in women may reveal a pelvic mass from the bladder or reproductive organs, or urethral prolapse or caruncle.

Rectal examination in men for tenderness (prostatitis) or prostatic enlargement, whether benign or malignant, may occasionally give rise to haematuria, possibly associated with vertebral tenderness from metastases.

Investigations

Urine. Haematuria found on dipstix may be false positive and can be confirmed by microscopic examination for red cells. Phase contrast microscopy of red cell morphology can distinguish medical from surgical causes. Urine culture is necessary to confirm infection when white cells are found in the urine, and three early morning samples are necessary to exclude tuberculosis when no organisms are seen with white cells. Cytological examination may indicate malignant cells. Proteinuria with casts found on microscopy may indicate glomerulonephritis. Crystals (calculi) or ova (schistosomiasis) may be seen on microscopy.

Blood. Full blood count, ESR, and electrolyte (especially potassium), urea and creatinine (for hydration) levels should be assessed. In children, antistreptolysin-O (ASOT) titres should be carried out and complement lev-

els measured because of suspected glomerulonephritis. Coagulation screen and sickle cell testing should be performed for bleeding disorders.

Intravenous urography (IVU). This is mandatory for all patients with haematuria. An ultrasound scan with a plain abdominal radiograph may be substituted in those few patients at risk of severe allergic reactions. The urogram may show calculi or abnormalities of the kidney or upper tracts.

The KUB (kidneys, ureters, bladder) radiograph may show opacities due to calculi. The patient may be bent to one side because of pain. The bones and soft tissues may reveal evidence of metastases or an absent renal shadow due to extravasation following trauma.

Ultrasound scan. Space-occupying lesions of the kidney found on IVU are scanned to determine if they are cystic or solid; the latter are suggestive of tumour. Occasionally, invasion of the renal vein may be seen. A CT or MRI scan may be necessary for solid lesions.

Cystoscopy. This detects tumours of the lower urinary tract and is mandatory even with a normal or abnormal IVU or ultrasound scan, because bladder tumours must be excluded. If investigations are all negative, further follow-up is controversial. Patients may be discharged immediately or followed up for 3 years.

ACUTE MICTURITION DIFFICULTY

It is especially important to be vigilant for two emergencies requiring immediate treatment:

- acute painless retention due to spinal cord compression, which is present without a history of voiding symptoms following, for example, disc prolapse or metastasis, which may not be associated with back pain and can be detected by neurological examination
- anuria and acute retention, which is possible even if urinary catheterisation yields urine; therefore, check urine output postcatheterisation, plus blood, urea and electrolyte levels.

History

Voiding symptoms in a patient older than 50 years often indicate benign prostatic hyperplastic (BPH) or prostate cancer. A urethral stricture is possible when there is a history of instrumentation or sexually transmitted diseases. Constipation can precipitate acute retention in patients with mild bladder outflow obstruction.

Haematuria may cause clot retention (which may be because of haemorrhage after prostatectomy). Previous urinary tract surgery, injury or instrumentation suggests a stricture.

Previous lower para-aortic lymph node dissection (aortic aneurysm repair), pelvic operation, (abdominoperineal resection) or anorectal surgery may damage autonomic nerves and lead to lower motor neurone bladder dysfunction. Other causes include:

- drugs: autonomic nervous system depressants
- lower urinary tract infection
- neurological disorders, e.g. Parkinson's disease, multiple sclerosis.

Examination

General. Check for signs of chronic renal failure in the presence of acute-on-chronic renal failure.

Abdominal. A tender bladder indicates acute urinary retention. A large non-tender bladder with dribbling from the penis suggests acute-on-chronic retention or a hypocontractile/atonic bladder due to detrusor failure.

A tight phimosis, meatal stricture or scars on the penis from previous sinuses suggest a sexually transmitted disease.

Rectal examination. Evidence of malignancy or BPH of the prostate should be sought. The size of the prostate is overestimated when in acute urinary retention.

CNS. Abnormal sacral sensation (S_{234}), loss of ankle reflexes or reduced anal sphincter tone and contractility may indicate a neurological cause.

Management

Simple measures include appropriate pain control, a hot bath, the sound of a running tap and relief of constipation.

Alternatively, *urethral catheterisation* should be performed, as follows. Under clean conditions, the narrowest possible catheter (usually 12 Fr Foley catheter) is passed about 1 or 2 minutes after analgesic lubrication of the urethra. The balloon is inflated sufficiently to maintain the catheter in the bladder and avoid bladder irritation, which might lead to detrusor contractions and bypassing of urine around the catheter. Usually only 8 ml is required for this purpose. The bladder is emptied completely and the residual volume is noted. If haematuria is present, it may be necessary to pass a large bore three-way catheter so that the bladder can be irrigated and clots removed. A saline intravenous infusion should be started if there is upper urinary tract obstruction as decompression is followed by a sodium-losing diuresis. Careful fluid balance (which can be monitored by daily weighing) and observation of urea and electrolytes are needed. If urethral catheterisation is difficult in spite of adequate lubrication, a suprapubic catheter should be inserted, but only if an enlarged bladder is definitely palpable. This can be confirmed by flexible cystoscopy or ultrasound scan. An introducer for the urethral catheter should only be used in experienced hands.

LOWER URINARY TRACT SYMPTOMS

There are multiple causes, and symptoms can be divided into those of voiding and filling. It is not always possible to distinguish the cause from the clinical features, so special investigations are often needed.

CAUSES

Physical obstruction. This can occur as a result of:

- benign prostatic hyperplasia (BPH)
- carcinoma of the prostate
- bladder neck stenosis
- urethral stricture, including meatal stricture
- penis disorders, e.g. phimosis
- congenital disorders, e.g. urethral valves, polyp or stricture
- calculi (bladder, urethra)
- external compression, e.g. loaded colon, pelvic tumour.

Functional causes include detrusor–sphincter dyssynergia, e.g. multiple sclerosis and underactive or atonic detrusor.

Other causes of lower urinary tract symptoms include lower urinary tract infection and changes in diurnal secretion of antidiuretic hormone (ADH), which can give nocturia.

DISTINGUISHING BETWEEN 'VOIDING' AND 'STORAGE' SYMPTOMS

In the new terminology, what were known as 'obstructive' symptoms have been renamed 'voiding' symptoms, and 'irritative' have been renamed 'storage' symptoms. These changes have been necessary because symptoms relate poorly to aetiology; the clinical picture needs to be complemented by appropriate investigations.

Voiding symptoms include:

- weak urinary force
- hesitancy (especially with a full bladder which suggests obstruction)
- terminal dribbling
- feeling of incomplete emptying.

Storage symptoms include:

- urinary urgency – this is divided into sensory, which is without detrusor contractions and so rarely associated with incontinence (e.g. urinary tract infection), and motor, which is with detrusor contractions and possibly incontinence (e.g. post-CVA)
- frequency
- nocturia
- incontinence/overflow following chronic retention, not necessarily with bladder outflow obstruction (e.g. in women after operation).

When a patient presents with symptoms, the following investigations are the minimum required:

- 24 hour frequency/volume chart recorded over 7 days with the time and volume of urine passed
- urine microscopy and culture
- serum creatinine and electrolyte levels
- urinary flow rate and voiding pattern (Fig. 35.1)
- ultrasound scan to show postmicturition residual urine or the presence of upper tract dilatation.

Flow rates and residual urine ultrasound should be repeated three times for reliable data, as patients may be embarrassed or nervous, preventing representative recordings to be made.

Further investigations include:

- micturating cystogram (in boys with suspected urethral valves); in children with urinary tract infection

(UTI) and suspected reflux, a renogram may be better
- pressure/flow cystometry (see below)
- ascending urethrogram – identifies strictures
- cystourethroscopy – detects stricture, bladder trabeculation, sacculation, diverticula, tumours
- prostate specific antigen (PSA) for estimation of prostate cancer risk is performed in some centres (see below).

Pressure/flow cystometry is an invasive investigation of the pressure/flow relationship of bladder function, which is indicated: to distinguish low flow rates due to detrusor hypoactivity without obstruction from low flow rates with obstruction and a normal detrusor; in men less than 55 years with low flow rates; in men with symptoms of outflow obstruction and a normal flow rate; and post-surgery for BPH. Pressure transducers are placed in the bladder via a urethral catheter and in the rectum. Detrusor activity ('pressure') is derived from these measurements by subtracting bladder pressure from rectal pressure, which is a measure of intra-abdominal pressure. The pattern of detrusor contraction during filling of the bladder with fluid and during voiding together with urinary flow rate gives information on detrusor contractility, stability and the extent of outflow obstruction (see Fig. 35.1).

EFFECTS OF OBSTRUCTION

The detrusor muscle hypertrophies to overcome the obstruction and can contract inappropriately, giving symptoms of urgency and frequency (detrusor instability). Inefficient emptying may follow, leading to chronic retention and the risk of infection.

Changes in the bladder wall can produce vesicoureteric reflux and obstruction to the ureters, resulting in hydroureter. This can compromise renal function, leading to voiding nephropathy. Complications from obstruction include infection, calculus formation and rarely bladder cancer (squamous cell carcinoma), e.g. with a stricture. Typically, infravesical obstruction leads to bilateral ureteromegaly, and supravesical obstruction produces unilateral ureteromegaly.

BENIGN PROSTATIC HYPERPLASIA (BPH)

BPH is part of the natural ageing process and is not a disease in itself. Similar lower urinary tract symptoms are

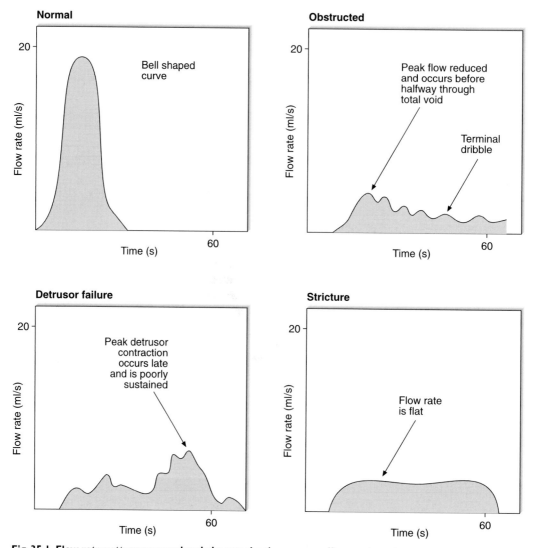

Fig. 35.1 Flow rate patterns: normal and abnormal, using pressure/flow cystometry.

experienced by both men and women with ageing, but in men the symptoms are usually attributed to BPH. This is not usually true. Prostate enlargement is detectable from age 30 years and reaches 80% by age 80. In the USA, approximately 25% of men aged 70 years or older have symptoms from BPH, but only about 10% in the UK need prostatectomy for relief of voiding symptoms.

PATHOLOGY

The prostate gland is a zonal structure comprising glandular tissue in a fibromuscular stroma divided into the central, peripheral and transition zones. Growth is regu-

lated by many factors, but notably by androgens. With time, the structures within the transition (periurethral) zone enlarge and form adenomas. These may grow outwards, compressing the peripheral zone and leading to a false capsule. Importantly, adenomas may grow inwards leading to urethral obstruction and symptoms. It is the symptoms that are important, and the overall size of the prostate bears little relation to the extent of symptoms or obstruction. BPH can contribute in two ways to bladder outflow obstruction:

- a static component due to the bulk of cells/stroma, which can be altered by operation

- a dynamic component arising from the smooth muscle tone within and around the urethra, which is susceptible to medical interventions.

The smooth muscle tone of the prostatic fibromuscular stroma, bladder neck and trigone contributes to obstruction of the urethra.

CLINICAL FEATURES

Patients are usually over 50 years and present with either voiding or filling symptoms, retention of urine or complications (e.g. infection, calculi). Examination is consistent with these features, but usually non-contributory. Nevertheless, it is essential to exclude chronic retention requiring urgent intervention. Rectal examination may reveal a carcinoma of the prostate.

INVESTIGATIONS

Peak urine flow rates are reduced compared to normal for the volume of urine voided, which can be read off a nomogram (minimum acceptable void = 150 ml). The pattern of flow over time shows a peak rate that diminishes slowly and a prolonged voiding time (Fig. 35.1).

Pressure/flow cystometry may be indicated as described above.

TREATMENT

A guide to treatment is the severity of the symptoms and the trouble these cause in patients with BPH. These can be assessed objectively by commonly used symptom scores. Indications for treatment include the presence of demonstrable outflow obstruction with either:

- absolute indications
  - acute or chronic retention of urine
  - renal dysfunction
  - complications (calculi, infection)
- relative indication
  - interference in lifestyle.

The commonest cause for frequency and nocturia is drinking excessively. With age, the bladder contracts, giving the desire to void at lower volumes than earlier in life. Patients bothered by nocturia as shown by the frequency/volume chart may be helped simply by fluid restriction at night and 3 hours before going to bed.

Frequency during the day may be reduced by drinking less overall. Conservative treatment should be tried for 3 months, as many will improve spontaneously.

Further treatment choices are now broad and controversial. Best results are obtained if voiding symptoms predominate. Storage symptoms may persist in 25% at 1 year, especially if there has been preceding chronic retention.

Medical

Alpha-blockers (e.g. prazosin, indoramin). By relaxing smooth muscle in the prostate, these drugs produce a small increase in flow rate. After about 4–6 weeks, this may be enough to alleviate symptoms sufficiently and will have the additional benefit of lowering blood pressure in patients with hypertension. However, adverse symptoms (postural hypotension, drowsiness) have been appreciable, though less frequent with highly selective blockers (α_{1c}, e.g. tamsulosin).

5-Alpha-reductase inhibitors. These block conversion of testosterone to its active metabolite dihydrotestosterone. Prostate size reduces and flow rates may improve marginally, but usually only after several months (e.g. finasteride).

Surgical

Prostatectomy. The adenoma obstructing the urethra is removed and a channel is created. A transurethral resection of prostate (TURP) is the conventional treatment of choice instead of open operation because of a lower mortality rate. Complications are usually minor, but can be troublesome.

Intraoperative complications include haemorrhage and hyponatraemia ('TUR syndrome'). The latter results from absorption of irrigation fluid during dilution of the blood. It is treated by fluid restriction.

Postoperative complications include:

- urinary tract infection and septicaemia
- retrograde ejaculation – this is common, so that patients must be warned pre-operatively
- urethral stricture
- bladder neck stricture
- incontinence (from sphincter damage, should be rare with skilled surgeons) – exclude UTI and diminish fluid intake; usually settles over time and may benefit from anticholinergic therapy

- impotence, especially if borderline performance pre-operatively
- secondary haemorrhage (10–20 days postoperatively) due usually due to infection; the patient needs to be warned before going home
- hypoactive detrusor, e.g. because of chronic retention or Parkinson's disease.

Laser prostatectomy is frequently performed with results almost as good as TURP and often with less morbidity. Open prostatectomy is indicated if the prostate is very large or if there are associated bladder complications (e.g. stones, diverticula). It can be carried out by the retropubic or transvesical route, but is uncommonly performed today.

New treatments. Vaporisation of the prostate has recently been introduced, with similar results to laser and TURP but without long-term data. Minimally invasive therapies such as transurethral needle ablation (TUNA) or transurethral microwave therapy (TUMT) produce modest changes and are still being evaluated. Prostatic stents have been tried in patients who are unfit for TURP but have several problems such as encrustation, blockage and migration. The stent may require removal, which is often difficult.

PROSTATE CANCER

AETIOLOGY AND EPIDEMIOLOGY

Prostate cancer is now the commonest cancer and the second or third commonest cause of death from cancer in men in the Western world (≈9000 deaths/year in the UK). This fact is in part due to the increasing age of the population, but also to other factors that are difficult to explain. Interestingly, about 30% of men aged 50–60 years have histological evidence of ('latent') prostate cancer, and this figure rises to almost 80% of men aged 80. The death rate is lower amongst the Japanese and higher in North America, where American Blacks present with more advanced disease than Caucasians. Prostate cancer is hormone-dependent, and part of the racial differential is explained by the lowest testosterone level in Asians and the highest in Blacks. Most men affected with 'clinical' prostate cancer (i.e. with clinically important cancer) are in the 65 to 85 year age group. Those with one first degree relative affected have twice the risk of developing the disease. Distinguishing between 'clinical' and 'latent' prostate cancer is the focus of much research.

SURGICAL PATHOLOGY

More than 90% of prostate tumours are adenocarcinomas, and they are often multifocal. Approximately 70% of them arise in the peripheral zone, 20% in the transition zone, and 10% in the central zone. Cancers in the fibromuscular stroma usually arise because of invasion from neighbouring zones. One of the most useful grading systems is the Gleason system. Five patterns of differentiation are recognised, and the worst two areas on histological examination are given a score. The sum of these two (2–10) is inversely proportional to the prognosis.

Spread of the cancer is staged according to the TNM classification (Table 35.1). Although direct extension of prostatic tumours is common, microscopic metastases frequently occur before evidence of local invasion; this makes treatment decisions difficult. Tumour cells may spread by the lymphatics to the pelvic lymph nodes or through the circulation to the axial skeleton. Hepatic and pulmonary metastases occur less commonly. Although direct rectal involvement is usually prevented by the fascia of Denonvilliers, prostate cancer can encircle and obstruct the rectum, requiring a colostomy.

Complications

These relate to local growth leading to bladder outflow obstruction producing bilateral (occasionally unilateral) upper urinary tract obstruction, haematuria and distant metastases, e.g. vertebral collapse causing spinal cord compression.

Table 35.1	TNM classification of prostate cancer
Stage	Extent of cancer
T_{is}	Carcinoma-in-situ
T1	Incidental finding of tumour at operation or on biopsy
T2	Intracapsular tumour with deformation of prostatic contour
T3	Extraprostatic extension possibly into the seminal vesicles
T4	Tumour fixed in the pelvis or invading neighbouring structures
N0	No evidence of lymph node involvement
N1–N4	Involvement of one homolateral lymph node to juxtaregional lymph nodes
M0	No evidence of metastases
M1	Distant metastases

Prognostic features

Cancer stage and Gleason score are the most useful indicators of the likely prognosis.

CLINICAL FEATURES

Despite the many men with latent prostate cancer, relatively few have symptoms, especially in the early stages. Approximately one-quarter of patients have symptomatic metastases at presentation and another quarter have asymptomatic metastases. Patients present with either lower urinary tract symptoms or complications of the disease. Symptoms may resemble BPH, which is often present simultaneously but is not related to the pathogenesis of prostate cancer.

Patients usually present with long-standing symptoms of outflow obstruction, and occasionally with haematuria, perineal pain, haematospermia (blood in the semen) and, rarely, renal failure. Acute urinary retention may also occur. In patients with advanced disease, skeletal pain may be a presenting symptom in about 1 in 8, as well as general symptoms of malignancy such as weight loss and fatigue.

With widespread availability of PSA testing, many patients are found with asymptomatic prostate cancer who might never have presented with symptoms. Similarly, prostatic biopsies or operation for outflow obstruction presumed to be due to BPH often yield cases of incidental carcinoma.

Signs

On digital rectal examination, palpable prostate tumours can be discrete hard nodules or may involve the entire prostate as a large, irregular and hard mass. Signs of local spread, distant metastases or cachexia may be present and indicate a poor prognosis.

SCREENING

Recently, screening for prostate cancer has occurred in some centres. Screening can be done by PSA measurement, digital rectal examination and transrectal ultrasonography combined with biopsy. The value of screening remains controversial until there is evidence that the treatment offered (radical prostatectomy/radiotherapy/hormonal manipulation) reduces either mortality or morbidity rates.

SPECIAL TESTS

Prostate specific antigen (PSA)

PSA is a serine protease produced by normal prostatic epithelial cells and in greater quantities by prostatic cancer and BPH. Absolute serum levels discriminate unreliably between BPH and cancer and rise normally with age. A variety of derivatives of PSA (PSA density, age-corrected PSA, PSA rate of rise, etc.) have been developed which are better but still unreliable. The ratio of free PSA to total PSA is a promising new tool. Serum PSA measurement is an easily accessible test which can be used as an aid to diagnosis or follow-up of patients after treatment.

Acid phosphatase

Historically, this was the first serum enzyme to be used in the diagnosis of prostate cancer. It has been superseded by PSA, but remains of value for the monitoring of metastatic disease if required in patients with confirmed carcinoma.

Transrectal ultrasound scan-guided biopsy

Transrectal ultrasonography can demonstrate areas of carcinoma in prostate and so help diagnose palpable prostatic abnormalities. It can guide biopsies of suspected tumours, which otherwise are performed blind and less reliably. Prostatic biopsy can be associated with septicaemia and should be accompanied by broad-spectrum prophylactic antibiotics. Haematuria is a common complication thereafter.

Bone scan

If bony pain is present and metastases are suspected, isotope scans may help to show the presence of secondary deposits. Up to 20% of patients with a negative skeletal survey (complete radiography of the skeleton) may prove positive by this technique.

TREATMENT

Given the vast numbers of patients with asymptomatic carcinoma of the prostate and the uncertain natural history of the disease, treatment has to be tailored according to the patient's life expectancy and general health, as well as to the grade and stage of the tumour.

In those with acute retention or bladder outflow

obstruction, a transurethral resection of the prostate is indicated to relieve the obstruction. This may be all that is necessary in some cases.

Local disease

The treatment of the cancer itself is controversial. In those with incidental carcinoma (T1 N0 M0), i.e. impalpable tumours that occupy a small proportion of the gland, probably no treatment is required; few patients ever develop further problems. If the cancer is more diffuse or multifocal, then more extensive treatment such as external beam radiotherapy may be offered. When the tumour is larger and palpable without extraprostatic extension (T0 N0 M0), radical prostatectomy may also be considered. For the latter, success is only possible if there is no invasion or distant spread, and preliminary lymphadenectomy may be necessary to exclude this. In this operation, the prostate and seminal vesicles are removed, with anastomosis of the urethra to the bladder; it is often followed by incontinence, impotence, and occasionally strictures. Up to 30% of patients may need further modalities of treatment postoperatively.

Following extraprostatic extension, cure is impossible and pelvic irradiation is often given.

Metastatic disease

Androgen deprivation (AD) of the prostate is usually offered when symptomatic metastases are present. It is uncertain whether AD before symptoms may improve the natural history. Ninety per cent of androgens are released by the testes, and 10% by the adrenal cortices. AD is carried out either surgically (orchidectomy) or medically. Luteinising hormone-releasing hormone (LHRH) analogues (e.g. goserelin) reduce LH release from the pituitary and subsequently diminish the release of testosterone from testicular Leydig cells. There may be an initial testosterone flare that may be complicated by a clinical exacerbation (e.g. spinal cord compression), and this can be prevented by an anti-androgen. Adrenal androgens are not affected by LHRH antagonists and can also be blocked by anti-androgens (e.g. flutamide) which interfere with the binding of dihydrotestosterone to its cytoplasmic receptor. The combination of anti-androgens and LHRH analogues is known as total androgen blockade; it may lead to a small survival advantage. Painful bony metastases are treated best by irradiation, but may benefit from hypophysectomy (rarely performed).

Complications

Tumour spreading into the bladder or ureters can obstruct the ureters, which can be relieved by either insertion of double-J stents or nephrostomy. These measures are usually indicated only when awaiting the results of hormonal therapy and not in later stages of the disease. Spinal metastases may collapse and produce acute spinal cord compression, which requires urgent decompression if recovery of neuronal function is to be achieved.

OTHER CAUSES OF VOIDING AND STORAGE SYMPTOMS

URETHRAL STRICTURE

Most strictures follow urethral instrumentation (iatrogenic), urethritis (gonococcal, non-specific urethritis, tuberculous) or perineal trauma. Other causes include inflammation (balanitis xerotica obliterans), neoplasia (squamous carcinoma, transitional cell carcinoma, adenocarcinoma) and congenital stricture.

Clinical features

Patients present at any age and complain predominantly of a weak urinary force, amongst other symptoms of obstruction. There may be a history of an aetiological factor. In men aged 20–40 years, congenital strictures present with UTIs. A life-long reduction in flow rate is usually present and may be overcome partially by detrusor compensation.

Investigations

The peak flow rate is reduced and the duration of flow is prolonged.

Treatment

Optical urethrotomy. The stricture is cut endoscopically with a knife under direct vision. The recurrence rate can be reduced by clean intermittent self-catheterisation with specially lubricated catheters.

Urethral dilatation. Periodic dilatation with metal sounds or plastic bougies under local anaesthetic is now rarely performed in the Western world. It is occasionally suitable for patients unfit for operation, but should be preceded by flexible cystoscopy.

Urethroplasty. Open reconstruction of the urethra may be necessary for recurrent strictures or for dense fibrotic strictures. It is usually performed in specialist units.

Meatotomy/meatoplasty may be necessary for strictures at the external meatus.

BLADDER NECK STENOSIS

Typical symptoms of outflow obstruction that occur after prostatic or bladder neck surgery may be caused by a fibrous stenosis of the bladder neck. Treatment is by incision of the bladder neck with a diathermy knife.

BLADDER NECK DYSSYNERGIA

When the bladder contracts during voiding, the bladder neck normally relaxes, but it fails to do so or actively contracts in this condition. The aetiology is unknown.

Clinical features

Patients present at age 20–50 years with a life-long history of frequency and poor stream. Neurological examination is normal. Urinary tract infections may be present.

Investigations

Videocystourethrography is the investigation of choice.

Treatment

Alpha-adrenergic blockers. These relax the bladder neck smooth muscle (see above).

Bladder neck incision. This is the most effective means of reducing obstruction, but leads to retrograde ejaculation. This problem may make it unacceptable to younger patients.

CHANGES IN THE PATTERN OF DIURNAL ADH SECRETION

Usually, more antidiuretic hormone (ADH) is secreted during the night than during the day, which prevents the bladder from overfilling at night and disturbing sleep. When ADH secretion decreases at night, urine output over 24 hours is more even, so nocturia may occur. This

can be detected by a frequency volume chart. It is common in infancy and bed-wetters and may occur again in the elderly. Treatment is by fluid restriction and/or administration of DDAVP, which is an ADH analogue. Complications of fluid retention and hypertension must be avoided.

LOWER URINARY TRACT SYMPTOMS IN WOMEN

Urethral stenosis

This occurs occasionally because of atrophic urethritis and should be treated by urethral dilatation or Otis urethrotomy and hormone replacement therapy.

Detrusor failure

This leads to chronic retention and follows prolonged bladder overdistension (e.g. prolonged labour >24 hours or postoperatively, when bladder overdistension is not noticed because of wound pain). Clean intermittent self-catheterisation is the treatment of choice every 4–6 hours and often works within 4 days. Drugs to increase bladder contractility occasionally help, but urethral dilatation is rarely effective.

UROTHELIAL TUMOURS

Transitional epithelium extends from the tips of the renal papillae to the navicular fossa in men, and halfway along the urethra in women. Tumours can occur anywhere along the epithelium, either singly or multifocally.

EPIDEMIOLOGY

Peak incidence occurs at age 65 years, and there are 9000 new cases per year in the UK. Transitional cell carcinomas (TCCs) are more common in the developed world, whereas squamous cell carcinomas are more common in the undeveloped world. Aetiological factors include:

- smoking (two- to fourfold risk)
- occupational exposure to aniline and aromatic amines (10% of patients)
- drugs, e.g. phenacetin, cyclophosphamide
- associated diseases, e.g. schistosomiasis
- endogenous carcinogens, e.g. tryptophan metabolites and nitrosamines

- chronic inflammation, e.g. in bladder outflow obstruction + infection, or stones in a diverticulum.

PATHOGENESIS

Premalignant conditions include:

- squamous metaplasia due to exstrophy, chronic bladder inflammation and schistosomiasis
- bladder leukoplakia.

About 90% of tumours are malignant transitional cell carcinomas. Squamous carcinomas occur in 10% due to chronic inflammation or schistosomiasis. Adenocarcinomas usually arise from urachal remnants in the vault of the bladder. Carcinoma-in-situ (CIS) describes malignant change that is confined to the bladder or upper urinary tract mucosa. It is more aggressive and invades early.

Histopathological staging of bladder tumours is vital to the prognosis and treatment, as well as the grade of the tumour (Fig. 35.2, Table 35.2).

CLINICAL FEATURES

Modes of presentation of urothelial tumours are as follows:

- painless haematuria (70–90%)
- malignant cystitis (dysuria, frequency, urgency, perineal pain) with (40%) or without (15%) proven bacterial infection
- incidental finding on cystoscopy (10%).

Less commonly, patients may present with features of bladder outflow obstruction, ureteric obstruction or metastatic disease (anaemia, bone pain, hepatomegaly, pyrexia).

INVESTIGATIONS

Urine. Microscopy indicates the presence of red cells in the urine. Cytology indicates the presence of malignant cells and is usually positive in the presence of CIS. The presence of leucocytes without infection on culture may also indicate a tumour.

Intravenous urography. In the ureter or renal pelvis, tumours appear as filling defects. Distortion or loss of calyces is seen in renal TCC. If the ureters are obstructed by a tumour arising within the bladder, then the tumour has invaded muscle, but a tumour within the ureter may still be superficial at this stage. Antegrade or retrograde ureterography may be necessary.

Table 35.2	Staging of urothelial tumours
Stage	**Extent**
pT_a	Confined to epithelium
pT_1	Invasion of subepithelial connective tissue
pT_2	Invasion of superficial bladder muscle
pT_{3a}	Invasion of deep muscle not beyond bladder wall
pT_{3b}	Invasion beyond bladder wall
pT_{4a}	Invasion of prostate, uterus or vagina
pT_{4b}	Fixation to the pelvis

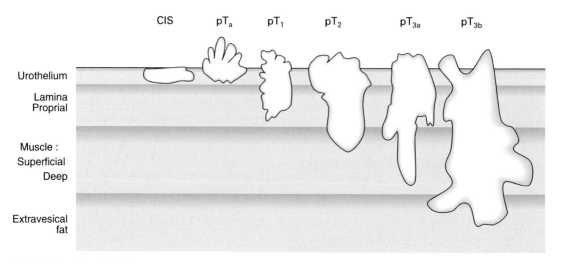

Fig. 35.2 Staging of bladder cancer.

Cystoscopy and examination under anaesthesia.
Inspection of the mucosa and biopsy of abnormalities are
carried out. It is essential to include bladder muscle in the
biopsy for accurate staging. Examination allows the clinical stage of the tumour to be determined.

MANAGEMENT

Bladder cancer is traditionally subdivided into two main
groups: 'superficial' and 'invasive'. The former consists
of the pT_a and the pT_1 category, whilst the latter are any
tumours that invade the detrusor muscle or deeper. pT_1
tumours are invasive in that they penetrate the basement
membrane. It has now been established clearly that the
behaviour of pT_a and pT_1 are quite distinct. Once pT_a
tumours are treated, between 50% and 70% of patients
will develop new tumours, almost invariably at the same
stage, but only 5% will eventually develop a new muscle-invasive tumour. The behaviour of pT_1 tumours is
quite different: once treated, up to 50% (especially if
they are poorly differentiated) will eventually develop
muscle-infiltrating tumours.

In the first instance, these 'superficial' tumours are
usually treated by transurethral resection. Some clinicians advocate the early use of intravesical cytotoxic
agents to reduce the development of new tumours and,
particularly with pT_1 tumours, immunotherapy with
intravesical BCG has been recommended and may
reduce the risk of subsequent muscle-invasive disease.
Some urologists think that the G_3pT_1 tumour may require
radical therapy including cystectomy. Muscle-infiltrating
tumours can be treated by either radiotherapy or systemic
chemotherapy, with salvage cystectomy or primary cystectomy. There is usually little point in offering cystectomy to patients with extravesical disease as these are
incurable, but rarely there is a role for palliative cystectomy.

The 5-year survival results of radiotherapy and cystectomy are broadly similar but, as with all these interventions, those advocating a particular therapy more
strongly are usually the proponents of that particular procedure. Accurate and careful staging before definitive
treatment is therefore of paramount importance. Five-
year survival following radical biopsies for invasive
bladder cancer is in the region of 40–50%.

RENAL ADENOCARCINOMA

This accounts for about 2% of all tumours and mainly
affects men aged between 65 and 75 years. Tumours may
occur bilaterally in about 3% of patients. The only
known risk factor is cigarette smoking, but an association
exists also with von Hippel–Lindau disease.

PATHOLOGY

There is solid tumour within the kidney, often with satellite nodules next to the primary tumour. Spread may
occur:

- to the perirenal fat and adjacent organs
- through the renal vein and inferior vena cava to produce
  metastases in the lung, liver, brain and bones
- via the lymphatics to the para-aortic nodes.

CLINICAL FEATURES

The classic triad of haematuria, flank pain and a palpable abdominal mass occurs in 10–15% of patients.
Patients may have metastases on presentation and may
complain of bone pain, dyspnoea and cough. In a variable number paraneoplastic syndromes may be present,
e.g. blood test abnormalities, weight loss and fatigue,
and pyrexia.

INVESTIGATIONS

Urine. Haematuria and occasionally pyuria are seen.

Blood tests. These may reveal anaemia, raised ESR,
abnormal liver function tests, hypercalcaemia and polycythaemia.

IVU. A space-occupying lesion distorting renal outline
or calyceal pattern may be seen.

Ultrasound scan. This will show a solid lesion with
possible involvement of the renal vein and inferior vena
cava.

CT scan confirms IVU and ultrasound diagnosis of
space-occupying lesion. It also helps pre-operative staging by providing information on local spread (through
renal capsule), regional node enlargement, tumour in the
renal vein or IVC. A CT scan of the chest detects metastases in the mediastinum and lung fields.

MRI. This will give similar information to a CT scan.

Angiography may help in uncertain cases. Embolisation may be performed simultaneously, although this is controversial.

Chest radiography. Lung metastases may be found.

MANAGEMENT

In the absence of metastases, a radical nephrectomy is performed. The kidney is removed together with the upper ureter, adrenal gland and surrounding perinephric fat within Gerota's fascia, plus any enlarged para-aortic lymph nodes or thrombus extending into the renal vein or IVC. In patients with a solitary kidney, a partial nephrectomy should be performed, if possible; otherwise renal replacement therapy will be required. When a single metastasis is present, occasionally nephrectomy combined with removal of the metastasis is performed (e.g. lobectomy with lung metastasis). There have been reports of metastases regressing following removal of the primary tumour, but this is very rare.

Palliative radiotherapy or radiological embolisation may be effective for patients with intractable symptoms such as bleeding or pain associated with the primary tumour. Symptoms from distant metastases may resolve with palliative local radiotherapy. There is some success with progestogens and biological response modifiers (BCG, interferon), but these still need to be evaluated in randomised controlled clinical trials.

PROGNOSIS

Prognosis in individual patients depends on the grade and stage of the tumour. For tumours confined to the kidney, the 5-year survival is 70–80% and overall survival is 30–50%. Occult metastases can become apparent at any stage following removal (but recurrence is not influenced by involvement of the IVC, provided that the tumour is removed without dissemination of emboli.)

NEPHROBLASTOMA (WILMS' TUMOUR)

This type of tumour is responsible for 10% of all childhood tumours, with a peak incidence at 2–4 years. Tumours are bilateral in 5% of children at the time of presentation. There is an association (15%) with congenital disorders, hemiatrophy of the body and aniridia.

PATHOLOGY

The tumour is soft and pale on cross section and often large enough to distort the rest of the kidney. There is commonly a mixture of both epithelial and mesenchymal elements with connective tissue components. The tumour may invade locally and form distant deposits within the lung, liver, bone or brain.

CLINICAL FEATURES

Patients present with vague pain in the loin or abdomen, and occasionally haematuria and non-specific complaints (anorexia, weight loss, anaemia and pyrexia). On examination, approximately 90% of patients have a palpable smooth abdominal or flank mass, and about 50% may be hypertensive. A proportion of patients present with bilateral tumours. There may be symptoms from metastases, which are present in 20% of patients, and a history of a congenital abnormality.

The differential diagnosis includes benign causes of kidney enlargement, mesoblastic nephroma or sarcoma, and retroperitoneal tumours such as neuroblastoma or lymphoma.

INVESTIGATIONS

Urine. Microscopic or macroscopic haematuria will be present. A 24 hour urine collection to determine catecholamine production will enable one to distinguish Wilms' tumour from neuroblastoma.

IVU. This will show distortion of the calyceal pattern by the tumour.

Ultrasound scan of the kidney distinguishes solid from cystic lesions and liver scan identifies metastases.

CT of abdomen and pelvis. This will enable pre-operative staging of the tumour.

Chest radiograph. This will detect any metastases.

Needle biopsy is used for diagnosis before chemotherapy.

TREATMENT

At laparotomy, a nephrectomy is performed for a solitary

tumour. If bilateral tumours are found, a nephrectomy is performed on the larger kidney and a partial nephrectomy on the other, if possible.

Chemotherapy is indicated in the presence of metastases or as adjuvant therapy. Overall response rates are greater than 75% in producing prolonged survival.

PROGNOSIS

Most patients with early disease can be cured by operation, and patients with advanced disease respond well to chemotherapy, giving overall 5-year survival rates of greater than 75%. A worse prognosis is associated with anaplastic, rhabdoid and clear-cell sarcoma pathological subtypes.

STONES

Calculi in the upper tracts are common in the USA and Europe and affect higher socioeconomic groups, but they are comparatively rare in Africa (unlike vesical calculi). The age distribution is bimodal. One peak occurs in the third decade and predominantly affects men, while the second peak occurs in the sixth decade and predominantly affects women.

PATHOGENESIS

The geographic distribution of the disease suggests that a diet low in dietary fibre may be important. Stones form when solutes in the urine become supersaturated and natural inhibitors of crystallisation (citrates) are deficient. The most common stones contain calcium (70%).

Risk factors include:

- metabolic, e.g. idiopathic hypercalciuria, hyperoxaluria, hyperuricosuria, cystinuria
- hormonal imbalances, e.g. hyperparathyroidism
- anatomical abnormalities leading to chronic infection or urinary stasis
- urinary infection with urease producing bacteria, e.g. *Proteus, Pseudomonas*
- idiopathic
- chemotherapy
- dehydration.

CLINICOPATHOLOGICAL SYNDROMES

Clinical features are related to the position and composition of the stone and the associated complications (Fig. 35.3).

Stones in the kidney that cause obstruction lead to continuous colicky loin pain, otherwise they may be picked up on an incidental radiograph or in the investigation of haematuria. When in the ureter, loin pain radiating to the groin or inguinal region may be felt; in men, pain radiates to the testicles or the tip of the penis. The loin may be tender on examination. Stones at the ureterovesical junction may create symptoms of bladder instability. Usually there is accompanying pyuria and macroscopic haematuria. Pyrexia and rigors occur with infection.

On examination, the patient appears extremely restless, sweaty, in pain and may be hypotensive.

Careful distinction from a leaking abdominal aortic aneurysm is necessary, as well as from diverticulitis, appendicitis and pyelonephritis.

MANAGEMENT

Acute phase

Urine. Haematuria, white cells and crystals of uric acid, calcium oxalate or cystine may be seen. A pH <5.5 suggests uric acid stones and a pH >8 suggests an infectious stone. Culture may reveal infection. Infection in the

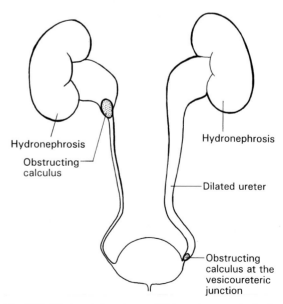

Fig. 35.3 Obstructed ureter and kidney from a calculus in the upper ureter and at the vesicoureteric junction.

presence of complete obstruction may lead to a negative MSU.

Full blood count, urea and electrolytes should be assessed.

Plain abdominal radiograph. Over 90% of stones are radio-opaque, with calcium-containing stones having the density of contrast and cystine stones of ground glass.

IVU. Early films show a dense nephrogram and often a delayed pyelogram. The ureter is dilated and visible in a continuous line to the level of obstruction. Occasionally, there is dilatation below the stone in partial obstruction.

Initial treatment is expectant. Adequate pain relief is essential with either opiates or non-steroidal anti-inflammatory drugs (ketorolac, diclofenac). Previously, a high fluid intake was encouraged and given intravenously if necessary, but this is probably ineffective and may damage the kidney.

Post-acute phase

Further investigations after repeated episodes include:

- 24 hour urine collections for calcium and phosphate assay
- stone analysis.

In the case of the latter, stones are collected by sieving the urine. This is useful to identify unsuspected constituents such as urate, xanthine and cystine.

Further treatment depends on the composition and position of the stone. Ninety per cent of stones in the distal ureter that are <4 mm in diameter will pass spontaneously, as well as 50% of those that are 4–6 mm and only 20% of stones >6 mm. Stones in the proximal ureter are less likely to pass.

Absolute indications for intervention are:

- infection
- obstruction in a solitary kidney
- impaction
- colic unresponsive to medication.

Extracorporeal shock-wave lithotripsy (ESWL) successfully shatters 90% of renal stones. Stones in the lower and midureter respond less well than those higher

up and may need to be pushed back into the upper ureter ('push bang'). Alternatively, *ureteroscopic removal* is possible, but stones larger than 6 mm need to be fragmented before extraction.

Ureterolithotomy is used rarely and usually only when ESWL or ureteroscopic techniques fail. Infectious stones in the kidney ('staghorn calculi') eventually lead to loss of kidney function and must be removed.

PREVENTION

This depends on the type of stone.

Calcium oxalate stones

The patient should have a high fluid and dietary fibre intake and should avoid oxalate-containing foods (tea, nuts). Hypercalciuria is treated by diuretics that decrease urinary calcium excretion (hydrochlorothiazide). Hypocitraturia responds to citrate supplements.

Uric acid stones

High fluid intake and low purine diet (red meat, peanuts, chicken) are indicated. Bed rest should be avoided and urine should be alkalised to between pH 6.5 to 7.0 using sodium bicarbonate or potassium citrate. Uric acid secretion should be reduced with allopurinol.

Cystine stones

In this case, high fluid intake, urine alkalinisation, cystine solubilisation by penicillamine and D-alpha-mercaptopropionylglycine are indicated.

Infectious stones

The nidus for infection or the anatomical abnormality must be removed and the urinary tract infection treated. This can be achieved by a combination of ESWL and percutaneous lithotripsy.

INFECTION

Infection arises in the kidney either by the retrograde ascent of bacteria from the bladder or by haematogenous spread. The lower 5 cm of urethra is colonised with bacteria in men and women, but UTIs are more common in women because this is the total length of the urethra. Colonisation of the perineum with gut bacteria is common. The commonest organisms are *Escherichia coli* and *Enterobacteriaceae* sp.

ACUTE RENAL INFECTIONS

These are infections of the renal parenchyma or cortical system.

Pathogenesis

Predisposing factors include ureteric stasis (obstruction, pregnancy, megaureter), vesicoureteric reflux and immunosuppression (diabetes mellitus). A renal carbuncle may occur by haematogenous spread from an infected skin lesion (staphylococcal) and results in an abscess of the renal cortex alone. Infection within the kidney that continues unchecked produces a pyonephrosis and eventually complete destruction of the kidney.

Clinical presentation

Typically, patients complain of loin pain, rigors and fevers, as well as nausea and vomiting. On examination, there is tenderness in the loin, intermittent fever and tachycardia. A mass may be palpable if the infective process has led to abscess formation. Depending on the severity of infection, there may be paralytic ileus and septicaemia. Distinction must be made from renal colic, cholecystitis, pancreatitis, appendicitis and diverticulitis.

Investigations

There are pus cells in the urine and occasionally organisms, especially if acute pyelonephritis is a result of ascending infection. Urine cultures are usually positive, and microscopic or macroscopic haematuria may be present. A neutrophilia and raised creatinine secondary to dehydration are commonly found. Urine and blood cultures are essential to guide further management.

A KUB (kidneys, ureter, bladder) radiograph may show a stone causing obstruction. There may be a delayed and weak nephrogram on IVU as well as evidence of a space-occupying lesion from a renal carbuncle. If the IVU shows obstruction, urgent decompression is indicated.

Treatment

Antibiotics (third generation cephalosporins, fluoroquinolones) given intravenously and then orally for up to 8 weeks are essential. These are changed according to the bacterial sensitivities. Rehydration and treatment of septicaemic shock may be necessary. A renal carbuncle or pyonephrosis must be drained under either ultrasound or CT guidance, but formal surgical drainage with antibiotic cover may be needed for these and perinephric abscesses. If infection is present with upper tract obstruction, insertion of a nephrostomy under ultrasound control is mandatory. Following resolution of the acute episode, the cause of the infection must be established and any anatomical abnormalities corrected.

CHRONIC PYELONEPHRITIS

This describes an entity comprising renal scarring in the presence of intermittent urinary tract infection. The danger is the possible complication of end-stage renal failure. Chronic pyelonephritis follows repeated episodes of acute pyelonephritis with continuous bacteriuria or in childhood secondary to vesicoureteric reflux.

Patients present with either recurrent UTI of bacteriuria on routine testing or in the investigation of renal failure. The diagnosis is confirmed by infection in the urine plus an IVU that shows cortical scarring over a deformed calyx.

Treatment is based on eradicating infection and preventing further renal damage. Long-term low-dose antibiotics may be required in some patients with repeated infections. Depending on the degree of damage to the kidney, nephrectomy or partial nephrectomy may be also required with long-term follow-up by renal physicians.

TUBERCULOSIS

This has become less common in the UK but remains important to diagnose, so as to avoid long-term sequelae. The organism reaches the urinary tract through the blood from a primary focus, often within the lung, and sometimes many years later. Infection may settle in any part of the genitourinary tract. Patients may be asymptomatic or complain of frequency, dysuria, and symptoms from complications of disease (e.g. loin pain from hydronephrosis, hypertension, renal failure).

There may be a sterile pyuria or calcification of the

urinary tract seen on radiography. Three early-morning urine specimens are cultured in Lowenstein–Jensen medium for 6 weeks to make the diagnosis, or occasionally acid-fast bacilli are seen on an immediate Ziehl–Neelsen stain. Cystoscopy may show superficial granulations, inflammation or gaping ureteric orifices due to fibrosis around the orifices and the bladder wall.

Chemotherapy (pyrazinamide, rifampicin, isoniazid) to eradicate infection is the mainstay, while monitoring the ureters to check for fibrosis that might be complicated by a stricture. Steroids can reduce fibrosis, but reconstructive surgery may be necessary.

LOWER URINARY TRACT INFECTIONS

'Cystitis' means inflammation of the bladder, of which bacterial infection is only one cause among many, e.g. allergy (rubber, alloys), *Candida*, trauma ('honeymoon cystitis'). Unconfirmed UTIs should not be treated.

Acute bacterial lower urinary tract infection

This affects up to 50% of women at least once in their lifetime. Men may develop problems because of an abnormality of the urinary tract. Clinical features are frequency, urgency, dysuria and occasionally haematuria. There may be some tenderness in the suprapubic region, but usually there is little to find unless there are systemic complications. Proteinuria and haematuria may be found on urinalysis. Microscopy must show >10 white cells/high power field with $>10^5$ organisms/ml grown on an MSU. Patients are started on an antibiotic (e.g. trimethoprim), which may be changed when bacteriological sensitivities are known. A high fluid intake and urine alkalinisation with potassium citrate or sodium bicarbonate may hasten recovery.

Further investigations should be performed in men with one proven UTI and in women with two proven UTIs, to search for an aetiological factor. Investigations include cystoscopy, KUB radiograph and ultrasound scan. Asymptomatic bacteriuria may be present in 2% of schoolgirls and should be tested.

Chronic and recurrent bacterial lower urinary tract infection

Recurrent infection may lead to a chronically inflamed bladder with cystic changes and the development of squamous metaplasia, with a very low risk of malignant change. Investigations are limited unless there are signs of upper tract involvement. Treatment includes long-term low-dose antibiotics (e.g. trimethoprim 100 mg b.d.) which is carried on for 6–12 months, and in some cases cystoscopy to exclude an abnormality.

Interstitial cystitis

This condition is poorly understood and probably has a multifactorial aetiology including autoimmune factors. Clinical features comprise frequency, nocturia, dysuria, suprapubic pain and tenderness. Patients have a small capacity bladder with mucosal erythema that bleeds on emptying. Treatment includes steroids, dimethyl sulphoxide and hydrostatic bladder distension; the results are unreliable.

Prostatitis

Symptoms are consistent with inflammation or infection of the prostate, including:

- pain in the perineum, sacrum, suprapubic area or the groin
- increased micturition frequency, terminal dysuria
- occasionally haematospermia and pain on ejaculation.

The prostate may be tender, swollen and oedematous. Depending on the extent of the disease, an abscess or epididymitis may be present. Signs of an acute systemic disturbance are manifest in *acute bacterial prostatitis*.

Diagnosis is established by culture of expressed prostatic secretions (EPS) obtained after prostatic massage which confirms bacterial prostatitis (*Escherichia coli*, *Enterobacter*, *Proteus*, *Klebsiella*, *Pseudomonas* spp.). The initial part of an MSU taken after EPS shows a higher cell and bacterial count than before massage. In *nonbacterial prostatitis*, EPS culture is negative but there are pus cells in the urine. In *prostadynia*, both EPS and urine culture are negative.

Further investigations are necessary to exclude anatomical abnormalities, outflow obstruction and urethral stricture. The partner may need to be tested for *Chlamydia* and bacterial infections of the vagina and cervix in cases of recurrent prostatitis.

Treatment with antibiotics (ciprofloxacin, tetracycline, trimethoprim) for 6–12 weeks is necessary because of the generally poor penetration of the prostate. Abscesses need to be drained surgically, usually by TURP. Nonbacterial prostatitis and prostadynia may respond to antibiotics also because of unsuspected *Chlamydia* infection. These drugs are combined with anti-inflammatory agents and occasionally alpha-adrenergic blockers. Recently, transurethral microwave thermotherapy has been found to be of benefit.

PENIS

BALANITIS

This is inflammation of the foreskin, which may also extend to the glans penis. The mainstay of treatment is scrupulous hygiene, but antibiotics may help to resolve the problem. If persistent, circumcision should be considered.

PHIMOSIS

This is a persistently tight foreskin that cannot be retracted behind the glans. The natural history of the foreskin is to begin to separate at the age of 3 years and to be completely retractile by 6 years. The foreskin may expand on micturition before this, but does not usually lead to retention. Therefore, circumcision is not indicated, even if it is requested, unless the tight foreskin causes bladder outflow obstruction, infections or other local problems.

Adults may a develop a phimosis because of balanitis xerotica obliterans. The foreskin becomes thickened and pale, and these changes may extend to the glans penis with constriction of the urethral meatus. Circumcision is indicated for this condition and meatotomy for meatal stenosis.

PARAPHIMOSIS

A retracted foreskin that cannot be returned to its natural position over the glans is a paraphimosis. This usually follows urethral catheterisation after the foreskin is pulled back, but it may also occur after erection. The glans becomes progressively congested the longer it is constricted by the tight foreskin. Manual reduction can be attempted, but it is usually too painful. After a regional block, the glans is compressed to reduce the swelling and the tight ring of foreskin drawn over the glans. The foreskin is extended to its full length and observed to make sure it does not retract again. Circumcision or dorsal slit is indicated after the acute episode has settled to avoid recurrence.

CANCER OF THE PENIS

The incidence of this cancer is 1 per 100 000 of the male population. It is rare among men who are circumcised at infancy. Predisposing factors include chronic irritation by retained smegma and concomitant infection that accompanies poor hygiene with an intact foreskin. The human papilloma virus and infection by genital herpes have also been associated with a higher incidence of carcinoma.

Premalignant lesions

The most common are leukoplakia, erythroplasia of Queyrat and Buschke–Loewenstein tumour. Approximately 30–40% of patients with squamous cell carcinoma of the penis have a history of premalignant lesions.

Clinical features

Penile cancer presents as a persistent sore or ulcer of the glans, a painless sore or a warty growth of the glans which the foreskin may conceal. A concealed tumour may progress so that it is first noticed when it is painful or because of a bloody or offensive discharge. The tumour spreads to the inguinal lymphatics, and inguinal lymphadenopathy is found in 50% of all patients at presentation. Enlarged nodes are due either to secondary deposits or to the spread of infection, in which cases they reduce in size on antibiotic treatment.

Histologically, this is a squamous cell carcinoma.

Staging

Diagnosis is made by biopsy of the lesion, careful examination of the inguinal nodes and, if necessary, CT scan of the pelvic and abdominal lymph nodes. The tumour can be staged by the TNM system.

Treatment

This is by either radiotherapy at an early stage or penectomy at an advanced stage. More advanced tumours may require radical amputation or palliative radiotherapy. Early stage lesions of the glans or foreskin have almost a 100% survival rate at 5 years or more. In North America, operation usually includes a superficial lymph node dissection and is followed by chemotherapy.

PEYRONIE'S DISEASE

A palpable plaque or scar is present, usually on the dorsum of the penile shaft, although it can occur anywhere or multifocally. Sometimes, there is an association with Dupuytren's contracture of the hand or a history of trauma. Peyronie's disease gives rise to a curvature on erection, which can be painful. It may progress to erectile failure because of associated venocclusive dysfunction. The process takes place over 6–18 months and sometimes regresses spontaneously. Treatment is indicated for painful erections, in which case Nesbitt's procedure is performed – shortening of the tunica albuginea diametrically opposite the plaque. In the presence of erectile dysfunction, insertion of a prosthesis may help.

PRIAPISM

This is an erection lasting longer than 4 hours. It represents a urological emergency. It is characterised by erection of the corpora cavernosa, but not of the corpus spongiosum. The danger lies in the progressive hypoxia, hypercapnia and sludging of the blood within the corpora progressing to cavernosal fibrosis and irreversible erectile failure.

Aetiology

The commonest cause is now iatrogenic and usually follows administration of intracavernosal agents such as papaverine or alprostadil.

Changes in blood viscosity may also be responsible, e.g. in leukaemia, myeloma and sickle cell anaemia.

Treatment

Simple measures such as cold showers and climbing stairs are rarely effective. First-line treatment is aspiration of blood from one of the corpora with a 19–21 gauge butterfly needle (20–50 ml) until the penis detumesces. If this fails, a 200 mcg/ml solution of phenylephrine should be made, and 0.5–1 ml injected every 10 minutes to a maximum dose of 1 mg until the erection subsides. The final procedure is to create a shunt between the erect corpora cavernosa and the glans penis or corpus spongiosum.

MALE ERECTILE DYSFUNCTION

This is defined as the inability to initiate or maintain an erection sufficient for penetration until ejaculation. Impotence is extremely common, affecting at least 10% of men and causing them great distress. The precise mechanism giving rise to an erection is poorly understood. The autonomic nervous system controlled by the brain initiates vasodilatation of the arteries to the corpora, cavernous smooth muscle relaxation and venous occlusion.

Aetiology

The causes of male erectile dysfunction include:

- diabetes mellitus
- arterial disease, e.g. Leriche syndrome
- psychogenic factors
- local penile problems, e.g. venous leaks, failure of cavernous smooth muscle relaxation, Peyronie's disease and cavernosal fibrosis post-priapism
- drugs, e.g. antihypertensives
- surgery, e.g. rectal excision, abdominal aortic aneurysm repair and radical prostatectomy
- endocrine causes, e.g. hypogonadism.

The distinction between psychogenic and non-psychogenic impotence is usually suggested by the sudden loss of erection prior to or at the onset of penetration with normal erections in the morning or on masturbation. Venous leaks are indicated by erections that are sufficient for initial penetration that fade during intercourse.

Investigations

These include:

- free androgen levels, especially if features are hypogonadal
- prolactin levels, especially if libido is low
- LH/FSH levels – raised in primary testicular failure
- Doppler ultrasound, to show the state of penile arterial circulation
- cavernosometry.

More tests than these are used, but they vary from centre to centre.

Treatment

A period of psychotherapy is appropriate for patients with psychological problems, and androgen supplements may be given providing androgen deficiency is proven.

Medical treatments are divided between the use of vacuum devices and intracavernosal injections of either alprostadil or papaverine (beware priapism, see above). If these fail, penile prostheses can be inserted.

EJACULATORY DYSFUNCTION

This commonly occurs in patients following bladder neck surgery, para-aortic dissection (e.g. for testis cancer), abdominoperineal excision of the rectum and prostatectomy. Patients have an orgasm, but semen passes into the bladder instead of through the penis. Fertility is affected in younger men, but sperm can be recovered from urine, washed and used to inseminate the partner successfully.

Other forms of ejaculatory dysfunction are primarily psychogenic, e.g. premature or retarded ejaculation, and respond to psychological intervention.

MICTURITION AND CONTINENCE

Micturition and continence depend on a complex interaction between the muscles and sphincters of the bladder and urethra coordinated by the neurological system. *Continence* depends mainly on the distal intrinsic sphincter mechanism which lies within the membranous part of the intraprostatic urethra in men, and between the bladder neck and the external meatus in women. The sphincter comprises a circular layer of striated muscle (the rhabdosphincter) designed for tonic contraction (slow-twitch) and innervated via somatic nerves from S_{2-4}. In men, a circular layer of smooth muscle at the bladder neck (proximal intrinsic sphincter) innervated by the sympathetic nervous system ($T_{10}-L_2$) contracts during ejaculation and prevents retrograde ejaculation. This contributes to continence in males but is poorly developed in females, in whom it is unimportant. Incontinence occurs when urethral resistance is exceeded by bladder pressure, which is constituted by intra-abdominal pressure and detrusor activity.

To enable *micturition*, sensory fibres from the bladder and urethra pass in the pelvic parasympathetic nerves through S_{2-4} to the spinal cord and up the spinothalamic tracts to the pons and cerebral cortex. Some fibres also pass through the sympathetic nerves to the hypogastric plexus. The detrusor contracts in response to parasympathetic (S_{2-4}) (cholinergic) stimulation through the pelvic nerves to the pelvic ganglia, which distribute nerve endings to the detrusor muscle. Sympathetic nerves from $T_{10}-L_2$ pass through the hypogastric nerves and the pelvic plexus and stimulate the proximal intrinsic sphincter. The sympathetic nervous system also synapses with the parasympathetic nerves in the pelvic ganglia, which can inhibit detrusor contractions. The rhabdosphincter is supplied by somatic fibres from S_{2-4} which travel with autonomic fibres in the nervi erigentes.

Many treatments are based on the pharmacology of continence and micturition system (Table 35.3).

INCONTINENCE

This is the involuntary loss of urine and affects about 5% of the female population. True incontinence represents continuous urine loss from an abnormal extra-urethral site, e.g. an ectopic ureter opening into the vagina.

PATHOPHYSIOLOGY

Urge incontinence

This is incontinence associated with a strong desire to void. It may be due to motor dysfunction because of bladder disease or uninhibited detrusor contractions, which are either neuropathic (detrusor hyperreflexia) or not (idiopathic detrusor instability).

Stress incontinence

This is incontinence with no concomitant rise in detrusor

Table 35.3	Pharmacological basis of incontinence and bladder dysfunction treatment				
Site	Nerve supply	Synapse	Stimulants	Relaxants
Detrusor	Parasympathetic S_{2-4}	Cholinergic	Bethanechol	Oxybutinin
Bladder neck	Sympathetic $T_{10}-L_2$	Noradrenergic	Ephedrine	α-blockers

pressure. True stress incontinence occurs when vesical pressure exceeds urethral resistance. Coughing, Valsalva manoeuvres and sneezing raise intra-abdominal pressure and intravesical pressure. Reductions in urethral resistance occur because of obesity, multiparity or childbirth in women and prostatectomy or pelvic fracture in men. Detrusor contractions can also be stimulated by raised intra-abdominal pressure (e.g. coughing) and so can mimic true stress incontinence ('stress-induced detrusor instability').

Overflow incontinence

Overflow incontinence arises because the bladder overdistends and the intravesical pressure exceeds urethral sphincter resistance. This occurs because of either bladder outflow obstruction or detrusor failure.

CLINICAL ASSESSMENT

It is important to check for a history of voiding symptoms in addition to filling symptoms and to be aware of chronic retention with overflow. Women may be aware that leakage is not from the urethra but is arising from a fistula in the vagina. Neurological features may also affect bowel function or sexual function in men. Constipation and faecal impaction may precipitate incontinence in the elderly. Past medical history (multiple sclerosis, diabetes mellitus, urethral surgery) and medication must be considered.

INVESTIGATIONS

An objective assessment of symptoms is made using a frequency/volume chart.

MANAGEMENT

Urge incontinence

This condition may resolve after treatment of local intravesical pathology or by drug therapy, such as anticholinergic or smooth muscle relaxant. Drugs are effective, although side-effects can be limiting (dry mouth, constipation, blurred vision), and should be accompanied by bladder training (i.e. graduated increase in time between voids).

Otherwise, treatment is by:

- hydrostatic bladder distension under general or epidural anaesthesia

- partial denervation of the bladder or cystoplasty; clean intermittent self-catheterisation is often necessary to completely empty the bladder after cystoplasty, which may be complicated by excessive mucus production leading to obstruction
- indwelling catheter or penile sheath
- urinary diversion (e.g. ileal conduit, Kock pouch).

Stress incontinence

Treatment of this condition is by:

- pelvic floor exercises in women and weight reduction if overweight
- oestrogens (local/systemic) in women with atrophic urethritis
- alpha-adrenergic agonists to increase urethral tone
- surgery – surgical elevation and support of the bladder neck above the pelvic floor
- endoscopic injection of Teflon around the bladder neck or para-urethral injection of collagen
- inflatable artificial urinary sphincter.

NEUROPATHIC BLADDER DYSFUNCTION

Urodynamic studies are usually necessary for accurate classification and as a guide to treatment. The common scenarios, as related directly to the urinary system, are as follows:

- Upper motor neurone lesions
  - *detrusor hyperreflexia*: an overactive detrusor gives symptoms of bladder irritability, which may result in urge incontinence (e.g. post-CVA) from uninhibited contractions
  - *detrusor–sphincter dyssynergia*: the detrusor contracts onto a closed sphincter, which may lead to upper tract dilatation (e.g. multiple screrosis, spinal cord injury, spina bifida).
- Lower motor neurone lesions
  - *detrusor hypoactivity*: an underactive or atonic detrusor produces voiding symptoms and may lead to chronic retention with its associated complications
  - *urethral sphincter incompetence*: underactive urethral closure can lead to stress incontinence.

The clinical picture may be mixed, and there may be features of both LMN and UMN lesions.

SPECIAL INVESTIGATIONS

Micturating cystogram. The bladder is filled with contrast for X-ray imaging during micturition to evaluate the bladder neck and urethra and to detect vesicoureteric reflux.

Urodynamic investigations. Cystometry allows assessment of residual urine, bladder sensation and bladder capacity and shows normal or uninhibited detrusor contraction. A high detrusor pressure indicates obstruction, and the site of obstruction (bladder neck or distal sphincter) can be found on radiological imaging (video-urodynamics). Urethral sphincter activity can be assessed by urethral pressure profilometry and pelvic electromyography.

KUB radiography and ultrasound may help to detect chronic complications, e.g. calculi and upper tract dilatation.

TREATMENT

Neuropathic incontinence

Treatment depends on the cause of the incontinence.

Detrusor hyper-reflexia. Anticholinergic agents (e.g. oxybutinin) or smooth muscle relaxants should be administered, but the side-effects are limiting. Surgical treatments are based on partial denervation of the bladder, bladder transection or increasing the functional capacity of the bladder (clam cystoplasty).

Incompetent sphincter. Drugs to increase outflow resistance (e.g. ephedrine) are occasionally effective. Implantation of an artificial urinary sphincter is possible in some patients. Women may benefit from a colposuspension, but retention can result requiring self-catheterisation.

If these treatments fail, consideration should be given in men to a penile sheath or an indwelling urethral catheter. Catheters may be complicated by a urethral or vaginal fistula in women and, if an indwelling catheter fails, urethral closure and a suprapubic catheter may be necessary. Urinary diversion may be possible in either sex providing the patient has sufficient dexterity to manage the stoma.

Neuropathic retention of urine

Usually this occurs because of detrusor failure (atonic detrusor), but occasionally it occurs because of detrusor–sphincter dyssynergia.

Detrusor failure. Voiding can be precipitated by abdominal straining and suprapubic pressure (Crede manoeuvre). Smooth muscle stimulants (e.g. bethanechol) or cholinesterase inhibitors (e.g. distigmine) are also helpful. Clean intermittent self-catheterisation can be used providing incontinence does not occur because the bladder capacity is too small.

Urethral overactivity. Urethral resistance can be lowered by alpha-adrenergic antagonists (e.g. indoramin). Self-catheterisation is used in women and sphincterotomy in men with the application of a condom device.

If these fail, urinary diversion can be considered to prevent complications.

COMPLICATIONS

Upper tract dilatation with renal failure may occur because of elevated detrusor pressure and chronic retention because of functional outflow obstruction. Outflow resistance can be lowered as above, and bladder emptying achieved by self-catheterisation. Other complications include infection and calculus formation.

FURTHER READING

Blandy J 1989 Lecture notes on urology, 4th edn. Blackwell Science, Oxford

Blandy J, Fowler C 1996 Urology, 2nd edn. Blackwell Science, Oxford

Bradshaw C et al 1997 Guidelines and management of men with lower urinary tract symptoms suggesting bladder outlet obstruction. Royal College of Surgeons, London

Chamberlain J et al 1997 Report prepared for the health technology assessment panel of the NHS Executive on the diagnosis, management, treatment and costs of prostate cancer in England and Wales. British Journal of Urology 79 (suppl 3): 1–32

Chisolm G, Fair W (eds) 1989 Scientific foundations of urology, 3rd edn. Heinemann, London

George S J R, Sambrook P 1990 Diagnostic picture tests in urology. Wolfe Publishing Ltd, Aylesbury

Gillenwater J Y et al (eds) 1995 Adult and paediatric urology, vols I and II, 3rd edn. Mosby-Yearbook, St Louis

Pagano F, Fair W R (eds) 1996 Superficial bladder cancer. ISIS Medical Media, Oxford

Vascular surgery

36

Arterial disease and amputations

John Wolfe   Gerard Stansby

OVERVIEW

Atherosclerosis is ubiquitous in Western populations. It can affect every artery in the body and can lead to either occlusion or dilatation of the vessel. Acute arterial occlusion can also be caused by embolism from a proximal site, especially in atrial fibrillation. This chapter considers the pathogenesis of atheroma and related conditions such as diabetes, together with its effects on the arterial circulation, whether occlusive or aneurysmal. It ends by discussing the indications for amputation and the types of operation available for patients with unreconstructable disease.

Successful arterial surgery became possible with the development of techniques for suturing vessels together and graft materials that could be used to bypass occlusive disease or replace aneurysmal arteries. Surgeons have always been concerned with the management of severe limb ischaemia. Now their role has extended to encompass the management of less severe ischaemic conditions such as intermittent claudication and aneurysms, for example those of the aorta and popliteal arteries, as well as operations on the carotid and other arteries.

SURGICAL PATHOLOGY OF ARTERIAL DISEASE

The causes of arterial disorders are:

- atheroma with or without diabetes
- embolism
- aneurysms

- systemic causes of small vessel disease – polyarteritis nodosa, systemic lupus erythematosus
- major vessel arteritis – seen most commonly in the tropics, and the Middle and Far East
- vasospastic conditions, e.g. Raynaud's syndrome
- Buerger's disease
- vascular trauma (see Ch. 16).

Atheroma

This is the major cause of arterial vascular disease in Western countries. Whilst the patient may present with arterial disease relating to the limbs, the process is usually part of a more general disorder involving cardiac, cerebral and carotid arteries amongst others. The lesions can take the form of: atheromatous plaque with secondary thrombotic occlusions, weakening of the wall leading to aneurysm, or ulceration with thrombosis and/or distal embolisation. Risk factors include:

- positive family history
- heavy cigarette smoking
- hyperlipidaemia or hypercholesterolaemia
- diabetes mellitus
- obesity
- hypertension.

Atherosclerosis usually affects major vessels. However, in some patients, particularly diabetics, small vessels at digital level may be affected alone or in combination with larger vessel disease. The distinction may influence the therapeutic options.

The classical sites for major arterial occlusion are:

- The aorto-iliac region where there is most often diffuse involvement of the terminal aorta and common iliac arteries, often with calcification. Much less frequently the disease is localised at the aorta or common iliacs with relatively normal vessels above and below.

- The superficial femoral artery in the thigh, particularly near the adductor hiatus.
- The popliteal artery.
- The bifurcation of the common carotid artery.

Embolism

Common causes of embolism are:

- atrial fibrillation (Fig. 36.1) – usually the result of
  — mitral valve disease
  — thyrotoxicosis
  — atheromatous coronary artery disease
- myocardial infarction and mural thrombus
- detachment of thrombi from an atherosclerotic plaque, e.g. at the bifurcation of the aorta or of the common carotid artery
- detachment of thrombus from aneurysms.

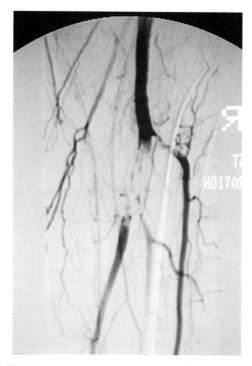

Fig. 36.1 Distal Subtraction Angiogram showing embolus in distal popliteal artery in patient with atrial fibrillation.

Less common causes are:

- septic endocarditis, in which case the embolus is also septic and a mycotic aneurysm may result at the site where it lodges
- atrial myxoma
- paradoxical venous embolism from deep veins of legs entering the arterial circulation through a septal defect.

The effects of an embolus are principally related to the capability of blood to get round the point of obstruction, and they range from nil where the collateral circulation is adequate to death of tissue when the vessel involved is an end artery.

Aneurysms

These are classified into two types: true aneurysms and false aneurysms.

In the case of the former, there is dilatation of the arterial wall. The majority of true aneurysms are due to arteriosclerotic degeneration of the media. The fact that some patients develop aneurysmal disease and others occlusive disease may be due to differences in collagen types. Occasionally, aneurysms may result from a congenital defect in the media (e.g. Marfan's syndrome, 'berry' aneurysms of the circle of Willis, Ehlers–Danlos syndrome and Behçet's disease).

In false aneurysms, the arterial wall is breached and the blood is contained by clot and surrounding tissues. They usually follow trauma, operation or arteriography. They are also being seen increasingly in drug addicts following intra-arterial injections, when they may be mycotic (i.e. infected).

The common sites of aneurysm (Fig. 36.2) are:

- the aorta
- the popliteal arteries – these are usually involved bilaterally and in association with abdominal aortic aneurysm
- the common femoral arteries – the commonest site of false aneurysm
- the visceral arteries – splenic, renal and coeliac.

Around 95% of *aortic aneurysms* involve the infrarenal aorta and its bifurcation. Fortunately, the disease usually spares the first 2 cm below the renal arteries, simplifying reconstructive surgery. Aneurysms extending above the renals are termed thoraco-abdominal aneurysms, or thoracic aneurysms if they are confined to the chest.

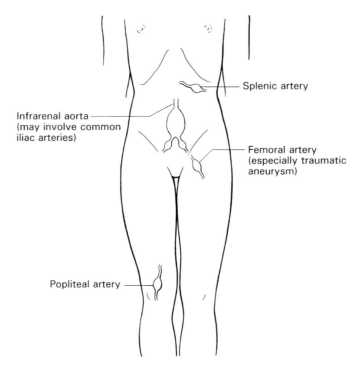

Fig. 36.2 Common sites for aneurysm.

Splenic artery

Infrarenal aorta
(may involve common
iliac arteries)

Femoral artery
(especially traumatic
aneurysm)

Popliteal artery

Systemic (collagen-vascular) diseases

Diseases such as scleroderma usually produce very distal disease which resembles that seen in diabetes. They are often also associated with a tendency to vasospasm.

Major arteritis

This is an ill-defined group of patients in which the supra-aortic arteries (Takayasu's disease) or the abdominal aorta may be involved by a dense inflammatory process, sometimes with giant cells. The peri-aortic inflammation may also affect the coeliac, superior mesenteric and renal arteries.

Vasospastic conditions

Only the smaller arteries can undergo sufficient spasm to produce significant ischaemia. Attacks of digital vasospasm are termed Raynaud's phenomenon, which is discussed below.

Buerger's disease (thromboangiitis obliterans)

The condition is a combination of inflammation and obliteration of arteries. It frequently affects the arms as well as the legs and may be associated with thrombophlebitis. It starts in the distal small vessels and spreads relentlessly proximally. A strong relationship with tobacco smoking is established, and it appears to be more common in some areas of the world, suggesting either genetic or environmental factors in its aetiology. Buerger's disease is confined to young people and is rare in Western societies, although it continues to be seen in developing communities where 'raw' tobacco is widely used.

CLINICAL FEATURES OF OCCLUSIVE VASCULAR DISEASE

SYMPTOMS

Pain is of two types:

- intermittent claudication
- rest pain.

Intermittent claudication

Claudication literally means limping (Latin: *claudicare*, to limp) and is used to label pain that is experienced in the limb on exercise and is relieved by rest. It is nearly always a lower limb symptom, although it can occur in the arms as a result of subclavian or innominate disease. The commonest site where pain starts is in the calf muscles, although claudication may also be experienced in the buttock or thigh and occasionally in the foot.

Surgical physiology. Pain produced in a limb on exercise is directly related to ischaemia of muscles in the region and is presumably caused by the liberation of pain-inducing metabolites.

The resting blood flows in both a normal limb and a limb with diseased vessels are usually about the same. On exercise the muscle bed dilates and blood flow is usually increased up to 10-fold. This increase cannot happen in a limb with a significant arterial stenosis.

The pain of intermittent claudication is characteristically cramp-like and varies from an ache to acute severe pain that arrests the patient's walking. The pain must be related to exercise to qualify for the description and must be relieved rapidly by rest. Useful information to be sought relates to the following.

Duration of symptoms.

Severity of symptoms. In mild claudication, the patient may be able to continue walking after the onset of pain, although they may have to slow down. In more severe claudication, the patient is forced to stop by the severity of the pain.

Progression or regression. In many cases it is not possible to assess accurately the rate or direction of progression of the disease without observation over many months. Claudication will often improve as collaterals open up.

Site. The distribution of pain often provides an indication of the site of major vessel occlusion.

Buttock pain means internal iliac occlusion, and calf pain is usually caused by a block of the superficial femoral artery in the thigh. Pain in the calves radiating up into the thighs is often due to aorto-iliac or generalised iliac artery disease. However, the patterns are not constant.

Claudication distance. The distance travelled before pain occurs is often an unreliable guide in that it is directly related to the amount of exercise performed and therefore depends on whether the patient is walking on flat ground or uphill. Patients usually state that pain occurs after they have walked a definite distance, e.g. 100 or 200 m, but the distance walked may vary from day to day. Also, claudication in one leg may be so severe as to mask milder claudication in the other.

Relief. When pain in the leg is due to occlusive vascular disease, it will always be relieved by rest. The relief is usually complete, though some patients complain of an ache that continues after the cramp-like pain has abated.

Rest pain

Rest pain is characteristically boring, gnawing and severe, often worse at night. It is felt in the foot or toes, not in a muscle group as in the case of claudication pain. Many patients complain of various types of discomfort at rest, but true rest pain will wake them from sleep, requires analgesia and is relieved by hanging the foot over the edge of the bed. If the ischaemia is severe enough, the rest pain will become continuous. It may not then be relieved, even by opiate analgesia. Rest pain (or the onset of necrosis or ischaemic ulceration) indicates threatened loss of the limb. This state is referred to as critical ischaemia.

Symptoms of generalised arterial disease

General symptoms of arterial disease are present in about 50% of patients with intermittent claudication and should always be sought by enquiry. Cardiovascular disease may cause angina, shortness of breath and swelling of the ankles. Cerebral vascular disease may be associated with a past history of strokes or transient attacks of visual disturbance or limb weakness.

SIGNS

There are both general and local signs.

General

It is of particular importance to search for pulse irregularities such as atrial fibrillation, hypertension, evidence of cardiac failure, bronchitis and emphysema, anaemia or polycythaemia. The carotid and subclavian vessels should be auscultated for bruits, indicating stenotic disease, and both radial pulses should be palpated at once to ensure they are synchronous. The abdominal aorta must be palpated for evidence of aneurysm.

Local

Inspection. Ischaemia of the lower limb may be associated with a dry pale skin, loss of hair, fissuring of nails, moist or infected interdigital clefts, ulceration and gangrene. There may be venous 'guttering', the veins being empty due to the inadequate circulation. Elevation of the affected limb will often cause pallor and blanching, which may be accentuated by rapid ankle and toe movement. When the limb is lowered below heart level it will regain its colour more slowly than on the healthy side, and after a few minutes it may become brick-red and congested (Buerger's test).

Palpation. Palpation of the peripheral pulses is the most valuable clinical observation. In many instances, the extent and position of the arterial disease can be estimated by this simple examination with a fair degree of accuracy. It is unusual for a patient with atherosclerosis to complain of symptoms before pulsation of one or more of the peripheral arteries has disappeared. If a pulse is absent at any point, there must be a proximal block of the vessel concerned. Thus, if the common femoral pulse is not palpable in the groin, the occlusion will be in the aorta, common iliac or external iliac arteries. If the femoral pulse is present but the popliteal and ankle pulses are absent, a portion of the superficial femoral or popliteal arteries will be occluded. The popliteal pulse may be difficult to detect and it should be sought with the knee slightly flexed. If it is very prominent, a popliteal aneurysm should be suspected. Foot pulses may also be difficult to feel; the dorsalis pedis pulse is absent in about 10% of normal individuals and the posterior tibial pulse in about 5%.

Palpable collateral vessels may occasionally be detected when major vessels are occluded. A pulse over the medial side of the knee joint may indicate a wide-open geniculate artery. Palpation of the superficial veins of the leg may reveal the presence of thrombosis, which accompanies thromboangiitis obliterans in 30% of patients.

Palpation for skin temperature may show marked change close to the site of a complete obstruction. Although patients with severe ischaemia will have a reduced skin temperature in the affected areas, the estimation of these temperatures is often unreliable, particularly if both limbs have not been equally exposed to the air. A warm knee may be found in patients with a good collateral circulation.

Auscultation. A systolic bruit over a main vessel indicates the presence of stenosis at that level or possibly higher up. Bruits from a stenotic aorta or iliac vessel may be heard anywhere from above the umbilicus to the groin.

The effects of exercise on the appearance of the limb and the distal pulses may be observed. In major vessel disease, pallor ensues and both weak and normal pulses can disappear.

SPECIAL TESTS

Electrocardiography, chest X-rays and blood examination (taking a particular note of polycythaemia, thrombocythaemia, hyperlipidaemia and impaired renal function), together with an examination of the urine for glycosuria, are standard investigations in the general assessment of patients with occlusive disease.

The measurement of ankle pressure before and after a standard exercise using sphygmomanometer and Doppler ultrasound blood velocity detector over the posterior tibial or dorsalis pedis arteries offers an objective quantitative measurement and a functional assessment of the severity of the disease. This test will save many patients with normal ankle pressures from unnecessary angiography, because it demonstrates the anatomical extent of the disease and the feasibility of reconstruction.

Arteriography is by far the most important of all special tests and will give information concerning the level and degree of obstruction, the condition of the collateral circulation and the state of vessels above and below the obstructed or stenotic site. Arteriography is safe in experienced hands, but it is still not without possible complications such as haemorrhage, damage to the arterial wall and dissecting aneurysm formation. Therefore, arteriography should only be carried out only if clinical assessment indicates that reconstructive surgery or angioplasty is likely to be of benefit. Digital subtraction angiography allows a very small volume of intra-arterial contrast material to be used or even an intravenous injection. It is thus safer than routine arteriography.

If symptoms are severe and incapacitating with signs of impending gangrene as indicated by rest pain, skin changes and ankle pressure measurements, then arteriography should be done urgently, because arterial reconstruction is the only way of saving the limb.

DIFFERENTIAL DIAGNOSIS IN INTERMITTENT CLAUDICATION

Sciatica

This may be confused with pain from arterial occlusive

disease. The pain of intermittent claudication occurs after walking some distance, while sciatic pain is usually precipitated by stooping, straining or heavy lifting. The ankle pressure after exercise is increased or unchanged in the absence of arterial disease.

Osteoarthritis of the hip

Degenerative disease of the hip joint may cause diagnostic confusion, particularly as its symptoms are most likely to occur after exercise and may be referred to the knee. However, the absence of local signs of peripheral arterial disease in the presence of restricted hip movements should be enough to warrant an X-ray examination of the hip, after which the diagnosis should be apparent. Again, ankle pressure measurements will determine the presence or absence of arterial disease.

Cauda equina claudication

This is due to compression of the cauda equina within the spinal canal. The symptoms may be similar to true claudication, but the pulses are all present.

MANAGEMENT OF OCCLUSIVE VASCULAR DISEASE

Managing the *underlying causes* of occlusive vascular disease includes, where appropriate:

- cessation of smoking
- dietary manipulation
- weight reduction to reduce the burden on the affected lower limbs and the taking of regular exercise
- control of diabetes
- treatment of cardiac failure
- specific therapy for diseases such as polyarteritis or lupus erythematosus.

Cessation of smoking is the single most important factor in the control of outcome both before and after surgical intervention.

Dietary manipulation is of use in patients with marked disturbance of cholesterol or lipids. Such strategies will help only in the long term. They may be supplemented by agents that lower cholesterol or triglycerides.

MANAGEMENT OF THE LIMB

General

Patients should be reminded that they have a limb or limbs that are at risk and that minor injury or infection may lead to gangrene. Specifically:

- the feet must be kept clean and dry
- the feet must be kept warm, and overheating and possible blistering must be avoided
- the toenails must be carefully trimmed
- corns, papillomas and fungal infection must be properly treated
- shoes should be soft and well-fitting
- minor trauma should be avoided.

Vasodilators. Many have been tried and none are of much use in critical ischaemia when the distal circulation is usually already maximally dilated.

Hypervolaemia. In patients with Buerger's disease who are having an exacerbation of the process, dextran 70 infusion may temporarily increase perfusion. Prostaglandins may also be of benefit, especially the more stable synthetic analogues of prostacyclin.

Specific

Claudication. Many patients with claudication can live within their distance. There is rarely any threat to the limb; only 10% of patients progress to rest pain. The mainstay of treatment is to give up smoking and to exercise as much as possible. In selected patients, when claudication is incapacitating, direct surgery or percutaneous balloon angioplasty should be considered (see below); sympathectomy is not helpful.

Major ischaemia from a proximal block with rest pain and impending or established gangrene. In this case, remove any remediable cause such as an embolus and then try to restore blood flow by direct methods. In aorto-iliac disease this restoration is usually by a Dacron bypass graft from aorta to iliacs or femorals, but radiologically guided balloon angioplasty or surgical thromboendarterectomy (disobliteration), in which the diseased intima and media are cored out, are also options. Below the inguinal ligament, some form of bypass graft is usually used, as angioplasty produces poorer results; saphenous vein is the best conduit.

Polytetrafluroethylene (PTFE) grafts can be used if the patient has no suitable veins. Direct arterial surgery can only be carried out if there are patent vessels distally (i.e. a good 'run off') as established by arteriography. Distal reconstructions to vessels at the ankle are now being attempted with success, although in general the longer the bypass, the lower the success rates.

In the complete absence of run off, sympathectomy may help but is unlikely to influence outcome.

Dead tissue should be amputated or occasionally allowed to separate. When the block is proximal and cannot be relieved, major amputation is usually required.

Ischaemia from distal block. By definition this is an end artery obstruction, and therefore direct bypass surgery will be inapplicable. Conservatism should be practised; provided the dead tissue is dry, it can often be left to separate spontaneously. Sympathectomy or prostaglandin infusions may be helpful.

Local treatment of gangrene due to arterial disease (see p. 392).

SPECIAL CONSIDERATIONS

DIABETES MELLITUS

Diseases associated with diabetes mellitus are:

- major atheroma
- small vessel disease
- combinations of major atheroma and small vessel disease
- neuropathy with or without major atheroma or small vessel disease.

The first three have been dealt with. It is important that the fourth is also recognised. Neuropathy is common in diabetes, although its nature is largely unknown. When a patient presents with a septic/necrotic lesion (Fig. 36.3) on the foot, it is important to try and assess the proportions of neuropathy and vascular disease that are separately responsible.

Vascular disease is characterised by:

- system involvement – retina, kidney
- predominantly cutaneous and gangrenous lesions.

Neuropathy typically has:

- ulceration and gangrene in the presence of foot pulses
- sepsis
- perforating ulcers
- spreading sepsis in fascial plane involving necrosis of fascia and tendons in spite of what appears to be a good blood supply
- clinical features of loss of sensation and position sense.

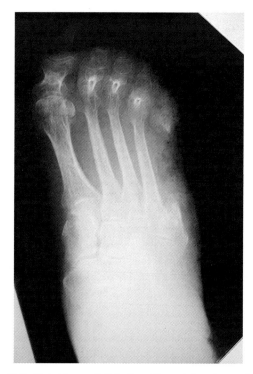

Fig. 36.3 Plain X-ray of diabetic with peripheral vascular disease and neuropathy showing osteomyelitic destruction of fifth metatarsal and gas in the tissues.

Management

The septic/neuropathic foot can be treated by local surgery. Often this has to be radical, involving removal of digits that have been destroyed by infection and by the local arteritis that occurs. Wide excision of dead fascia may be required. However, major amputation can usually be avoided. Clearly, advice on subsequent management for the patient must be rigorous.

VASOSPASTIC DISEASES

Raynaud's phenomenon is characterised by attacks of pallor and pain in digits (nearly always the hand) followed by cyanosis and then rubor as the condition relents. The phenomenon is seen in:

- Raynaud's disease, when it occurs without other cause, usually in females
- both sexes, as a manifestation of some other disorder, the most important of which are
  — scleroderma (systemic sclerosis)
  — the prolonged use of vibrating tools

— cold hypersensitivity associated with a positive Coombs' test, when the lesion is probably 'sludging' of red cells in the capillaries.

Proximal major arterial disease may present as Raynaud's phenomenon. This should be especially suspected in unilateral Raynaud's. Cervical ribs may damage the intima of the subclavian artery with resulting distal embolisation. Arteritis (Takayasu's disease) may also present with cold fingers but can be differentiated by the lack of pulses and reduced blood pressure.

Management

This is obviously related to cause.

Raynaud's disease. Cervical sympathectomy is of little value. Vasadilatory and alpha-adrenergic blocking agents such as thymoxamine and nifedipine may be of value, and prostacyclin infusions can be used for the more severely affected. The main pillar of treatment is the prevention of cold by maintaining the core temperature, electrically heated gloves and avoidance of cold immersion of the hands.

Raynaud's phenomenon. Some patients with an underlying collagen disorder respond to steroids or cyclophosphamide.

CAROTID ARTERIAL DISEASE

Typically atheroma affects the bifurcation of the carotid artery. In recent years it has been realised that up to 30% of strokes result from emboli from or disease in major extracranial vessels. Two forms exist:

- emboli from an ulcerated plaque at the common carotid bifurcation (approximately 90% of cases)
- occlusion of the carotid bifurcation when circle of Willis perfusion is inadequate, either anatomically or because of contralateral disease (approximately 10% of cases).

Both pathological situations may cause established strokes or 'transient ischaemic attacks' (TIAs, i.e. neurological events lasting by definition less than 24 hours); these result in sudden loss of vision (amaurosis fugax), fleeting paraesthesias in limbs, temporary paralysis and loss of cerebral functions such as speech. Patients who suffer TIAs should be investigated by tests to ascertain

the degree of carotid stenosis. Duplex Doppler ultrasound and angiography are the most widely used investigations.

Management

Antiplatelet therapy confers a 12% advantage in preventing major stroke. *Carotid endarterectomy* is indicated for greater then 70% symptomatic stenosis, providing the surgical risk is low and the life expectancy good.

The management of moderate (30–70%) symptomatic stenosis and asymptomatic stenosis remains uncertain.

ANEURYSMS

The natural history can be benign enlargement, possibly with spontaneous resolution by thrombosis; thromboembolism, especially with popliteal aneurysms; or rupture. This last is uncommon in abdominal aneurysms less than 5 cm in diameter. Beyond 5 cm, the incidence of rupture increases progressively. Some common sites for aneurysm are shown in Fig. 36.2.

Symptoms can be due to:

- Pressure on surrounding structures, e.g. duodenum, lumbar spine, iliac vein or ureter.
- Rupture – sudden onset of pain and shock. Radiation of pain in rupture of an aortic aneurysm may be to the loin or groin, mimicking renal colic. Prompt diagnosis and urgent transfer to the operating theatre is vital.
- Fistula formation into adjacent structures such as the vena cava or intestine.

Management of abdominal aortic aneurysms

Asymptomatic and less than 5 cm in diameter. Observe regularly, control hypertension if present and monitor the size of the aneurysm with annual ultrasound scan.

Symptomatic or greater than 5 cm in diameter. Operative treatment is usually indicated. In the elective case, CT scan (Fig. 36.4) is helpful in defining the proximal extent in relation to the renal arteries.

The operation involves clamping the aorta below the renal arteries and clamping the iliac arteries distal to the aneurysm. The aneurysm sac is opened longitudinally and the aortic segment is replaced with either a straight

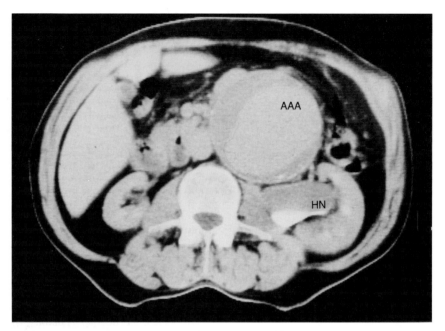

Fig. 36.4 CT scan showing a large aneurysm of the abdominal aorta (AAA). The left hydronephrosis (HN) was an incidental finding.

or a bifurcation synthetic graft. The graft is laid inside the aneurysm, which is then closed over it. It is now possible to repair some aneurysms endoluminally by passing a prosthetic graft up from the femoral arteries under radiological control. The graft is then held in place using a metal stent, which can be dilated using a balloon catheter. As this is a new technique, its precise indications and longer-term results are still unclear.

The operative mortality rate for ruptured aneurysms remains at about 50%, whereas for elective resections it is about 5%.

AMPUTATIONS

In civilian surgical practice, amputations are required most often for lower limb peripheral vascular disease.

INDICATIONS FOR AMPUTATION

A dead limb

The life of a limb (or part of it) may be destroyed in several ways.

It can be destroyed by *trauma*, when major blood vessels have been involved, or by *atherosclerotic occlusive vascular disease* of major vessels, usually of the lower limb when gangrene of the foot or digits has occurred. In the case of the latter, a mid-thigh or sometimes a below-knee amputation will usually be indicated unless successful direct arterial surgery has been performed, in which case a major amputation may be avoided.

Limb destruction may also result from *diabetes mellitus*, when gangrene of the foot is usually the result of a combination of factors (atherosclerosis, infection and peripheral neuritis). In these patients, a limited amputation of toes or the foot is often successful when only small vessel thrombosis has occurred and when major and more proximal limb vessels are unaffected.

Pyogenic infection, in the presence or absence of diabetes, can also destroy the life of a limb; progressive sepsis or gangrene of the foot or digits will require conservative amputation.

A lethal limb

The life of the patient may be threatened if the limb is retained under the following conditions.

An osteogenic sarcoma. Amputation of the whole of the affected bone is indicated if there remains no evidence of metastases after supervoltage radiotherapy.

Subungual malignant melanoma. This requires amputation of the digit. Amputation of a limb may be justified on some occasions to remove a foul fungating tumour which is not treatable by other means.

Gas gangrene. Amputation of all or part of the affected limb will be required if all or most muscle groups are involved by spreading myonecrosis (see also Ch. 16).

Acutely ischaemic limb. This can be life-threatening in cases where restoration of the circulation may precipitate renal failure.

A useless limb

The affected limb may be considered inferior to an artificial limb or to no limb at all because it is:

- paralysed as the result of poliomyelitis or some other nerve lesion
- repeatedly infected, by osteomyelitis
- intractably painful, when amputation is occasionally considered for such conditions as postoperative or postradiotherapeutic brachial neuralgia which have failed to respond to less drastic measures; or for rest pain that cannot be controlled by reconstructive arterial surgery.

TYPES OF AMPUTATION

Provisional

This is performed when it is anticipated that primary healing is unlikely to occur because of infection or ischaemia. The amputation is performed at the lowest possible site so that if further amputation is necessary, it will result in a stump of adequate length.

Technique. Skin and deep fascia flaps are raised as with definitive amputations, but the wound is left open to allow delayed primary healing. This method is commonly used when the blood supply to the stump is doubtful or when dead tissue and sepsis are present distally.

Definitive

Toe amputations. A racquet incision is used around the base of the toe and onto the upper surface of the foot,

whereby no incision is made on the sole of the foot. Often the metatarsal head is also removed to enable the wound to be closed without tension (ray amputation).

Forefoot amputations. Bone section is usually at the mid-metatarsal level. The principle should be to resect sufficient bone to enable closure without tension. Flaps should be constructed such that the plantar flap is longer and the thick plantar skin is used to cover the bone ends.

Transtarsal amputation (Chopart's and Lisfranc's amputations). This is an amputation through the tarsal bones. It is rarely used because it results in an equinovarus deformity due to unopposed tendon action and an unsatisfactory stump for weight-bearing.

Syme's amputation. This entails an initial disarticulation through the ankle joint; the tibia and fibula are then divided at the level of the joint and their ends are covered with a single flap of skin from the heel. The operation is performed very rarely, and most commonly for trauma.

Below-knee amputation. Bone section is through the tibia and fibula a minimum of 9 cm below the knee joint. Two main techniques, either with a long posterior flap or with equal skewed flaps can be used (Fig. 36.5). The aim should be to produce a conical stump without too much muscle bulk suitable for use in a non-end bearing prosthesis.

Gritti–Stokes amputation. This is a supracondylar amputation in which the femur is cut across at the level of the adductor tubercle; the patella is then placed over the cut end to form a broad base for an end-bearing prosthesis.

Above-knee amputation. In this case the weight is borne largely by the ischial tuberosity and the muscles of the thigh. Usually equal anterior and posterior flaps are used. The site of section of the femur should not be closer than 12 cm from the knee joint to allow room for the knee joint in the prosthesis.

Operative technique. The following procedure should be followed:

1. Avoid a tourniquet if the amputation is for peripheral vascular disease.
2. Measure the site of amputation.
3. Cut appropriate skin flaps and raise them with some thickness of fascia and/or muscle.

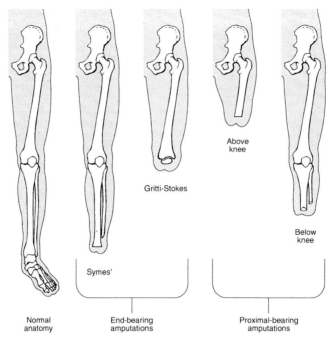

Fig. 36.5 Different types of below-knee amputation.

4. Divide soft tissue at the level of the proposed bone division.
5. Secure vessels as they are encountered.
6. Divide nerves above the level of the proposed bone division to avoid a painful neuroma.
7. Avoid redundant skin flaps.
8. Insert subcutaneous drain tubes to amputation site.
9. Carefully apply a dressing.

PRE AND POSTOPERATIVE CARE

This entails consideration of the patient, the amputation stump and the prosthesis.

The patient

The pain should be controlled until amputation can be undertaken. There is evidence that improved pre-operative pain control may reduce the incidence of phantom limb pain postoperatively.

Other diseases should be controlled, but note that diabetes is not likely to be stable until dead or infected tissue is removed.

Any spreading infection should be limited. Operative contamination must not be allowed to become a serious infection, particularly in bedridden or diabetic patients; this is achieved by the use of perioperative antibiotics. The commonest cause of gas gangrene in civilian life is clostridial infection of an above-knee amputation because of faecal contamination.

The patient should be encouraged to maintain an optimistic outlook about rehabilitation.

The stump

Management of the amputation stump must include:

- resting the stump on a pillow
- placing a bed cradle over the stump
- preventing flexion deformities of the hip and knee joints by suitable exercise and splints
- avoiding major change of stump dressings for 5–7 days unless excessive oozing occurs or signs of infection are apparent
- removing drain tubes from the amputation site by 24–48 hours
- removing skin sutures between 10 and 14 days
- encouraging stump muscle and joint exercise with the help of supervised physiotherapy.

The prosthesis

This is fitted when the following situations prevail:

- the stump is well healed and conical
- the scar is stable
- the patient's general and mental condition is optimal.

In some major specialised centres, immediate fitting is used, but the technique has only limited application.

SPECIAL COMPLICATIONS OF AMPUTATION

The following complications may arise as a result of amputation:

- haemorrhage – reactionary or secondary
- sloughing flaps
- skin eczema, callosities, ulceration, redundancy, adherent scar
- stump muscle wasting
- painful neuroma
- osteomyelitis and ring sequestrum
- phantom limb pain.

FURTHER READING

1991 Symposium on Amputations. Annals of the Royal College of Surgeons of England 73: 133–177

Greenhalgh R M, Mannick J A 1990 The cause and management of aneurysms. Bailliere Tindall, London

Halliday A 1995 Surgical management of carotid stenosis. Annals of the Royal College of Surgeons of England 77: 323–324

McPherson G A D, Wolfe J H N 1992 Acute ischaemia of the leg. In: ABC of vascular diseases. BMJ Publishing, London

MacSweeney S T R, Powell J T, Greenhalgh R M 1994 Pathogenesis of abdominal aortic aneurysms. British Journal of Surgery 81: 935–941

Stonebridge P A, Murie J A 1993 Infrainguinal revascularisation in the diabetic patient. British Journal of Surgery 80: 1237–1241

Thompson M M, Sayers R D, Beard J D, Bell P R F 1993 Femerodistal bypass procedures. Hospital Update Feb: 90–99

37

Venous and related conditions of the lower limb

John Wolfe   Gerard Stansby

OVERVIEW

By far the commonest venous condition is varicose veins, which develop because of incompetence or destruction of the valves that normally prevent blood escaping from the deep into the superficial venous system. Varicose veins are the commonest cause of leg ulcer, others being arterial insufficiency, sensory denervation and trauma, infection and neoplasia. The cause, diagnosis and treatment of deep venous thrombosis are covered, together with its potentially lethal sequel, pulmonary embolism. The chapter ends with an account of lower limb swelling including lymphoedema.

Four conditions are considered:

- varicose veins
- lipodermatosclerosis and ulceration of the leg
- venous thrombosis and pulmonary embolism
- swelling of the lower limb.

VARICOSE VEINS

Varicose veins (varices) can be defined as dilated, lengthened and tortuous veins. In the superficial venous system of the leg, they are usually associated with incompetent (i.e. non-functioning) venous valves.

SURGICAL ANATOMY

Superficial venous system – the system of veins in the subcutaneous tissues superficial to the deep fascia

The long saphenous vein arises from the dorsal venous arch on the medial aspect of the foot. It passes in front of the medial malleolus as it travels up the medial aspect of the leg and thigh, before emptying into the femoral vein after passing through the fossa ovalis. It contains more than 12 valves. Just before its junction with the femoral vein, the proximal end of the long saphenous vein usually receives four tributaries: the superficial circumflex iliac, the superficial epigastric and the superficial and deep external pudendal veins. However, considerable variations may occur; any of these tributaries may empty directly into the femoral vein, and additional tributaries may be present. The long saphenous vein may also be duplicated and may occasionally course up the leg deep to the deep fascia (Fig. 37.1).

The short saphenous vein arises from the dorsal venous arch on the lateral border of the foot behind the lateral malleolus and runs upwards superficial to the deep fascia in the midline of the calf before piercing the deep fascia and entering the popliteal vein. It receives tributaries which pierce the deep fascia from the calf muscles. Again, there are many variations in its course, in its communications with the long saphenous system, and in particular in the precise level at which it enters the popliteal vein (Fig. 37.2).

Perforator system

The perforating or communicating veins are veins which pass through the deep fascia and connect the superficial and deep venous systems. Usually they contain valves and under normal conditions allow blood to flow only from the superficial to the deep system. Incompetence of the valves guarding the perforators allows transmission

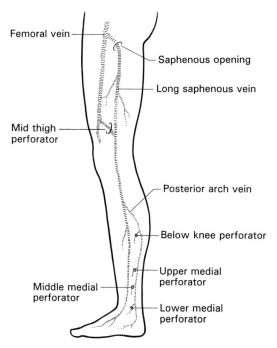

Fig. 37.1 Long saphenous and perforating veins. Medial side of the leg.

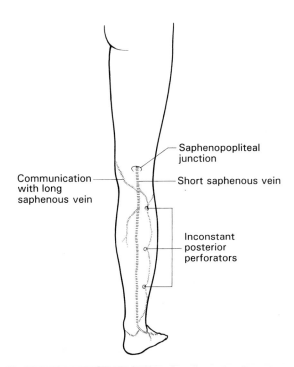

Fig. 37.2 Short saphenous and perforating veins. Posterior aspect of the leg.

of pressure from deep to superficial systems, particularly during exercise.

Deep venous system – the system of veins beneath the deep fascia

This consists of the femoral and popliteal veins, veins (venae comitantes) accompanying the anterior tibial, posterior tibial and peroneal arteries, as well as the valveless blood lakes in the calf muscles. The system communicates with the superficial system at the following sites:

- saphenofemoral junction in the groin constantly
- subsartorial canal by inconstant perforators on the medial aspect of the thigh
- short saphenopopliteal junction constantly
- medial aspect of the lower leg by constant perforators via the posterior arch vein (Fig. 37.1)
- posterior aspect of the leg by inconstant perforators.

Internal iliac vein and veins of round ligament

Gluteal veins run back from the labia and perineum and upper and inner aspects of the thigh, and pass beneath the lower fold of gluteus maximus to enter the pelvis and internal iliac venous system. Veins accompanying the round ligament drain the labia majora and converge into the inguinal canal to enter the ovarian veins.

In pregnancy, vulval varicosities are a common occurrence; they are a combination of gluteal veins, round ligament veins and superficial and deep external pudendal tributaries of the long saphenous system.

SURGICAL PATHOLOGY

At rest there is little difference between the pressure in the superficial and deep systems. However, on exercise in the normal limb, the muscle pump propels blood centrally, pressure falls in the deep system and blood is sucked in from the superficial system so that pressure also falls in that system. By contrast, if the valves protecting the superficial system are incompetent, the muscle pump forces blood into the superficial system, preventing the normal fall in pressure. Thus, the superficial veins become engorged and varices become apparent.

Most varicose veins arising outside pregnancy have no definite cause. However, the potential causes of incompetent valves leading to varicose veins are:

- Congenitally weak or absent valves.
- Thrombosis in either the superficial or the deep system. Valves proximal to the thrombosis may be disrupted by back pressure. In addition, those in recanalised deep veins will often be damaged.
- Back pressure from venous obstruction such as caused by pelvic malignancy.
- Hormones of pregnancy (progesterone and relaxin), which dilate not only uterine veins but also lower limb veins, causing valvular mechanisms to become incompetent. This hormonal effect is maximal in the first 3 months, i.e. before the uterus is capable of producing mechanical obstruction to the iliac veins.
- An occupation involving prolonged standing is believed by some to predispose to varicose veins.

CLINICAL FEATURES

Symptoms

Symptoms in relation to the cause include:

- pregnancy
- deep vein thrombosis
- pelvic obstruction

Patients with unilateral swelling or a 'white leg' in pregnancy may be unaware that they had an iliac vein thrombosis. Fracture of the tibia and fibula always leads to calf vein thrombosis.

Symptoms from the veins and subsequent venous hypertension are:

- cosmetic disfigurement
- pruritus which may be associated with venous eczema
- ache or pain, which may occasionally be 'bursting' and severe in nature; the pain is often noticed after a period of standing
- occasionally spontaneous bleeding can occur from a superficial varix.

Signs

These can be divided into signs related to the causes of varicose veins and those related to the effects.

Causes. Pregnancy, pelvic tumours, previous deep venous thrombosis or a healed lower leg fracture may be apparent.

Effects. Inspection of the anatomical distribution of varicosities is indicative but can be misleading. A medial venous 'flare' suggests long saphenous or medial calf perforator incompetence, and a lateral 'flare' suggests short saphenous incompetence.

Lipodermatosclerosis is usually associated with damage to the deep venous system and the calf perforating veins. This induration and pigmentation (haemosiderin from lysed red cells) of the cutaneous and subcutaneous tissue are a result of chronic venous hypertension. Some of these patients eventually develop venous ulceration. Because the common site for calf perforators is medial, lipodermatosclerosis and venous ulceration are most commonly seen on the medial side of the calf above the medial malleolus.

Sites of perforators may be marked by a varix or a palpable pit, although these clinical signs can be misleading.

Suprapubic varicosities are a vital clue to previous iliac vein thrombosis and act as important collateral venous drainage.

Tap test. The long saphenous vein is found and percussed above the knee, with the other hand feeling the transmitted thrill in the groin. This thrill is entirely normal but identifies the termination of the long saphenous vein. The test is then reversed: the groin is percussed and the transmitted thrill is felt above the knee. This finding is abnormal and implies a single column of blood (i.e. no valves) between the upper and lower hands.

Cough thrill. This is the complementary test to the tap test. The fingers are placed over the saphenofemoral junction and when the patient coughs, a thrill is palpable if there are no valves between the right atrium and the examining hand (i.e. saphenofemoral incompetence).

Tourniquet test (Trendelenburg test). The limb is elevated, the varicosities are emptied and a tourniquet is applied below a suspected incompetent site. If the vein wall remains empty when the patient stands, there are no incompetent communications below the level of the tourniquet. Some perforator sites are more accurately controlled by a finger than by a tourniquet.

Special tests

Directional Doppler ultrasound can confirm the presence of saphenofemoral or short saphenous incompetence by detecting reflux on release of manual compression of the calf. It will also confirm deep valvular incompetence by demonstrating reflux in the popliteal vein despite digital compression of the short saphenous vein behind the knee.

Duplex Doppler (combining both ultrasound imaging and flow measurements) can accurately assess sites of both deep and superficial venous reflux. Unfortunately it is not available in all centres.

Deep to superficial venography is useful in outlining the site of calf and thigh incompetent perforators and can confirm or exclude coexisting occlusion of the deep veins. A pedal vein is injected with contrast medium, while the superficial veins are occluded with a tourniquet at the ankle. Leakage of contrast through the perforating veins indicates incompetence.

Measurement of ambulatory venous pressures (with a needle in a vein on the foot), while a tourniquet controls the superficial veins, will confirm deep venous incompetence and venous hypertension.

TREATMENT

Three methods of treatment are available.

Support hosiery or bandages

The indications for this method are:

- deep venous insufficiency
- elderly patient
- pregnancy
- those who are unfit for, or who refuse, operation.

Although bandages can be used, the support of choice is a well-fitting graduated compression elastic stocking which includes the heel. It should be applied before getting out of bed in the morning and worn for the whole day. This is the treatment of choice in most patients with deep venous insufficiency.

Injection sclerotherapy

Indications for this type of treatment are:

- postoperative recurrences
- troublesome vulval varicosities
- as an alternative to operation.

Technique. A sclerosant solution such as 3% sodium tetradecyl sulphate is injected into an empty varicose tributary. Compression is maintained over the site by rubber pads and elastic bandaging for a few weeks in the hope that clotting can be avoided and intravascular granulation tissue will form, which will later become fibrous and obliterate the vein lumen permanently. If intravascular clotting occurs, the vein will recanalise and varicosities re-form. For this reason, the method is unsuitable for major perforator sites, such as the saphenofemoral junction, since the vein cannot be adequately compressed. The injections can be repeated at various sites in the leg, but the total amount of sclerosant should not exceed 10–12 ml, otherwise haemolytic effects may occur. Also, the injections must always be intravascular or skin ulceration can follow. Even well-performed injection sclerotherapy is less effective than operation in the presence of major venous incompetence.

Operation

The principles of operation are:

- ligation of incompetent perforator sites
- removal of varicosities.

Operative treatment for long saphenous varicose veins entails a dissection of the saphenofemoral junction with division of its tributaries and ligation of the saphenous vein flush with the femoral vein. Likewise, short saphenous incompetence is treated by ligation of the short saphenous vein flush with the popliteal vein. Because of the variable position of the saphenopopliteal junction many surgeons employ either Duplex scanning or venography to mark the site precisely. Other incompetent perforator sites (if present) should also be isolated and ligated. Lengths of varicose systems may be removed with the aid of wire strippers.

Stripping of the long saphenous vein is commonly performed, but it should be stripped from groin to knee rather than from groin to ankle as the risk of damage to the saphenous nerve is lower. Smaller varicose tributaries may be avulsed, ligated or injected. Postoperative recurrence of varicose veins is unfortunately common and may reflect either poor surgical technique (i.e. missed tributaries or sites of incompetence) or the development of new sites of incompetence.

ULCERATION OF THE LEG

Ulceration of the leg is a common problem. Chronic venous leg ulceration affects 3.5% of patients in the over 65 year age group at some time and throws enormous burdens on the health service in terms of both dressing costs and staff time. Disorders of the venous system account for about 75% of cases of leg ulcers, but there are a number of other possible causes to be considered:

- arterial
  - ischaemic, due to major vessel disease
  - vasculitic, due to small vessel disease, e.g. rheumatoid arthritis
- neuropathic – most traumatic ulcers have a neuropathic element, e.g. alcoholism, peripheral neuropathy, diabetes, tabes dorsalis and syringomyelia
- traumatic
- systemic disease, e.g. pyoderma gangrenosum
- primary infective – usually related to malnutrition
- neoplastic
- self-inflicted.

VENOUS ULCERATION

Surgical pathology

Leakage of blood under high pressure from the deep veins into the superficial system, particularly in the region of constantly placed perforators over the medial side of the leg, results in venular dilatation (ankle flare) and leathery induration and pigmentation of the skin as the result of stagnation of the circulation (lipodermatosclerosis) and eventually ulceration. It has been suggested that the deposition of fibrin outside the capillary wall and the trapping of white cells in the microcirculation are responsible for impairing the transport of oxygen and nutrients to the tissues, resulting in the pathological changes found. Trauma and infection may be associated factors.

Clinical features

Patients may have a past history of deep vein thrombosis, and they may have visible varicosities of the superficial system. In addition, many patients will be shown on investigation to have had a previous unrecognised deep vein thrombosis or venous hypertension owing to deep venous valve incompetence.

Signs of venous ulceration include:

- varicose veins
- perforator incompetence
- lipodermatosclerosis
- the ulcer itself – in over 90% of cases the ulcer will be situated in the distal third of the leg on the medial side.

Treatment

Treatment is either conservative or operative.

Conservative. This is the initial treatment of choice once it has been ascertained that the ulcer is venous. To this end, all patients with an apparent venous leg ulcer should have their arterial foot pressures measured with a hand-held Doppler probe and a sphygmomanometer cuff to exclude arterial insufficiency. Likewise if the ulcer fails to heal, a biopsy should be taken to exclude malignancy.

Method. The conservative (i.e. non-operative) treatment of venous leg ulcers can be summarised as follows:

- correct any general disorder, in particular obesity, cardiac failure, anaemia, vitamin deficiency or any debilitating illness
- apply appropriate dressings to the ulcer
- apply compression bandaging or hosiery
- elevate the limb.

Except in sloughy or very infected ulcers, in which antiseptics or desloughing agents may be indicated, modern ulcer dressings rely on producing a moist environment over the ulcer. This technique encourages maximal rates of epithelial regrowth. Dressings should be changed at an interval determined by the amount of exudate produced, but they can often be left for up to a week. Changing dressings too frequently may impair epithelial regrowth.

The use of local antibiotics should be avoided; these are usually unnecessary and may be dangerous if a sensitivity reaction or resistant organism develops. Systemic antibiotics are required only in the presence of cellulitis, lymphangitis or lymphadenitis. A positive bacteriology swab does not in itself require treatment since all ulcers are colonised by bacteria which will disappear as the ulcer heals.

The purpose of compression and elevation is to reduce venous hypertension. Compression can be achieved by carefully applied elastic bandages, perhaps in several layers. Patients should also be encouraged to elevate the leg for as much time as possible. Most ulcers can be treated on an outpatient basis, but occasionally admission for bed rest is necessary. The foot of the bed is elevated about 60 cm (2 feet). This treatment will heal the majority of ulcers not complicated by peripheral arterial disease, although it is not always practicable and may require a prolonged hospital stay.

Once the ulcer has healed, the patient should be instructed to wear an efficiently fitted graduated compression elastic stocking. The heel should be included and it must extend from the bases of the toes to just below the knee. For maximum benefit, the stocking should be applied before rising each morning. It may be discarded at night, provided the foot end of the bed is elevated.

Operative

Skin grafting. Indications for this treatment are failure of conservative treatment or the presence of extensive ulcers that would require prolonged conservative treatment before healing occurred.

Perforator ligation. This method is indicated when incompetent medial calf perforators are demonstrated on venography or Duplex scanning with normal deep veins. Contraindications to this method are:

- incompetent deep venous system
- severe ulceration and wide area of severe lipodermatosclerosis where incisions would have to be made through diseased skin.

Long and short saphenous ligation. Venous ulceration may be associated with superficial incompetence alone, and ligation of the sites of incompetence is then indicated.

OTHER LEG ULCERS

Surgical pathology

Arterial ulcer. Such ulcers are caused by skin ischaemia, usually in association with atherosclerotic peripheral vascular disease. Ulceration occurs commonly on the toes, dorsum of the foot, anterior tibial area or heel, and appears as patches of dry gangrene. Buerger's disease (thromboangiitis obliterans), a disease of men aged between 20 and 40 years, may also be associated with skin gangrene. Small vessel vasculitis may also cause ulceration in patients with rheumatoid arthritis and other collagen disorders.

Neuropathic ulcers. Ulcers occurring in association with diseases of the nervous system which result in sen-

sory loss are called 'neuropathic' or 'trophic'. The mechanism of their production is one of repeated injury or pressure which is allowed to occur because of loss of appreciation of pain in the area.

Conditions that underlie neuropathic ulceration include diabetic and alcoholic peripheral neuritis, tabes dorsalis and syringomyelia.

The ulcers commonly occur on the sole of the foot or the heel, where they may penetrate to bone or joint levels.

Note that ulceration in association with diabetes mellitus may be precipitated by atherosclerosis, infection, peripheral neuritis or a combination of all these factors. The toes and feet are commonly affected.

Traumatic ulcer. This is most likely to occur where skin is closely applied to bony prominences (e.g. the shin, malleoli and back of the heel). Plaster sores and bedsores may be included in this group. A common lesion, particularly in the elderly, occurs when a flap of skin is raised by trauma with its base distally. If it is replaced, it often undergoes necrosis.

Infective ulcer. There are three types of infective ulcer.

Pyogenic ulcer. Inoculation with staphylococcal organisms may be so potent as to result in abscess formation and skin necrosis.

'Bairnsdale ulcer'. A chronic inflammatory response in the skin to *Mycobacterium ulcerans* results in the formation of an irregular ulcer with widely undermined edges and pale, 'watery' granulation tissue in its base. Smears reveal many acid-fast bacilli. Such lesions are now also occurring in HIV-positive patients.

Syphilitic ulcer. Gummatous ulceration of tertiary syphilis is rare in developed countries. It tends to occur on the outer side of the leg as the result of necrosis of a chronic granuloma of muscle. It is typically a painless punched-out ulcer with vertical edges and a sloughing base.

Neoplastic ulcer. Metastases from a distant primary source can lodge in the skin and ulcerate, but this is rare.

Primary tumours of the skin (e.g. squamous cell carcinoma or malignant melanoma) can also present as ulcers. Malignant change may occur in long-standing venous ulcers, in the scars of old ulcerated burns or in chronically discharging osteomyelitic sinuses (Marjolin's ulcer).

Neoplastic ulcers are usually recognised by their heaped-up and proliferative edges. The diagnosis should be suspected in non-healing ulcers and a biopsy taken.

Cryopathic ulcer. Cryopathy is a term used to describe a condition resulting from cold.

Chilblains. These are probably the result of intense vaso-constriction of skin arterioles in areas exposed to cold and blisters. Ulceration can occur, particularly on the feet.

Cold injury. Immersion of the foot in the wet at just above freezing temperatures can result in ischaemic changes in the skin and subcutaneous tissues, which may result in superficial gangrene (trench foot).

Exposure to freezing temperatures results in crystalli-sation of tissues and probable denaturation of intracellu-lar protein and destruction of enzyme systems (frostbite). This causes gangrene of at least the full thickness of the skin.

Self-inflicted ulcer. Injury to the skin by scratching, cutting or the injection of substances occurs most often in those who are psychologically abnormal or hope for some personal gain.

Clinical features

These can be considered under the following headings.

The ulcer. Any ulcer should be described according to its site, size, shape, floor, edge, base, exudate and the nature of the lymph field draining the area. Whenever reasonable doubt exists as to the nature of the ulcer, a biopsy is required.

Venous ulcer. This occurs typically over the lower and medial aspect of the leg.

Arterial ulcer. This occurs on the toes, dorsum of the foot or heel.

Traumatic ulcer occurs anywhere, but when associated with plasters or prolonged bed rest it is closely related to bony prominences.

Neuropathic ulcer. This occurs on the sole or heel of the foot.

Syphilitic ulcer has a punched-out appearance.

Primary infective ulcer. This has a widely undermined edge and watery granulation tissue.

Neoplastic ulcer has heaped-up edges.

The cause

Arterial insufficiency. This may be evident from a history of intermittent claudication or rest pain or from the pres-ence of ischaemic changes in the limb (e.g. dry pale skin, loss of hair, fissuring of nails and absence of peripheral pulses).

Systemic manifestations of any of the causes given above. Thorough clinical examination is mandatory.

Other. In about 10% of cases, no cause is apparent and *special tests* will be required:

- urinalysis – particularly if diabetes is suspected
- full blood examination – if anaemia is suspected
- autoimmune blood screen if vasculitis is suspected
- culture of ulcer discharge – for organisms including mycobacteria
- biopsy of edge of ulcer – particularly if malignancy is suspected
- Duplex scanning or venography – if suspicion of deep vein thrombosis persists
- ankle Doppler pressures and arteriography – if there is suspicion of peripheral arterial disease
- plaster immobilisation of affected part – if self-inflicted ulcer is suspected.

Treatment

Arterial ulcer. The presence of an ulcer usually means that there is a severe degree of ischaemia (i.e. critical ischaemia). Local treatment to the ulcer is therefore unlikely to be effective unless the arterial supply can be improved.

Relief of pain is necessary; this may be severe so that regular analgesics are required. If a patient continues to smoke against strong advice, it may be because he is not getting enough analgesic.

Simple dressings are used. A dry gangrenous part should be exposed. Obviously loose slough may have to be removed and pus drained.

Antibiotics are prescribed and circulation is restored.

This is done by one of two methods:

- direct arterial surgery
- lumbar sympathectomy.

The possibility of being able to restore flow by circumventing a block in a major vessel is best assessed by arteriography. Every effort should be made to carry out direct arterial surgery, perhaps combined with angioplasty, as otherwise a major amputation is likely.

Lumbar sympathectomy dilates skin vessels and may possibly dilate collaterals around a major axial block. It is rarely effective alone in the severe problem of arterial ulcer or gangrene.

Neuropathic ulcer

Treatment of the cause. This is necessary in, for example, diabetes or alcoholism.

Treatment of the limb. Clawing of the toes due to intrinsic muscle paralysis is treated with a well-fitted shoe and inner sole. When the toes become flexed, amputation may be necessary.

Treatment of the ulcer. Trophic ulcers are best treated by rest and simple dry dressings; healing will occur unless infective or ischaemic factors are also present. Careful chiropody, soft shoes, thick socks and sponge rubber inner soles may retard the development of further ulcers.

Persistent trophic ulceration will require either amputation of an affected toe, or excision of a heel or sole ulcer together with underlying bony prominences. The defects are closed by primary suture or skin graft.

Neoplastic ulcer. Wide excision and skin grafting will be indicated for epithelioma or malignant melanoma, and excision of regional lymph nodes, radiotherapy or chemotherapy may also be required.

VENOUS THROMBOSIS AND PULMONARY EMBOLISM

Venous thrombosis most commonly affects the lower limbs. It may result in serious complications which include pulmonary embolism, deep venous and perforator incompetence due to recanalisation of veins, and venous claudication if venous outflow from the limb is obstructed. Occasionally the acute occlusion may lead to superficial gangrene.

CLASSIFICATION

Superficial vein thrombosis may occur in:

- varicose veins
- veins used for intravenous therapy
- apparently normal veins
  — hidden malignancy (Trousseau's syndrome)
  — Buerger's disease (thromboangiitis obliterans)
  — altered constituents of the blood.

Deep vein thrombosis may affect the following vessels:

- upper limb
  — superior vena cava
  — axillary vein
- lower limb
  — soleal sinuses (calf vein thrombosis)
  — superficial femoral vein thrombosis
  — iliofemoral thrombosis (occasionally this leads to phlegmasia alba dolens).

SURGICAL PATHOLOGY

Predisposing factors

There are three commonly accepted predisposing factors to clot formation (Virchow's triad), all of which may interact in any single instance.

Stasis. Slowing of the circulation allows the central stream of platelets to become more peripheral and therefore able to become attached to the endothelial lining of the vessel.

Stasis is likely to occur in the following situations:

- heart failure
- confinement to bed, which leads to reduced muscle pump activity and a slow rate blood flow in the legs
- pelvic mass, for any reason, causing compression of iliac veins.

Endothelial trauma. In arteries, it is well known that the intimal damage that occurs with atherosclerosis may predispose to clot formation. In veins, endothelial trauma may occur in the following situations:

- rough handling of an unconscious patient
- pressure on unprotected calf muscles from unpadded operating tables or their fixtures
- intravenous therapy in association with trauma to the vein from a cannula or needle

- nearby infection associated with inflammation of the vein wall
- trauma to limb especially involving fractures.

Altered constituents of the blood. These include:

- increased viscosity of the blood resulting from loss of water from the circulation, as in dehydration, or an increase in the cellular elements of the blood, as in polycythaemia, leukaemia and malignancy
- increased 'stickiness' of platelets after operation and parturition
- increased fibrinogen levels after operation
- protein C, protein S, and antithrombin III deficiency
- activated clotting factors IX, X and XI after operation
- other changes (largely unknown) associated with the contraceptive pill and malignancy.

Thrombus formation

The features of thrombus formation are as follows.

Platelet deposition. A finely granular coral-like mass of platelets ('coraline clot' or 'white thrombus') is deposited on the endothelium. The proportion of white thrombus in any particular clot varies, but it predominates in the arterial tree. It is known that anticoagulants have little effect on platelet aggregations but that aspirin is effective.

Deposition of other blood elements. Fibrin becomes interlaced between platelet clumps to strengthen and anchor them. Red and white cells are trapped in the mass, and a complex structure develops which may occlude the vessel.

Wave of clotting. A red tail streams away from the head of the clot in the direction of the blood flow. This tail is smooth, slippery, non-adherent and particularly likely to break up to form emboli. This is the 'propagative' or 'consecutive clot' or 'red thrombus' of phlebothrombosis, and there is little or no adherence to the vessel wall. The slower the blood flow, the larger is the clot. Anticoagulants are of considerable value in preventing the formation of this type of clot.

Chemical inflammation. This is probably the result of release of substances from disintegrating elements in the clot, or more frequently of some extraneous sub-

stance (e.g. bacterial breakdown products). An inflammatory reaction occurs in the wall of the vessel and the clot becomes adherent and therefore less dangerous. This is the stage of thrombophlebitis and is associated with symptoms and signs of inflammation. In a superficial vein, a red, warm and painful cord is produced; in a deep vein, calf pain and an elevated temperature occur.

CLINICAL FEATURES

The predisposing cause

A history of varicose veins, malignancy or recent intravenous therapy may indicate a cause for superficial vein thrombosis, while a history of a recent operation, confinement to bed, heart failure, dehydration or polycythaemia may account for a deep vein thrombosis.

Massive deep vein thrombosis (phlegmasia caerulea dolens – literally painful swollen and blue) and superficial thrombosis occurring in apparently normal veins must always raise suspicion of a hidden malignancy, such as carcinoma of the bronchus or pancreas.

The stage of phlebothrombosis

Because the clot is propagative and not attached to the vein wall, there are no local signs to indicate its presence. If the patient has had one or more moderate or large pulmonary emboli, its existence will be known, but its exact site of origin may be impossible to determine without special tests.

The inadequacy of clinical assessment has led to the development of objective tests to detect deep vein thrombosis before clinical features are manifest. These tests include the following.

Doppler ultrasound. A hand-held Doppler can identify reduced or obstructed flow in major veins. By listening over the femoral vein and manually compressing the calf, an augmented signal can be heard if the axial vessels (popliteal, femoral, external iliac) are patent. Absence of augmentation implies occlusion. Confusing results may be obtained when a thrombus is only partially obstructing or when extensive collateral flow is present.

Duplex ultrasound. This combines ultrasound imaging with flow measurement. Colour Duplex allows cod-

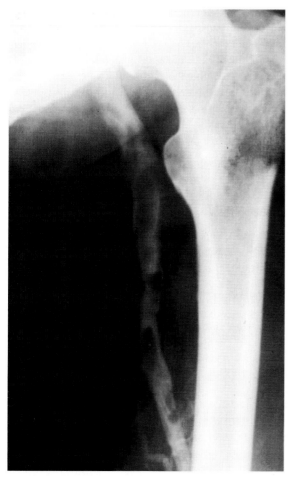

Fig. 37.3 Venogram showing thrombus in the left superficial femoral vein.

ing of the direction of flow using arbitrary colours. Colour Duplex is a very accurate method for diagnosing deep venous thrombosis and can give results comparable to venography in experienced hands.

Venography (phlebography) (Fig. 37.3) is probably the most accurate and widely available test. The phlebographic diagnosis of deep vein thrombosis is based on the presence of well-defined filling defects in opacified veins.

Labelled fibrinogen uptake. Radioactive iodine-labelled fibrinogen is taken up and incorporated as fibrin into any new thrombus, and this uptake can be detected with a scintillation counter. The test is performed by firstly blocking the uptake of iodine by the thyroid gland with sodium or potassium iodide and then giving 100 mCi of ^{125}I-labelled fibrinogen intravenously and counting the radioactivity at fixed points down the legs. If count rates show an unexpected and persistent elevation, deep vein thrombosis can be confidently diagnosed.

The test is reliable when compared with venography, but it is of doubtful value in the upper thigh and of no value at levels above the inguinal ligament. There is also a delay of 24–48 hours after administering fibrinogen before the counts are of diagnostic value. The test is therefore limited to those patients who are being screened for a deep venous thrombosis, having blocked the thyroid gland pre-operatively.

The stage of thrombophlebitis

Superficial vein. A tender, cord-like thickening is easily palpable over part of the course of the vein. The skin over the site is reddened, and temperature and pulse may be elevated.

Deep vein. Calf tenderness and an elevated temperature are constant features. Passive dorsiflexion of the foot produces calf pain (Homan's sign), and later swelling of the limb occurs with pitting oedema. In the event of a massive deep vein thrombosis, severe shock may accompany oedema of the entire limb and the lower abdominal wall. In this situation, pain may be agonising, and the limb can assume a dusky purple colour which persists on elevation, while subcutaneous veins are turgid and peripheral arterial pulses may be impalpable. Phlegmasia caerulea dolens is the severe end of this spectrum and can progress to venous gangrene. Venous gangrene is uncommon and results in superficial tissue loss but not usually loss of the limb. Phlegmasia alba dolens is another variant where the leg is pale and pulseless because of arterial compression due to massive oedema.

TREATMENT

Superficial vein thrombophlebitis

Treatment is either prophylactic or curative.

Prophylaxis. This includes treatment of varicose veins and careful intravenous therapy techniques. The lower limb should not be used for an intravenous drip.

Curative treatment. If spontaneous thrombosis

occurs in an apparently normal vein, consideration must be given to hidden cancer or Buerger's disease. In the common situation, superficial thrombosis occurs in a varicose vein, and there are two methods of treatment available: conservative or operative.

Conservative. Supportive bandaging is prescribed for comfort and the patient is encouraged to remain ambulant. Simple analgesics and local heat are given, and the foot end of the bed is elevated by about 23 cm (9 inches) at night. Anti-inflammatory agents such as phenylbutazone may be prescribed for their analgesic and anti-inflammatory effects.

There is usually no place for antibiotics because the thrombotic process is basically one of chemical inflammation and not infection. However, in the event of a thrombosis occurring in an arm or leg vein being used for intravenous therapy, the possibility of inoculation and bacterial infection cannot be dismissed; in this situation a broad-spectrum antibiotic is justifiable after a blood culture has been taken.

It is doubtful whether anticoagulants have any place in the routine treatment of superficial vein thrombosis. However, they may be advisable in the uncommon event of the phlebitic process rapidly extending to the region of the saphenofemoral junction, at which time there is a danger of propagation into the deep venous system.

Operative. If the thrombotic process is seen early and is localised, and the patient has gross varicose veins, then the clot may be ignored and the varicosities treated on their merits.

Ligation of the saphenofemoral junction should be considered in the unusual event of rapid propagation proximally of the thrombotic process.

Deep vein thrombosis

Superior vena caval thrombosis with its attendant chest wall collaterals is virtually always secondary to obstruction and is largely a problem of diagnosis of the cause (usually malignancy) rather than treatment; it will not be discussed further. Axillary vein thrombosis occurs spontaneously, after excessive exertion in young adults or in association with the contraceptive pill or thoracic outlet syndrome. It is attended by swelling and blueness of the upper limb. It is an unusual condition which responds readily to general supportive therapy, although now the possibility also exists to treat it with fibrinolytic agents.

Deep venous thrombosis of the lower limb is far more prevalent. These episodes probably begin in the soleal sinuses in most cases, but primary iliofemoral thrombosis is responsible for about one-third of postoperative cases.

In deep vein thrombosis, when the clot is confined to the lower leg veins (principally the soleal sinuses), little harm ensues. It is when an axial vein becomes blocked that long-standing trouble is likely. The thrombotic process leads to either of the following:

- permanent occlusion of the vein, which is relatively uncommon
- damage to the valves both in the deep veins and at the communications between deep and superficial perforating veins.

In either event there is venous hypertension distal to the site of thrombosis, which may lead to venous ulceration.

Prophylaxis. This involves both general and specific measures and is tailored to the patient's risk of thromboembolism as assessed preoperatively (Table 37.1).

General. Pre-operative weight is reduced if the patient is grossly overweight. Pre-operative and postoperative graduated compression stockings are placed on the legs of all patients undergoing major surgery, particularly those with a past history of deep vein thrombosis, myocardial disease or varicose veins with major perforator incompetence.

During an operation, the leg veins are protected with an adequately padded operating table and fittings, in addition to stockings, and on completion of operation, a paralysed patient must be carefully handled.

Postoperatively, the foot of the bed is elevated by 9 inches (23 cm). The patient should wear elasticated stockings and should be advised against sitting out of bed with the legs dependent and against crossing the legs. Frequent leg exercises are necessary and early ambulation after operation.

Specific. Antithrombotic agents such as subcutaneous heparin (5000 units every 12 hours for 7–10 days) or dextran 70 are administered during and after operation.

Peroperative mechanical prophylaxis is performed, such as intermittent electrical stimulation of the calf muscles or pneumatic calf compression.

Conservative treatment. The limb is supported with elastic stockings and the foot end of the bed is elevated.

Pharmacological treatment is with anticoagulant and fibrinolytic drugs.

Table 37.1   Risk categories for thromboembolism in surgical patients

High risk
General and urological surgery in patients over 40 years with a recent history of DVT or PE
Extensive pelvic or abdominal surgery for malignant disease
Major orthopaedic surgery of lower limbs

Moderate risk
General surgery in patients over 40 years lasting 30 minutes or more
General surgery in patients below 40 years on contraceptive pill

Low risk
Uncomplicated surgery in patients under 40 years without additional risk factors
Minor surgery of less than 30 minutes' duration in patients over 40 years without additional risk factors

Anticoagulant drugs. These will not unblock a totally occluded vein, but they will reduce the extent of the consecutive thrombus and the incidence of pulmonary embolism.

At present it appears that the best routine is to give 5000–10 000 units of heparin as a 'loading' dose by intravenous injection. This is followed by a continuous intravenous infusion of heparin in a dose of 1000–2000 units/hour. At 6 hours the clotting should be checked and the infusion adjusted to maintain an activated partial thromboplastin time of 1.5 times normal. Thereafter the clotting time is estimated daily. Some patients are heparin-sensitive while others may be resistant, and therefore less or more of the drug may have to be given. The method is relatively safe even in the early postoperative period provided the treatment is carefully controlled. It is probably best avoided in the presence of active peptic ulceration or late pregnancy, while dosages may have to be reduced if liver or renal disease is present.

The major complications are haemorrhagic. A falling platelet count may indicate heparin-induced thrombocytopenia. Heparin therapy should be continued for 5–10 days, but once local symptoms and signs in the leg have begun to improve, the patient is allowed to ambulate with the legs in support stockings. Near or at the end of heparin treatment, oral anticoagulants (usually warfarin) may be introduced and continued for 3–6 months. Dosages are adjusted so as to keep the prothrombin time between 2 and 2.5 times control.

All patients with major deep vein thrombosis should persevere with support stockings for at least 6 months.

Fibrinolytic drugs such as streptokinase, urokinase and tissue plasminogen activator (t-PA) have an increasing role in the treatment of major deep venous thrombosis. They can completely dissolve thrombus if given within 3 days of onset, but have a higher risk of haemorrhagic complications than heparin alone. Rapid clearance of thrombus may, however, preserve venous valve function and reduce the occurrence of the postphlebitic limb syndrome of deep venous insufficiency. t-PA has the advantage of being less likely to produce allergic reactions.

Operative treatment. The place of operative treatment in deep vein thrombosis of the lower limbs remains controversial and the vast majority of patients are best managed non-operatively. Methods available include the following.

Inferior vena caval plication. This has largely been superseded by the development of umbrella filters. Traditionally it was considered if pulmonary emboli continued despite adequate anticoagulation or if anticoagulant therapy was contraindicated. It may also be considered as an adjunct to pulmonary embolectomy for acute and massive pulmonary embolism. Caval plication has an appreciable mortality rate when performed on a very sick patient, and about 30% of survivors subsequently experience trouble with chronic venous stasis.

Caval umbrella filters. Under local anaesthesia, the internal jugular vein is exposed and a collapsed umbrella filter attached to a flexible lead is inserted and threaded through the superior vena cava, the right heart and on into the inferior vena cava under X-ray control. The umbrella is then opened out so that it impinges against the caval wall above the thrombotic process, and the flexible lead is unscrewed and withdrawn through the neck.

The results with the use of such umbrella filters are encouraging, but their precise place has yet to be established. Indications are as for caval plication but morbidity is significantly lower.

Thrombectomy. When thrombosis of the iliofemoral segment is seen within the first 48 hours, the clot can be sucked out or pulled out with a balloon catheter through a groin incision. In addition, venograms can be performed on the operating table to establish the completeness of the clot removal. Surgical thrombectomy may also be combined with a temporary arteriovenous fistula to help improve patency.

PULMONARY EMBOLISM

Massive pulmonary embolus can be fatal. Under these conditions, emptying of the right heart is obstructed and circulatory failure rapidly develops. However, in most cases, pulmonary embolism occurs between the seventh and tenth postoperative days as a continuing process and not as a single and dramatic episode.

The lungs have a remarkable ability to dispose of emboli, and even repeated emboli may be symptomless and/or completely lysed. Massive emboli may cause rapid death, however, and repeated smaller emboli may cause pulmonary hypertension as progressively more of the pulmonary vasculature is blocked off.

Clinical features

A large part of the pulmonary circulation can be occluded by emboli without any demonstrable alteration of pulse, blood pressure, chest X-rays or electrocardiographic tracings.

In addition, there may be no features of a deep vein thrombosis present in a lower limb, indicating that the clot may have arisen in the iliofemoral segment.

Symptoms and signs. These fall into three categories based on severity:

- *massive and fatal* – sudden collapse, severe dyspnoea and marked cyanosis before death
- *less severe* – retrosternal pain, circulatory collapse with lowered blood pressure, tachypnoea, tachycardia, cold blue extremities, elevation of central venous pressure and haemoptysis
- *small* – these lodge in the periphery of the lung causing pleuritic pain and a pleural rub.

Special tests

Chest X-ray. This may look normal; alternatively, there may be paucity of vascular markings, a peripheral wedge opacity or basal collapse.

Electrocardiogram. This is a useful test to exclude myocardial infarction. A normal ECG does not exclude pulmonary embolism. T wave inversion in the right precordial leads is the most common change, although it does not always occur immediately; evidence of right atrial enlargement or the development of right bundle branch block are helpful features. All the ECG changes are usually transient.

Lung scintiscan. This test cannot be used in the massive and severe cases of pulmonary embolism because the patient is too ill to be moved and positioned in front of the gamma camera. However, it is helpful both in diagnosis and in assessing progress in less massive instances. ^{131}I-or technetium-labelled macro-aggregates of human serum albumin can be injected intravenously; scanning the lung fields will detect areas of poor perfusion as less radiodense portions of the scan. This finding could be due to an embolus or pulmonary collapse (infection). A ventilation scan will, however, be normal in the case of a pulmonary embolus (a ventilation–perfusion mismatch).

Pulmonary angiography. In suspected massive pulmonary embolism, pulmonary angiography is very useful in making the diagnosis and in determining the distribution and severity of obstruction before considering operative removal of the clot. An infusion catheter can also be inserted for the administration of thrombolytic therapy.

Arterial blood gases. Major pulmonary embolism is associated with arterial hypoxaemia and often severe metabolic acidosis.

Tests for the diagnosis of deep vein thrombosis ^{125}I-fibrinogen test, Duplex scanning and venography). These are negative in 15–20% of patients with confirmed pulmonary embolism. The source of the thrombus may have been the internal iliac veins, which are not well seen on venography, but positive venography is most useful in planning treatment.

Treatment

Prophylaxis: as for deep vein thrombosis.

Treatment

General support. This includes the use of analgesics for pain, the treatment of shock by inotropic agents and the administration of oxygen.

Anticoagulants. Heparin therapy is begun immediately the diagnosis is suspected.

Thrombolysis. For major pulmonary embolism thrombolysis with t-PA, streptokinase or urokinase can be tried. These agents can be given as an intravenous bolus, but if pulmonary angiography is to be performed they can be administered by catheter directly into the thrombus.

Pulmonary embolectomy. Angiographic facilities are required to confirm the diagnosis and heart–lung bypass is necessary to carry out the operation. A vena caval filter should be inserted at the end of the procedure.

SWELLING OF THE LOWER LIMB

Swelling of the lower limb is often due to medical conditions such as heart failure and renal disease, but the surgeon is more concerned with peripheral causes, most of which are venous or lymphatic in origin.

CLASSIFICATION OF CAUSES

Causes can be classified into central and peripheral causes.
Central causes are:

- Cardiac
  — congestive cardiac failure
  — constrictive pericarditis
- Renal
  — acute nephritis
  — nephrotic syndrome
- Hepatic
- Nutritional
  — protein lack or loss as in protein-losing enteropathy
  — thiamine lack
- Hormonal
  — Cushing's syndrome
  — Myxoedema.

Peripheral causes include:
- Venous disease
  — incompetent valves in the deep venous system
  — deep venous thrombosis
- Lymphoedema
  — primary, usually the result of inadequate lymphatics: at birth, this can be due to lymphoedema congenita and, when familial, Milroy's disease; later onset is usually in adolescence or pregnancy, but sometimes later
  — secondary, usually the result of absent or inade-

quate lymph nodes: previous excision, radiotherapy, malignant infiltration, inflammation, parasitic infestation (filariasis)
- Miscellaneous
  — lipoedema
  — erythrocyanosis frigida
  — arteriovenous fistulas
  — tight bandage or plaster
  — injuries: fracture, and muscle contusion
  — infection: cellulitis, abscess.

SURGICAL PATHOLOGY

Venous disease

Engorgement of the venous system of the lower limb, due to deep venous incompetence or extensive thrombosis, allows the hydrostatic capillary pressure of blood to exceed its colloid osmotic pressure, with the result that fluid of low protein content collects in the extravascular tissues causing pitting oedema of the limb.

Thrombosis of the inferior vena cava may occur as an extension from an iliofemoral thrombosis; it may also occur in association with abdominal cancer, puerperal sepsis or other infective processes.

Oedema is seen in its most extensive form, involving the whole leg, after massive thrombosis throughout most of the deep venous system of the leg and the iliofemoral veins (phlegmasia caerulea dolens).

Primary lymphoedema

This results from obstruction to lymphatic flow because of developmental subcutaneous lymphatic channel defects when the lymph vessels fail to remove protein molecules adequately from the tissues. An increase in the tissue colloidal osmotic pressure takes place, which increases filtration of fluid across the capillary membrane and decreases reabsorption. As a result, fluid of a high protein content collects in the tissues and pitting oedema becomes evident.

Lymphangiographic studies have enabled primary lymphoedema to be subdivided into four groups:

- distal obliteration (60%), causing mild below-knee oedema, frequently bilateral and usually in females
- pelvic obstruction (30%), causing severe whole leg oedema, usually unilateral; males are affected as frequently as females

- thoracic duct occlusion (50%), causing bilateral oedema of the whole leg
- refluxing megalymphatics (5%), causing chyle-filled skin vesicles, chylous ascites and occasionally chylothorax or chyluria.

Secondary lymphoedema

This is more common than primary lymphoedema.

Whichever of the listed causes precipitates lymphoedema, the skin and subcutaneous tissues thicken as the condition becomes chronic. Attacks of cellulitis occur, often caused by beta-haemolytic streptococci, which accentuate the changes; pitting is lost. Later still, the skin becomes hyperkeratotic or horny and vesicular eruptions appear.

Miscellaneous causes

Lipoedema. This is an abnormal accumulation of fat, particularly around the thighs, buttocks, and ankles.

Erythrocyanosis frigida. This is exposure to cold combined with some constitutional susceptibility. It may cause the skin of the lower third of the legs of adolescent females to become cold, blotchy, blue and blistered (chilblains). The legs are fatter than normal, and subcutaneous fat necrosis may result in the formation of hard, tender nodules. The condition presumably arises as the result of a hypoplastic microcirculation through the skin.

Arteriovenous fistulas. Congenital arteriovenous fistulas in the lower limb may be localised or diffuse. The latter are often associated with a giant swollen limb, superficial angiomas, varicose veins and varicose lymphatics in the adolescent.

Traumatic arteriovenous fistulas follow penetrating injuries, when the limb gradually swells and becomes associated with varicose vein formation. Swelling is usually minor.

DIAGNOSIS

The cause of swelling of the lower limb can usually be established from a consideration of the following questions.

Is it central in origin?

Central causes for generalised oedema such as cardiac, renal, or hepatic disorders must be excluded by history and examination.

Is it unilateral in distribution?

Unilateral swelling of the limb indicates that there must be a local cause, which is of venous or lymphatic origin in most cases.

Is it venous or lymphatic in origin?

Venous. Most often, some of the following features will be apparent.

There may be a history of deep vein thrombosis after pregnancy, operation or confinement to bed, with the subsequent development of a painful and swollen leg. Occasionally, deep vein thrombosis may occur for no apparent reason; then hidden malignancy or the contraceptive pill may have to be considered as possible predisposing factors.

There may also be a history of an acute episode of severe pain over most of the limb in association with marked shock, rapidly developing extensive oedema, cyanotic skin, turgid subcutaneous veins and superficial skin ulceration. This would indicate a massive deep vein thrombosis (phlegmasia caerulea dolens).

The presence of varicose veins, perforator incompetence (blow-outs, fascial pits, ankle flares), varicose dermatitis and varicose ulceration indicates chronic venous insufficiency.

Oedema of the leg may be present, which may be pitting in the early phase but non-pitting when chronic and associated with skin and subcutaneous thickening.

Lymphatic. Oedema of lymphatic origin, in contradistinction to that of venous origin, is rarely painful at any stage; in addition, the skin of a lymphoedematous limb remains remarkably healthy for many years apart from recurrent attacks of cellulitis. Skin pigmentation and ulceration, which are typical of chronic venous stasis, are not apparent.

Primary lymphoedema. There is a family history in 20% of cases, and it is unilateral in 50% of cases. It is of gradual onset and apparently worse in warm weather. It is a soft pitting oedema in the early stages but, like chronic oedema of venous origin, it becomes non-pitting in the chronic phase when skin and subcutaneous thickening are present.

After many years, hyperkeratotic, horny and vesicular changes may occur, which lead to ulceration and discharge of lymph.

Secondary lymphoedema. This differs from primary lymphoedema in being of rapid onset and unilateral in distribution; most often there is an obvious cause for its occurrence.

Is it arteriovenous in origin?

On rare occasions when central and local causes are not apparent for the oedema, an arteriovenous abnormality will have to be considered. Features suggestive of arteriovenous fistula formation vary according to whether it is localised or diffuse, congenital or traumatic.

Local. Features include:

- gigantism of the limb, which may occur if the fistula is congenital or if it is acquired before completion of epiphyseal fusion of limb bones
- distended superficial veins
- superficial angiomas (congenital fistulas)
- warmth, thrill and bruit (machinery murmur) over a fistula
- coolness of the limb below the fistula
- muscle wasting below the fistula
- Branham's sign – the patient develops a bradycardia when the fistula is occluded with the thumb.

Systemic. Features are:

- elevated pulse pressure
- cardiac enlargement and later cardiac failure.

Special tests

When the diagnosis is still in doubt, the following special tests may be of value.

Venography (phlebography). The injection of radio-opaque contrast medium into an ankle vein or femoral vein will outline the site and extent of a thrombotic process.

Lymphangioscintigraphy. An isotopic study of lymphatic clearance is diagnostic of lymphoedema, but anatomical detail is lacking. Occasionally, a lymphan-

giogram using intralymphatic radio-opaque solution is indicated.

Arteriography. This a valuable test when arteriovenous fistula formation is suspected.

TREATMENT

Deep vein thrombosis

The treatment of deep vein thrombosis is discussed on page 396.

Primary lymphoedema

Treatment is either conservative or operative.

Conservative. This is indicated for mild oedema (90% of cases) and includes:

- limb massage with a pneumatic compression boot
- limb elevation at night
- application of well-fitting elastic stockings
- bed rest and antibiotics for attacks of cellulitis.

Operative. This is indicated for severe disabling cases of oedema not responding to conservative measures or for chronic neglected cases with recurrent cellulitis. It is only necessary in approximately 5% of patients.

The operations are based on the principle of wide excision of the subcutaneous tissue to reduce the volume of the leg, since the disease is confined to the skin and subcutaneous tissue. If the skin is healthy, flaps are raised (Homan's operation), but in elephantiasis split-skin grafts are placed on the raw surface (Charles' operation). Lymphaticovenous anastomoses are occasionally useful.

Secondary lymphoedema

Conservative treatment is by limb massage, elevation and bandaging, as above.

When the causative condition is inactive and lymphoedema is severe and incapacitating, a wide variety of operations has been considered, but results are not encouraging.

Arteriovenous fistulas

Traumatic fistulas. Immediate operation and arterial

and venous reconstruction, with or without arterial or venous graft, will prevent limb swelling. Alternatively, a delayed operation and arterial and venous reconstruction or quadruple ligation may be performed when the collateral circulation is well established (3 months).

Congenital and diffuse fistulas. Embolisation of the fistula under radiological control is the most satisfactory treatment but is sometimes disappointing.

Limb-shortening operations, such as bone resection or epiphyseal stapling, are not always satisfactory.

FURTHER READING

Angle N, Bergan J J 1997 Chronic venous ulcer. British Medical Journal 314: 1019–1023

Belcaro G, Nicolades A N, Veller M 1995 Venous disorders – a manual of diagnosis and treatment. W B Saunders, London

Bergqvist D, Comerota A J, Nicolaides A N, Scurr J H (eds) 1994 Prevention of venous thromboembolism. Med-Orion, London

Nicolaides A N, Sumner D S 1991 Investigation of patients with deep vein thrombosis and chronic venous insufficiency. Med-Orion, London

Ruckley C V 1988 A colour atlas of surgical management of venous disease. Mosby-Wolfe, London

Tibbs D T 1994 Venous disorders, vascular malformations and chronic ulceration in the lower limbs. In: Morris P J, Malt R A (eds) Oxford textbook of surgery, Oxford University Press, Oxford

Verstraete M 1997 Prophylaxis of venous thromboembolism. British Medical Journal 314: 123–125

General disorders

External hernias

Bruce Waxman

38

OVERVIEW

External hernias, particularly the more common types – inguinal, femoral and umbilical – are a significant cause of morbidity. This chapter covers the principles of the surgical anatomy and pathology of hernias, both of which are dealt with in some detail as students often find the anatomy of hernias difficult to understand. All different types of external hernia are discussed, with an emphasis on correlating the surgical anatomy with the principles of surgical treatment and the different operations for hernia repair, including the impact that the use of mesh has had in surgery for inguinal hernias.

A hernia is a protrusion of the whole or part of a viscus from its normal position through an opening in the wall of its containing cavity.

An external hernia is a protrusion of a viscus from the peritoneal cavity into an abnormal position, the commonest site being inguinal.

CLASSIFICATION

Hernias can be classified into:

- inguinal
- femoral
- umbilical and para-umbilical
- epigastric
- incisional
- obturator
- Spigelian
- lumbar
- gluteal
- sciatic
- perineal
- hiatus.

The *commoner hernias* are inguinal, femoral, umbilical and para-umbilical.

PREDISPOSING FACTORS

All hernias occur at the sites of weakness or potential weakness of the abdominal wall which are acted on by a continued or repeated increase in abdominal pressure. Frequently such sites are where blood vessels and other structures enter or leave the abdominal or thoracic cavity.

Congenital defect

A congenital peritoneal sac predisposes to hernia formation in early life and can result in:

- persistence of processes vaginalis allowing indirect inguinal hernia formation
- incomplete obliteration of umbilicus allowing umbilical hernia formation
- patent canal of Nück allowing indirect inguinal hernia formation in females
- persistent communication between abdominal and thoracic cavity allowing diaphragmatic hernia formation (see p. 241).

Acquired defect

Weakness of the anterior abdominal wall can result from surgical incisions causing incisional hernia, and muscle weakness as a result of obesity with fatty infiltration, pregnancy, wasting diseases, normal ageing processes, poliomyelitis and nerve division (e.g. an increased incidence of right inguinal hernia following appendicectomy caused by an ilio-inguinal nerve injury).

PRECIPITATING FACTORS

Herniation occurs when the intra-abdominal pressure is rapidly and repeatedly raised by such factors as:

- chronic cough
- straining at defaecation
- bladder neck or urethral obstruction
- pregnancy and parturition
- vomiting
- severe muscular effort
- the filling of an existing sac by ascitic fluid, which renders it obvious.

SURGICAL PATHOLOGY

THE SAC

An external abdominal hernia usually has a peritoneal sac with a neck, body and fundus which completely contains any extruded contents. However, a sliding hernia incompletely contains its contents when sigmoid colon, caecum or bladder is involved; in this variety the sac is deficient posteriorly or, put another way, the posterior wall of the sac is formed by the viscus.

THE CONTENTS

The contents may comprise:

- omentum
- bowel
- portion of circumference of bowel (Richter's hernia)
- Meckel's diverticulum (Littre's hernia)
- two loops of bowel (Maydl's hernia)
- bladder.

The contents may be reducible, irreducible, obstructed or strangulated.

Reducible contents can be completely emptied from the sac by external pressure.

Irreducible contents cannot be completely emptied from the sac. This may be caused by adhesions formed between the contents and the peritoneal sac; retention of faeces in large bowel in the sac (incarceration), or fibro-

sis and constriction of the neck of the sac. The term 'incarcerated', which may also be used to describe either irreducible or obstructed hernia, is probably best avoided.

Constriction of the neck of the sac causes a mechanical obstruction of the contents (e.g. small bowel obstruction) but the contents remain viable.

Strangulated contents occur when the blood supply of the contents is impaired, rendering gangrene imminent; this is the end stage of irreducibility and obstruction.

PRINCIPLES OF TREATMENT OF HERNIAS

These principles apply to the treatment of uncomplicated (reducible) hernias.

NO TREATMENT

This will be indicated in elderly patients with severe debility who refuse surgery. Operation is the most satisfactory treatment and should be advised wherever possible.

TRUSS

In infants up to 1 year of age, reducible indirect inguinal and umbilical hernias may occasionally be treated with a truss in the hope that by keeping contents out of the sac, the normal obliterative processes will proceed. However, natural closure of a sac is no longer possible after 1 year or if the hernia reappears during the trial with the truss. The method is not strongly recommended.

In adults with easily reducible inguinal hernias, a truss is indicated only if operation is refused or contraindicated because of general debility. A truss used in healthy young adults has disadvantages in being an encumbrance and in being associated with pressure atrophy of the inguinal muscles and of causing the development of adhesions between the sac and its contents.

PRINCIPLES OF OPERATIVE MANAGEMENT

Pre-operative

Precipitating factors should, whenever possible, be controlled, in particular: obesity, constipation, bladder neck obstruction, chronic cough and smoking. Instruction in breathing exercises is a valuable measure aimed at improving the patient's general health and reducing the risk of a recurrent hernia postoperatively.

Operative

The following manoeuvres are used alone or in combination.

Herniotomy. This is simply excision of the sac at its neck. For indirect inguinal hernias in infants or children, this is all that is necessary. For direct hernia in adults, with a diffuse bulge of the posterior wall, herniotomy is undesirable and may lead to bladder injury.

Herniorrhaphy. This is closure of the defect with local tissues. The defect may be the deep inguinal ring, the posterior wall of the inguinal canal (transversalis fascia), or the femoral ring.

Hernioplasty. This strictly means the strengthening of a defect with a patch or inlay of living material such as fascia lata, but it has come to include the repair of a defect by an inlay or darn with some absorbable or non-absorbable foreign material (e.g. polypropylene mesh).

Postoperative

At this stage, management involves the continued avoidance of pre-operative factors which might precipitate hernia recurrence.

PRINCIPLES OF OPERATIVE REPAIR

The strength of a hernia repair depends in particular on four factors.

Reconstitution of anatomy. Hernias disturb the normal anatomy, which should be reconstructed to as near normal as possible (e.g. reconstitution of transversalis fascia in inguinal hernia).

Apposition of fascial, aponeurotic or tendinous structures. Scar tissue formation is promoted when fibrous structures are apposed by sutures. Suturing muscle to fascia neither promotes sound healing nor reconstitutes anatomy.

The absence of tension. The function of any suture material, whether absorbable or non-absorbable, is one of approximation only. When sutures are inserted under tension, they cut through the tissues and the tissues separate and return to their original positions weakening the repair.

Suture material and fibroblastic reaction. Suture material must retain its strength until the formation of healthy scar tissue, as the ultimate strength of the repair is dependent not on the suture but on the laying down of collagen by fibroblasts.

Absorbable sutures stimulate a brisk inflammatory response which subsides when they fragment and are absorbed after 3–4 weeks. This is insufficient time for consolidation of strength. Non-absorbable monofilament material, on the other hand, is walled off by fibroblasts, and multifilament material is walled off and invaded by fibroblasts, while an open mesh becomes part of the permanent fibrous tissue reparative process.

Monofilament materials (polypropylene or nylon) have an additional advantage in that they cause neither local trauma nor an acute inflammatory response, and they do not have crevices in which bacteria can lodge. Thus they are the materials of choice.

CAUSES OF RECURRENT HERNIA

PRE-OPERATIVE

These include any factor that predisposes to faulty or delayed healing.

Operative

Operative causes include any factor involving faulty technique, with failure to:

- follow the principles of operative repair
- identify an indirect sac and ligate it at its neck
- perform a herniorrhaphy in the presence of a defect
- repair a defect adequately, particularly transversalis fascia
- achieve adequate haemostasis, so predisposing to wound haematoma and infection
- close the medial corner of the posterior wall of the inguinal canal between the conjoint tendon, pubic tubercle and inguinal ligament; failure to do this predisposes to a direct hernia recurrence.

Postoperative

Causes of recurrent hernia at this stage include the persistence of pre-operative factors, wound haematoma and wound infection.

INGUINAL HERNIA

This is the commonest type of hernia in both males and females.

SURGICAL ANATOMY

The inguinal canal is an oblique passage or intermuscular split about 4 cm long in the lower part of the abdominal wall, passing downwards and medially from the internal inguinal ring to the external inguinal ring. Through the canal passes the spermatic cord in the male and the round ligament in the female.

The external ring is formed by a V slit in the external oblique aponeurosis and is situated 1 cm above and lateral to the pubic tubercle (Fig. 38.1). It transmits the vas deferens, the testicular artery (branch of the aorta on the right and renal artery on the left), the artery of the vas (branch of the inferior vesical), the cremasteric artery (branch of the inferior epigastric), the pampiniform plexus of veins, the ilio-inguinal nerve, the genital branch of the genitofemoral nerve, the processus vaginalis when present and the cremaster muscle.

The anterior wall of the inguinal canal is made up of the arching fibres of the internal oblique muscle laterally and the aponeurosis of the external oblique medially (Fig. 38.2). Both structures are covered by superficial (Scarpa's) fascia, subcutaneous fat and skin.

The floor of the inguinal canal is formed by the gutter of the inguinal ligament laterally and the lacunar ligament (Gimbernat's ligament) medially.

The roof of the inguinal canal is formed by the lower borders of the internal oblique and transversus abdominis muscles (Fig. 38.2).

The posterior wall of the inguinal canal consists of the conjoint tendon medially (the fused common insertion of the internal oblique and transversus abdominis muscles into the pubic crest) and the lateral umbilical ligament, the inferior epigastric artery and the fascia transversalis laterally (Fig. 38.2). The triangular area bounded by the inferior epigastric artery, the inguinal ligament and the lateral border of the rectus abdominis muscle (Hesselbach's triangle) is a thin and weak part of the posterior wall which is covered only by transversalis fascia and peritoneum (Fig. 38.3).

The internal ring lies about 1.5 cm above the inguinal ligament at the midinguinal point (midpoint between the anterior superior iliac spine and the symphysis pubis), being a U-shaped condensation of the fascia transversalis (Fig. 38.2).

The internal ring transmits the same structures as the external ring, although the coverings are different.

The intergrity of the inguinal canal depends on the strength of the anterior wall in its lateral part when contraction of the external oblique narrows the external ring;

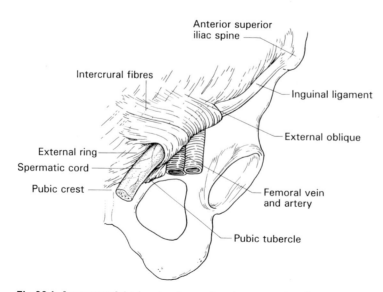

Fig. 38.1 Anatomy of the inguino-femoral region – anterior view.

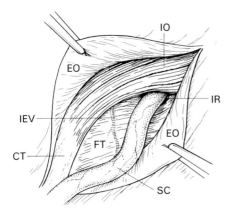

Fig. 38.2 Internal oblique and inguinal canal (external oblique aponeurosis reflected). EO, reflected external oblique aponeurosis; IO, arching muscle of internal oblique; CT, conjoint tendon; FT, fascia transversalis; IEV, inferior epigastric vessel; IR, internal inguinal ring; SC, spermatic cord.

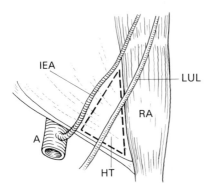

Fig. 38.3 Hesselbach's triangle – posterior view. HT, Hesselbach's triangle; IEA, inferior epigastric artery; LUL, lateral umbilical ligament (obliterated umbilical artery); RA, rectus abdominis; A, femoral artery.

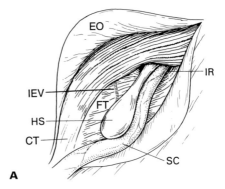

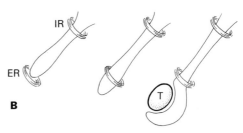

Fig. 38.4 Indirect inguinal hernia. A. External oblique reflected: EO, external oblique; IEV, inferior epigastric vessels; FT, fascia transversalis; CT, conjoint tendon; HS, hernial sac; SC, spermatic cord; IR, internal ring. **B.** Hernial sacs: (from left to right) bubonocele, funicular, complete (scrotal). ER, external ring; IR, internal ring; T, testis.

Indirect inguinal hernias are usually congenital in origin and they may be subdivided into:

- bubonocele
- funicular
- complete or scrotal (Fig. 38.4B).

The coverings of an indirect inguinal hernia are:

- peritoneum
- extraperitoneal fat
- internal spermatic fascia (derived from the fascia transversalis at the internal ring)
- cremaster muscle and fascia (derived from the muscle of internal oblique and transversus abdominis and the areolar tissue between these muscles)
- external spermatic fascia (derived from the crura of the external ring – external oblique aponeurosis)
- superficial fascia and skin.

the strength of the posterior wall in its medial part when contraction of the internal oblique and the transversus abdominis muscles straightens the conjoint tendon; and the upward and lateral movement of the U-shaped internal ring.

TYPES OF INGUINAL HERNIA

Indirect

This enters the inguinal canal through the internal inguinal ring lateral to the inferior epigastric vessels and transverses the full length of the canal in front of the cord (Fig. 38.4A).

Direct

This type of hernia is usually a diffuse bulge of the

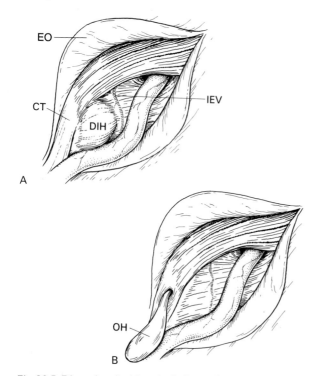

Fig. 38.5 Direct inguinal hernia. A. External oblique reflected: EO, external oblique; IEV, inferior epigastric vessels; CT, attenuated conjoint tendon; DIH, direct hernial sac. **B.** Congenital direct hernia (Ogilvie's hernia) (OH).

medial portion of the posterior wall of the inguinal canal (Hesselbach's triangle) medial to the inferior epigastric vessels and which is behind, above, or below the cord (Fig. 38.5A). Direct inguinal hernias are acquired, with the exception of a rare type in which there is a rigid circular defect in the conjoint tendon (Ogilvie's hernia, Fig. 38.5B).

The coverings of a direct inguinal hernia are:

- peritoneum
- fascia transversalis
- conjoint tendon (if the hernia passes medial to the lateral umbilical ligament)
- external oblique aponeurosis
- superficial fascia and skin.

Indirect and direct hernia (dual hernia, pantaloon hernia or saddle bag hernia)

This presents with dual sacs straddling the inferior epigastric vessels.

Sliding

This is caused by a laxity of the parietal peritoneum and a hollow viscus sliding underneath. The posterior wall of the sac therefore includes not only peritoneum but also an abdominal viscus – sigmoid colon on the left, caecum on the right and occasionally bladder.

CLINICAL FEATURES

Indirect inguinal hernias occur at all ages, and when caused by a persistence of the processus vaginalis they present soon after birth or in adolescence.

Direct inguinal hernias occur most often in the middle-aged or elderly as an acquired condition.

Sliding inguinal hernias occur almost exclusively in men and more commonly on the left side, being large and globular extending into the scrotum and are often irreducible.

Symptoms

A lump. This appears in the groin, sometimes after a bout of strenuous exercise and disappears on lying down unless irreducible.

Discomfort or pain. Discomfort in the groin is common and is probably the result of stretching of the neck of the sac, but severe pain in the lump or in the abdomen usually indicates obstruction or strangulation.

Vomiting. This suggests obstruction or strangulation.

Signs

General. Special attention must be paid to the following:

- precipitating factors, especially chronic lung disease, urinary obstructions, colonic disorders and previous appendicectomy
- signs of obstruction or strangulation, particularly dehydration, shock and peritonitis.

Local. The following are noted on *inspection* with the patient standing and coughing: an indirect inguinal hernia passes downwards and medially towards the scrotum, whereas a direct inguinal hernia protrudes directly forwards in the inner part of the inguinal canal.

On *palpation* with the patient lying down, an indirect

inguinal hernia, when reducible, returns in an upward and lateral direction and is prevented from returning by pressure over the internal ring at the midinguinal point.

A small inguinal hernia (bubonocele) may not be detectable unless the little finger invaginates the scrotum and is passed into the external ring: an impulse will be felt when the patient coughs. This is an uncomfortable examination and should be carried out only if there is doubt.

A direct inguinal hernia is seldom large enough to enter the scrotum and, when it is reducible, it returns directly backwards. Since it lies medial to the internal ring, it cannot be controlled by pressure over this site, and with a finger in the external ring the cough impulse is directed forwards.

Whether the hernia is indirect or direct, it is important to assess the nature of the contents of the sac; intestine gurgles on reduction of the hernia but omentum does not.

When making a local assessment of an inguinal hernia it is important to remember the following three points:

Firstly, it is sometimes not possible to decide clinically whether an inguinal hernia is direct or indirect.

Second, a tense, tender, irreducible hernia (most often an indirect hernia) in the absence of abdominal pain is simply irreducible. However, when persistent pain, loss of cough impulse and perhaps oedema and reddening of the skin over the hernia are present, together with other signs of intestinal obstruction, strangulation of bowel must be suspected. An obstructed hernia cannot always be distinguished clinically from a strangulated one; the distinction can only be made at operation which, in the presence of symptoms and signs of bowel obstruction, is an urgent requirement.

Finally, an absent cough impulse alone does not indicate strangulation of bowel as the hernia sac may be plugged with omentum. Omental strangulation is likely when a tense, tender, irreducible hernia is present in the absence of features of bowel obstruction.

Differential diagnosis of a groin lump

Femoral hernia. A femoral hernia appears in the groin below the medial end of the inguinal ligament, lateral to the pubic tubercle, and enlarges upward over the inguinal ligament, medial to the pubic tubercle.

Inguinal lymph nodes. When inguinal lymph nodes are palpable, they may be confused with an irreducible inguinal or femoral hernia, but they are usually multiple and associated with constitutional symptoms of fever and malaise.

Saphena varix. This is associated with varicosities of the long saphenous vein. The varix lies below the inguinal ligament and disappears when the limb is elevated; it imparts a thrill and bruit when the patient coughs (Cruveilhier's sign).

Femoral aneurysm. This is usually caused by atherosclerosis but it may follow trauma, especially false aneurysm after femoral puncture for angiography. The aneurysm lies below the inguinal ligament and is associated with expansile pulsation.

Psoas abscess. This is a fluctuant tender swelling arising below the inguinal ligament, with general signs of toxicity. Signs of the primary inflammatory condition in the bowel or lumbar spine may be present.

Encysted hydrocele of the cord. This appears as a tense irreducible swelling anywhere along the cord. It moves downwards when traction is exerted on the testis.

Hydrocele of the canal of Nück. This appears as an irreducible, tense, cystic swelling in the superficial ring of a young female, and is a cyst replacing the distal round ligament.

Lipoma of the cord. This may produce features similar to those of an encysted hydrocele, or it may be indistinguishable from an irreducible hernia.

An incompletely descended testis emerging from the external ring. This appears as an uncomfortable, mobile lump, with an upper limit, associated with an absent testis in the scrotum. An inguinal hernia is usually present.

Ectopic testis. A testis situated in the superficial inguinal pouch or at the root of the penis may cause confusion, but again the absence of a testis from the scrotum indicates maldescent.

Complicated inguinal hernias

Obstructed or strangulated inguinal hernias require urgent operation. A short period of pre-operative resuscitation with intravenous fluids is indicated when dehydration is present.

At operation one of the three following situations will be encountered:

- the hernia reduces on opening the external oblique and dividing the external ring
- the hernia reduces spontaneously under general anaesthetic
- the hernia is not reduced after dividing the external ring.

The first situation is the commonest occurrence. After the sac is opened, the involved loop of bowel is found and assessed for viability. When it is not viable, resection is performed; the hernia is then repaired in the usual manner.

In the second situation, where the hernia reduces spontaneously, the operation is continued, and on opening the hernia sac the loop of bowel or portion of omentum which has been involved in the hernia is most often located just deep to the internal ring through which it can be delivered and its viability assessed.

When the involved bowel loop cannot be located, and provided there are no perioperative signs of peritonitis, no bleeding or faeculent fluid present on opening the sac, the hernia is simply repaired in the usual manner. When the viscus cannot be located, but when there are pre-operative signs of peritonitis or there is discoloured peritoneal fluid, or blood is present in the sac, then a formal laparotomy must be performed to locate the involved bowel.

The third situation, in which the hernia is not reduced after dividing the external ring, usually occurs because of a tight neck of the sac or adhesions; the constriction ring causing the tightness plus the adhesions must be divided, the contents of the sac dealt with as necessary and repair of the defect performed.

Operations on complicated hernias are best covered with a broad-spectrum antibiotic, to reduce the incidence of wound infection should a bowel resection be necessary.

TREATMENT

Uncomplicated inguinal hernias

The general principles outlined on page 405 apply to inguinal hernias.

Operation is the most satisfactory treatment and should be advised whenever possible.

Operation may be performed with either general anaesthesia or local/regional anaesthesia. The procedure may be performed either on an inpatient basis or in well-informed, healthy patients in a day surgery setting. The patient should be able to return to pre-operative physical activity and employment 2–6 weeks after surgery.

There are three groups of patients.

Indirect inguinal hernias in children and adolescents. In these, there is a normal posterior wall to the inguinal canal, and if there has been no stretching of the internal ring, herniotomy alone is sufficient (Fig. 38.6A).

Indirect inguinal hernias in healthy adults. These patients have good inguinal musculature and an intact posterior wall of the inguinal canal, but when the internal ring is stretched and widened then the following steps are required:

- herniotomy
- herniorraphy
- hernioplasty
- laparoscopic hernia repair.

Herniotomy. See Figure 38.6A.

Herniorrhaphy. The Shouldice operation incorporates all the principles of operative repair, closing the hernial defect with local tissues. All three layers of the abdominal wall are strengthened using monofilament non-absorbable sutures (stainless steel wire or polypropylene). The transversalis fascia is divided and reconstituted by imbrication (double breasting, Fig. 38.6B), the fascia of the conjoined transversalis and internal oblique is approximated to the inguinal ligament by imbrication and the divided external oblique is similarly closed by double breasting. Recurrence rates of less than 1% at 5 years illustrate the effectiveness of this repair.

Hernioplasty. The two common procedures performed are insertion of mesh or a darn. The *mesh procedure*, popularised by Lichtenstein, has become the most common form of inguinal hernia repair, but is also particularly useful for hernias with a large posterior wall defect and recurrent hernia. The mesh, a criss-cross lattice of synthetic monofilament material, usually polypropylene, is fashioned into a 'fish-like' shape, with a defect near the tail for the spermatic cord.

The mesh is placed underneath the cord, the 'head' end is sutured to the pubic tubercle and the 'body' is sutured

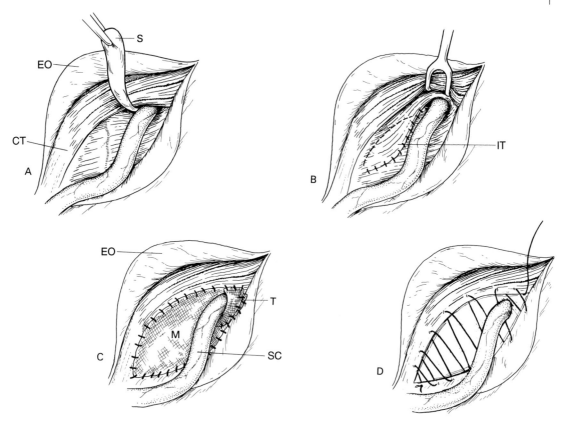

Fig. 38.6 Inguinal hernia repair. A. Herniotomy: S, indirect sac; EO, reflected external oblique; CT, conjoint tendon.
B. Herniorrhaphy – Shouldice operation: IT, imbrication of transversalis fascia (first of three-layered repair) with continuous
suture. **C.** Hernioplasty – mesh repair using polypropylene mesh (M) cut in 'fish-like' shape, sutured in position and 'tail' of mesh
(T) wrapped around the cord (SC). **D.** Hernioplasty – darn repair with continuous suture.

to the internal oblique aponeurosis and conjoint tendon superiorly and the inguinal ligament inferiorly. The two components of the tail are wrapped around the cord, crossed over and sutured in place laterally. Staples may also be used to fix the mesh in place (Fig. 38.6C). Because the mesh is foreign material, the use of prophylactic antibiotics is recommended.

The *darn* involves either interlocking or continuous 'figure of 8' non-absorbable monofilament sutures incorporating posterior wall plication and approximation of the conjoint tendon to the inguinal ligament (Fig. 38.6D).

Laparoscopic hernia repair. This technique uses a percutaneous peritoneal or intraperitoneal approach using the laparoscope, video camera, and other laparoscopic retractors and instruments. Several small incisions are made in the lower abdomen for access of this equipment. The repair involves excising or reducing the hernia sac and insertion of a mesh which is either stapled or sutured in position. The alleged advantages of this procedure are small wounds and earlier return to work.

Large indirect, direct sliding and recurrent hernia. In these, there is a weakened and often attenuated posterior wall of the inguinal canal and the following are required.

Herniotomy. This is performed except for direct hernial bulges when the sac is inverted, or for sliding herniae when it is impossible to excise the sac completely.

Herniorrhaphy. In most instances after establishing the anatomy and excising cremaster, a Shouldice repair can be performed.

Hernioplasty. An inlay of mesh or a darn with monofilament nylon is used to reinforce or replace the weakened and attenuated posterior wall of the canal.

Orchidectomy. In very large indirect (scrotal) or recurrent hernia in the elderly male, excision of the cord and testis may be necessary to allow obliteration of the internal ring and prevent further recurrence.

FEMORAL HERNIA

The majority of femoral hernias are acquired and occur more frequently in middle-aged and elderly females in whom increased abdominal pressure during pregnancy was probably an initiating factor. However, in females the prevalence of inguinal hernias is greater than femoral hernias.

SURGICAL ANATOMY

The femoral sheath is composed of a funnel-shaped prolongation of the fascia transversalis in front and the fascia behind, and it contains the femoral vessels. The sheath is separated from the medial side of the femoral vein by a space, the femoral canal, which contains fat, lymph channels from the deep inguinal glands, the lymph gland of Cloquet and, under abnormal conditions, a femoral hernia. The canal is about 2 cm long.

The femoral ring is the abdominal end of the femoral canal and is bounded anteriorly by the inguinal ligament (Poupart's ligament), medially by the crescentric edge of the lacunar ligament (Gimbernat's ligament), posteriorly by the pectineal line of the horizontal ramus of the pubis and the pectineal ligament (of Astley Cooper), and laterally by the femoral vein All these boundaries are rigid except for the femoral vein.

In 30% of cases the pubic branch of the inferior epigastric artery replaces the obturator artery when there is a 10:1 chance of it passing medial to the neck of a femoral hernia. In this position it is vulnerable if the lacunar ligament is divided to widen the femoral ring.

The femoral hernia orifice is the superficial end of the femoral canal. It is well formed only in the presence of a femoral hernia when condensation of the fascia lata of the thigh at the saphenous opening becomes more apparent.

When a femoral hernia enlarges, it passes through the saphenous opening of the fascia lata, then up over the inguinal ligament in the subcutaneous plane superficial to the superficial fascia (Scarpa's fascia).

The coverings of a femoral hernia are:

- peritoneum
- extraperitoneal fat
- fused transversalis fascia, and fascia lata
- superficial fascia
- subcutaneous fat and skin.

OTHER TYPES OF FEMORAL HERNIAS

The majority of femoral hernias pass through the femoral canal but rare types occur and these are described below.

Prevascular hernia. This passes in front of the femoral artery and is sometimes associated with congenital dislocation of hip (Narath's hernia).

Pectineal hernia. This passes behind the femoral vessels between the pectineus muscle and its fascia (Cloquet's hernia).

External femoral hernia. This passes lateral to the femoral artery (Hesselbach's hernia).

Lacunar hernia. This passes through the lacunar ligament of Gimbernat (Langier's hernia).

CLINICAL FEATURES

Patients present in one of two ways:

- with a lump
- with obstruction or strangulation.

The lump is usually a small globular swelling situated below and lateral to the pubic tubercle. It is apparent on standing or straining but may disappear on lying down.

In the case of obstruction or strangulation, the femoral ring is small and narrow and is surrounded by rigid structures with the exception of the femoral vein. The anatomical arrangement predisposes to irreducibility and strangulation of hernial contents. The obstructing agent is either the neck of the sac or the femoral ring itself.

The lump becomes tense, tender and irreducible and the overlying skin may be oedematous when strangulation is present.

In addition the features of a small bowel obstruction are apparent with abdominal pain and vomiting.

It should be remembered that an obstructed femoral hernia, particularly with a Richter's type of strangulation, may be extremely difficult to detect in an obese patient and it may be overlooked unless a very careful search is made.

Differential diagnosis

This is the same as for inguinal hernias (p. 410).

TREATMENT

There is no place for conservative treatment of femoral hernia for two reasons: no truss can be fitted to control the femoral ring; and there is always a risk of strangulation.

Operation

This may be performed by one of three methods.

Supra-inguinal. A midline vertical (Henry's incision), a vertical pararectal (McEvedy's incision) or a transverse incision in the skin crease above the inguinal ligament is used, and an extraperitoneal approach is made behind the inguinal canal to the fundus of the sac, which is opened and emptied of its contents. The sac is then reduced from the groin into the abdomen where it is excised.

A herniorrhaphy is performed by suturing the inguinal ligament to the pectineal ligament.

The operation has the advantages of providing optimum conditions for dealing with gangrenous bowel and for repair of the femoral ring; it has, however, a disadvantage in that there is imperfect access to the fundus of the sac, which may make its removal difficult.

These approaches are recommended for obstructed and strangulated femoral hernias, as they provide optimal circumstances for dealing with the contents of the sac, especially ischaemic bowel, access to the peritoneal cavity, access for herniorrhaphy, and exposure of an aberrant obturator artery.

Inguinal (Lotheissen operation). A transverse inguinal incision is used as for an inguinal hernia operation, the inguinal canal is opened and its posterior wall incised (with or without division of the inferior epigastric vessels). An extraperitoneal approach is then made to the sac and the femoral ring which are then dealt with in the same way as in the supra-inguinal operation.

The operation has the disadvantage that the inguinal canal is transgressed and inguinal herniorrhaphy is also required.

Subinguinal (Lockwood operation). A transverse incision is made directly over the swelling in the groin and the sac is separated from its layers of fat and fascia and then opened, emptied and tied off. A herniorrhaphy is performed by suturing the inguinal ligament to the pectineal fascia; alternatively a purse-string suture may be used, starting at the inner end of the inguinal ligament and picking up Gimbernat's ligament, pectineal fascia and the lateral side of the saphenous opening and its fascia lata. A plug of mesh sutured in place is another alternative.

The operation has the disadvantage of making it difficult to resect bowel when gangrene is present, or to ligate the sac at its neck. In addition, there is a largely theoretical disadvantage of possible damage to the abnormal obturator artery if incision of the lacunar ligament is performed to facilitate reduction of the contents of the hernial sac.

The operation has the advantages of being speedy, simple and may be performed with ease under local anaesthesia, and it remains popular with most surgeons.

UMBILICAL HERNIA

EXOMPHALOS

This is a rare neonatal condition caused by an anomaly of the second stage of gut rotation when the midgut loop fails to return into the abdominal cavity during the 10th week of fetal life and presents at birth as two types: minor and major.

Exomphalos minor. The sac is small and the umbilical cord attached is at its summit. Treatment involves twisting the cord, so facilitating reduction of the sac, and this is maintained by a firm dressing for 2 weeks.

Exomphalos major. The sac is large and contains the small and large bowel and often part of the liver, whilst the umbilical cord is at the inferior margin of the sac. Surgical repair is urgent as rupture and subsequent peritonitis are liable to occur. Principles of repair involve constructing skin flaps or using synthetic material to cover the defect and definitive repair performed at a later date but the prognosis is often poor.

UMBILICAL HERNIA OF INFANCY

This occurs through a defect in the umbilical cicatrax during the first few days of life. A hernial sac protrudes as a small knob at the umbilicus and it is most apparent when the child cries or strains.

Umbilical hernias are reducible and rarely strangulate.

Treatment is conservative as most disappear within 12–18 months; in the meantime they may be retained by a simple pad. Occasionally they persist after this period and operation is then recommended. The sac is excised through a transverse subumbilical incision and the small fibrous defect is closed with a few interrupted sutures.

PARA-UMBILICAL HERNIA

In the majority of cases this occurs as an acquired condition in middle-aged, obese, multiparous women in whom there is often an initial small defect in the linea alba just above the umbilicus. The peritoneal sac is often preceded by the extrusion of a small knuckle of extraperitoneal fat through the tendinous fibres of the linea alba.

As the hernia enlarges, the peritoneal sac cannot enlarge indefinitely because of the fixation of the peritoneum about the umbilicus. It splits and the contents, which are most often omentum and, in a very large hernia, transverse colon and small bowel, become loculated and adherent. For these reasons a large para-umbilical hernia is seldom reducible and strangulation is likely to occur.

Treatment is operative because of the risk of complications, particularly when the hernia is irreducible. The standard practice is to perform Mayo's operation, which entails a transverse elliptical incision with excision of the umbilicus, redundant skin and the fibroperitoneal sac and then to incise the rectus sheath on each side of the defect. Closure is effected by overlapping the upper and lower flaps with interrupted mattress sutures. Large defects may be closed with mesh.

EPIGASTRIC HERNIA

This is a midline protrusion of extraperitoneal fat, and occasionally a small peritoneal sac, through a defect or defects in the linea alba, usually in fit, muscular males under 40.

It presents as a small irreducible hernia often situated midway between the xiphisternum and the umbilicus and is usually felt more easily then it is seen.

Many epigastric hernias are symptomless but pain, discomfort or digestive disturbances occur and simulate peptic ulceration or gall bladder disease.

Treatment entails excision of the knuckle of fat and any associated hernial sac and repair of the defect by lon-

gitudinal suture or by a transverse overlap operation of the Mayo type if the defect is large.

INCISIONAL HERNIA

This is discussed in Chapter 8.

HIATUS HERNIA

This is discussed in Chapter 24.

MISCELLANEOUS HERNIA

OBTURATOR HERNIA

This is an acquired hernia through the fibro-osseous obturator canal, which is situated between the obturator groove on the lower surface of the horizontal ramus of the pubis and the upper border of the obturator membrane. The hernia is commoner in women and usually occurs after the age of 50 years.

Intestinal obstruction is the common mode of presentation and the diagnosis is established at laparotomy. Occasionally a lump is recognisable in the upper and medial aspect of the thigh when pain may be referred to the inner aspect of the knee by the geniculate branch of the obturator nerve.

At operation, the sac and its contents are reduced into the abdomen but herniorrhaphy is impossible because of the rigid nature of the canal and the presence of the obturator nerve. The defect may be covered with mesh.

SPIGELIAN HERNIA

This is a herniation through the linear semilunaris at the outer border of the rectus abdominis muscle, which occurs about halfway between the pubis and umbilicus (at about the level of the semilunar fold of Douglas).

It is probably an acquired condition and may be confused with a direct inguinal hernia, although it is usually situated higher and more medial.

Treatment is operative as the hernia is liable to strangulate.

LUMBAR HERNIA

This is either an incisional hernia following a loin incision or a spontaneous occurrence through the inferior lumbar triangle of Petit bounded by the iliac crest, the posterior edge of the external oblique and the anterior edge of the latissimus dorsi; or through the superior lumbar space bounded by the 12th rib, the lower border of serratus posterior inferior, the anterior border of sacrospinalis and the internal oblique. Hernias through these anatomically weak places are wide-necked and reducible, and are usually controlled by a surgical belt although they are best treated surgically.

GLUTEAL HERNIA

This occurs through the greater sciatic notch, either above or below pyriformis muscle. Most often it is diagnosed at laparotomy for patients presenting with a mechanical small bowel obstruction; rarely as a palpable gluteal swelling.

Treatment is operative.

SCIATIC HERNIA

This is a protrusion through the lesser sciatic notch and is usually discovered at operation for bowel obstruction; very rarely does it present as a gluteal swelling or cause pain in the distribution of the sciatic nerve.

PERINEAL HERNIA

Most often this occurs as an incisional hernia following an abdominoperineal excision of the rectum. Primary perineal hernias are rare but may be anterolateral, presenting in women as a swelling of the labia majora, or posterolateral, presenting as a swelling in the ischiorectal fossa.

Treatment is by a combined abdominoperineal repair.

FURTHER READING

Devlin H B 1988 Management of abdominal hernia. Butterworths, London

Dunn D C, Menzies D 1996 Hernia repair: laparoscopic approach. Blackwell Science, Oxford

Kingsnorth A N 1995 Modern hernia management. In: Johnson C D, Taylor I (eds) Recent advances in surgery 18. Churchill Livingstone, Edinburgh, p 159–178

Lichtenstein I L, Schulman A G, Amid P K et al 1989 The tension-free hernioplasty. American Journal of Surgery 157: 188–193

Nyphus L M, Condon R E 1996 Hernia, 4th edn. Lippincott, London

Skin conditions

Bruce Waxman

Numerous conditions of the skin are of surgical interest. Only the commoner ones will be discussed.

CLASSIFICATION

Skin and related conditions discussed are as follows:

- Cysts
  - pilar (sebaceous)
  - dermoid: inclusion, implantation
  - ganglion
- Dermatofibroma
- Kerato-acanthoma
- Keloid
- Lipoma
- Dupuytren's contracture
- Epidermal tumours
  - papilloma
  - seborrhoeic keratosis
  - senile keratosis
  - Bowen's disease
    - basal cell carcinoma
    - squamous cell carcinoma
    - pigmented naevi
    - malignant melanoma
    - Kaposi's sarcoma.
- Conditions of the toenails.

CYSTS

A cyst is a pathological term for a cavity filled with fluid and lined by either epithelium or endothelium.

PILAR (SEBACEOUS) CYST

The term 'sebaceous' misrepresents this very common lesion, which actually consists of a cyst lined by epidermis and filled with keratinous debris – an offensive, creamy, 'toothpaste-like' material – not sebum. Pilar cysts are particularly common on the scalp, neck, scrotum and face, but they can occur anywhere on the skin. The diagnosis is readily established from the typical features of a firm spherical swelling which is always in the epidermal layer of the skin and often associated with a punctum.

Treatment

Excision is recommended for cosmetic reasons and to prevent possible complications such as infection, ulceration, calcification or keratinous horn formation. Meticulous excision of all the epidermal lining will reduce the common tendency for recurrence.

DERMOID CYSTS

Inclusion (sequestration) dermoid cyst

This occurs at sites of closure of embryonal fissures and may appear at the inner or outer angles of the orbit, the midline of the neck, abdomen or on the scalp.

There is a firm or tense unilocular cyst, not attached to skin; it differs from an implantation dermoid in that its wall contains hair, hair follicles, sweat and sebaceous glands.

Treatment. Excision is recommended to prevent infection or for cosmetic reasons.

Implantation dermoid (epidermoid) cyst

This occurs commonly in the palm of the hand or fingers as a subcutaneous cystic swelling which is sometimes associated with a scar from a precipitating injury. Gardeners who prune roses are one particularly prone group.

An implantation dermoid contains white greasy material which is surrounded by a wall of stratified squamous epithelium. Hair, hair follicles, sebaceous glands and sweat glands are absent.

The mode of development of an implantation dermoid is uncertain but explanations offered include:

- implantation of epidermal cells beneath the skin by a puncture injury
- Epithelialisation of a haematoma by cells from adjacent sweat glands, in the absence of a puncture wound.

Treatment. Excision is recommended to prevent infection or for cosmetic reasons.

INFECTION OF SKIN CYSTS

As has been implied, secondary infection is frequent in epidermoid or dermoid cysts. If the consequent abscess is merely drained, then recurrence is inevitable. It is better at the time of incision to curette the abscess under antibiotic cover so as to remove or destroy the lining of the cavity. Almost always such an approach is adequate.

GANGLION

Though not of cutaneous origin, ganglions are commonly mistaken for epidermoid cysts, but lie deep to skin and in the vicinity of joints. There is a tense unilocular cystic swelling lined by compressed fibrous tissue and containing gelatinous fluid which lies in close relation to or communicates with the synovial membrane of a joint or a tendon sheath. It occurs most frequently on the dorsum of the wrist or foot but occasionally is related to the long flexor tendons in the palm or the peroneal tendons at the ankle.

The pathogenesis of this lesion is uncertain; it may represent a leakage of synovial fluid with secondary fibrous encapsulation, myxomatous degeneration of connective tissue, or an extrasynovial benign synovioma.

Ganglia may cause pain or discomfort or interfere with the function of tendons.

Treatment

The ganglion is excised under regional or general anaesthetic and bloodless field (with tourniquet). This is the most certain method of treatment but recurrence is still common, perhaps because the source of the synovial leak is difficult to identify.

DERMATOFIBROMA (histiocytoma)

This presents as a firm nodule 0.5–2 cm in diameter, fixed to the epidermis but freely mobile. The lesion is usually found on the lower leg, is often singular and is thought to result from minor trauma such as an insect bite which causes a reactive proliferation of histiocytes leading to fibrosis and scarring.

Treatment is excision for cosmetic reasons.

KERATO-ACANTHOMA (molluscum sebaceum)

An affliction of adults who are usually over the age of 50 years, it occurs exclusively on hair-bearing areas, particularly those exposed to sunlight, such as the face, neck and dorsal surfaces of the hands and forearms.

The lesion grows rapidly over 1 or 2 months to appear as an elevated dome-shaped swelling with smooth sides and central umbilication containing a keratotic plug which can be peeled off with difficulty to reveal a bleeding granular floor.

Untreated, the lesion gradually regresses over 6–9 months to leave finally an irregular depressed scar.

The aetiology is unknown but it probably arises from

hyperplasia of hair follicle epithelium and metaplasia of sebaceous glands.

Treatment

Excision is usually recommended as it is often difficult to distinguish a molluscum sebaceum from an epithelioma.

When the diagnosis is certain, curettage of the central keratin plug and the floor of the lesion will hasten regression; the alternative is to do nothing and allow it to disappear spontaneously.

KELOID

This is an irregular hypertrophy of vascularised collagen forming a raised ridge on the site or scar of previous injury. Individual and racial predisposition is an important factor in keloid formation, but in ordinary circumstances the condition occurs more in burns and wounds that heal by secondary intention. Spontaneous keloid may occur over the sternum.

Ridges of keloid often form 'claw-like' projections invading the surrounding skin outside the borders of the original scar, thus differentiating it from a hypertrophied scar.

Treatment

Inevitable recurrence follows excision; however, repeated monthly injections of triamcinolone acetonide into the lesion for 6 months generally give satisfactory results.

LIPOMA

This is the commonest of all benign tumours, occurring in any situation where there is fat but particularly in the subcutaneous tissue of the trunk and limbs. Lipomas also occur in subperiosteal, subperitoneal (retroperitoneal), subfascial and subsynovial planes and in the submucosa of the bowel.

They usually appear in adult life as soft lobulated, fluctuant tumours and have definite and definable edges when subcutaneous in position.

Calcification is an occasional occurrence in a lipoma but it is rare for liposarcomatous changes to occur.

Adiposis dolorosa of Dercum is a term applied to diffuse or nodular painful deposits of fat in women.

Sclerosis with loss of blood supply can make a lipoma painful but may be followed by shrinkage or even disappearance.

Treatment

Excision is recommended if lipomas are large, unsightly or troublesome.

Subfascial lipomas may extend through intermuscular planes and create difficulties if the operation is performed under local anaesthetic.

DUPUYTREN'S CONTRACTURE

This condition is not strictly of cutaneous origin but is included here for convenience. There is thickening of the palmar fascia resulting in flexion contractures of the fingers of the hand with particular involvement of the ring and little fingers. The cause is unknown but it is thought to be familial and the incidence is increased in those of Celtic origin, alcoholics, diabetics and epileptics treated with phenytoin. The condition is more common in males. Some patients have similar contractures of the penis, associated with bowing of the penis (Peyronie's disease), or involvement of the plantar fascia of the feet. There is no clear association with trauma. Microscopically there is a fibroblastic proliferation without special features.

Clinical features

The first signs are nodules in the palm at the base of the affected finger, followed by a thick palpable cord with subsequent contraction leading to flexion of the digit.

Treatment

Surgical treatment is the only effective form of therapy and is indicated when the palm of the hand and fingers can no longer be placed flat on the table. Local excision of the affected palmar fascia with a multiple Z-plasty closure of overlying skin is most commonly practised, allowing sufficient opening of the hand but minimizing the risk of complications such as digital nerve injury or skin necrosis.

Postoperatively, the hand is immobilised in a firm wool and crepe dressing with gentle mobilisation commencing after the first week.

EPIDERMAL TUMOURS

PAPILLOMA

This is a common benign, sessile or pedunculated and sometimes pigmented tumour composed of squamous epithelium.

The common wart (verruca vulgaris) is a papilloma which probably arises from a virus infection. It may be single or multiple, and may disappear spontaneously. When the lesion occurs on the sole of the foot, it may be difficult to differentiate from a corn which is a localised horny plug of epithelial cells in the epidermis. However, if it is pared down until tiny haemorrhagic spots are seen emanating from the finger-like projections of hyperplastic prickle cells of the papilloma, the distinction will be made.

Treatment

Papillomata are usually excised for cosmetic reasons. However, plantar warts often demand removal because of pain; they may be treated with silver nitrate, curettage or excision.

SEBORRHOEIC WART (seborrhoeic keratosis)

This is a common benign and sessile condition of the elderly which appears as a dark brown raised area on the face, limbs or trunk. It is a hyperplastic condition of the basal cell layer of the skin with laminated pearls of keratinised material or dendritic melanin-forming cells. The lesion is typically 'greasy' to touch but may occasionally be impossible to distinguish from a melanoma.

Treatment

Excision is indicated when melanoma cannot be excluded.

SENILE (SOLAR) KERATOSIS

This is a hard scaly condition of the elderly occurring particularly on the parts of the skin exposed to sunlight. It is composed of hyperkeratotic areas with mitotic figures in the basal layers of the epidermis.

Treatment

Malignant change to squamous cell carcinoma occurs in about 25% of cases and excision is therefore recommended as a prophylactic measure.

BOWEN'S DISEASE

This is a slowly growing premalignant reddish-brown lesion with well-defined margins affecting the middle-aged and elderly. It tends to form crusts and ulcerate; multiple lesions, which tend to coalesce, are common.

Microscopically there is hyperkeratosis with mitotic activity in the basal layers, where multinucleated giant cells and large clear cells are seen.

Treatment

Malignant change to squamous cell carcinoma may occur after many years and excision is therefore recommended.

BASAL CELL CARCINOMA (rodent ulcer)

This is particularly liable to occur in fair and dry-skinned people constantly exposed to sunlight. Elderly subjects are usually affected and the majority of lesions occur on the face above the line joining the angle of the mouth and the lobe of the ear, but no part of the skin is exempt.

Macroscopically the tumour begins as a pearly nodule with tiny venules coursing across the surface; it later proceeds to central ulceration with a raised, rolled or beaded edge.

Microscopically the typical features are densely packed islands of uniform cells continuous superficially with the basal layer of the epidermis. The cells of the periphery of the islands are more deeply staining and have a palisade arrangement perpendicular to the surrounding connective tissue; cell nests (keratinised cores) are absent.

Direct spread superficially or deeply may be so extensive as to destroy the nose and eyes and erode through the skull, but the tumour rarely metastasises.

A benign variant is a cylindroma which arises from basal cells of hair follicles or sweat glands of the scalp. These may be multiple (inherited as autosomal dominant) and cover the scalp (turban tumour – epithelioma adenoides cysticum).

Treatment

Radiotherapy. Superficial radiotherapy will cure over 90% of lesions.

Surgery. Excision and suture repair for small lesions. Wide excision and skin grafting are indicated in the following circumstances:

- recurrence after radiotherapy
- involvement of muscle, cartilage, or bone
- occurrence close to cartilage or the eye.

SQUAMOUS CELL CARCINOMA (epithelioma)

Like basal cell carcinoma, this lesion occurs particularly in elderly fair-skinned people exposed to sunlight.

Predisposing factors

These include:

- senile (solar) keratosis
- Bowen's disease
- exposure to sunlight or irradiation
- chronic irritation
  - leukoplakia
  - burn scar, varicose ulcer, osteomyelitic sinus (Marjolin's ulcer)
- genetic
  - xeroderma pigmentosa
  - albinism
- geographic
  - Kangri cancer of Kashmir – from charcoal heater on abdominal skin
  - Kang cancer of NW China from oven bed, on skin of legs and buttocks
- other
  - lupus vulgaris (tuberculosis of the skin)
  - erythroplasia of Queyrat (penis)
  - Paget's disease of skin (vulva, anus, axilla, breast).

Macroscopically the lesion may appear as a warty growth or as a malignant ulcer with raised and everted edges.

Microscopically there are solid clumps of epithelial cells extending into the dermis with finger-like projections. Cell nests or epithelial pearls with central keratinised cores and surrounding cells arranged in 'onion-skin' fashion are characteristic, while intercellular bridges and small round cell infiltration of the dermis are usually present.

Direct spread to surrounding structures is slow and, while lymphatic involvement is usually late, it is an ever-present danger.

Treatment

Radiotherapy. Superficial radiotherapy will cure over 80% of early lesions.

Surgery. Wide excision is indicated for the same reasons as those pertaining to basal cell carcinoma. Lesions on the hands, feet, perineum and vulva are ideally treated by surgery.

Lymph nodes. If the regional lymph nodes are clinically involved, a block dissection is indicated, and when the primary lesion and the nodes are closely approximated, a dissection in continuity is preferable.

PIGMENTED NAEVI

Surgical pathology

Pigmented naevi (moles) are composed of proliferations of melanocytes at different layers of the skin. Melanocytes are probably derived embryologically from neural crest elements of ectoderm that migrate into the skin and are capable of forming melanin from dioxyphenylalanine (DOPA). Melanin may be transferred from melanocytes to other cells. Melanocytes reside mainly in the basal layer of the epidermis and numerically are in constant ratio with the prickle cells of the basal layer but may migrate into the dermis or less often the epidermis. The deeper the collection of melanocytes, the bluer is the naevus.

Pigmented naevi of benign nature are of five types:

- junctional naevus
- intradermal naevus
- compound naevus
- blue naevus
- spindle cell naevus.

Junctional naevus. This is a smooth, flat or elevated naevus of all shades of brown, which can occur anywhere on the body from birth to later life. When naevi occur on the palm, soles, digits, or genitalia, they are always junctional in type.

Microscopically there is a proliferation of melanocytes at the epidermodermal junction. The cells have clear cytoplasm, dark nuclei and varying amounts of melanin. Junctional naevi rarely become malignant, but nevertheless it is from this group that 90% of malignant melanomas occur.

Increased 'activity' of a junctional naevus, which indicates malignant change, is evidenced by:

- increase in size
- increase in pigmentation
- ulceration, crusting or haemorrhage
- satellite pigmented spots
- microscopic evidence of hyperchromasia, anaplasia, mitotic figures and subepithelial spread.

Intradermal naevus (common mole). When junctional activity ceases, the naevus cells lie within the dermis and form a mature pigmented lesion which is rare in children but commoner with increasing age. It is light or dark brown in colour and may be papillary, flat or warty; it is often raised and hairy and occurs anywhere on the body except the palms, soles and genitalia; it never becomes malignant.

Microscopically the overlying epidermis appears normal and the dermal naevus cells are arranged in characteristic alveoli or ribbons. The cells have lost the typical features of clear cells but some of them coalesce to form giant cells.

Compound naevus. Junctional cells migrate into the dermis so that both junctional and intradermal components are present. The latter is inactive and incapable of multiplication or pigment production, but the junctional component is responsible for this lesion being potentially malignant.

Blue naevus. This is a flat hairless bluish lesion devoid of surface elevation which is seen on the face, dorsum of the hands and feet, and the buttocks of babies (Mongolian spot).

The blue naevus is not premalignant, and when occurring in babies it usually disappears before the age of 5 years.

Microscpically there are spindle-shaped and melanin-containing melanocytes in ribbon-shaped masses or whorls in the dermis.

Spindle cell naevus. Malignant melanoma is a very unusual occurrence before puberty, but a pigmented hairless and warty naevus occurring at this time and pursuing a benign course may have all the microscopic features of malignant melanoma. Junctional activity is marked with prominent mitotic figures and segregation of bizarre-looking multinucleate giant cells. There is, however, no dermal invasion and the outcome is always favourable.

Treatment of naevi

Naevi appearing at birth are innocent tumours and are removed only for cosmetic reasons.

Naevi appearing before puberty are mainly flat juctional naevi and, since malignant melanoma does not occur in this age group, their removal is again indicated for cosmetic reasons only.

Naevi appearing after puberty should be removed if they are:

- situated in potentially dangerous areas (soles of feet, palms of hands and genitalia)
- subjected to repeated trauma from clothes, braces, belts and razors
- showing signs of malignancy.

Naevi appearing at birth or before puberty can be excised close to their margins.

Any excised naevus must be subjected to careful histological study.

MALIGNANT MELANOMA (melanoma)

This forms about 2–3% of all skin malignancies, and in Australia the incidence has increased fourfold in the last 30 years. Around 90% of melanomas arise from junctional elements of pre-existing naevi and in 10% of cases the lesion arises de novo.

Women are said to be affected more often than men, particularly in the age group 20–40 years, but this is probably not true. A melanoma is more likely in the lower extremity of a woman and the trunk or arm of a man. Celtic ancestry and exposure to the sun are well-documented predisposing factors. Black-skinned people are relatively resistant to melanomas, although these may occur on their palms, soles or mucous membranes.

Melanoma is one of the most malignant and dangerous forms of cancer and, although occurring most often on the skin, it can arise in other parts of the body, especially the eye and beneath the nail (subungual melanoma). Occasionally, widespread metastases present without the primary site being discovered.

Surgical pathology

Macroscopic features. Malignant change in a pre-existing innocent mole will manifest itself by an increase in size with elevation above the surface, an increase in pigmentation, nodularity, haemorrhage, ulceration or satellite pigmentations.

Microscopic features. There is marked junctional activity and invasion of the dermis and deeper structures. The cell structure and arrangement vary considerably; it may appear like a carcinoma in which cells are epithelial in character and arranged in alveoli, or it may appear like a sarcoma in which spindle cells predominate.

Spread. There may be lymphatic spread by emboli, to regional lymph nodes, or by permeation, to produce secondary nodules in the vicinity of the primary lesion. Dissemination by the bloodstream to any part of the body is usually a late development.

Special features. There is no doubt that malignant melanoma incites an immune response and this may account at least in part for the remarkable variation of the clinical course.

Classification and prognosis

Histological grading. The depth or level of invasion of the skin and the thickness of the lesion are two factors that indicate the invasiveness of the tumour and are useful for grading, determining appropriate treatment and indicating prognosis.

Level of invasion. Clark divides the skin into five levels for purposes of staging melanoma (see Fig. 39.1) the deeper the invasion the worse is the prognosis:

- level I – intra-epidermal (in situ, premalignant)
- level II – invasion into the papillary layer of the dermis
- level III – invasion into the junction of the papillary and reticular dermis
- level IV – invasion of the reticular dermis
- level V – invasion of the subcutaneous fat.

The 5-year survival for level II is greater than 90%, whereas for level V it is less than 50%.

Tumour thickness. Breslow expresses invasiveness in terms of thickness in millimetres as measured histologically and this scheme correlates well with prognosis. Tumours less than 0.75 mm rarely metastasise, whereas approximately 30% of those between 0.76 and 1.5 mm will metastasise, and for lesions greater than 3.0 mm in thickness more than 80% will metastasise.

General prognostic features. Other pathological features indicating a poor prognosis are:

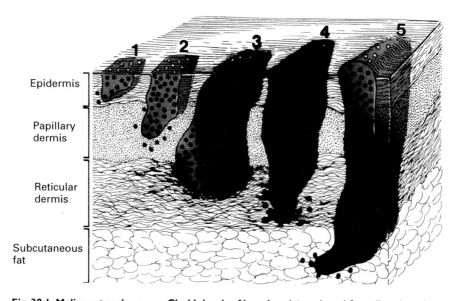

Fig. 39.1 Malignant melanoma – Clark's levels of invasion. 1, intradermal; 2, papillary dermal; 3, papillary–reticular interface; 4, reticular dermal; 5, subcutaneous fat.

- ulceration
- amelanosis
- poor lymphocytic reaction
- satellitosis – tiny deposits away from the main growth
- high mitotic index.

Lesions of the extremities have a good prognosis compared with those of the trunk. Melanomas in women have an overall better prognosis than those in men, which is partly related to the different distribution of site.

Education programmes aimed at the public and the medical profession result in greater awareness, earlier presentation and better overall outcome, as illustrated in Queensland, Australia.

Clinical patterns

Five clinical patterns of melanoma are recognised.

Lentigo maligna (Hutchinson's freckle). This presents on the malar region of the face in middle-aged women and is the least malignant type. The lesion is flat, rounded in shape with an irregular edge and uneven pigmentation. Melanocytes invade the dermis but the tumour is not very thick (usually less than 0.75 mm). Treatment is local excision with a narrow margin and prognosis is excellent.

Superficial spreading (Pagetoid melanoma). The commonest form of melanoma, this occurs in any area exposed to the sun. The lesion is raised, has an irregular edge and a variegated coloration. All levels of invasion exist but epidermal invasion predominates and lymphatic infiltration is prominent.

Nodular melanoma. The melanoma is elevated, convex or even pedunculated, occurring at sites not exposed to the sun, and is often amelanotic. This is the most ominous form of melanoma with extensive dermal invasion, rapid growth and early metastases.

Acral-lentiginous (acral: of the extremities). These are melanomas occurring on the palm of the hands, soles of the feet and under the nails of hands and feet (subungual melanoma). The prognosis is poor, similar to that of nodular melanoma.

Amelanotic. This is a special form of nodular melanoma but with a worse prognosis. There is loss of pigment especially in the central part of the tumour which is quite pink in colour.

Treatment

Cooperation between the pathologist and surgeon is vital for the diagnosis and treatment of melanoma. Although paraffin sections are the safest means of making a histological diagnosis and grading the tumour, advances in interpretation of frozen sections of melanomas enable excision biopsy and definitive surgery to be performed at the one operation.

Recent developments in surgical treatment of melanoma have questioned accepted dogma (especially the need for wide margins of excision and split-skin grafting from the contralateral limb) as neither compromising the width of excision nor taking skin from the same limb increases local recurrence.

Early cases

Primary lesion. A wide local excision of the melanoma is performed, with a margin of 1–3 cm and as deep as the deep fascia. The thicker the melanoma (according to Breslow), the wider is the margin.

The defect may be closed primarily or with a split-skin graft taken from whichever site is convenient.

Regional lymph nodes. There is no universal agreement on the treatment of the regional lymph nodes, but in general it is dependent on whether or not the nodes are clinically involved.

When the regional nodes are *not clinically involved*, the following approaches may be used:

- immediate 'prophylactic' block dissection
- delayed 'prophylactic' dissection
- regional perfusion combined with surgery
- close observation
- treatment based on histological grading.

All agree that if a block dissection is to be performed, it should be in the form of an en bloc excision of the primary lesion, the intervening lymphatics and the first echelon of lymph nodes, whenever this is anatomically possible. A lesion of the thigh can be removed in continuity with the ilio-inguinal lymph nodes, but for a lesion below the knee, excision of intervening tissues and lymphatics is unnecessary.

A delayed block dissection of the regional lymph nodes may be performed 2–3 weeks after adequate excision of the primary. A possible benefit of the delay is to allow time for any malignant cells in lymphatics to travel to regional lymph nodes.

Block dissection, whether immediate or delayed, is associated with a significant morbidity (swollen limb and flap necrosis).

The rationale behind regional perfusion combined with surgery is that tumour cells are constantly en route to the regional nodes and must be destroyed by a high local concentration of cytotoxic agent. This can be achieved by isolating the circulation of the limb and perfusing with melphalan, using a pump oxygenator. The lesion is then excised. The 5-year survival in lower limb melanoma is improved by this approach, but unfortunately its use is limited to special centres.

Some surgeons consider that the results of immediate or delayed 'prophylactic' node dissection do not justify its use and that nothing more than continued observation is required. Block dissection is performed if the nodes become clinically involved.

Treatment based on histological grading is a somewhat more rational approach. Melanomas of level I or II and less than 0.75 mm thick require excision only, because metastases are rare. Lesions of level IV or V and greater than 3.0 mm in thickness have a poor prognosis and may benefit from a combination of prophylactic lymph node dissections and limb perfusion. The best choice of treatment for the intermediate group level III or IV and thickness 0.76–1.5 mm has not yet been established, but the combination of excision and limb perfusion has gained in popularity.

In cases of malignant melanoma where the regional nodes are *clinically involved*, the prognosis is very poor and only 5% of these patients survive 5 years.

The methods of treatment available are as follows:

- immediate block dissection
- endolymphatic therapy plus block dissection
- perfusion and block dissection.

When using endolymphatic therapy plus block dissection, the block dissection should be performed about 4 weeks after the intralymphatic injection, at which time the isotope has had time to decay to safe level. The operation can, however, be technically more difficult if more than 4 weeks have been allowed to elapse. The disadvantage of the treatment is that it can only be performed in a specialised radioisotope unit.

Advanced cases. When the lesion is locally irremovable or when metastases are present, systemic combination chemotherapy, including imidazole carboxamide (DTIC), may be employed but response is not universal. BCG vaccination, either intralesionally for recurrent melanoma or by multiple intradermal injection, has been used to stimulate an immunological response but the results have been disappointing.

Amputation of a limb may occasionally be justified on some occasions to remove a foul, fungating tumour.

KAPOSI'S SARCOMA

This is an angiosarcoma involving capillary and perivascular connective tissue cells. The cells are probably activated by an oncogenic cytomegalovirus (CMV). The tumour may be indolent or aggressive.

The indolent form affects elderly men especially in central Europe or Ashkenazic Jews. It carries a good prognosis with a median survival of 10 years.

The aggressive form affects immunosuppressed patients especially with HIV infection (AIDS) or following organ transplantation. There is also a high incidence in Africa, especially in the Bantu of Uganda where there is also a common association with Burkitt's lymphoma. In this form, the tumour grows rapidly often coalescing with other lesions and the median survival is only 12 months.

The Kaposi's lesions affect mainly the skin but may also affect the gastrointestinal tract, including the mouth and anus. The tumours affecting the skin are usually flat and deep purple to red in colour and affect the extremities and the torso.

The results of treatment are variable but responses have been achieved with local radiotherapy or systemic interferon.

TOENAILS

These may be the site of various surgical conditions. Apart from paronychia and glomus tumour, which usually occur on fingers, most nail abnormalities are found on the great toe.

CLASSIFICATION OF TOENAIL DISORDERS

These are classified into:

- 'ingrown' toenail (onychocryptosis)

- 'overgrown' toenail (onychogryphosis)
- nail bed lesions
  — subungual haematoma
  — subungual exostosis
  — melanoma
  — glomus tumour.

SURGICAL PATHOLOGY

'Ingrown' toenail

The basic defect is a pressure necrosis of the nail wall and nail sulcus due to persistent contact with the edge of the nail plate. Subsequent ulceration, inflammation and suppuration cause the nail wall and nail sulcus to swell and develop exuberant granulation tissue which in turn exaggerates the contact with the nail plate.

Factors which predispose to abnormal pressure between the nail plate and the nail wall and sulcus are as follows.

Soft tissue abnormalities. A toenail cut short and curved allows the unsupported pulp of the toe to roll over the nail edge when upward pressure is exerted on walking (Fig. 39.2).

A soft and lax pulp, which may result from debilitating diseases and hyperhidrosis, rolls easily over the nail plate edges.

A crowded foot in an ill-fitting or pointed shoe may cause pressure to be exerted between the nail wall and nail plate of the first or second toe.

Nail abnormalities. These include a congenitally hypercurved nail or a secondarily hypercurved nail. The latter may result from peripheral arterial disease, pulmonary disease or ageing.

Bone abnormalities. These include subungual exostosis and upward tilt of the tip of the distal phalanx.

These defects may cause the nail plate to become domed and allow abnormal pressures to be exerted between the nail plate edge and the nail wall.

'Overgrown' toenail

Excessive growth of the nail plate occurs by proliferation of the cells in the germinal matrix. This causes the nail to thicken, lengthen and pile up, to form a nail which is said to resemble a ram's horn.

Nail-bed lesions

Subungual haematoma. This is a tense and painful haematoma beneath a nail as the result of a crushing injury.

Subungual exostosis. This is a small overgrowth of bone on the dorsal surface of the distal phalanx which may enlarge and deform the nail and destroy the nail bed.

Subungual melanoma. This acral-lentiginous form of melanoma has a poor prognosis, but may be mistaken for a haematoma, although it usually lifts the nail causing a distortion of the nail bed.

Glomus tumour. This is an extremely painful and well-encapsulated tiny bluish tumour. It is benign and arises from the neural tissue of specialised subcutaneous arteriovenous anastomoses which are concerned with heat regulation. Most of these tumours occur in the upper extremities and about 30% are subungual, but the subungual regions of the lower extremities are not excluded.

Microscopically there is a tangled mass of blood vessels surrounded by a musculoendothelial or neuromatous stroma.

TREATMENT

'Ingrown' toenail

Treatment is either conservative or operative.

Conservative. This should be adopted initially in all cases, and includes:

- correct trimming of the nail so that pulp is unable to roll over the nail plate edge (Fig. 39.2)

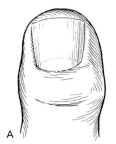 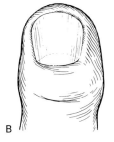

Fig. 39.2 Toenail trimming. A. Correct. **B.** Incorrect.

- the wearing of clean socks and the use of foot baths when excessive sweating is present
- the careful application of dusting powder to the toe and web spaces, making sure that the nail sulcus is not 'caked'
- the placing of cotton wool beneath the nail plate edge and along the sulcus to facilitate the separation of these structures
- thinning of the central portion of the nail with a razor blade, sandpaper or file, to make it more pliable and able to give way more readily to the forces applied during walking
- control of exuberant granulation tissue on the nail wall with silver nitrate
- advice regarding correctly fitting shoes.

Operative. This is indicated when pain or discomfort persists despite conservative treatment or when drainage of pus is necessary.

The operations available are discussed below.

Nail plate operations. Simple avulsion of the nail is indicated when it is essential to establish free drainage of pus. Wedge excision of portions of the nail only serves no permanently useful function.

Nail wall operations. Excision of most of the soft tissue from the side of the toe with or without pedicle grafts is not popular, but can be justified when pulp migration is considered the initiating factor.

Nail bed operations. Excision of all or part of the nail bed concerned with nail growth (germinal matrix) is the most popular operation because by preventing regrowth of the nail, recurrence is uncommon.

The two operations that are usually employed can be performed using a digital nerve block and tourniquet, assuming circulation to the toe is normal.

The first is *wedge resection* (Watson–Cheyne operation), in which a partial excision of the nail and subjacent matrix is performed with excision or currettage of the nail skin fold (Fig. 39.3). Matrix removal may be incomplete and phenolisation or cryoprobe treatment of the matrix is now used in some centres.

The second is *Zadik's operation* (nail bed ablation). This operation produces excellent and long-lasting results. The incisions are planned to contain adequately any swollen or granulating nail wall and two proximal extensions are made from the edges of the nail fold

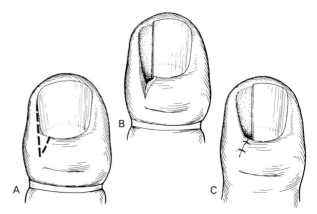

Fig. 39.3 Wedge resection operation for ingrowing toenail. **A.** V-shaped cut to excise nail fold granulation tissue and expose corner of germinal matrix. **B.** One-quarter of nail and germinal matrix excised. **C.** Skin flap sutured and raw area left to granulate.

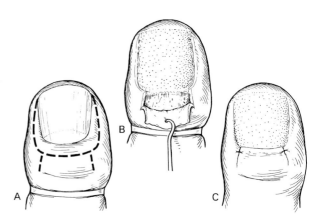

Fig. 39.4 Zadik's operation for ingrown toenail. A. Line of incision. **B.** Nail removed, flap raised, germinal matrix excised and phalanx exposed. **C.** Flap replaced and sutured to non-germinal growth.

towards the distal interphalangeal joint, so that a wide flap of skin can be raised to allow access to the nail root and the matrix. The nail is removed, the limits of the matrix are dissected out, and a block of tissue containing the matrix is excised to leave bare phalanx. The flap is then replaced and sutured to the proximal edge of the remaining nail bed (Fig. 39.4).

'Overgrown' toenail (onychogryphosis)

Conservative treatment by repeated trimming with heavy cutters may keep the condition under control.

A nail bed ablative procedure is the only permanently effective cure.

Nail bed lesions

Subungual haematoma. Relief of pain is obtained by evacuating the clot through a hole made in the nail with a trephine or the red-hot end of a paper clip.

Subungual exostosis. The nail is avulsed and the exostosis excised through the nail bed.

Subungual melanoma. Excision biopsy and histological confirmation are followed by ray amputation including the phalanx and distal metatarsal or metacarpal.

Glomus tumour. Excision is associated with dramatic and lasting relief of pain.

FURTHER READING

Macgregor I A, Macgregor A D 1995 Fundamental techniques of plastic surgery and their surgical applications, 9th edn. Churchill Livingstone, Edinburgh
Soutar D S 1996 The surgical management of cutaneous malignant melanoma. In: Johnson C D, Taylor I (eds) Recent advances in surgery 18. Churchill Livingstone, Edinburgh, p 215–234

Index